THE GOLD'S GYM BOOK OF BODYBUILDING

Other Books in the Gold's Gym series include:

Gold's Gym Training Encyclopedia
Solid Gold: Training the Gold's Gym Way

THE GOLD'S GYM BOOK OF BODYBUILDING

KEN SPRAGUE
BILL REYNOLDS

CONTEMPORARY
BOOKS, INC.
CHICAGO

Library of Congress Cataloging in Publication Data

Reynolds, Bill.
Gold's gym book of bodybuilding.

Bibliography: p.
Includes index.
1. Bodybuilding. 2. Bodybuilders—Biography.
I. Sprague, Ken. II. Title.
GV546.5.R49 1983 646.7'5 [B] 82-19904
ISBN 0-8092-5694-0
ISBN 0-8092-5693-2 (pbk.)

Exercise photos by John Balik
Exercises printed by Isgo Lepejian, Burbank, CA

Exercise models: Tom Platz, Casey Viator, Maria Gonzalez, Cheryl Howard, Valerie Mayers, Ricky Valente, Charles Glass, Janaire O'Hara, Bob Jodkiewicz, Mike Armstrong, Andreas Cahling, Dean Tornabene, Corrine Cunningham, Eric Sternlicht.

Published by Contemporary Books, Inc.
180 North Michigan Avenue, Chicago, Illinois 60601
Manufactured in the United States of America
Library of Congress Catalog Card Number: 82-19904
International Standard Book Number: 0-8092-5694-0 (cloth)
0-8092-5693-2 (paper)

Published simultaneously in Canada by
Beaverbooks, Ltd.
150 Lesmill Road
Don Mills, Ontario M3B 2T5
Canada

This book is dedicated to Frank Wainwright, Heinz Sallmayer, Cesar Juliani, and other bodybuilders who have gone before, but are still with us.

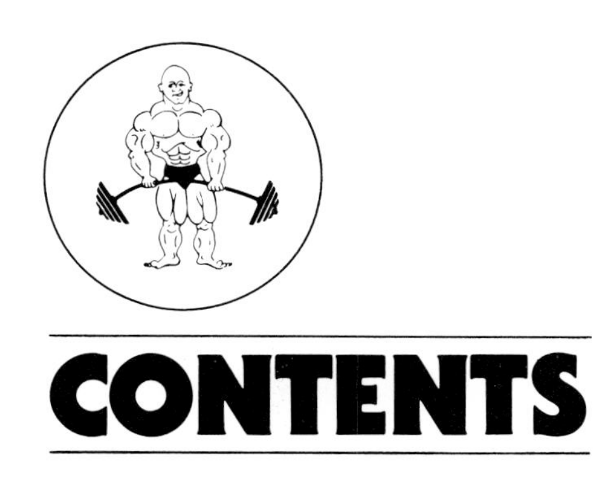

CONTENTS

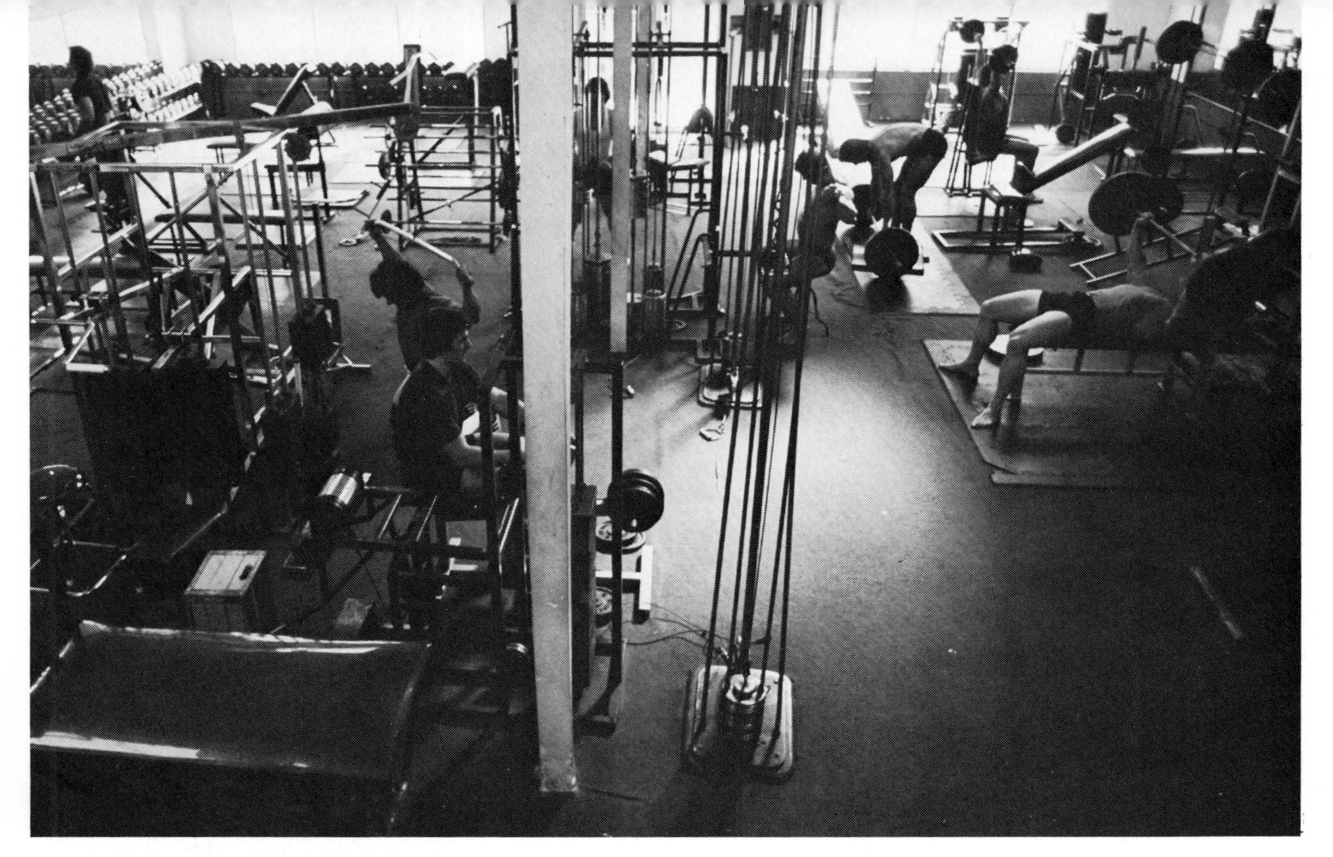

Interior of the original Gold's Gym located on Pacific Avenue in Venice, California. It became known as "The Hall of Champions" as Schwarzenegger, Columbu, Zane, Waller, Nubret, Szkalak, and a large number of other international stars trained there.

Lou Ferrigno really attracts a crowd at Gold's II for a photo session supervised by Joe Weider (right) and conducted by Craig Dietz. *(Photo by Art Zeller)*

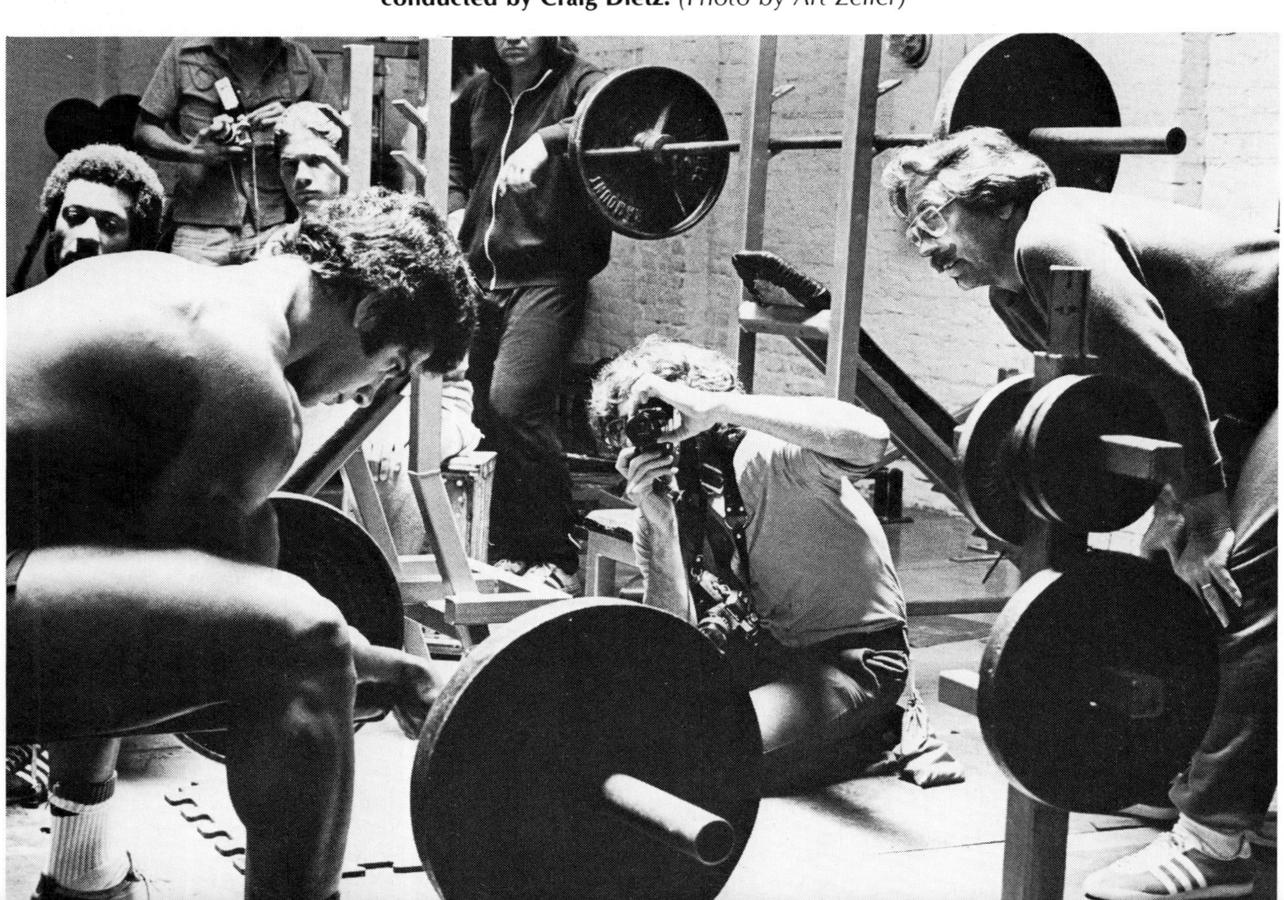

Interior of Gold's Gym III, the present huge building located in Venice, California. *(Photo by Mike Neveux)*

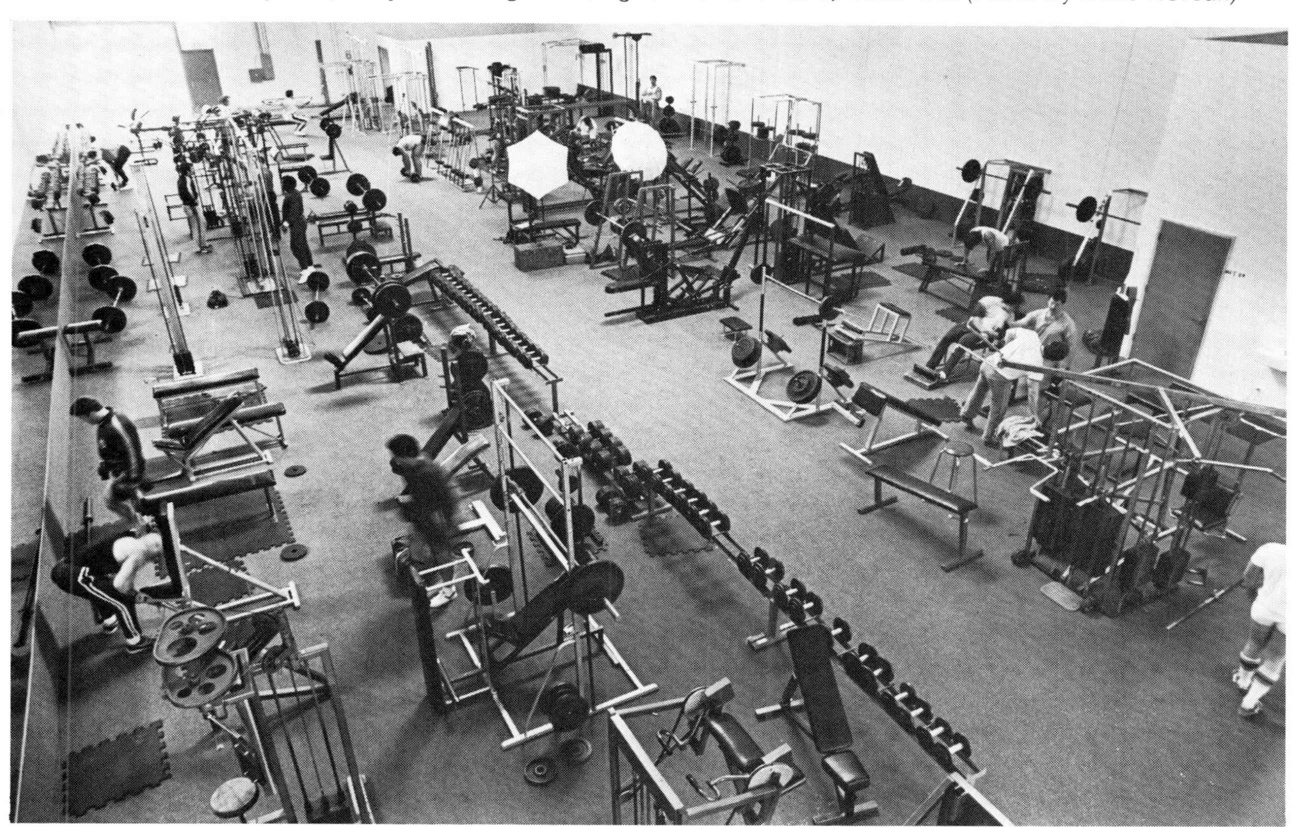

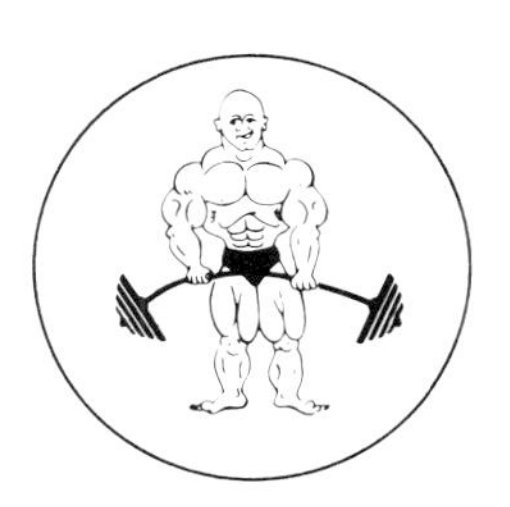

1 BODYBUILDING, GOLD'S GYM STYLE

In recent years bodybuilding has become one of the world's fastest-growing sports. Hundreds of thousands of men and women have flocked into gyms from California to New York, from Montreal to Buenos Aires, from Sydney to Tokyo, and from Mexico City to Cairo. So many bodybuilders and national bodybuilding federations have affiliated themselves with the International Federation of Bodybuilders (IFBB) that our sport is now the fifth most popular worldwide.

Gold's Gym has now been at the vanguard of the international bodybuilding movement for 15 years. Virtually every bodybuilding superstar of recent years has either trained exclusively at Gold's Gym or worked out there periodically. As a result, Gold's has become so popular that there are now nearly 100 Gold's Gym franchises in operation all over the world.

Every Mr. Olympia and Ms. Olympia winner has trained at Gold's Gym. Some of the best-known bodybuilders who have worked out at Gold's include Arnold Schwarzenegger, Lou Ferrigno, Lisa Lyon, Dr. Franco Columbu, Kike Elomaa, Chris Dickerson, Laura Combes, Serge Nubret, Rachel McLish, Casey Viator, Boyer Coe, Larry Scott, Sergio Oliva, Lisa Elliott, Frank Zane, Tom Platz, Johnny Fuller, Dr. Lynne Pirie, Albert Beckles, Tony Pearson, Shelley Gruwell, Mohamed Makkawy, Tim Belknap, Carla Dunlap, Andreas Cahling, Scott Wilson, Gerard Buinoud, Stacey Bentley, Mike and Ray Mentzer, Jacques Neuville, Steve Davis, Dennis Tinerino, Jusup Wilkosz, Danny Padilla, Ali Malla, Samir Bannout, Ed Corney, Bob Jodkiewicz, Claudia Wilbourn, Lynn Conkwright, Robby Robinson, Ricky Wayne, Kal Szkalak, Ron Teufel, Greg DeFerro, Ken Waller, Dave Draper, Debbie Diana, Pete Grymkowski, Kent Keuhn, Candy Csencsits, Roy Callender, Valerie Mayers, Dave Johns, Dale Adrian, Clint Beyerle, Dr. C. F. Smith, Bill Grant, Bertil Fox, Kay Baxter, Mike Katz, Don Ross, Georgia Fudge, Bob Birdsong, Hubert Metz, Rod Koontz, Jorma Raty, Madeline Almedia, Tony Emmott, Roger Walker, and Gary Leonard.

Isn't this an impressive list? And it's only the tip of the iceberg in terms of a master list of all champion male and female bodybuilders who have at some point in time trained at Gold's Gym.

Brief profiles of all of these champions are presented in Chapter 10 of this book. Each miniprofile includes a photo and a workout

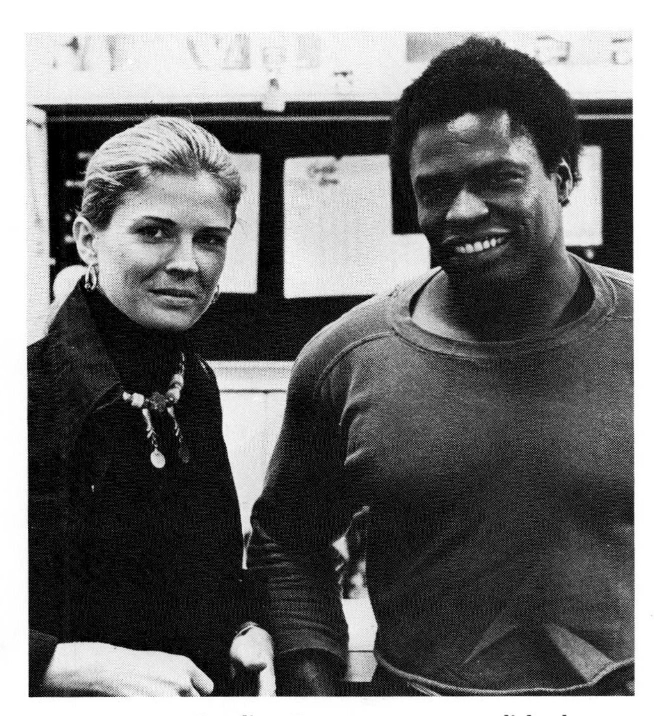

Actress Candice Bergen, an accomplished photographer, visited Gold's to document the growing bodybuilding movement (about 1977). Here she discusses the sport with Dave DuPre, Mr. California.

routine or valuable training or dietary tip from the profiled champ. Along with the other information included in this text, these short profiles will greatly assist you in reaching your goals as a bodybuilder.

What Is Bodybuilding?

Weight training—or the use of resistance apparatus such as barbells, dumbbells, and various exercise machines—encompasses several distinct categories:

1. *Bodybuilding*—The use of weight training to change the body's appearance.
2. *Strength Training*—Using weights to build maximum muscle power.
3. *Athletic Conditioning*—The use of weight training to improve athletic performance.
4. *Physical Fitness*—Using weights to increase general physical fitness, particularly strength.
5. *Injury Rehabilitation*—The use of weights to quickly regain normal strength in an injured joint or muscle group.

Bodybuilding in America is nearly a century old. Its popularity received a great boost at the turn of the century, when a German strongman named Erwin Muller performed widely on the vaudeville circuit under the stage name Sandow. He was so perfectly formed that a legion of men turned to weight training to improve their physical appearance.

A few years later Allan Calvert founded his Milo Bar-Bell Company in Philadelphia. Calvert began to manufacture adjustable barbell and dumbbell sets on which cast-iron discs could be fitted to increase or decrease the weight of the barbell or dumbbells. Prior to Calvert's innovation, barbells and dumbbells were cast in fixed poundages, so adjustable sets were a great advance. Calvert also sold his sets via mail order, making them accessible to men across America.

It should be noted that prior to the late 1960s and early 1970s few women would be caught dead near a barbell set. Women's bodybuilding is a recent phenomenon, competitive bodybuilding for women even a more recent happening. The first serious women's bodybuilding competition, a World Championships won by Lisa Lyon, was sponsored by Gold's Gym at the Los Angeles Embassy Auditorium in June 1979.

Lisa Lyon, the first World Women's Bodybuilding Champion, works her triceps at Gold's II. In the background to the left is Eddie Corney doing Roman Chair Sit-Ups. *(Photo by Craig Dietz)*

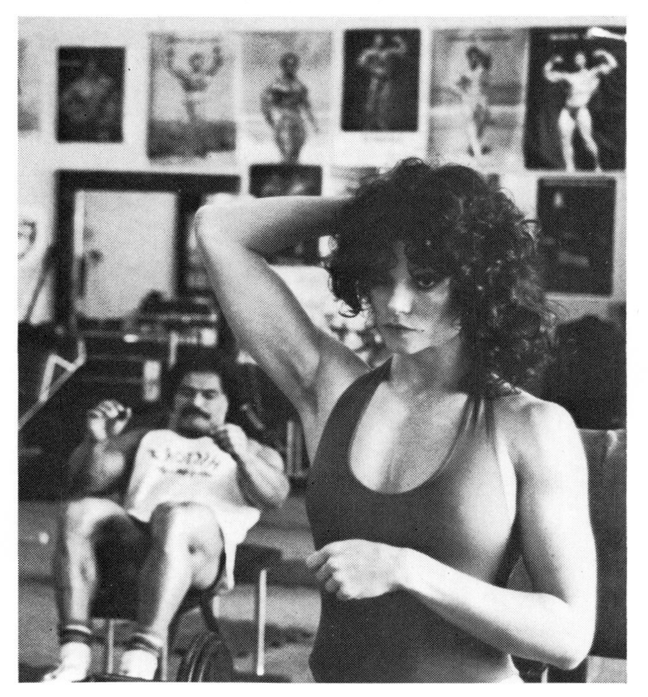

Since then, of course, women's bodybuilding has literally exploded in popularity.

During the 1920s bodybuilding was widely promoted by Bernarr MacFadden, author of numerous health and fitness books and publisher of *Strength* magazine. MacFadden sponsored a periodic physique contest through *Strength* and presented a medal to each winner. One such winner was an Italian immigrant named Angelo Siciliano. He is better known as Charles Atlas.

When *Strength* magazine failed during the early 1930s it was purchased by Bob Hoffman, who later became an Olympic weightlifting coach. Hoffman changed the magazine's name to *Strength & Health,* and his new magazine has been published continuously for the past 50 years.

Hoffman was primarily interested in competitive weightlifting, but he promoted bodybuilding widely via *Strength & Health.* He has employed John C. Grimek, the first Mr. America winner in 1940 and 1941, for nearly 40 years. Grimek is currently the editor of *Muscular Development,* a second Hoffman periodical, and he has appeared on more than 100 bodybuilding magazine covers over the years.

Without a doubt, the greatest driving force in publicizing bodybuilding has been Joe Weider, who began publishing *Your Physique* magazine in 1940. Now called *Muscle & Fitness,* this magazine has been published continuously since its inception, and it's so widely circulated that it's considered the bible of the sport.

In partnership with his brother Ben, president of the IFBB, Joe Weider has steadfastly promoted bodybuilding to the point at which it has become the world's fifth most popular sport. Numerous male and female professional bodybuilders can now make a handsome living from their sport. Truly, bodybuilding has reached the beginning of what could be a Golden Age.

Advantages and Disadvantages

There are a couple of minor disadvantages to bodybuilding training. The first of these is that the repetitious nature of weight workouts can make it somewhat boring. This is particularly true if you follow the same schedule of exercises for a relatively long period of time.

You will, however, be encouraged to change your training schedule from time to time, and this will prevent you from becoming bored. Additionally, the further you get into weight training and bodybuilding, the more intricate your task will become. When you are constantly monitoring all of your body's physiological responses to training, it is exceedingly difficult to become bored with your workouts.

Second, bodybuilding training doesn't provide your body with much cardiorespiratory fitness. Actual endurance training, such as running or cycling, is needed to accomplish this. The objective of bodybuilding, however, is to build muscle. And, as you become more advanced as a bodybuilder, you will be encouraged to do quite a bit of aerobic endurance training in addition to your weight workouts.

Arrayed against the disadvantages of bodybuilding training are four advantages. First, bodybuilding allows for total selectivity in training individual muscle groups, even small parts of each muscle mass. As a result, you can stress any muscle group you'd like to hit.

Second, in combination with diet, bodybuilding training allows you to gain or lose body weight at will. Markedly overweight or underweight individuals can fairly easily and quickly normalize their appearance through weight workouts and through a correct and persistent application of the dietary practices outlined in this book.

Third, when working out with weights you can very quickly gain exceptional strength. This by-product can actually be quite valuable to you. It makes many of your daily tasks easier. Also, you never know when a great degree of reserve physical power will come in handy. Strong arms, legs, and necks won't be broken as easily as weak ones, and an excellent physical condition can improve your chances of making it through a serious surgical operation and shorten recovery time.

Fourth, your strength will never outgrow the equipment you use. When you do calisthenics you are limited to the use of your body weight. Therefore, you will never grow any bigger or stronger than necessary to handle your body weight. With barbells, dumbbells, and the various bodybuilding machines, however, you can use up to a half-ton on most of your exercises.

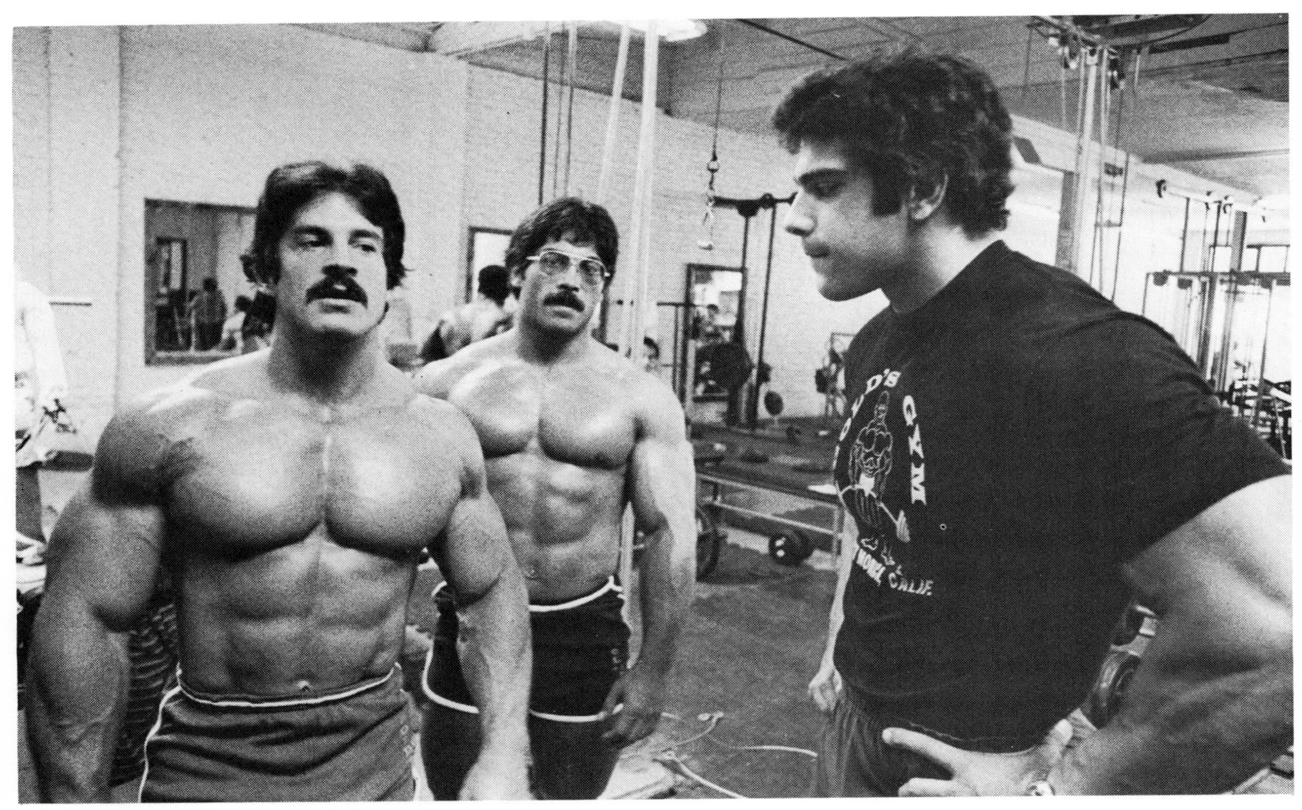

Lou Ferrigno discusses a bodybuilding technique with the Mentzer brothers. All three of these remarkable athletes have won Mr. America titles. *(Photo by Craig Dietz)*

Age Factors

Age has no bearing on whether or not you can train like a bodybuilder. It does, however, have a direct bearing on the speed with which you can gain muscle mass and quality. Prior to the age of about 14, young men and women generally aren't endocrinologically mature enough to make good gains. And after about age 45 the body is aging quickly enough to begin retarding the degree of improvement you can expect from your training. Practically speaking, then, the best bodybuilders are usually between the ages of 18 and 45.

If a young man or woman is quite dilligent in his or her training, it is possible to become an outstanding bodybuilder during the late teens. Casey Viator is probably the best example of this. At 18 he burst onto the national bodybuilding scene by placing third in the Mr. America contest behind Ken Waller and Chris Dickerson. Later that year he won the Teenage Mr. America and Senior Mr. USA titles. A year later, in 1971, he became history's youngest Mr. America winner. Casey is now about 30 and remains a staunch competitor in IFBB Pro shows.

Like fine wines, bodybuilders seem to improve with age. Most of the winners of men's professional titles in recent years have been over 35 years of age. At 50 Ed Corney still places respectably in the Mr. Olympia contest. Albert Beckles has won several pro titles at age 45, and Chris Dickerson (the all-time pro bodybuilding money winner) was over 40 before he won his first professional title.

You've no doubt noticed that we mentioned no very young or very mature female bodybuilders in this discussion. This is not to slight women bodybuilders. It is merely because the sport has not been in existence long enough to produce the same clear-cut age group examples of men's bodybuilding. There are, however, many good teenagers and past-40 contestants in women's competition. With time, the age parameters in women's bodybuilding will expand dramatically.

Men vs. Women

Your sex greatly influences the degree of strength and muscle mass that you can expect to attain. To build a great amount of muscle your body must have relatively large quantities of the male sex hormone testosterone. Both men and women secrete testosterone and the female sex hormone estrogen, but men secrete primarily testosterone and women primarily estrogen.

As a result, men can build strength and muscle mass more quickly and to a greater ultimate degree than women. Granted, some very muscular women have attained a relatively high degree of muscle mass (e.g., Laura Combes, Lisa Elliott, and Pillow), but they still look quite small next to such massive male bodybuilders as Tom Platz, Robby Robinson, and Franco Columbu.

A few women have relatively high androgenic (male hormone) levels in their bodies and have been relatively muscular all of their lives. Pillow and Lisa Elliott are good examples of women in the upper range of androgen production. Still, they have had to train exceedingly hard to develop balanced muscle proportions throughout their bodies.

Even women with low levels of androgens can become champion bodybuilders, though they generally must train for a somewhat longer period of time than the high-androgen women to become champions. Laura Combes and Rachel McLish are good examples of this type of low-androgen woman.

Due to the relatively low androgenic secretions of women (even in those we have called *high-androgen women*), they will be much weaker than men in a workout. But, generally speaking, women have a higher degree of physical endurance than their male training partners. They also usually have higher resistance to pain, so they can endure high-intensity workouts more readily.

Compared to men, women are stronger in the

Richard Baldwin and Laura Combes have frequently trained for extended periods of time at Gold's Gym. And the results are obvious—Richard has twice won his class at the Mr. America competition and Laura was the first Ms. America winner! *(Photo by John Balik)*

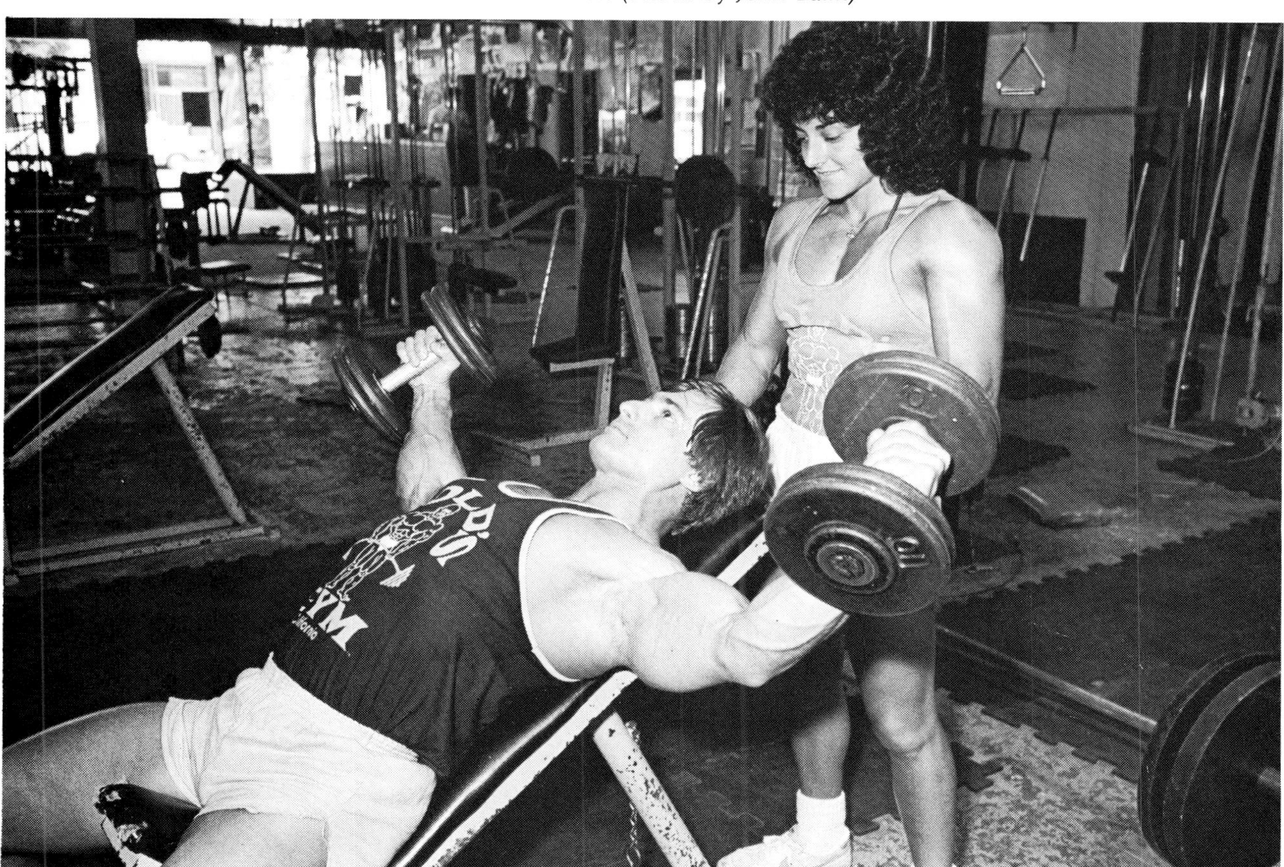

legs and weaker in the upper body. Some women can do leg exercises with weights comparable to those used by men of similar body weight. On arm, shoulder, chest, and back movements, however, they are comparatively weaker.

As will be discussed in much greater detail in Chapter 4, men and women make very compatible training partners. A woman can't handle a man's training poundages, while a man won't be able to do a woman's long and intense workouts. As a result, a man inspires a woman partner to train heavier, while she in turn inspires him to train longer and more intensely.

Bodybuilding Myths

At some point someone probably told you that working out with weights would make you muscle-bound or cause a woman to look like a man. Certainly, most good bodybuilders have been told that their muscles will turn to fat if they stop training.

There are six main "muscle myths" that must be exposed. In each case we will discuss the myth and then reveal the truth underlying it. This process should dispel any remaining doubts you might have about becoming a bodybuilder.

1. *Bodybuilding training will make you muscle-bound.* This is probably the most persistent muscle myth, and it suggests that working out with weights will make your body so tight and inflexible that you won't be able to scratch your own back or participate effectively in athletics.

Actually, scientists began investigating weight training and bodybuilding more than 30 years ago. They quickly discovered that weight workouts actually improve body flexibility. Indeed, almost all bodybuilders are far more flexible than the average person. Those who aren't have invariably been injured while participating in some other sport. As an example, a shoulder separation incurred while playing football can easily limit shoulder flexibility and function.

Speaking of football, superstar Walter Payton of the Chicago Bears has used progressive resistance weight training to build massive arms and shoulders. He can walk 50 yards on his hands, punishes anyone who tries to tackle him, and has never been seriously injured despite being near to the top of the NFL's "hit list" for several years. He's flexible *and then some!*

2. *All of your muscles will turn to fat once you stop working out.* It is physiologically impossible for muscle tissue to be converted to fat. What actually happens when you suspend your weight workouts is that your muscles gradually atrophy, or shrink in size and strength. This process takes about a year to run its course.

Then why are some former bodybuilders fat today? The answer to this question is true for *all* of the numerous athletes in any sport who have become fat after retiring from competition. When you train virtually every day for several hours you regularly burn up relatively large quantities of calories. As a result, you can consume more food than you can if you are physically inactive. But when you suspend training you no longer burn up so many calories. So, if you continue to eat the same amount as when you were working out every day, you will accumulate a caloric excess and gradually gain body fat. The obvious solution to this problem is to decrease your caloric consumption to compensate for the calories you are no longer burning off in your workouts. If you follow this advice, you will never grow fat after you cease heavy training with weights.

In actual practice, few bodybuilders ever stop training for very long. As they grow older they don't train as intensely as when they were competing, but they still hit the gym almost every day. Once you have iron fever, you're usually hooked for life.

3. *Bodybuilding will make a woman look like a man.* As noted in the foregoing section on men versus women, women don't secrete the same amounts of testosterone as do men. Therefore, they simply can't develop a man's muscle mass and quality. Additionally, a woman secretes large quantities of estrogen, which guarantees the integrity of her femininity. Unless she makes the disastrous mistake of taking male hormones, no woman will look masculine as a result of her bodybuilding training.

4. *Bodybuilding training can stunt your growth.* There are a somewhat disproportionate number of male and female competitive body-

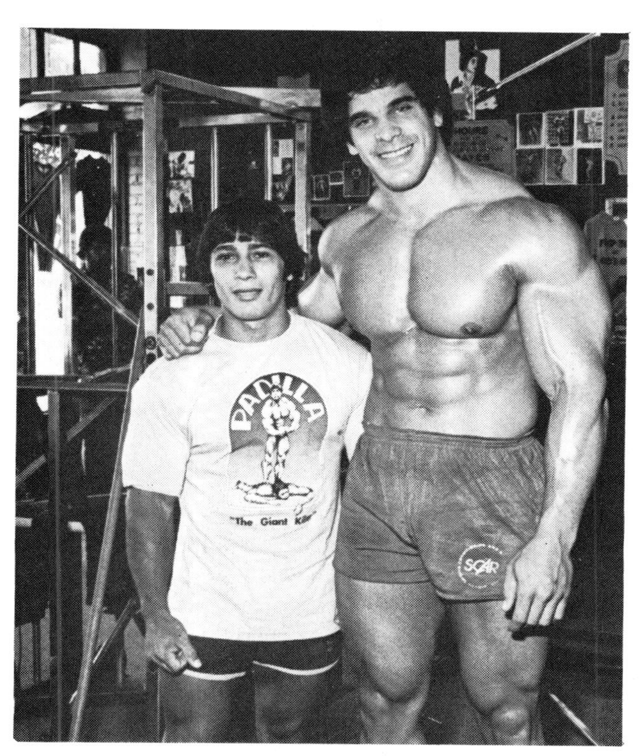

The long and short of Gold's Gym bodybuilders—6'5" Lou Ferrigno with his 5'3" buddy, Danny Padilla. Both athletes have won Mr. America and Mr. Universe titles. *(Photo by John Balik)*

builders who are below the national average in height, leading some individuals to conclude that bodybuilding workouts can stunt one's growth. Taller athletes are usually naturally selected for other sports in what could be called a sort of "sports Darwinism." Having a more compact torso and short limbs allows the bodybuilder to attain the proper proportions needed to win a contest. And as a result, bodybuilding tends to naturally select short or medium-statured men and women.

There are numerous tall bodybuilders, such as Lou Ferrigno (6'5") and Dr. Lynne Pirie (5'9"). Scientists have determined that any type of physical activity will tend to stimulate height increases rather than inhibit them. Proper diet can also result in height increase, and bodybuilders consistently follow health-promoting diets. Certainly, parents needn't worry that their sons and daughters will end up being short in stature simply because they decide to become bodybuilders.

5. *Bodybuilding training will wreck your back, knees, elbows, and other joints.* Such spinal or joint injuries are much more common in other sports than in bodybuilding. As long as you follow the warm-up procedures we will outline, and maintain the correct biomechanical (body) positions for each exercise, you needn't fear damaging your joints through bodybuilding training.

6. *Bodybuilding training can slow you down.* As with the myth about becoming muscle-bound, scientists proved more than 30 years ago that heavy weight training improves speed rather than detracting from it. Reaction time can't be improved through weight workouts, but a stronger muscle can contract faster and more strongly, thereby moving a limb more quickly. Sprint speed, for example, is a direct function of thigh and calf strength. In modern athletics, virtually all athletes include weight training in their overall conditioning regimens. They certainly wouldn't do this if heavy weight workouts inhibited their speed, because it would reduce their athletic ability.

Five Inspiring Success Stories

Every champion bodybuilder is a living success story. Each one—male and female—has conquered obesity, severe underweight condition, physical weakness, illness, and hopelessness. To conclude this chapter we will present the stories of five champions who have trained regularly at Gold's Gym. These case studies should inspire you to train like a superstar from your very first workout.

Tom Platz

In recent years Tom Platz has become the most incredible male bodybuilder on today's scene. Many aficionados of the sport feel that Tom has become the logical heir to Arnold Schwarzenegger's crown as the sport's dominant athlete.

Tom's father gave him a barbell set for Christmas when he was 13. Tommy had been overweight, and his father felt that physical activity would improve his health and appearance. Tom did train a little with his weight set, but it wasn't until two years later that he took to bodybuilding with a vengeance. "I felt a calling—the same as a priest feels one—to be-

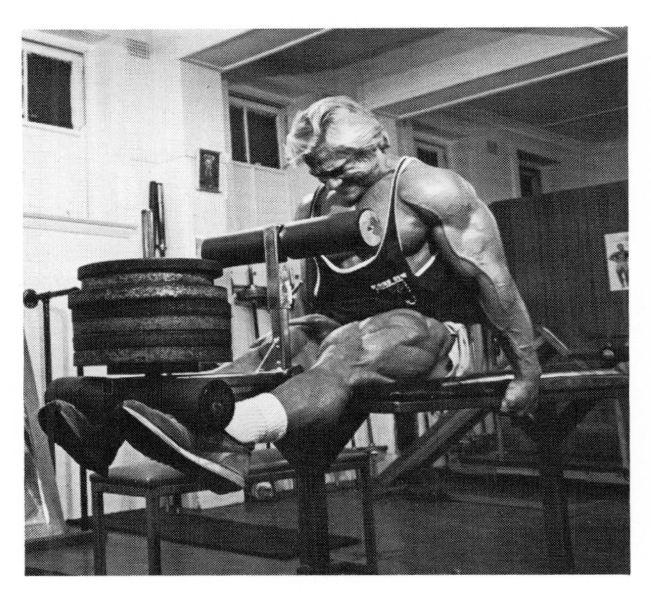

Tom Platz. *(Photo by Mike Neveux)*

come a champion bodybuilder," Tom stated.

Platz rapidly gained muscle, and before his 20th birthday he had placed second in the Teenage Mr. America competition and won the Mr. Michigan title. By 1977, he was good enough to place second in his class at the Mr. America competition. But his legs were dramatically superior to his upper body, and most bodybuilding experts predicted that Tom would go no further as a bodybuilder.

Tom never takes "no" for an answer, however, and he slaved away at Gold's Gym to improve his upper body. Platz had his efforts rewarded when he won the 1978 IFBB Mr. Universe title. Three years later he placed third in the Mr. Olympia contest, establishing himself as the man to beat in the Olympia in future years.

Stacey Bentley

Stacey was very overweight as a young girl. She was also the frequent victim of long depressions. Out of a sense of despair she joined a Nautilus fitness center. This began her dramatic transformation from overweight adolescent to champion bodybuilder.

"I hope that every fat girl out there decides she's had enough and that it's time to make a change," Stacey said. "It can be done, and I'm a good example of what bodybuilding can do for

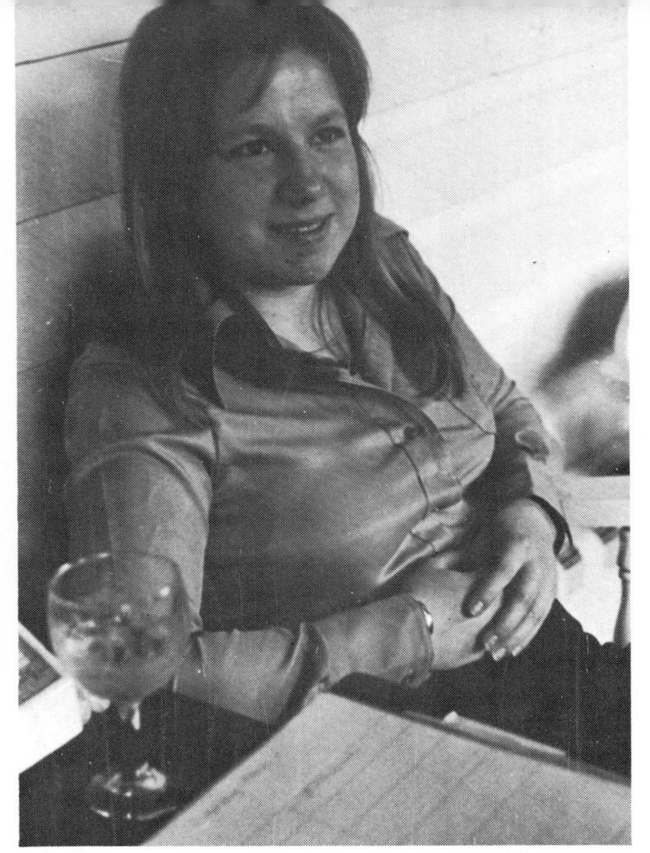

Stacey Bentley, above, was frequently depressed and overweight. Below, after weight training for a year, Stacey had shed the extra weight and the blues. *(Bottom photo by Peter Brenner)*

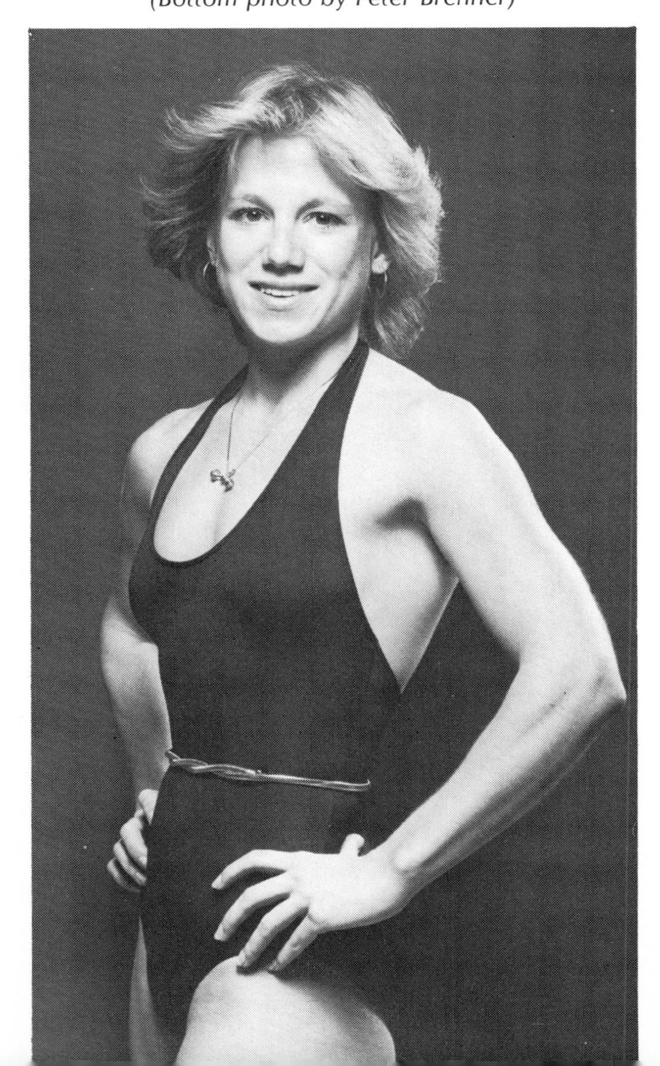

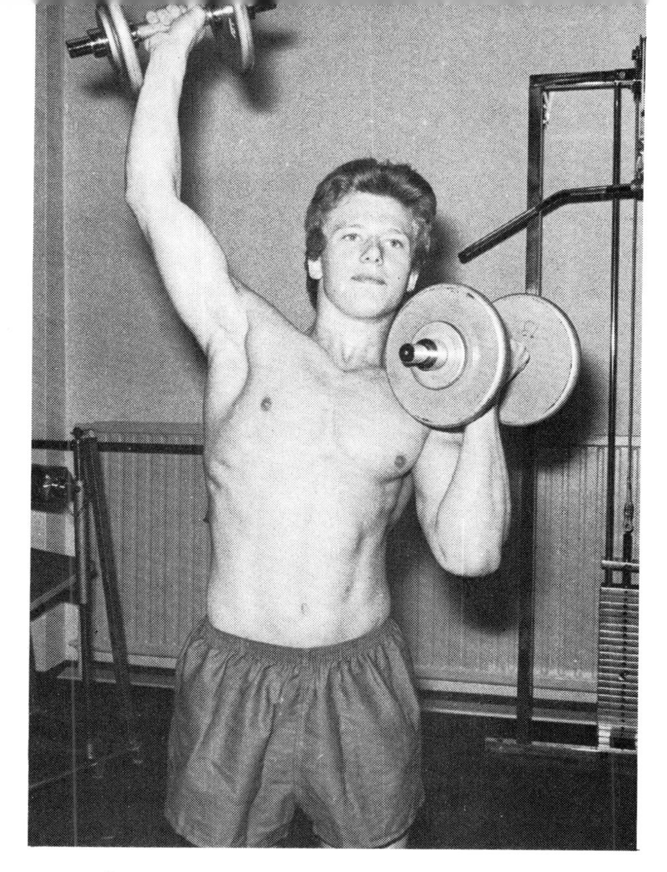

Andreas Cahling, above, looked like the original skinny kid, but he packed on plenty of muscle, below. *(Bottom photo by John Balik)*

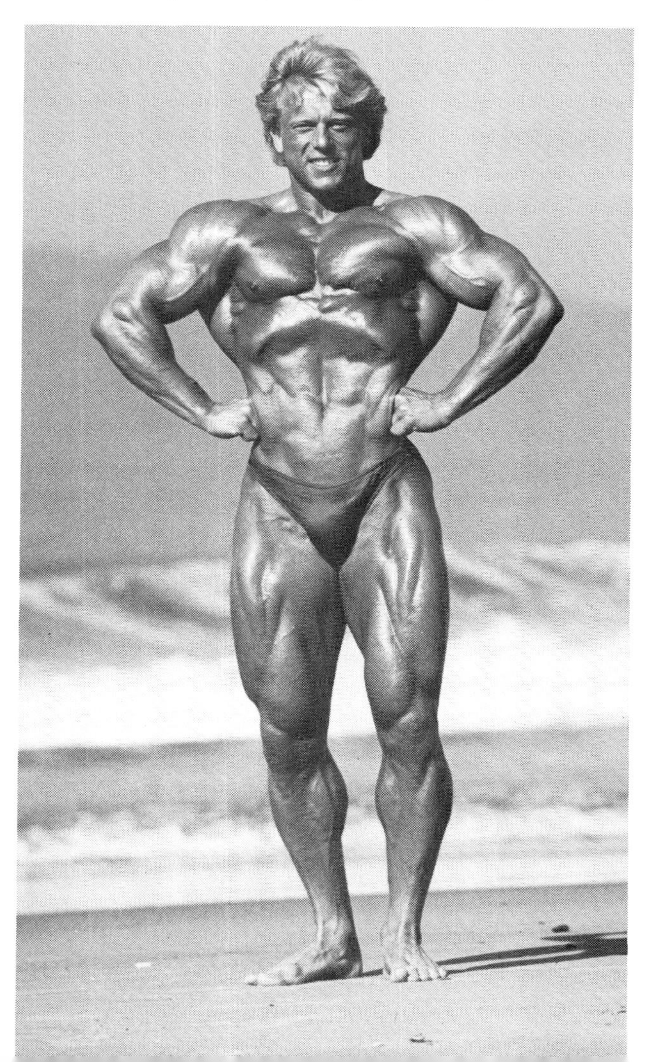

any woman. At 5′1″ in height, I once weighed between 140 and 150 pounds. Within a year of commencing training I had reduced my weight to 115 pounds and greatly improved my self-image. Another year and I was down to 105 pounds and beginning to place in bodybuilding competitions!"

Stacey proceeded to win the Zane Invitational Bodybuilding Championships and the World Couples Championships (with Chris Dickerson as her partner). She also placed in the top five in the first Ms. Olympia contest. She is currently retired from bodybuilding competition and pursuing a religious calling.

Andreas Cahling

Andreas is typical of the many international bodybuilders who have trained at Gold's through the years. With a strong background in wrestling and judo, a skinny Cahling landed in California for a vacation in 1975. He found the atmosphere there so congenial that he decided to stay and train at Gold's Gym.

From a base body weight of 155 pounds, Andreas slowly added solid muscle mass until, in 1980, he won the prestigious IFBB Mr. International title. He is now one of the world's most popular bodybuilders and a budding businessman. His success story is similar to those of Arnold Schwarzenegger, Franco Columbu, and numerous other international bodybuilders who have found a home at Gold's Gym.

Andreas Cahling's story is even more interesting because he has achieved his greatest bodybuilding successes as a lacto-ovo-vegetarian bodybuilder. He will give you a number of tips on vegetarian bodybuilding in Chapter 6 of this book.

Rachel McLish

Gold's member Rachel McLish is without a doubt the most successful woman bodybuilder to date. She has won the U.S. Championships, World Championships, and Ms. Olympia title. Rachel is also beginning to be successful as a model and in television commercials. And she is writing a book on women's bodybuilding. She feels that weight training can be used to develop beauty from the inside out.

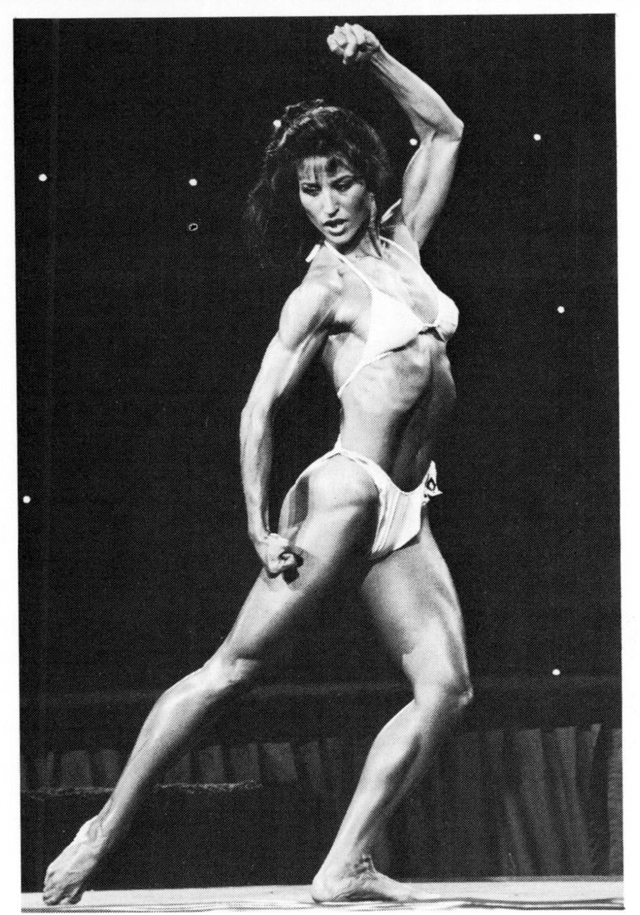

Rachel McLish, Miss Olympia 1982. *(Photo by John Balik)*

When Rachel began bodybuilding at the age of 19 she was somewhat underweight. At 26 she now weighs 118–120 pounds at a height of 5′6″. This is approximately 20 pounds more than she weighed initially. And as she gradually improves her body, Rachel becomes more and more beautiful.

"There's truth in the old adage that beauty comes from the inside out," Rachel McLish maintains. "The bodybuilding lifestyle—the training, diet, and regular habits—results in buoyant health, which translates into radiant beauty. I always look the best in the sense of feminine beauty on the day of a competition when I'm totally peaked out, so I'll still be bodybuilding when I'm 75. And I'll expect to look 39 at that age!"

Tim Belknap

Tim Belknap's success story is probably one of the most inspirational you will ever read. He literally rose from the dead to begin bodybuilding training, eventually won the Mr. America contest, and became one of the most respected new champion bodybuilders to come along in many years.

Belknap was so small, sickly, and weak as a youth—he was diabetic—that even the girls at his junior high school could (and regularly did) beat him up. One day he was rushed to a hospital in a diabetic coma and was actually pronounced dead on arrival at the emergency room, only to be revived subsequently. By the time he was finally released from the hospital Tim weighed only 95 pounds.

Resolving to pull himself up by the bootstraps, Tim Belknap joined a health spa and began regular and progressive bodybuilding workouts. Slowly at first, and then with gathering momentum, he began to make gains in muscle mass and health improvement.

Ultimately, Belknap built his body up to a relatively solid 215 pounds (he's 5′5″ tall). He developed phenomenal power and stamina, which allowed him to do Squats with 675 pounds 10 times and do Bench Presses with 505 pounds six times.

Tim Belknap is diabetic and will be so as long as he lives, but girls no longer pound him. From a sickly youth, this former pencil neck has grown to become one of the most herculean bodybuilders of all time!

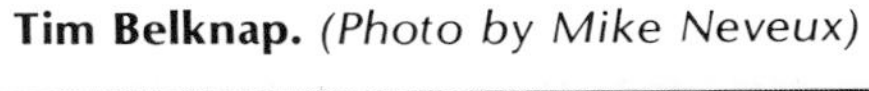

Tim Belknap. *(Photo by Mike Neveux)*

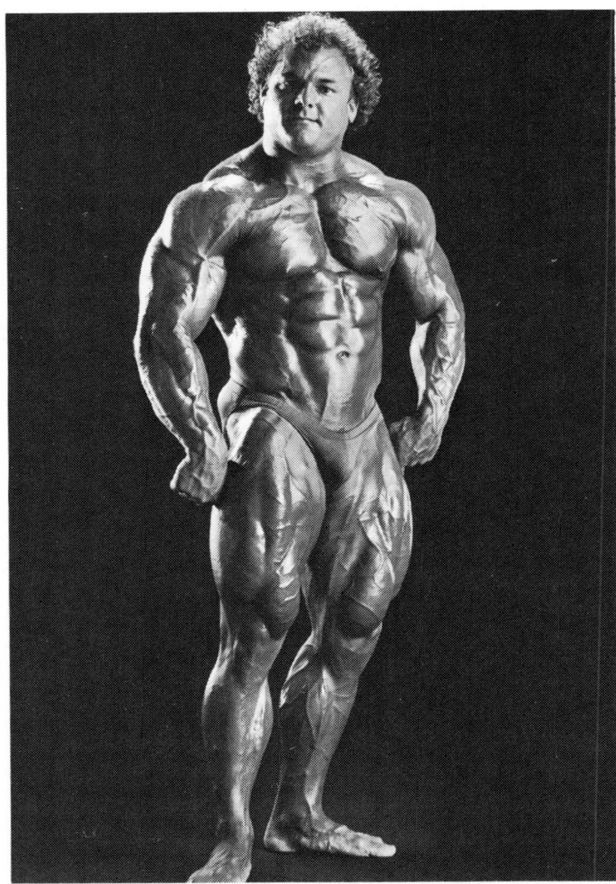

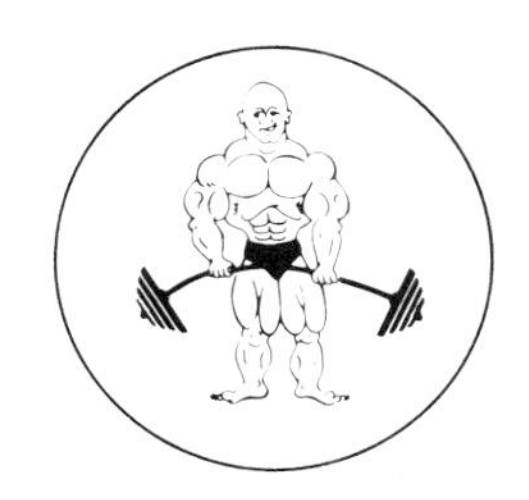

2 BODYBUILDING FUNDAMENTALS

Welcome to the fantastic world of bodybuilding! You are about to take the first steps on what may or may not be a long journey to success as a competitive bodybuilder. The road you follow will not be without hardship, but you have joined an elite group of men and women who thrive on hard work and self-sacrifice. We are confident that you will reach your goal by following the road map we begin to draw for you in this chapter.

First we will present a group of definitions; then you will be introduced to the tools of a bodybuilder's trade—the barbells, dumbbells, exercise machines, and other apparatus that you will use during each workout. Other topics to be covered include the importance of physical examinations; the physiology of muscle growth; the relationship between overloading a muscle and progression of resistance; where to train; how often to work out; how many counts to do of each exercise; the value of taking rest intervals; how to choose correct training poundages; how to break into a new workout and avoid muscle soreness; what to wear during a training session; some basic nutrition tips; the value of sleep, rest, and recuperation; how to keep accurate training journals; and how to warm up efficiently and productively before working out.

The information contained in this chapter is fundamental to every workout you will ever take as a bodybuilder, so it's essential that you master every technique discussed before stepping into a gym for your first training session. Don't be afraid to go over this chapter more than once, until you are certain that you know every technique and procedure forward and backward. Such a thorough mastery of the information contained in this chapter will make your workouts far more productive over the years.

Basic Terminology

Bodybuilding has spawned a unique jargon that can be confusing to any novice trainee. In this section we will define 10 fundamental terms, which when understood will sweep away 95% of your potential confusion. There also is a Glossary at the back of this book that will define most terms used in bodybuilding.

An *exercise* is each individual movement that you do when you train. Less frequently, an exercise is referred to as a *movement.* Sit-ups and Push-ups are calisthenic exercises, movements that use the weight of your body for resistance. Some of the most commonly performed bodybuilding exercises are Squats, Bench Presses, Barbell Bent Rows, and Barbell Toe Raises. These and numerous other exercises are illustrated and described precisely in chapters 3, 5, and 7.

A *repetition* is each individual count that you do of an exercise. Repetitions are often abbreviated to *reps.* Distinct groupings of reps (most commonly 6–12) are called *sets.* Normally, several sets (most commonly 3–5) are done of each exercise, with a *rest interval* of 60–90 seconds between sets. A rest interval gives you time to catch your breath and prepare yourself mentally for the next set.

The full schedule of sets and reps that you do of various exercises in one day is called a *routine,* a *program,* or a *training schedule.* Occasionally these terms refer to a specific routine that is written out on a card for reference while training, handwritten in a training journal, or printed in a book or bodybuilding magazine.

When you actually perform your routine, you will be taking a *workout,* or *working out* or *training.* A workout is occasionally referred to as a *training session.*

If you have a working knowledge of the foregoing terms—and are familiar with the pieces of training equipment described and depicted in the next section—no one will laugh at you if you walk into any of the Gold's Gyms located around the world. In fact, you'll speak "bodybuildingese" as well as Pete Grymkowski, Rachel McLish, Casey Viator, and all of the other famous alumni of Gold's Gym.

Bodybuilding Equipment

There are myriad pieces of bodybuilding equipment, most of which you will use regularly in your workouts. These pieces of equipment fall generally into four classifications: free weights (barbells, dumbbells, and related apparatus), Nautilus machines, Universal Gym machines, and Corbin-Pacific (formerly Corbin-Gentry) machines. The last three types of equipment are trade-named, and each manufacturer has a variety of resistance exercise machines available. There are literally hundreds of manufacturers and distributors of free weights and related apparatus throughout the United States, Canada, and the rest of the world.

Each type and individual piece of equipment will be described and depicted and its unique function and values given. Combining this information with the exercise descriptions in chapters 3, 5, and 7, you will be able to walk totally cold into any gym in America, recognize the various pieces of equipment, and use them correctly and safely.

Free Weights

Free weights are the most commonly used type of equipment throughout the world. In most home gyms free weights are the only type of equipment available to an aspiring bodybuilder. They are far and away the least expensive of the four major classes of bodybuilding equipment noted. For less than $200 you can equip a home gym sufficiently to allow a great workout for every muscle group in your body. Sufficient Nautilus, Universal Gym, or Corbin-Gentry equipment for an equivalent workout will cost between $3,000 and $50,000, however. The parent Gold's Gym in Venice, California, has an installation of all four types of equipment that cost more than $100,000!

A *barbell* is the most basic piece of free-weight equipment. It consists of a steel bar four to six feet in length to which flat metal or vinyl-covered concrete discs called *plates* are attached by means of clamps called *collars.* Most commonly, exercise plates come in sizes weighing 50, 25, 20, 15, 12½, 10, 7½, 5, 2½, and 1¼ pounds.

The bar of a common exercise barbell set is usually encased by a hollow metal tube called a *sleeve,* which allows the bar to rotate more freely in a bodybuilder's hands. Most sleeves are scored with shallow crosshatched grooves called *knurlings,* which allow a more secure grip on the barbell when a bodybuilder's hands are sweaty.

Inside collars keep the plates of a barbell from sliding inward against the hands. Inside collars are either welded permanently in place or attached semipermanently by means of *set* screws. *Outside collars* are attached outward of the plates to keep them from falling off. The set screw in the outside collars of an adjustable

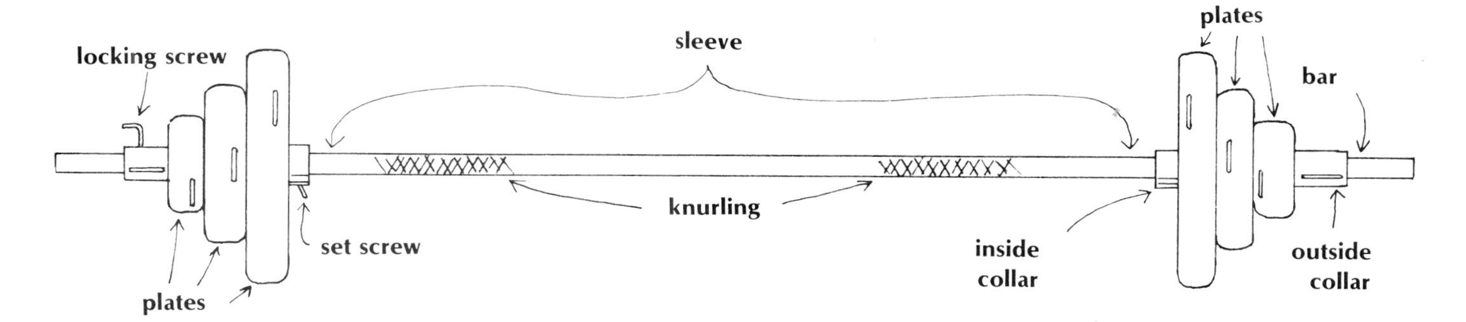

Figure 1

exercise barbell usually has a handle attached to it to allow for quick tightening and loosening of the collar. Figure 1, above, shows a common adjustable exercise barbell with all of its parts labeled correctly.

At a home gym barbells are usually adjustable, but in large commercial gyms there will be a wide variety of *fixed barbells* with the weights welded or bolted permanently in place. These *fixed weights* are provided in 5–10-pound increments from about 20 pounds up to 150 pounds or more. These barbells are placed on racks, and the correct weight of each one is painted clearly on the barbell's plates. When you use one of these fixed barbells it is good bodybuilding etiquette to return it to the correct rack as soon as you are finished with it.

With an adjustable set you must include the weight of the bar and its collars as a base poundage to which you add appropriate plates to form a desired exercise weight. An exercise bar, with its collars, normally weighs five pounds per foot of length. To be more precise, you can actually weigh your bar and its collars.

If you buy a barbell and dumbbell set for home use, you will find that the metal plates are more durable than the vinyl-covered ones. Some of the metal plates in use at Gold's/Venice are more than 10 years old, have been used hundreds of thousands of times, and are still as good as new. Vinyl-covered concrete plates are easy on bedroom floors, but with heavy use they will break open and lose their usefulness. Also, vinyl-concrete plates are much more bulky than metal ones, and to make up a respectable training poundage with them requires an exceedingly long bar.

You can use barbells to exercise literally every major musculoskeletal group of your body. Barbells are almost always used with two arms or two legs at once, and you can very quickly use substantial poundages in most barbell movements.

In any large commercial bodybuilding gym you will see a larger-than-usual barbell about seven feet in length called an *Olympic barbell.* This is an expensive, specially machined, and standardized barbell used in national and inter-

Sergio Oliva, "The Myth" and winner of three Mr. Olympia titles, warms up using an Olympic barbell at Gold's I. *(Photo by Art Zeller)*

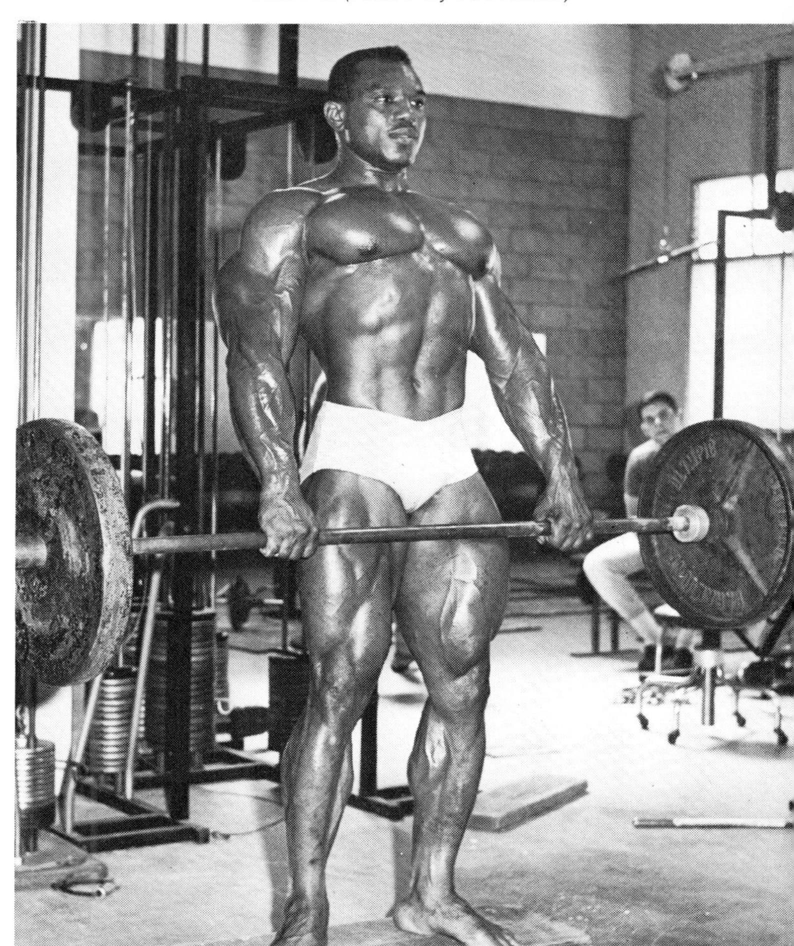

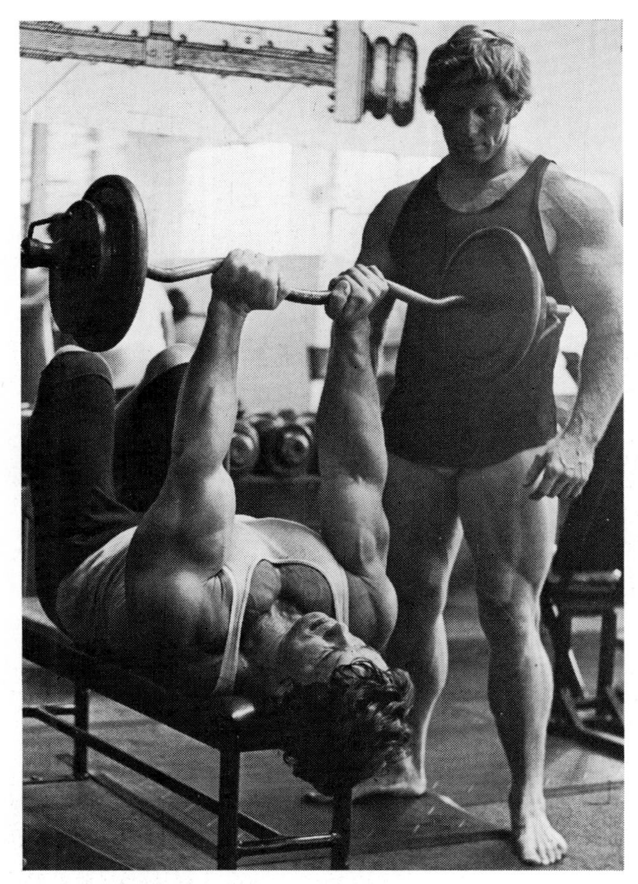

Kenny Waller (Mr. America, Mr. International, and twice Mr. Universe) spots Arnold Schwarzenegger for an intense set of Lying Triceps Extensions using an EZ-curl bar. *(Photo by Bob Freeman)*

national competitive weightlifting meets. Olympic bars are also used to load the body with very heavy poundages for such exercises as Squats, Bench Presses, and Deadlifts. These barbells can safely be loaded to 700 pounds or more, which is enough resistance to accommodate even the strongest bodybuilders.

Olympic barbells are standardized so that unloaded bars weigh either 20 kilograms (44½ pounds) or 45 pounds. Each adjustable collar weighs either 2½ kilos (5½ pounds) or five pounds. The most common metric plates used on these sets are 20, 15, 10, 7½, 5, 2½, and 1¼ kilograms. On nonmetric sets the most commonly used plates weigh 45, 35, 25, 10, 5, and 2½ pounds. Nonmetric sets are most commonly found in America gyms.

In organized gyms—as well as in some home gyms—you'll see a type of multicurved barbell bar that Roy Callender (Pro and Amateur Mr. Universe) calls "wiggly bars." These are more commonly referred to as *EZ-curl bars.* EZ-curl bars allow you to use a wider variety of hand grips than you can use on a normal straight barbell bar. You'll use an EZ-curl bar most frequently for arm exercises.

Dumbbells are shorter versions (usually 10–14 inches in length) of barbells. Each is intended for use in one hand, using one or both arms at a time. You can do dumbbell movements for all of the major musculoskeletal groups of your body. The nomenclature of a dumbbell is identical to that of a barbell. In a home gym you will use adjustable dumbbells, which often lack inside collars. At Gold's/Venice there are several racks of paired, fixed dumbbells in five-pound increments ranging in weight from five pounds apiece to 150 pounds apiece.

In any organized commercial gym you will find a wide variety of *exercise benches.* These include *flat benches, incline benches,* and *decline benches.* You lie an incline bench with

Mike Mentzer bombs his back for lat thickness at Gold's II with One-Arm Dumbbell Bent Rowing. *(Photo by Bill Reynolds)*

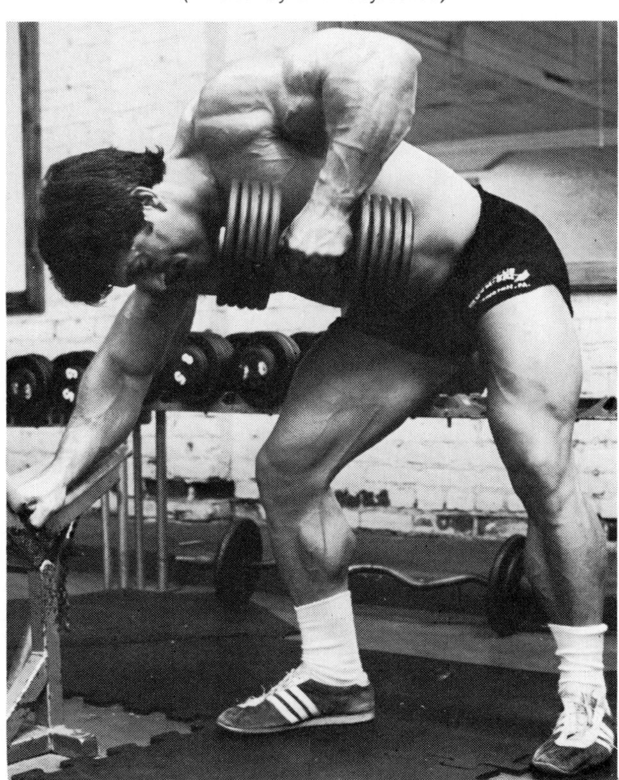

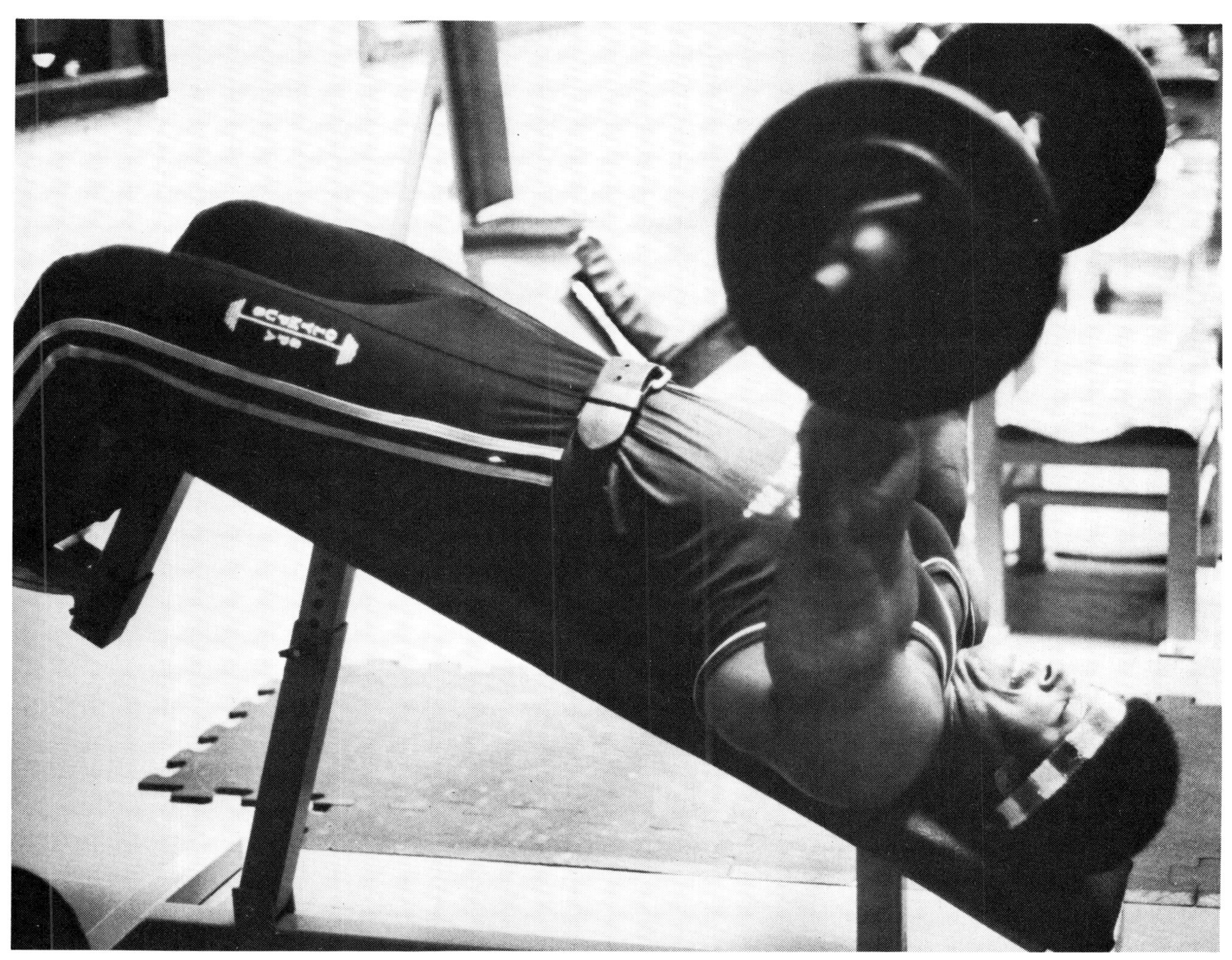

Bill Grant (Pro Mr. World and Pro Mr. America) adds to his triceps development with a super-intense set of Triceps Extensions on a decline bench. *(Photo by Bill Reynolds)*

your head at the top end, while you lie on a *decline bench* with your head at the bottom end. These benches are used for a wide variety of chest, shoulder, arm, forearm, and back exercises. The function of each bench will become crystal clear to you as you read the exercise descriptions in chapters 3, 5, and 7.

One specialized bench, called a *bench press rack* or *bench pressing bench,* has uprights at one end with weight-supporting hooks or cups attached to them. In the bodybuilding exercise called a Bench Press, you will quickly be able to use more weight than you can get into position for the movement unassisted. With this bench you can load up a heavy barbell while lying on the supports, then lift the weight off unassisted from the supports to do a set of Bench Presses.

A *squat rack* operates according to the same principle as a bench press rack. The muscles of a bodybuilder's thighs are so large that you will very quickly be able to do Deep Knee Bends (usually called *Squats* in bodybuilding parlance) with a much heavier barbell held across your shoulders than you can lift up to your shoulders. Several types of squat racks allow you to load up a heavy barbell that's supported at a level a little lower than your shoulders. Then you simply step under the bar, position it comfortably across your shoulders, straighten your legs to take the weight off the supports, walk backward one or two steps, correctly position your feet, and then do your set of Squats. Once you have finished your set you merely walk forward and place the barbell back on the rack.

The simplest type of squat rack consists of two vertical supports fastened to individual portable stands. At the top of these supports are welded hooks or cups like those on a bench press rack on which the weight rests. This type of squat stand is OK for home gym training, but in organized gyms you'll invariably find heavy-duty squat racks permanently bolted to the floor and gym wall. One such squat rack consists of two or more vertical steel pipes with two cross pipes welded to the top and bolted on the other end to the gym wall. This type of squat rack doesn't allow for individual trainee height variance, however, so you'll more often see a squat rack with two long angled steel pieces attached to the floor on one end and the wall on the other. To these pieces of steel are welded pins projecting out every two to three inches to hold the bar in position at a wide variety of heights.

Intensity is written all over the face of Lou Ferrigno (Mr. America, Mr. International, The Incredible Hulk, and Hercules) as he does Cable Side Laterals at Gold's II. *(Photo by Craig Dietz)*

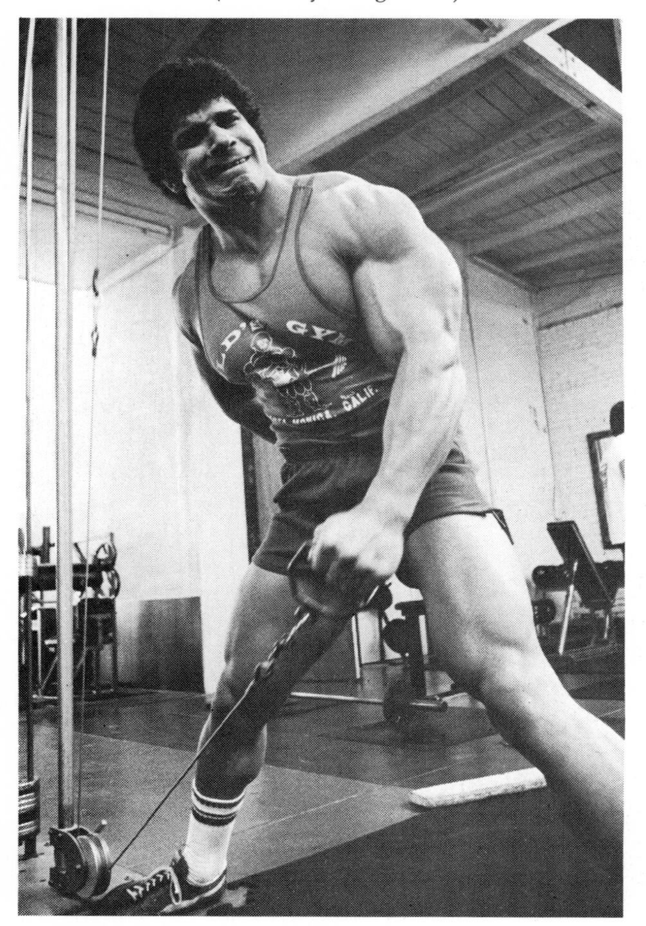

Squat racks are usually used to do heavy Squats and Front Squats, which develop the powerful thigh, hip, and lower back muscles. Occasionally, however, you'll see very strong bodybuilders use such a rack to avoid cleaning a heavy weight to the shoulders for Military Presses and Presses behind the Neck, two superb shoulder mass-building movements.

Most first-class commercial bodybuilding gyms will have a *Smith machine,* which consists of two upright runners along which you can slide a permanently attached barbell handle. The machine is also constructed in such a manner that you can stop the bar with hooks at six-inch intervals along the uprights. A Smith machine is excellent for doing Military Presses, Presses behind the Neck, and even Squats.

There are two types of *calf machines* in most bodybuilding gyms, a *standing calf machine* and a *seated calf machine.* Both machines are used to develop the powerful calf muscles along the back of your lower legs. In the early days of weight training and bodybuilding, the only calf-building movement most people used was a Calf Raise, done standing with a barbell held across the shoulders. Unfortunately, this movement had little value, because it was difficult to maintain balance while doing it. The standing calf machine was developed to combat this problem of balance. The machine consists of a yoke attached to an upright or to the wall by a large hinge. A weight is attached to the yoke. You simply place the yoke across your shoulders, in which position you can do Toe Raises with no worries about your balance during the movement.

The only way you can develop the soleus muscle, which lies under the gastrocnemius of your calf, is to do Calf Raises with your leg bent at a 90-degree angle. Originally, Seated Toe Raises were done with the knees bent at a 90-degree angle while sitting on a bench and holding a heavy barbell across the knees. Unfortunately, this movement is cumbersome in terms of getting the weight into position. A modern seated calf machine allows you to do Seated Toe Raises with a heavy weight resting comfortably and securely on your knees.

Various types of *leg tables* are available,

either combining *leg extension machines* and *leg curl machines* or featuring one or the other machine. A leg extension machine operates on a leverage principle to place direct isolated stress on the quadriceps muscles along the front of the thighs. A leg curl machine allows you to place the same type of direct isolated stress on the biceps femoris, or hamstring, muscles along the back of the thighs.

At Gold's Gym a wide variety of exercise *pulleys,* which consist of one of more pulleys, a steel cable, a handle on one end of the cable, and a weight on the other end, are available. You will become thoroughly familiar with these pulleys as you master the exercises depicted and described in chapters 3, 5, and 7. Cables are most frequently used to develop the chest, arm, and shoulder muscles.

A *preacher curl bench,* which is often called a *Scott curl bench* in honor of the man who pioneered its use, Larry Scott (the first Mr. Olympia winner), is an angled pad at the top of some type of support. By leaning over this pad and doing Barbell Curls or Dumbbell Curls, you can strongly stress your biceps muscles with no chance of cheating during the movement. This bench is used to develop a round, full biceps muscle, particularly biceps that are very full at the lower insertions. Bill Grant (Pro Mr. America and Mr. World) used this bench extensively at Gold's, and his biceps are incredibly full and round.

There are several types of *curl machines,* which are used to develop the biceps. The machines are excellent for biceps development, because they operate with a pulley apparatus that keeps tension on the biceps muscles throughout their full range of movement.

Holdovers from the gymnastics training that many early bodybuilders did are *chinning bars* and *dipping bars.* You may already be familiar with these pieces of equipment. Chinning bars are used to develop the latissimus dorsi muscles of the upper back, while dipping bars are used to develop the muscles of the chest, shoulders, and upper arms.

Beautiful Rachel McLish, Miss Olympia and Pro World Champion, gets serious with a heavy set of Seated Pulley Rows at Gold's III. *(Photo by Mike Neveux)*

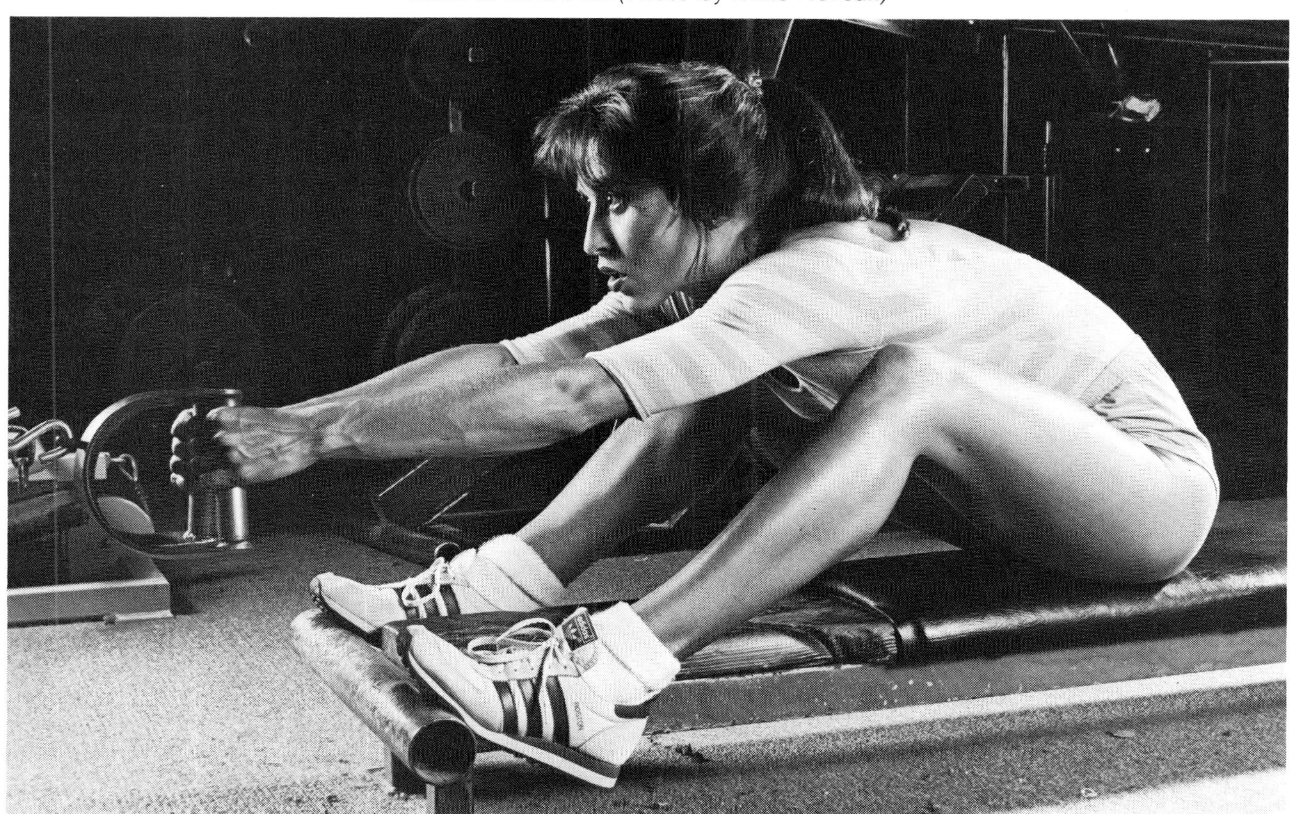

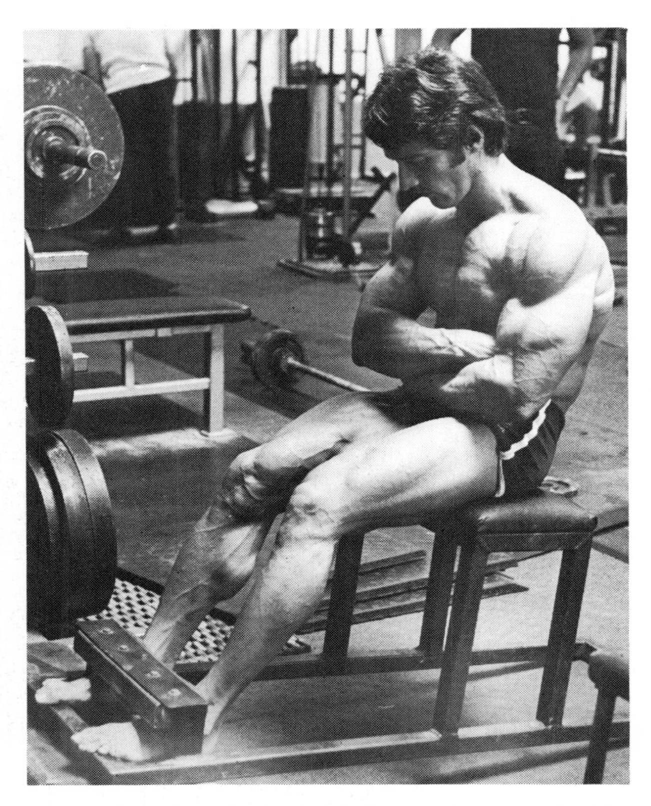

Lost in thoughts of winning his next Mr. Olympia title, Frank Zane does hundreds of Roman Chair Sit-Ups.

Several types of *hack machines* are intended to develop the front thigh muscles in relative isolation from the other muscles of the body, but without the spinal compression experienced when doing Squats. With one type of hack machine you grasp handles at the sides of your hips and lie back against a movable platform as you do the movement. On another type of hack machine, one that seems to be very popular at Gold's, you do the same type of movement with your shoulders resting against a pair of yokes attached to the movable part of the machine.

There are several types of *leg press machines* with which you can also do thigh exercise with very heavy weights without the type of spinal compression felt when doing Squats. The oldest type of leg press machine consists of vertical runners, along which is fitted a weighted platform. While lying on your back, you place your feet on that sliding platform and bend and straighten your legs against the weight. There is also a 45-degree-angled leg press machine that has become very popular at Gold's.

A *lat machine* consists of a bar attached to a cable running through one or more pulleys to a weight. By pulling this bar down to your body, you can simulate a chinning movement. With a lat machine you can use a weight much lighter than your body weight, so if you are unable to do a sufficient number of Chins, you can do a similar movement with a lat machine. The lat machine is used to build up the latissimus dorsi muscles of the upper back.

A *seated rowing machine* consists of a handle attached to a cable running through a low pulley, a higher pulley, and down to a weight stack. By sitting on the bench attached to the machine, you can do a movement similar to rowing a boat but with a very heavy weight. The seated rowing machine is used to develop the large latissimus dorsi muscles of your upper back.

An *abdominal board* consists of a padded board with a strap or set of roller pads attached to one end. The end with the pads usually has a sort of ladder arrangement with which the abdominal board can be adjusted at various angles. This apparatus is normally used to do Sit-ups and Leg Raises, movements that develop the front abdominal muscles.

A *Roman chair* can also be used to develop the front abdominal muscles. This apparatus consists of a padded seat and a toe bar. By sitting on the seat and placing your toes under the bar, you can do short-range Sit-ups to stress the front abs. The Roman chair has become quite popular among champion bodybuilders over the past few years.

You can use a *wrist roller* to develop the muscles of your forearms. This consists of a dowel-like arrangement around which you roll a cable or cord attached to a weight. You can roll up the cable either forward or backward. Some wrist rollers are used freehand, while others are attached to some type of support system bolted to the gym wall.

A *neck strap* consists of a head harness attached to a weight. By doing various head movements while wearing this neck strap, you can develop all of the muscles of your neck.

Universal Gym

A single Universal Gym machine incorporates exercise stations on which you can do movements for all of the major musculoskeletal groups of your body. As such, Universal Gyms are convenient and versatile units. They're especially good in school situations, because several students can work out on one machine simultaneously. And for the number of functions it allows, the machine is relatively inexpensive.

The drawback of Universal Gym machines—as well as of most other exercise machines—lies in the narrow range of individual movements that can be done for each muscle group. At most, only two or three movements can be done for each body part on a Universal Gym machine. And experienced bodybuilders would soon become bored doing such a small variety of exercises. Using free weights and related apparatus, in contrast, you can do 100 or more exercises for most muscle groups. With that much variety available in exercise routines, it's very difficult to become bored with your training.

At Gold's Gym virtually all of the better bodybuilders use a Universal Gym machine for at least one or two exercises in each workout. The floor pulley is seldom used, and the lat pulley is more often utilized to do Pulley Pushdowns for triceps development than Lat Pulldowns for back development. The bench pressing station is used more by good bodybuilders to do Incline Presses and Decline Presses than it is to do Bench Presses. And the leg press and overhead pressing stations are quite popular.

Newer-model Universal Gyms incorporate "variable resistance" into many of the movements that can be done on them. Generally speaking, your muscles are mechanically much weaker at the beginning of a movement than at the end of it. Universal Gyms have taken this into consideration by altering the geometry of their machines so the weight feels relatively heavier as you near completion of the movement. Variable resistance like this in an exercise can give you a greater degree of strength and muscular development.

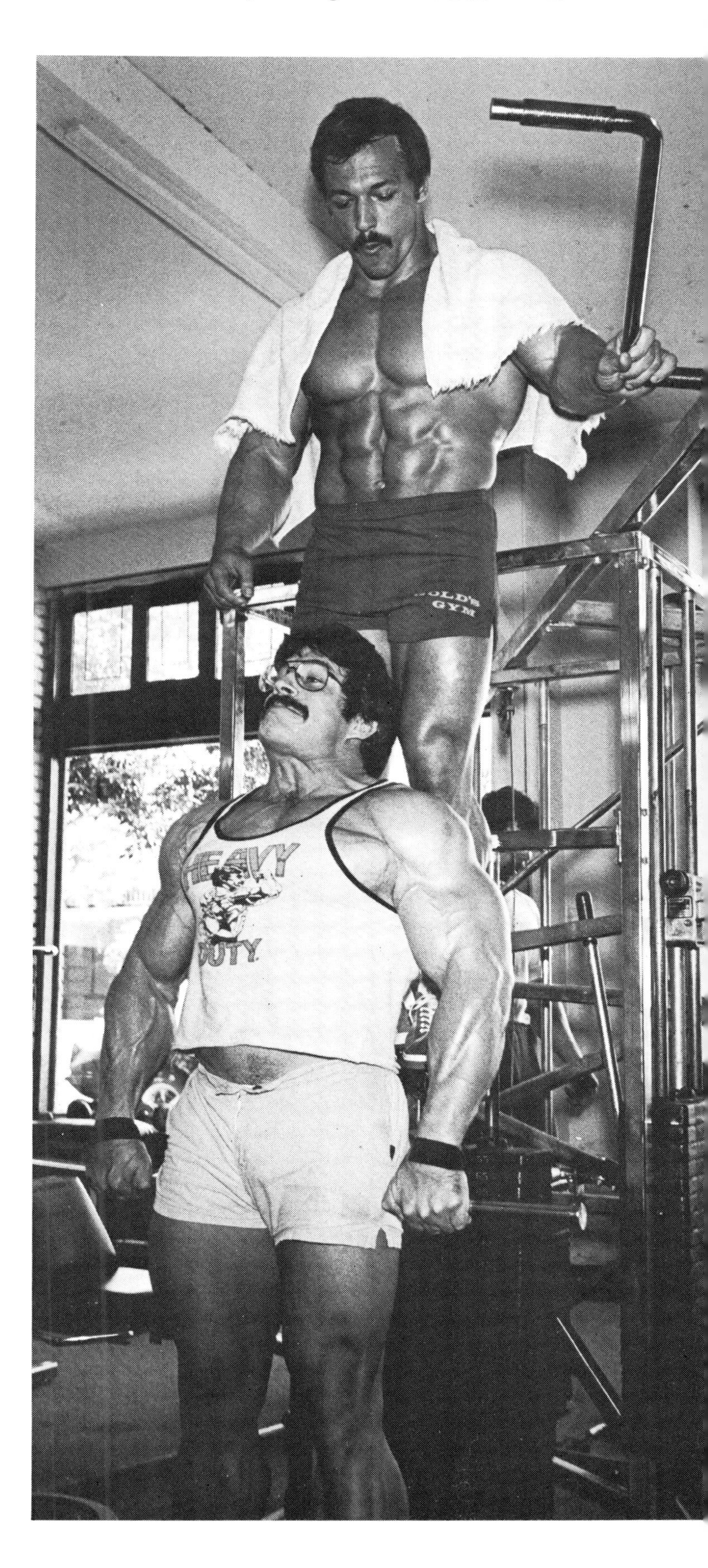

Mike Mentzer pumps some REALLY heavy iron, doing Shrugs with the entire weight stack of a Universal Gyms bench press station plus massive 220-pound Casey Viator! *(Photo by John Balik)*

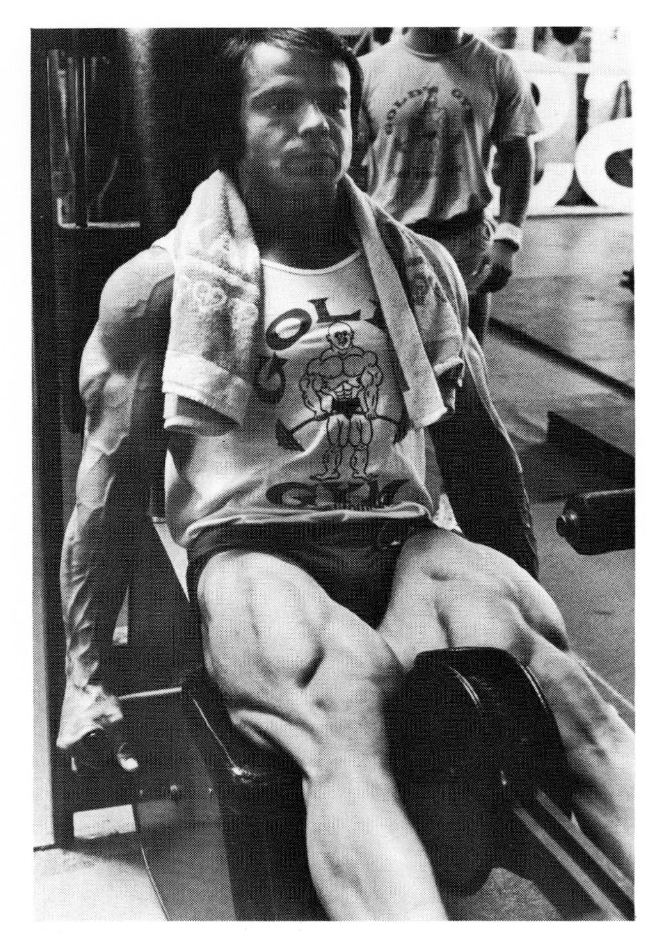

Petr Stach, the best Czech bodybuilder (winner of several Mr. Europe titles) reps out on a Nautilus Leg Extension machine at Gold's II.
(Photo by Bill Reynolds)

Nautilus Machines

Nautilus machines evolved during the late 1960s and early 1970s, and they have become popular with athletes and with some bodybuilders. Most bodybuilders, however, will incorporate only two or three movements using Nautilus machines into their routines. The leg extension, leg curl, and biceps curling machines seem to be the most popular with run-of-the-mill bodybuilding champs.

A few bodybuilders—most notably Casey Viator and Mike and Ray Mentzer—have at various times used a majority of Nautilus movements in their routines. Relatively short bodybuilders like Madeline Almeida and very tall bodybuilders like Lou Ferrigno don't seem to fit into many of the machines, however. Several top bodybuilders have also complained about developing joint soreness while using Nautilus machines.

The main advantage of Nautilus machines is that they are constructed to provide the most intense resistance to the working muscles. All of the machines provide resistance through a spiral cam (pulley), which applies continuous and direct tension to the working muscles. By varying the radius of that cam, Nautilus provides variable resistance to the muscles, and this resistance is balanced to conform exactly to the normal strength curve of the working muscles. Finally, Nautilus machines provide resistance over a full—even an exaggerated—range of motion for each muscle group. Because of these features, a bodybuilder can make each set so intense that a muscle group can be stimulated thoroughly after only three or four total sets.

There are two disadvantages to Nautilus machines—the low number of possible exercises and the high cost. No more than two or three movements can be done for each body part, quickly leading to training boredom. And the machines are exceedingly expensive, far too expensive for home-gym installation. Most machines cost about $5,000, and it would cost at least $50,000 to buy enough machines to train the entire body thoroughly. Still, these machines are popular enough for Gold's/Venice to have purchased a full line of them for use by members. And the machines are used quite heavily, even though few bodybuilders utilize them all.

Corbin-Pacific Machines

Corbin-Pacific came out with a line of bodybuilding exercise machines during the late 1970s. These machines also feature variable rotary resistance, and they are constructed to put a minimum of wear and tear on the body's joints. It's still a little early to determine conclusively how popular these machines will become with Gold's Gym members, but early reactions seem to be very positive. The rowing-type lat machine is particularly good, because a chest-supporting attachment allows you to do Bent Rowing movements with enormous weights without any possibility of lower back strain.

Physical Exams

It's important for anyone over the age of 30, anyone who has been physically inactive for at least a year, and anyone who is 20 pounds or more overweight to undergo a physical examination prior to commencing bodybuilding training. Anyone who is over 40 years of age, or who has a family history of heart disease, should make sure a stress test electrocardiogram (EKG) is included in this exam.

Bodybuilding training places great physical stress on the body, and under rare circumstances this stress can cause a breakdown or failure of the heart or circulatory system, and may contribute to complications in some other organ system. Your physician can often detect such physical vulnerabilities during your examination. If he does, be sure to follow his recommendations regarding exercise to the letter.

An orthopedist or chiropractor can also advise you as to how to treat minor joint and muscle injuries during a workout. In many cases bodybuilding training will improve a weak back or injured knee. In other cases, however, you might be forced to avoid certain exercises in your routines.

Why Muscles Grow

Although there is limited scientific evidence to support the opposite viewpoint, most physiologists agree that past a certain age the number of muscle cells and fibers in the human body no longer increases with exercise. Instead, as a response to physical stress, these individual muscle cells and fibers increase in size and mass, a process known as *muscle hypertrophy*.

A muscle will increase its degree of hypertrophy in response to the application of a perceived overload. And such an overload is provided by increasing the intensity of resistance applied to each muscle. Intensity is increased by increasing the weight used in an exercise, by increasing the number of repetitions done with a particular weight, by doing a set number of reps with a set weight in a shorter length of time, or by combining two or more of these variables. Ordinarily, bodybuilders use a combination of increasing reps and increasing weight, though close to a competition they will increase intensity by shortening the rest intervals between sets.

When a muscle is stressed heavily, then allowed to recuperate fully by being rested for at least 48 hours before it is stressed again, it will respond by growing a little in strength and mass. And by progressively increasing the intensity of resistance in each workout, a muscle can be coaxed into greater and greater hypertrophy over a period of time.

For many years bodybuilders believed that a weight workout broke down muscle cells, which then grew back larger and stronger while resting between training sessions. The study of cell metabolites, however, has led physiologists to believe that there is no muscle cell breakdown during heavy exercise. Still, an adequate period of rest between workouts, along with heavy exercise, is a vital requisite to muscle growth.

Progression

When you overload a muscle group it quickly adapts to the added stress by growing larger and stronger so that it can comfortably handle the added stress when called on to lift it again. As an example, let's say your back muscles are strong enough to lift a 50-pound sack of sugar with comfort and a 55-pound bag with some degree of difficulty. If you continually lift the 50-pound sack, the 55-pound bag will always feel a little heavy. But if you have to lift the 55-pound sack a couple of times, your muscles will soon be strong enough for the heavier sack to feel about as light as the 50-pound bag used to feel.

In bodybuilding training, muscle hypertrophy is encouraged by progressively putting more and more resistance on each muscle group. As soon as a muscle can comfortably lift 55 pounds, it is forced to lift 60. And once 60 pounds is easy to lift, that muscle is forced to lift 65. In this way the muscles are able to continue to grow in strength and mass.

As mentioned earlier, bodybuilders normally combine increasing the weight and increasing the reps in an exercise. If you flip ahead a few pages to the end of Chapter 3, you will note that in the exercise programs presented a range of repetitions (e.g., 8–12) is suggested for each

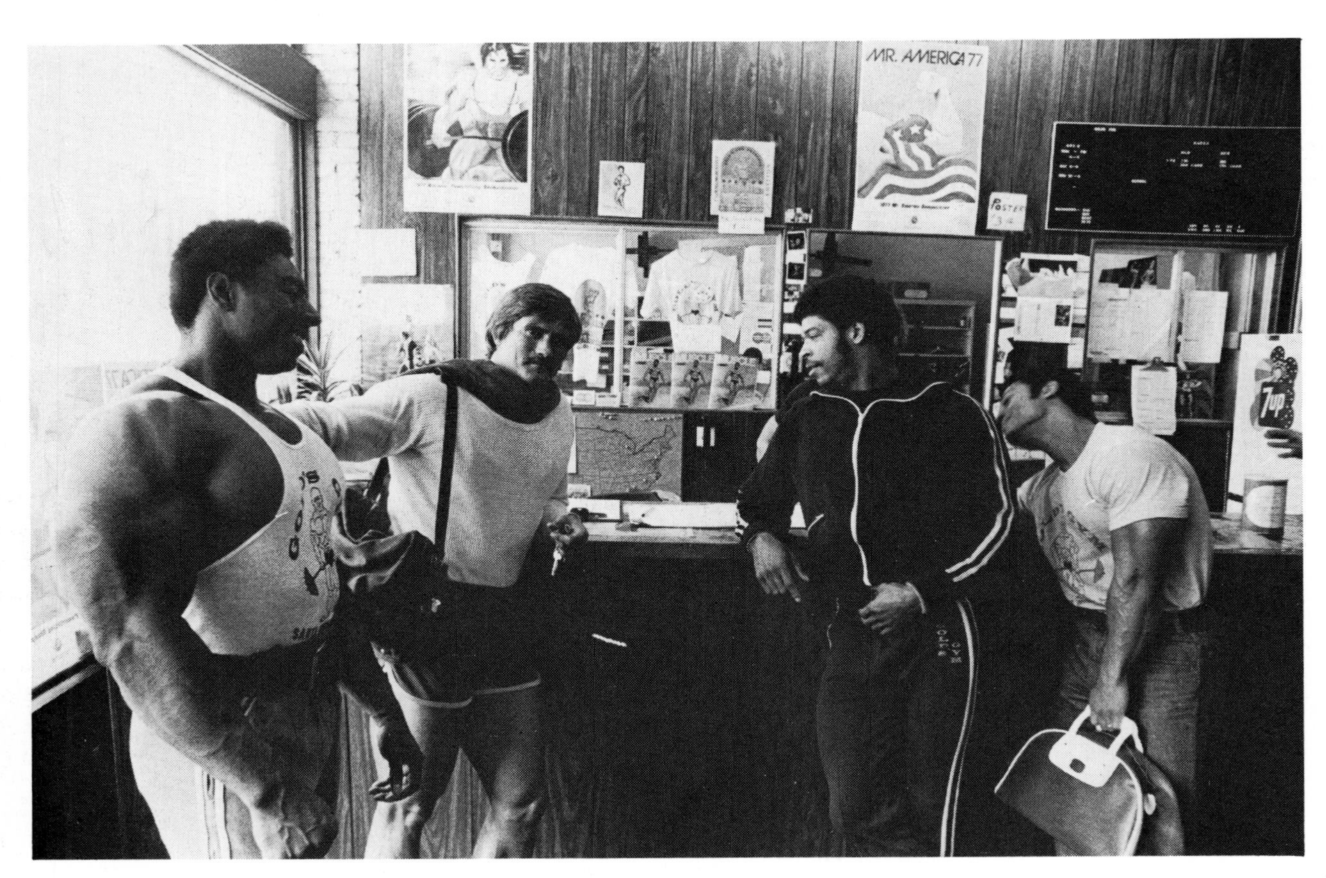

Group photo of some of the Gold's Gym champs after a heavy workout—(left to right) Dave Johns, Roger Callard, Bill Grant, and Mohamed Makkawy—was taken at Gold's II in Santa Monica, 1978. *(Photo by Peter Brenner)*

exercise. These figures are called *guide numbers.* In the case of 8–12, eight is a *lower guide number* and 12 is an *upper guide number.*

In your training routine you will begin by doing the lower guide number of reps with a certain weight. Then, during each workout, you will add one or two reps until you can comfortably do the upper guide number of reps. Once the upper guide number is reached you will add 5–10 pounds to the barbell, dumbbells, or machine you are using, drop the reps back to the lower guide number, and begin working up again. Increasing your training resistance in this progressive manner is very effective and at the same time does not excessively tax the muscle and the rest of the body.

Just so there will be no confusion, here is a chart of a typical resistance progression in the Military Press over a four-week period (note: "50 × 8" is a form of bodybuilding shorthand that indicates you are to do eight repetitions with 50 pounds:

	Day 1	Day 2	Day 3
Week 1	50 × 8	50 × 9	50 × 10
Week 2	50 × 11	50 × 12	55 × 8
Week 3	55 × 9	55 × 10	55 × 11
Week 4	55 × 12	60 × 8	60 × 9

Ordinarily you'll be able to add one or two new reps during each succeeding workout. The body does have natural up-and-down energy cycles, however, and on a down day you might not be able to add a new repetition to an exercise. Hang in there, though, and on an up day you'll probably be able to add two or three new reps. Generally speaking, you'll find it somewhat easier to add new reps during each successive workout when you are starting your training than when you are well into your bodybuilding career.

The amount of weight you can add on an

exercise once you've reached the upper guide number for reps varies as a function of your sex and the muscle group you are working. Men are naturally stronger than women, as discussed in Chapter 1. The legs and back are larger muscle groups than any others in the body, and so require larger jumps in resistance.

As a result of the foregoing factors, a male bodybuilder can usually add 10–20 pounds to leg and back exercises and 5–10 pounds to movements for other muscle groups. Female bodybuilders, on the other hand, can comfortably add 5–10 pounds to leg and back exercises and 2½–5 pounds to movements for other smaller body parts.

If you examine the routines at the end of Chapter 3, you will notice that multiple sets (e.g., three sets) are suggested for many exercises. When you use multiple sets of an exercise you should reach the upper guide number on each set before increasing your resistance.

To prevent any confusion, here is a chart illustrating four weeks of progression on Barbell Bent Rowing, assuming that you are required to do three sets of 8–12 reps of the movement during each workout:

	Day 1	Day 2	Day 3
Week 1	60 × 8	60 × 10	60 × 11
	60 × 8	60 × 9	60 × 9
	60 × 8	60 × 8	60 × 9
Week 2	60 × 12	60 × 12	60 × 12
	60 × 11	60 × 12	60 × 12
	60 × 10	60 × 11	60 × 12
Week 3	65 × 9	65 × 10	65 × 11
	65 × 9	65 × 9	65 × 11
	65 × 8	65 × 8	65 × 9
Week 4	65 × 11	65 × 12	70 × 8
	65 × 11	65 × 12	70 × 8
	65 × 10	65 × 12	70 × 8

The foregoing example of progression is the one that beginning and intermediate bodybuilders will use most frequently in their training. We will present advanced-level methods of progression in later chapters.

Where to Train

There are four main places in which you can train: (1) at Gold's Gym, at one of its franchises all over the United States and the rest of the world, and at other commercial bodybuilding gyms; (2) at home; (3) in a school or YMCA weight room; and (4) at a health spa, Nautilus facility, or comparable commercial exercise establishment. Let's discuss the pros and cons of working out in each of these environments.

Gold's Gym in Venice, California, is absolutely the best bodybuilding gym in the world, and hundreds of top bodybuilders from around the globe have moved to southern California over the years specifically to train at Gold's. Many hundreds more have visited the Hall of Champions for several weeks before a major competition to peak out better than they ever have before.

Not only is Gold's Gym superbly equipped, but it also attracts the best bodybuilders in the world. To work out with these champions is incredibly inspiring, and many visiting bodybuilders make such great gains at Gold's that they decide to stay. Bob Jodkiewicz was a young Mr. Virginia winner when he visited Gold's to peak for the Mr. America show. He was so blown away by the training atmosphere and made such good gains that he immediately moved to Los Angeles. Two years later he won the prestigious Junior Mr. America contest. Now he is one of the world's best bodybuilders.

There are numerous Gold's Gym franchises across America, and all of them are the best bodybuilding gyms in their particular areas. Besides these Gold's Gyms, numerous other commercial bodybuilding gyms of varying quality are available. You can find these gyms listed in the Yellow Pages of your telephone directory. If you have more than one gym to choose from, try a couple of workouts in each one and then choose one to join based on where you got your best workouts.

School and YMCA weight rooms vary widely in quality, but if you can find a well-equipped gym of this type, you can train pretty well there. Unfortunately, you ordinarily won't find top bodybuilders training there to inspire you and to answer your training questions, as is the case at Gold's. Still, you get back what you put into

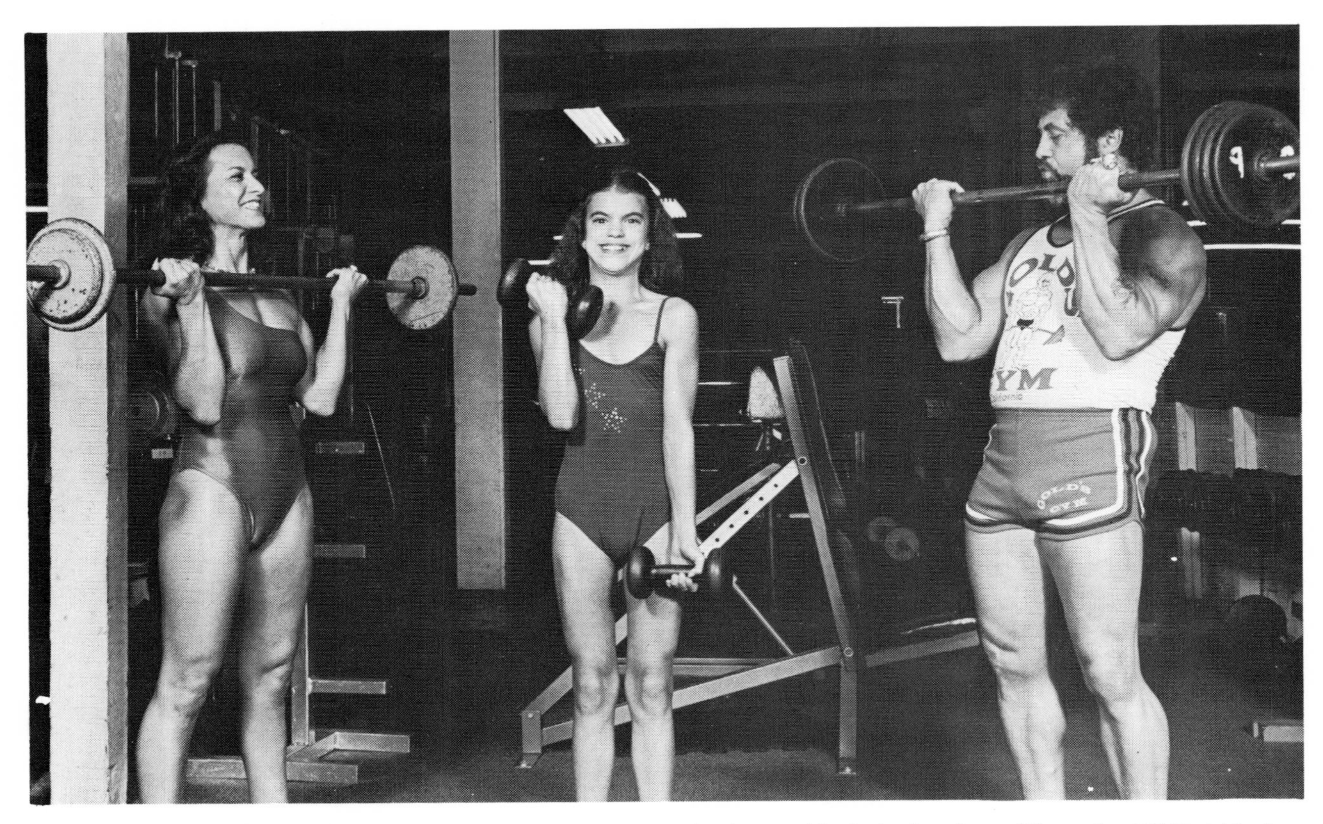

Family training is "in" at Gold's. Rita & Charlie Brown train there with their daughter. *(Photo by Bill Dobbins)*

your training, and you can get a pretty good workout at a well-equipped YMCA, high school, or college weight room.

Health spas, Nautilus facilities, and other commercial exercise facilities aimed for use by the general public are relatively poor places for an aspiring bodybuilder to work out. They are ill equipped, in terms of both equipment variety and the range of exercise weights available. Also, they are overcrowded, especially in the morning and early evening.

Home-gym training can be very beneficial, provided you have access to a well-equipped gym. You won't be tied down to established gym hours, as with a commercially run bodybuilding establishment. So, if you get the urge to do a couple of sets of chest training at 3:00 a.m., you can do it in your home gym rather than waiting until morning.

The disadvantage of home-gym training is a lack of camaraderie. It's easy to get bored with your workouts or burn out totally when training alone. Still, a number of champions have won high-level bodybuilding titles while training at home, and more than half of today's bodybuilding superstars took their first workouts at home.

To get the most out of your training in a home gym, you should strive to fully equip your workout quarters. The best way to do this is to buy used equipment at reduced prices through newspaper advertisements or at flea markets. You can also build many of your own benches and other apparatus. Once you have a full complement of equipment for your home gym, you can plunge into it to your heart's content at all hours of the day and night.

Training Frequency

At the beginning and early-intermediate levels of training you should train your entire body in one workout session on three nonconsecutive days per week. By allowing nearly one full day of rest between workouts, and then two days of rest before beginning the cycle anew, you give your body sufficient resting time between training sessions for full recuperation and hence for the fastest possible muscle growth.

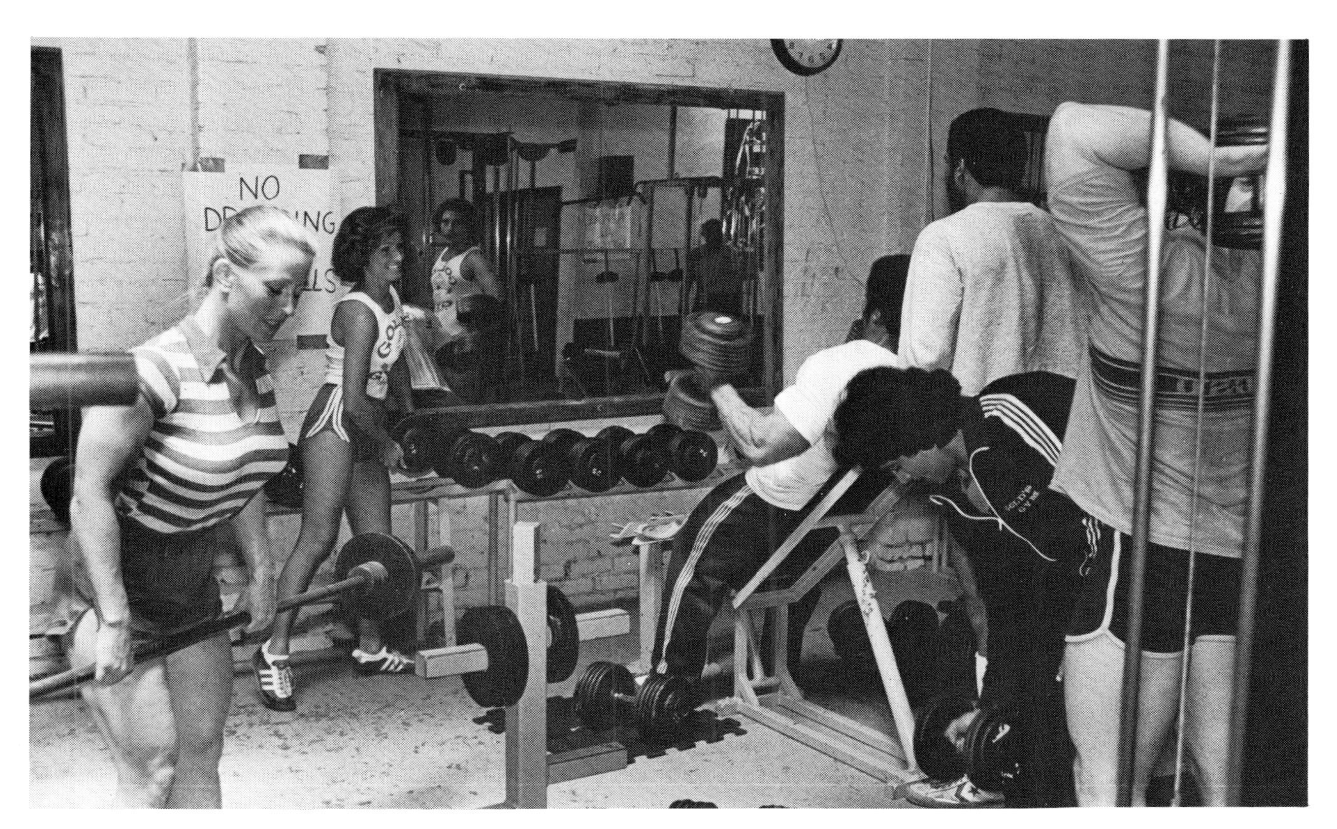

Group training photo at Gold's II in Santa Monica, taken about 1978. *(Photo by Peter Brenner)*

Normally you can train on Mondays, Wednesdays, and Fridays, which leaves your weekends free for family activities and recreational pursuits. You can, however, also work out on Tuesdays, Thursdays, and Saturdays or on any other combination of three nonconsecutive days per week that is convenient to you.

As you progress as a bodybuilder your workouts will eventually become too long to be done comfortably in one session. Then you can begin to train four, five, or six days per week on what is known as a split routine. On such a program you will work only a half or a third of your body in each workout, still allowing each muscle group approximately 48 hours of rest between training sessions before working it again.

How Many Reps

The numbers of repetitions you should do for each exercise in the various programs outlined in this book will be suggested, but you should also be aware of what the different repetition ranges will do for your muscles. For maximum strength you should do low repetitions (normally 1–3 reps), for muscle mass you should do medium repetitions (normally 5–8 reps), and for muscular definition and detail you should do high repetitions (normally 10–15 reps).

Different muscle groups respond best to different repetition schemes. Most of your body's muscles will respond best in a bodybuilding sense when stimulated with sets of 8–12 repetitions, while the calf and forearm muscles respond better to reps in the range of 15–25. The abdominals need even higher repetitions, in the range of 25–50.

Rest Intervals

The length of the rest intervals you take between sets is crucial. With too little rest your muscles won't recuperate enough to do justice to the next set. With too much rest your body will begin to cool off (blood will leave the muscles exercised), at which point you become increasingly susceptible to injury.

The normal rest interval is approximately

60–90 seconds between sets at the beginning and intermediate levels of training. Later, when you are training with very heavy weights to develop muscle mass, you can rest for up to two minutes between sets. Don't rest any longer than that, however, or you might incur an injury. Even later, when you prepare for a competition, you will take very short rest intervals of 20–30 seconds. For now, though, keep your rest intervals between 60 and 90 seconds.

Training Poundages

In the first workout program presented at the end of Chapter 3 you will be given suggested initial training poundages in terms of a percentage of your own body weight. These percentages are indicated in the two columns labeled "% Men" and "% Women." If the poundage you calculate is not a multiple of five (e.g., 43½ pounds), reduce the poundage to the next lowest multiple of five pounds (in this case, to 40 pounds).

These suggested beginning training weights are based on "average" strength levels for men and women. As you know, however, few individuals are really average. Therefore, you may need to raise or lower the suggested poundage after a workout or two. A set done with a correct training weight should be comfortably difficult to complete. If you must strain to complete it, or if you are completely unable to complete the assigned number of repetitions, the weight should be reduced. But if the set is easy to complete, the weight will need to be raised.

After you have been training steadily with weights for 4–6 weeks, you will easily be able to judge your own training weights. As a result, workout poundages are suggested only for the initial level of training. Since it is impossible to know readers' strength levels, to suggest further poundages would be presumptuous.

Program Break-In

Training with weights is such heavy work that your muscles will become severely sore for several days if you try to jump right into a full workout the very first day you touch a weight. To avoid such painfully sore muscles, you must break into doing a full program over a period of three or four weeks, slowly and progressively. With such a slow break-in, you will experience only the mildest form of muscle soreness.

For the first week of training you should do only one set of each recommended exercise. You should also avoid increasing the training weights until the second or third week of workouts, even if the barbells and dumbbells feel fairly light to you. Increasing workout weights too early can easily result in painfully sore muscles.

Beginning with the second week of training, you can do two sets of every movement in which you are required to do two or three sets. Finally, beginning with the third week, you can do the full program, gradually increasing the resistance you use for each movement as your muscles grow larger and stronger.

If you do get carried away, however, and your muscles become sore, the best way to relieve the soreness is to take frequent, long, hot baths. After a few of these hot baths you will be able to resume your workouts without additional discomfort.

Breathing Patterns

Beginning bodybuilders are always concerned about how to breathe during an exercise. In reality, you will find natural points during heavy exercises at which you can breathe comfortably. Otherwise, you will find it easiest to inhale during the lowering cycle of a movement and exhale during the exertion (raising) cycle.

You should *never* hold your breath during an exercise. Doing so will build up intrathoracic pressure, which will impede the blood flow to and from your brain, causing you to faint. Technically, this is called a Valsalva effect. If you black out while doing a heavy Bench Press, you could conceivably be killed as the bar crashes downward. As long as you breathe inward or outward during a bench press, however, you will never pass out.

Exercise Form

The form that you adopt when doing each exercise dictates how much of the resistance actually affects the working muscles. If you use sloppy exercise form, you deprive the working muscles of much of the resistance they should receive. But by using correct form, you transfer maximum resistance to the muscles intended to be stressed by any bodybuilding movement.

When using correct form you must confine movement to those parts of the body specified in the exercise descriptions in chapters 3, 5, and 7. Do not allow your knees to jerk, your back to bend unnecessarily, or your body to sway back and forth during a movement. Such extraneous motion is referred to as cheating, and it robs the muscles of much of the resistance they should be receiving from an exercise.

As you become more experienced as a bodybuilder, you will learn how to use cheating to make an exercise more difficult to do. At the beginning and intermediate levels of training, however, you will most likely cheat to remove stress from the muscles intended to be trained by a movement. Cheating should, therefore, be avoided at all costs.

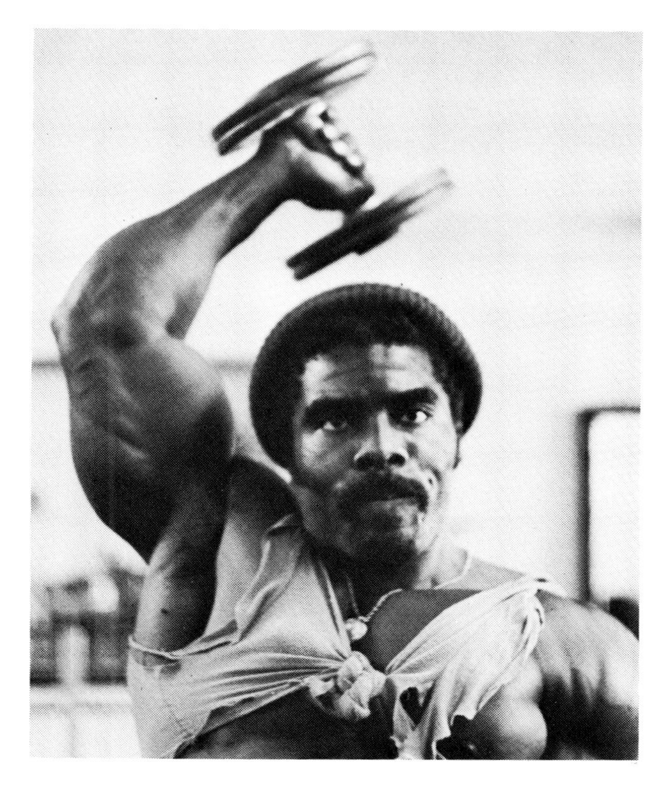

One of Robby Robinson's ardent fans offered "The Black Prince" $100 for the tattered workout shirt he wore for many weeks. Needless to say, a bargain was struck POST HASTE! *(Photo by Jack Neary)*

Exercise Cadence

The speed at which you raise and lower the weights that you use in a workout is also important. Raising and/or lowering the weight too quickly is a form of cheating, and it should be avoided.

When you raise the weight, do it relatively slowly to get the full effect of the weight on your muscles. Raising it fully should take you three or four seconds. You should lower the weight even more slowly, in four or five seconds. There is considerable benefit in lowering a weight slowly, so never simply allow the weight to fall. Resist its downward path, so the weight is lowered under full control and your muscles are stressed by the movement

Training Attire

In choosing what to wear while working out, pay attention to wearing clothing that allows your limbs a full range of movement, as well as clothing that is appropriate for the temperature in the gym in which you work out. In warm weather most bodybuilders wear shorts and a T-shirt or tank top. If it's a little colder, you can wear a warm-up suit, as long as it allows you full freedom of movement while you train.

In extremely cold weather you might be forced to wear more than one sweat suit. In such a case, keep in mind that several light layers of clothing will be much warmer than a couple of equally thick layers of heavier clothing. Layering traps insulating air between thicknesses of clothing, hence keeping your body heat from escaping. Instead of an extra warm-up suit, try wearing tights to insulate your legs and an extra T-shirt or two to keep your torso warm.

Beneath your outer clothing you can wear an athletic supporter or bra, depending on your gender. Neither of these items of clothing is mandatory, however.

We believe that every bodybuilder should wear shoes while training, as well as absorbent sweat socks to soak up perspiration. Shoes prevent your toes from being stubbed and protect your feet from dropped barbell plates. They

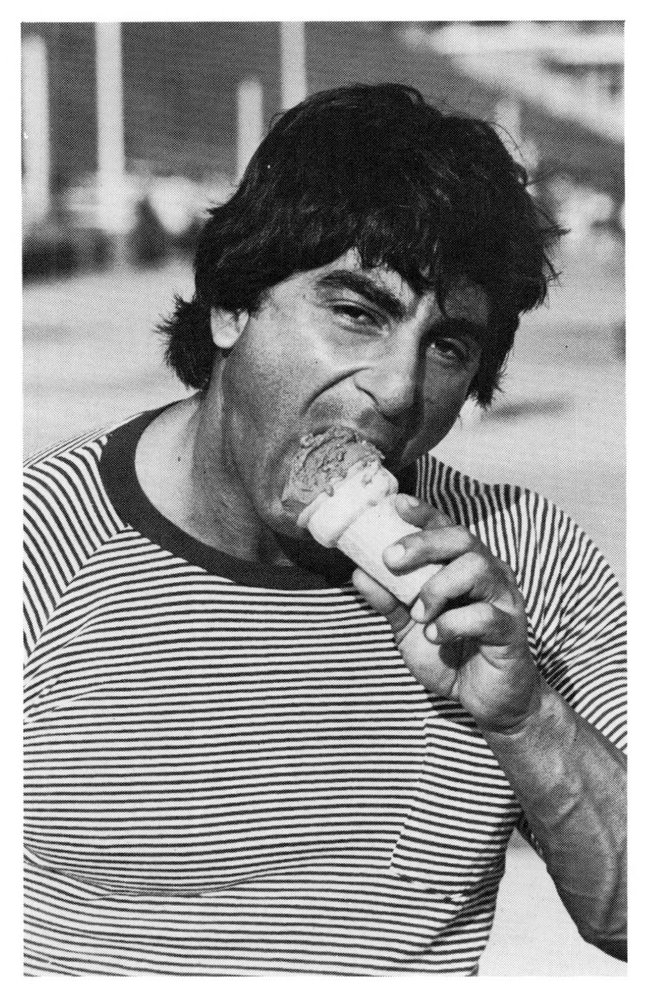

As Dennis Tinerino demonstrates, there's room for an occasional bite of junk food in a top bodybuilder's diet. Generally speaking, however, emphasis should be put on a balanced and health-promoting diet.
(Photo by Mike Neveux)

also protect the arches of your feet from compression injuries when you are lifting heavy weights in a workout. Running shoes are ideal for bodybuilding training, since they have built-in arch supports. Running shoes also have an excellent tread, which will come in handy when you do calf exercises standing on a block of wood.

Basic Nutrition

What you can eat can have a tremendous effect on how fast you progress as a result of your training. Indeed, many bodybuilders firmly believe that correct nutrition is responsible for up to 75%–80% of a bodybuilder's ultimate success. Bodybuilders feel that nutrition is particularly important during the last few weeks before a competition.

To guide you in your choice of foods, here are eight basic nutrition guidelines.

1. *Eat sufficient high-quality protein.* The muscles of your body are formed from protein. You should eat between one-half gram and one gram of protein per pound of body weight per day, spread among three or more meals each day. Animal protein is far more usable in the human body than vegetable protein. Egg white is the most assimilable of all proteins (nearly 90% of its protein is absorbed by the body), followed closely by the protein in milk and milk products. White meats (fish, poultry breasts, etc.) are generally much more assimilable than red meats (beef, pork, etc.).

2. *Avoid refined carbohydrates.* Foods such as white sugar and white flour—as well as anything containing these two elements (e.g., ice cream, cake, candy)—provide your body with useless calories, since they contain few other nutrients. Refined carbohydrates also adversely affect your energy levels by overloading your system with too much glucose. Since you can't immediately use so much glucose, the body turns what it can't use into fat. Carbohydrates are vital food elements, but you should get your supply of them from fresh and unrefined sources such as fruit, vegetables, and whole grains, which don't overload your system.

3. *Reduce your consumption of animal fats.* All types of fats contain more than twice as many calories as proteins and carbohydrates. One gram of fat yields nine calories when metabolized in the human body, while both protein and carbohydrates yield only four calories per gram. Animal fats, compared to vegetable fats, are harmful to the heart and circulatory system. To decrease your comsumption of animal fats, you can eat nonfat milk products, avoid eating the fatty yolks of eggs, and eat lower-fat meats such as fish and skinned poultry breasts, rather than higher-fat meats like beef and pork.

4. *Drink plenty of water.* Water is a good body cleansing agent, and you should drink at least 6–10 glasses of water per day. Distilled water is totally free from impurities (e.g., fluorine, chlorine) so it is preferable to tap water.

You can buy distilled water in any grocery store.

5. *Supplement your diet with vitamins and minerals.* One of the most convenient ways to supplement your diet with vitamins and minerals is to take one or two multipacks of such food supplements each day. These multipacks are cellophane packets containing several tablets and capsules of vitamins and minerals. Numerous companies market these multipacks, so check out your local health food store to see which ones are available. Keep in mind that you should always consume any vitamin and mineral supplements along with your meals. All supplements are assimilated more efficiently by the body when consumed with normal foods.

6. *Eat four or five smaller meals per day.* By eating frequent small meals, you allow your body to better digest and assimilate the nutrients you take in. Small meals are much easier for your body to digest than are large ones.

7. *Eat a great variety of foods.* Every food that you consume has a unique nutrient content, and most foods lack useful quantities of one or more nutrients. You can compensate for these deficiencies by eating another food that has an excess of the missing nutrient(s). Therefore, the more different foods that you eat, the better your chances of consuming a diet that is well balanced in nutrients.

8. *Avoid sodium-laden foods.* Sodium has a great affinity for water. Indeed, one gram of sodium will retain 50 grams of water in your body, and excessive water retention can bloat your body. Table or sea salt is the worst offender in terms of dietary sodium intake. You should avoid table salt, as well as artificial sweeteners, which contain sodium saccharide.

In order to give you a totally clear picture of how a bodybuilder will eat when following the guidelines just presented, the following is a typical menu for year-round, normal diet. The exact amounts will depend on sex, BMR, energy levels, and many other factors.

Meal 1 (8:00 a.m.)—three poached eggs, two slices of whole-grain toast (without butter), one piece of fruit, a glass of nonfat milk, food supplements.

Meal 2 (11:00 a.m.)—tuna salad with a minimum (just enough to wet it) of dressing, one or two pieces of fruit, iced tea with lemon.

Meal 3 (2:00 p.m.)—one whole broiled chicken breast (skinned before broiling), brown rice, green salad, a glass of nonfat milk.

Meal 4 (5:00 p.m.)—broiled fish, dry baked potato, one or two green or yellow vegetables, iced tea, food supplements.

Meal 5 (8:00 p.m.)—cold turkey breast, nonfat yogurt, piece of fruit.

In later chapters we will gradually refine the basic nutritional information presented in this section. For now, however, you can make great progress by following the guidelines just presented.

Sleep, Rest, and Recuperation

As mentioned earlier, your body must be allowed to recuperate fully if you are to achieve maximum muscle hypertrophy from your training. Proper sleep and rest are vital components of the recuperative cycle, so you will need to know how much sleep and rest to get each day.

It has been said that a physically and mentally healthy person should spend one third of life working, one third following personal pursuits, and one third sleeping. Eight hours of sound sleep has come to be accepted as the healthy standard. But individual sleep requirements will vary as much as two or three hours above or below this standard.

You should be guided mostly by how you feel during the day when choosing how long to sleep. If you feel tired and sleepy throughout the day you undoubtedly need more sleep. Be careful not to sleep too much, however, because oversleeping for just one night can disrupt your normal sleeping patterns for several days.

The amount of sleep that your mind and body require for full recuperation will vary as a function of both your training intensity and the proximity of a competition. The harder and longer you train, the more sleep you will require. When you are nervous before a competition, on the other hand, you will be able to function optimally on much less sleep.

You should seriously consider the value of a 15–20-minute nap in the late afternoon as an energy restorer. If such a short nap doesn't make it difficult for you to get to sleep at night, you will profit both mentally and physically from taking one. Such a refreshing nap is actually institutionalized in some societies.

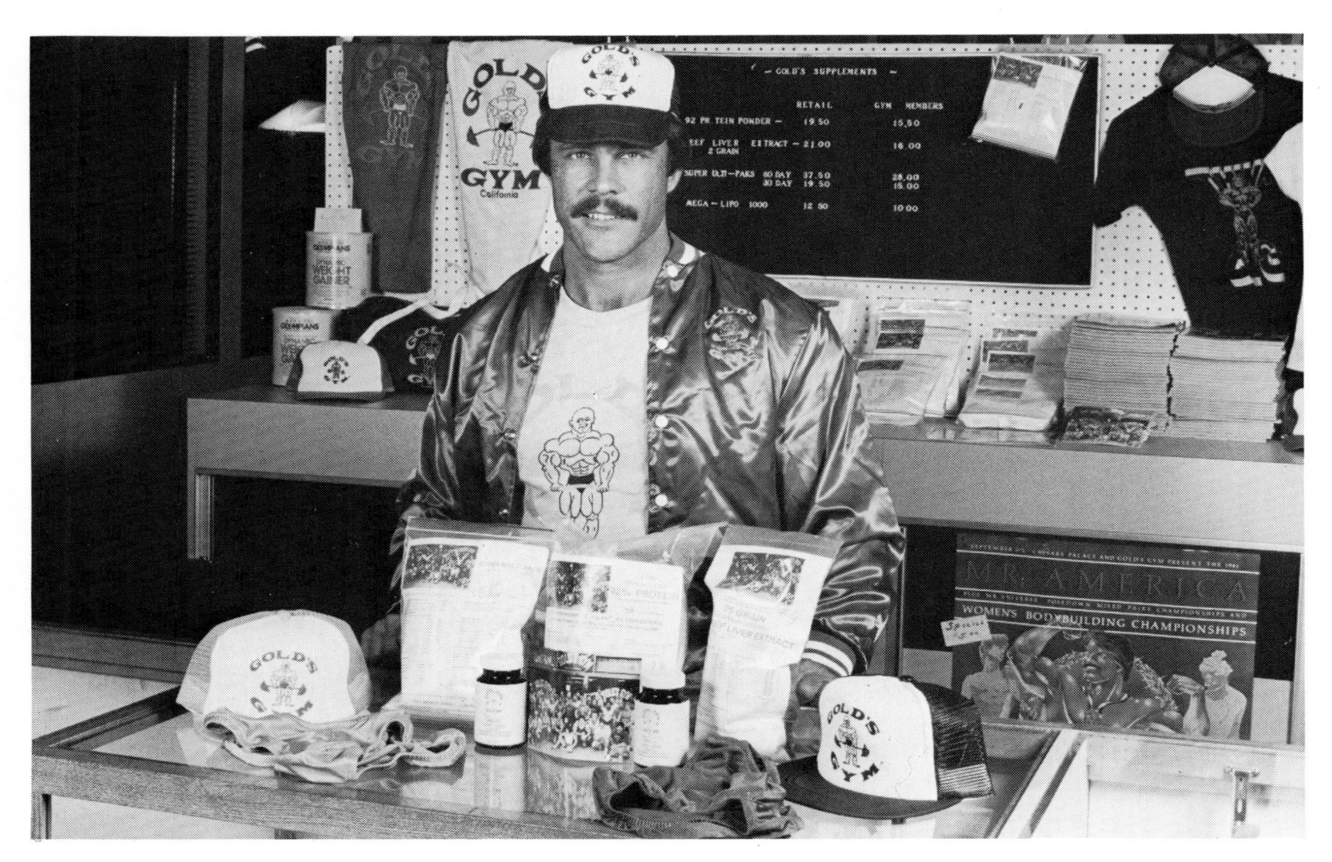

Pete Grymkowski, current owner of Gold's Gym, displays some of the wares he has for sale at the gym.
(Photo by Bill Dobbins)

Proper rest is nearly as important as sound sleep in the recuperative cycle. Unnecessary energy expenditures—and particularly expenditures of nervous energy—can disrupt your recuperative processes. Avoid excessive running, swimming, or other aerobic activity other than when peaking for a competition and be careful to plug all nervous energy leaks by avoiding emotionally draining situations.

Record Keeping

Most bodybuilders keep some type of training records, either mental or written, and it seems that the very best bodybuilders keep the most detailed written records. Frank Zane is a good case in point, since he has kept a detailed and accurate training journal for many years. He has won the Mr. America and Mr. World titles, three Mr. Universe titles and three Mr. Olympia titles, proving the value of his record keeping. Hulking Lou Ferrigno has kept such a training journal virtually since his initial workout, and his body shows the results as well. By studying these records, they have discovered what works and what doesn't work for them in terms of which exercises, how many sets and reps, and a variety of other factors that can affect their training.

At a minimum, a bodybuilder should record the date of each workout, along with the exercises, training poundages, sets, and reps done. These data can be entered in a loose-leaf or spiral-bound notebook or in some other type of bound book with lined pages on which you can write your workout. Also available is an excellent and inexpensive commercially printed log, developed by the editors of *Muscle & Fitness* magazine. It's on sale in most bookstores, and it can be ordered directly from the magazine. This training diary includes plenty of pages for record keeping, inspirational photos of the best bodybuilders, and a plethora of valuable training tips from the champs.

As you will recall from the discussion of progression earlier in this chapter, there is a standard form of bodybuilding shorthand for recording exercise weights, sets, and reps, and you should use this shorthand to enter each workout in your diary. To review, doing 10 repetitions with 250 pounds in a Squat would be recorded like this:

Squat: 250 × 10

You'll seldom do only one set of an exercise, however, so you'll need to know how to record multiple sets of a movement. If you used 100 pounds in a Barbell Curl for four sets of eight repetitions but only managed to do seven reps on your final set, your notation would look like this:

Barbell Curl: 100 × 8 × 8 × 8 × 7

Quite frequently bodybuilders will do their sets of a heavy basic exercise with different weights on each set. Let's say that on a Bench Press movement you did 12 repetitions with 135 pounds, 10 reps with 165, 8 reps with 185, 6 reps with 205, and 4 reps with 225 pounds. Your notation for this workout would be as follows:

Bench Press: 135 × 12; 165 × 10; 185 × 8;
205 × 6; 225 × 4

In recording each full workout, start with the date entered at the middle of the top of the page and then list all of your exercises in the order in which you do them. Be sure to include the weights, sets, and reps you use for each movement. Here is an example of how you might record a basic workout in your training diary.

9-20-82

1. Sit-ups 0 × 50 × 50 × 50
2. Standing Calf Machine 225 × 15 × 15 × 12
3. Bench Press 100 × 10, 120 × 8, 135 × 6
4. Incline Db Press 45 × 8 × 7
5. Bb Bent Row 110 × 8 × 8 × 8
6. Lat Machine Pulldown 120 × 10, 130 × 7
7. Squat 135 × 10, 155 × 8, 175 × 6, 185 × 5
8. Leg Curl 40 × 8 × 8 × 6
9. Side Lat Raise 20 × 10 × 9 × 9
10. Bent Lat Raise 25 × 7, 20 × 8 × 8
11. Bb Shoulder Shrugs 150 × 15 × 15
12. Bb Curl 70 × 8 × 8 × 8
13. Db Concentration Curl 30 × 12 × 11

In addition to training information, you can record in your diary the foods and food supplements you consume, how long and how well you sleep, your mental state, your energy levels, and any other factors that might have a bearing on your success as a bodybuilder. Clarence Bass, one of the best past-40 competitors, keeps a training diary as detailed as this. So does Debbie Diana, U.S. Women's Bodybuilding Champion.

Beginning bodybuilders should keep monthly records of their body measurements. Simply pass a tape measure around your neck, flexed biceps, forearm, expanded chest, waist, thigh, and calf. Then record these measurements in your diary. Take all of your body measurements "cold," i.e., before a workout. Postworkout (pumped-up) measurements are very misleading and thus of lesser value to a bodybuilder.

Once past the intermediate level of bodybuilding training, however, you will probably want to cease recording measurements. As Ken Waller (Mr. America, Mr. Universe) said, "The more advanced you become, the less value there is to taking measurements. Advanced bodybuilders are more concerned with the qualities of muscle shape, hardness, and definition, and these particular qualities don't show up on a tape measure."

Rather than taking measurements, you might profit from having photographs taken of yourself from a variety of angles each month or two. These photos can be pasted in your training diary to provide a visual record of your bodybuilding progress.

There are two main advantages of keeping an accurate training journal. First, by reviewing a detailed log you can isolate which training techniques, routines, and exercises work best for your unique body. Over the years you will be trying a wide variety of new training factors, and meticulously kept diary notes will greatly assist you in deciding which of these factors work best for you.

Secondly, reviewing your journal can give

you quite a boost in training enthusiasm. Nothing can jack you up as fast as seeing progress in your strength levels, because with increased strength comes increased muscle mass. Over the short haul you won't notice marked improvement in the training poundages you use. But by checking back six months or a year in your diary, you'll see incredible progress!

Safety Rules

If you follow the safety procedures outlined in this section, you will find bodybuilding training a totally safe activity. If you don't, however, you could be seriously injured—even killed—while training. In several instances very strong male bodybuilders have been killed while doing heavy Bench Presses without the benefit of a spotter.

Gold's Gym member Lou Ferrigno (Mr. America, Mr. International, twice IFBB Mr. Universe, and a noted film star) has taken a particular interest in weight training and bodybuilding safety. He has outlined the following 12 tried and proven bodybuilding training safety rules.

1. *Always use spotters.* You should use a spotter on all Bench Press movements and Squats whenever you are at or approaching your strength limit. (As a beginner, it would be wise to have a spotter right away.) An alert spotter can keep you from being pinned under a weight, which is particularly vital when you are doing Barbell Bench Presses. You will not need a safety spotter when using dumbbells or various exercise machines. While these machines may be expensive, they all have safety factors built into them that will prevent you from being pinned beneath the weight.

2. *Never train alone.* This is an offshoot of Rule 1. The majority of serious weight training accidents occur while a bodybuilder is training alone. Therefore, you should never train alone, even if you work out in your own home gym. Try to find a training partner or two and always train with one of them. Your training partner can spot you on all heavy movements, saving you from potential injury.

3. *Use catch racks.* Whenever possible, you should do your Squats on a Squat rack equipped with catch racks on which you can place the barbell if you can't get up with it. Most commonly this rack consists of a low set of horizontal bars, but occasionally it will consist of a lower set of pins on the horizontal members of the Squat rack. Some Bench Press racks also are equipped with either a catch rack or a set of the low pins as just described.

4. *Use collars on your barbell.* There is a natural temptation to leave the collars off an Olympic barbell when doing heavy exercises, particularly if you are frequently changing the weights. If you fail to use collars and one end of the bar dips significantly below the level of the other end, however, you can abruptly lose the plates off one end of the barbell. Then the loaded end will whip violently downward, potentially wrenching your lower back or some other body joint. Therefore, regardless of how inconvenient it might seem, you should always take the time to tightly fasten collars on each end of your barbell.

5. *Never hold your breath during an exercise.* As mentioned earlier in this chapter, holding your breath while you are exerting can cause you to faint. If you black out while you are Bench Pressing, the weight could come crashing down across your face or neck, resulting in a catastrophic injury. By breathing rhythmically as you exercise, you can totally prevent the occurrence of a Valsalva effect.

6. *Maintain good gym housekeeping.* Whenever the floor of a gym is littered with barbells, dumbbells, or loose plates it's probable that sooner or later someone will trip over the loose equipment. This will be especially disastrous if the person who trips happens to be holding a heavy barbell overhead at the time. It is both good etiquette and a good safety procedure to return all barbells, dumbbells, and loose plates to the proper storage racks immediately after you are finished using them.

7. *Train under competent supervision.* When training in a group situation it is best to have a knowledgeable supervisor. A good gym instructor can prevent the type of horseplay that will cause accidents. Such an instructor can also encourage the type of good exercise habits—and particularly proper body positions for each exercise—that will prevent injuries.

8. *Don't train in an overcrowded gym.* When a gym is packed with bodybuilders you will

probably be forced to rest too long between sets of each exercise. This can cause you to cool down enough to become vulnerable to injury. It would be much better to choose another time of the day to train, when the gym is less crowded.

9. *Always warm up thoroughly.* The subject of proper warm-ups will be covered in depth in the next section. In terms of safety, a thorough warm-up drastically reduces your chances of incurring a joint or muscle injury due to overstress. A proper warm-up also improves your neuromuscular coordination, making all of your exercises smoother and more coordinated.

10. *Use proper biomechanical (body) positions in all exercises.* These biomechanical positions will be explained in detail in the exercise descriptions in chapters 3, 5, and 7. Learn each body position thoroughly and be sure to use it at all times when you do the exercise that requires it. Deviating from the correct biomechanical position for an exercise while using a heavy weight can leave you vulnerable to injury.

11. *Use a weightlifting belt.* On all heavy leg and back exercises, as well as on overhead pressing movements, you should use a weightlifting belt. Such a belt, cinched tightly around your waist, will keep your lower back warm and will provide your midbody with added stability. The use of a weightlifting belt will cut the frequency and severity of lower back and abdominal injuries by more than 75%.

12. *Acquire as much knowledge as possible about weight training and bodybuilding.* The more you know about bodybuilding training, the less likely you are to incur injury. Be certain to master all of the information in this book as well as in all of the other bodybuilding books and magazines that you can lay your hands on. Become as thoroughly familiar as possible with every subject—biomechanics, kinesiology, physiology, biochemistry, etc.—related to bodybuilding. Armed with such knowledge, you can easily avoid potential injuries.

Warm-ups

Scientific investigators have determined that a proper warm-up performs several valuable functions for a bodybuilder or any other type of athlete. Essentially, these functions help prevent injuries, refine neuromuscular coordination, and prepare the body for greater strength efforts.

A good warm-up increases the heart rate and augments blood circulation. These changes make the body's muscles and connective tissues more supple and resistant to sudden physical stress. A proper warm-up also brings greater oxygen supplies to the muscles, making them capable of generating more force and expending more energy than normally possible. It has been scientifically demonstrated that warmed-up

Running in place.

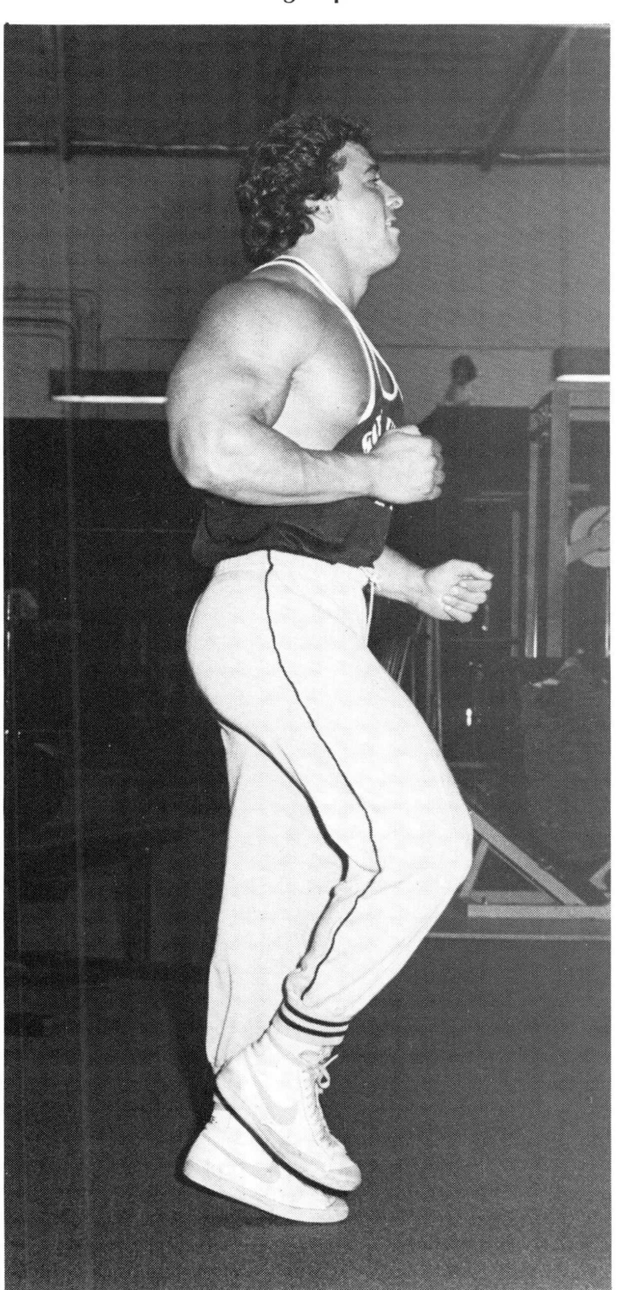

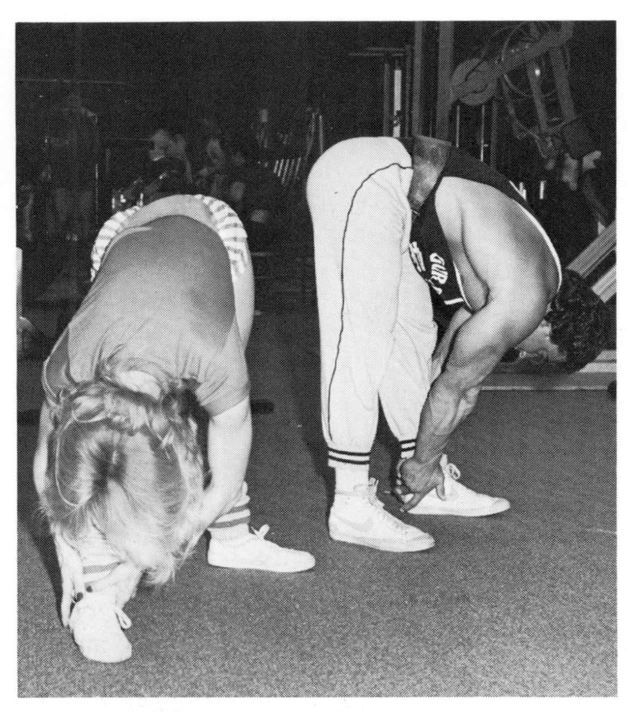

Back and hamstrings stretch.

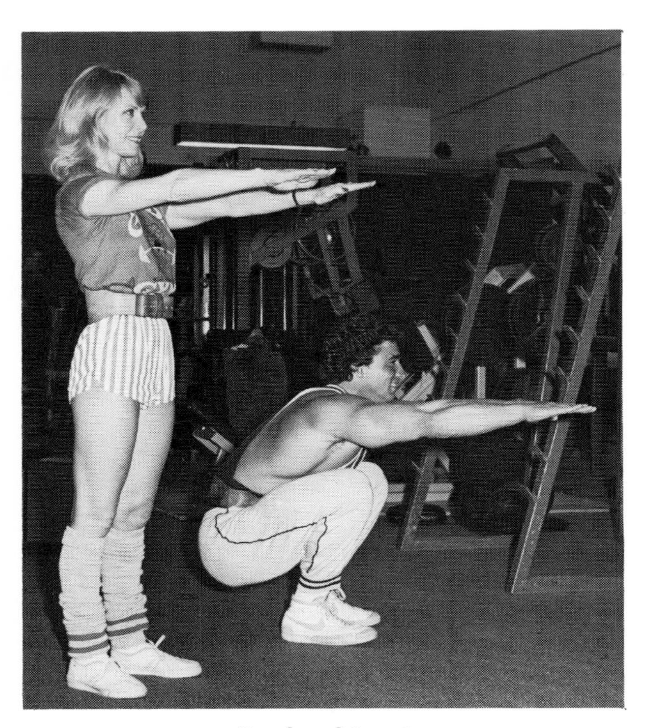

Freehand Squat.

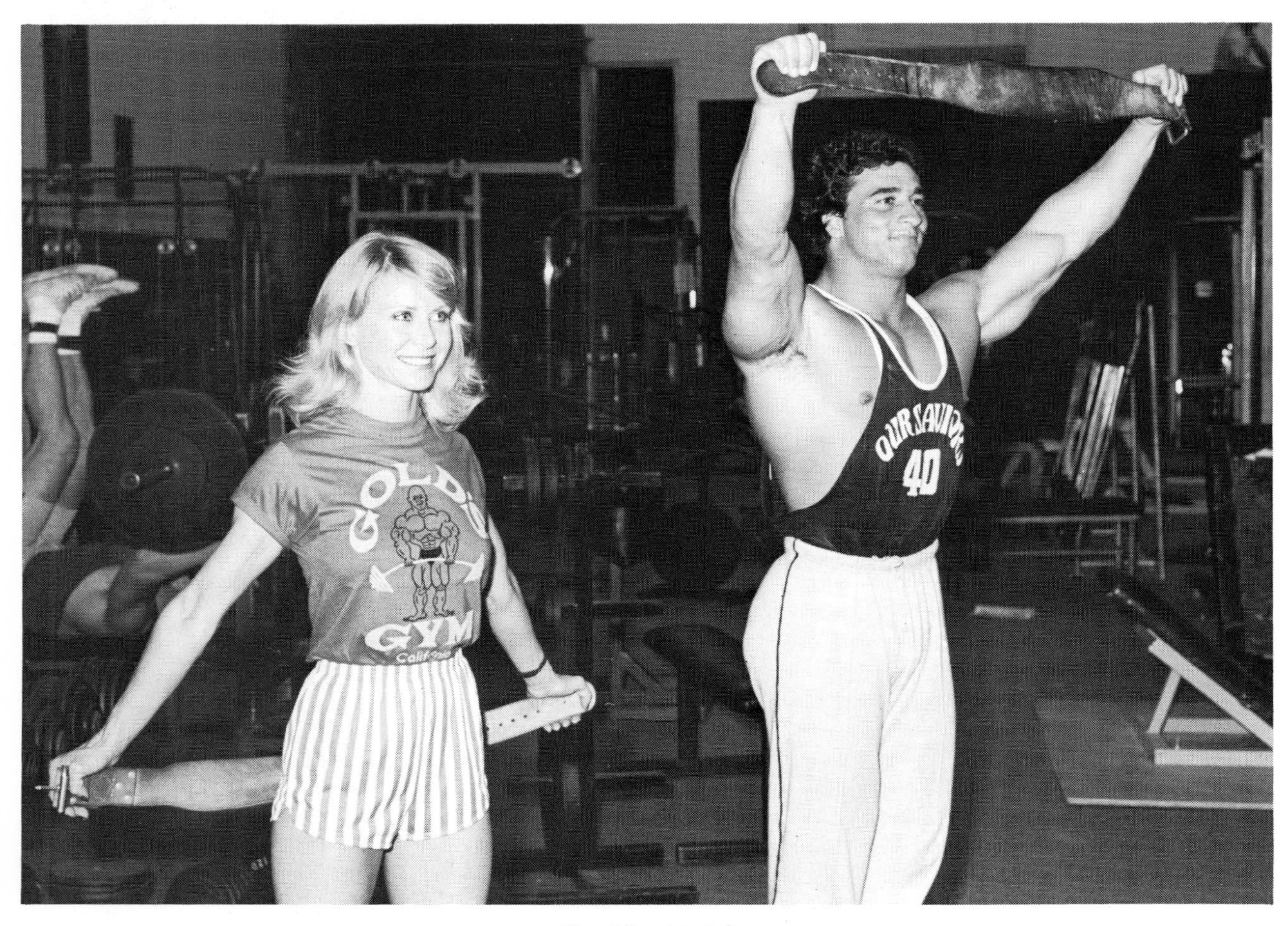

Shoulder Stretch.

muscles are significantly stronger than cold muscles. And the increased suppleness makes a working muscle and its connective tissues much more resistant to injury.

Scientific experiments have also demonstrated that a proper warm-up significantly improves neuromuscular coordination. In other words, with a good warm-up behind you, your body movements and coordination will improve greatly. This function is particularly important if you must perform complicated movements such as high jumping or Olympic-style weightlifting.

You must spend 10–15 minutes warming up prior to every bodybuilding session. Begin your warm-up with brief aerobic activity to stimulate your respiratory and circulatory systems. Then perform a variety of stretching and calisthenic movements. Conclude your warm-up by doing one or two lightweight sets of 15–20 repetitions on each exercise in your bodybuilding program before moving on to your heavy muscle-building sets.

We suggest that you do the following series of eight warm-up exercises prior to commencing your bodybuilding workout.

1. *Jogging in Place.* Spend two to three minutes either jogging in place or skipping rope. Begin by raising your feet, with a slow cadence, only a short distance from the floor. Then gradually speed up the tempo of the movement and augment the height to which you raise your feet on each step.

2. *Back and Hamstrings Stretch.* Spread your feet approximately 2½–3 feet apart and lock your legs straight. Bend forward and to your left, grasping your left ankle with both hands. Pull your shoulders and torso gently toward your left ankle until you feel a slightly painful stretching sensation in your lower back and the back of your left leg. Hold this stretched position for 20–30 seconds. Repeat the movement to the right side.

3. *Freehand Squat.* Place your feet at shoulder width and rest your hands on your hips. Slowly bend your knees and sink into a full squatting position. Straighten your legs and return to the starting position. Repeat this movement 20–30 times.

4. *Shoulder Stretch.* Grasp the ends of a towel and extend your arms over your head so they are straight and you have tension on the towel. Slowly move your hands to the rear, "dislocating" your shoulders and moving your hands downward and to the rear until the towel touches your lower back. Return your hands to the starting position by simply reversing the movement. Slowly repeat the movement four or five times.

5. *Jumping Jacks.* Stand erect with your feet together and your arms down at your sides. Dip your knees slightly and spring four to six inches from the floor. As you spring from the floor, simultaneously spread your feet to shoulder width and swing your hands in semicircles di-

Jumping Jacks.

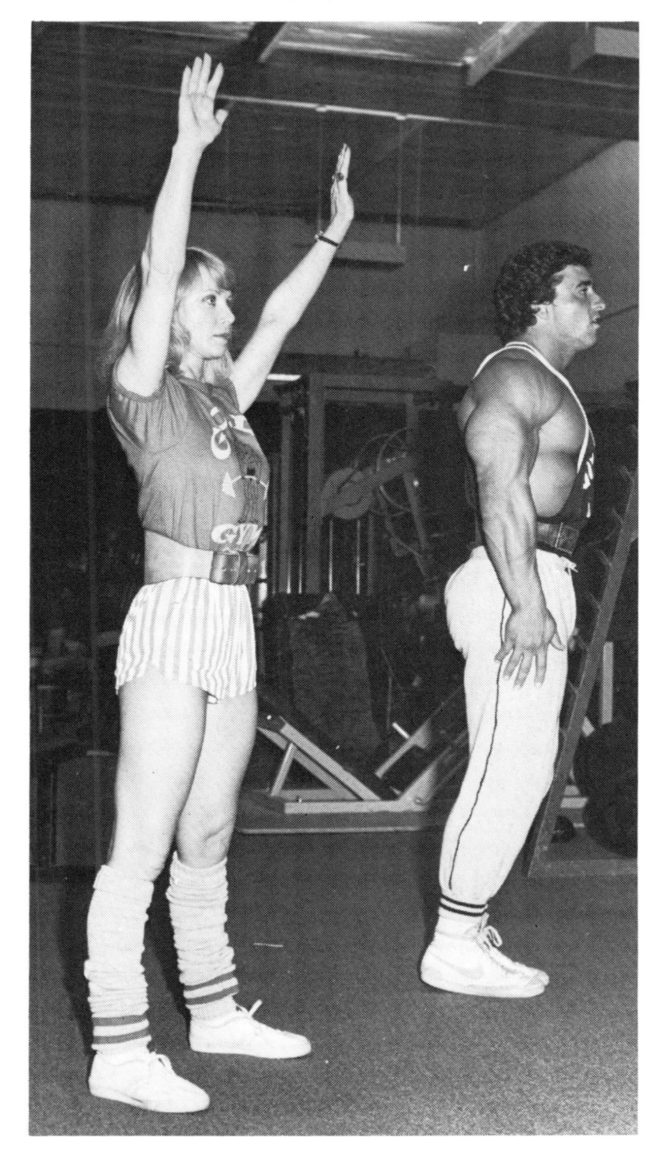

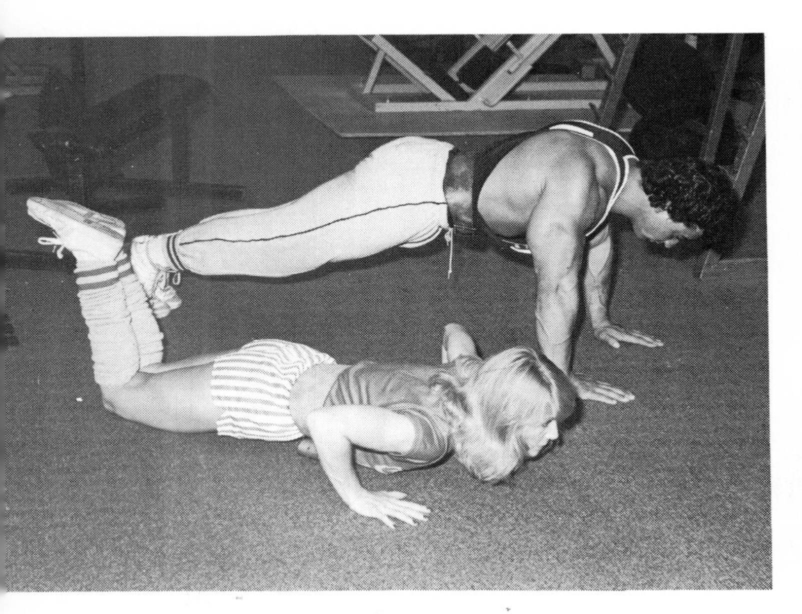

Push-up.

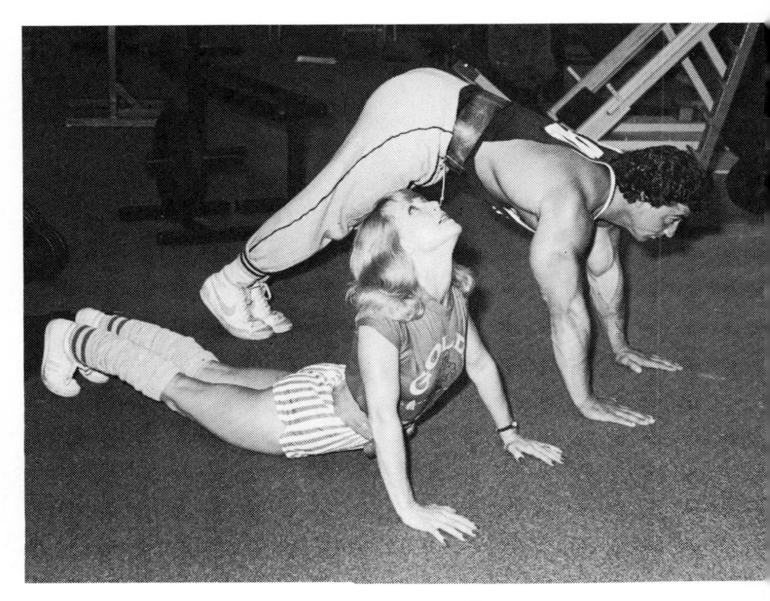

Torso Stretch.

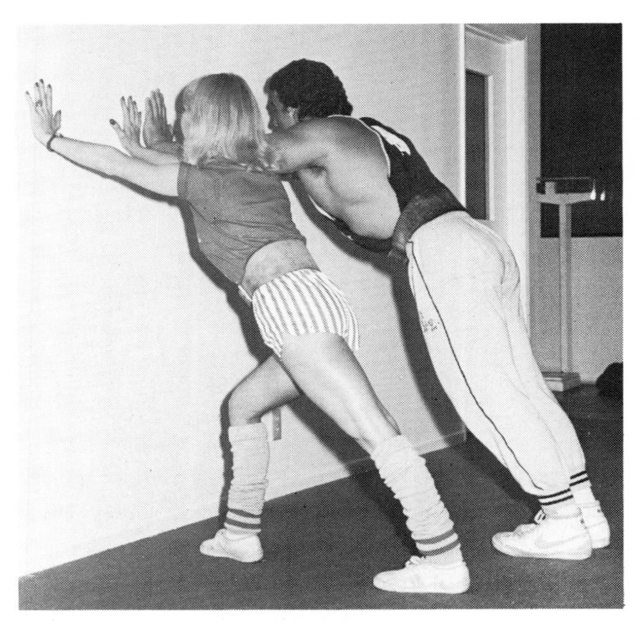

Calf Stretch.

rectly out to the sides and upward until they touch directly above your head just as your feet again touch the floor. Immediately spring back upward and return your hands and feet to the starting position. Do this movement rhythmically for 30–50 repetitions.

6. *Push-ups.* Assume a prone position with your torso and legs on a straight line and your weight supported on your toes and hands as illustrated (women can support their weight on their knees and hands). Bend your arms fully until your chest lightly touches the floor, then straighten your arms and return to the starting position. Repeat the movement for 20–30 repetitions.

7. *Calf Stretch.* Stand facing a wall with your feet about three feet back from the wall. Lean forward and place your hands on the wall at shoulder height. Keeping your torso and legs in a straight line, bend your arms slightly and attempt to force your heels to the floor. Hold the fully stretched position for 20–30 seconds.

8. *Torso Stretch.* Assume the same starting position as for a Push-up (women must assume the men's starting position). Keeping your arms and legs straight, bend at the waist and lift your hips as far from the floor as possible. Then—still keeping your arms and legs straight—lower your hips as close to the floor as possible. Hold this fully stretched low position for 20–30 seconds.

This warm-up should make you sweat slightly, and it will mildly accelerate your respiration and pulse rates. At this point, you can do a light, high-rep warm-up set of your first bodybuilding exercise, then launch directly into your full bodybuilding workout.

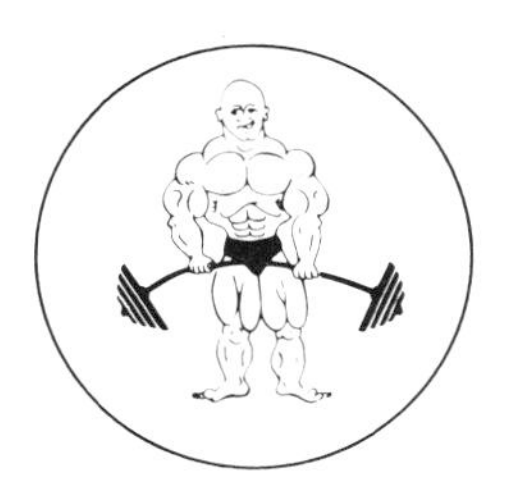

3 BEGINNING-LEVEL EXERCISES & WORKOUTS

Now that you have digested the rudiments of progressive bodybuilding training, it's time to learn several exercises for each of the body's seven major muscle groups. These are the thighs, calves, back, chest, deltoids (shoulders), arms, and abdominals. No direct neck exercises are included, since that body part grows sufficiently in size and strength simply as a consequence of doing upper back and shoulder exercises.

With each detailed exercise description in this chapter—as well as in subsequent chapters—we have included one or two photographs to depict the correct starting and finishing positions of the movement. By comparing the photos with the exercise description, you will be able to master each exercise without additional coaching.

As you learn each new exercise, practice it first with a very light weight until you can do it with good body coordination and you are confident that you are doing it correctly. Pay very close attention to each safety suggestion outlined in the exercise descriptions. Weight training is very heavy exercise, and it is relatively easy to injure yourself when training with an incorrect body position during an exercise. But by following the outlined performance directions to the letter, you will avoid the chance of injuring yourself while training.

If at any time you feel that you don't understand an exercise that is described and depicted in this and subsequent chapters, don't hesitate to consult a more experienced bodybuilder. It might even be a good practice to have such a man or woman watch your first two or three workouts, just to correct your exercise form before a mistake becomes ingrained as a bad habit.

Both male and female bodybuilders have been used in the photos for the various exercises. Since we sincerely feel that bodybuilding is suited to both sexes, we have tried to split the pictures evenly between the sexes. However, which exercises are illustrated with men and which with women was an arbitrary choice; it does not indicate that those exercises are intended only for one sex. All weight training and bodybuilding exercises can be used by both men and women.

At the conclusion of this chapter we have included several training routines that have been formulated using the exercises presented in this chapter. You can use the first of these programs

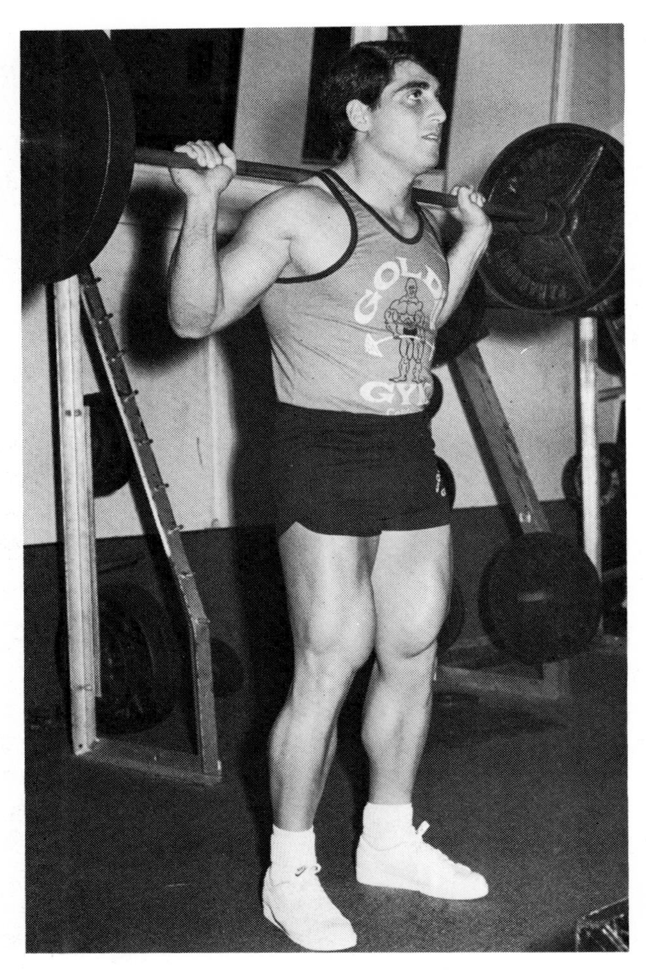

Squat—start.

for 4–6 weeks and then progress through the other routines in sequence, using each one for an additional 4–6 weeks. In this manner you can progress from rank beginner to the intermediate level of bodybuilding with little difficulty in five or six months.

Thigh Exercises

Squat

General Comments: Most champion competitive bodybuilders consider this movement the most valuable of all bodybuilding exercises. Certainly, it is unsurpassed as a front thigh and lower back movement. It also places secondary stress on the hamstring muscles at the backs of the thighs, the upper back, and the abdomen. And by following a program of heavy Squats you will beneficially stimulate the body's metabolism, edging it toward a tendency to add muscular body weight at a relatively fast pace.

Starting Position: Rest a loaded barbell across your shoulders behind your neck and grasp its handle out near the plates to keep it in this position. If you are careful to rest the barbell across your trapezius muscles, rather than over one of your cervical vertebrae, you will experience no discomfort when holding the bar in this starting position. If you do experience any pain, simply wrap the handle of the barbell with a thick towel to provide a cushion between the barbell bar and your body.

Once you have the bar across your shoulders, stand with your feet set at approximately shoulder width. Your toes should be pointed outward at about a 45-degree angle on each side. Stand erect and tense the muscles of your back and abdomen. Focus your eyes on a point at shoulder height on the wall in front of you and keep your eyes focused on this point

Squat—finish.

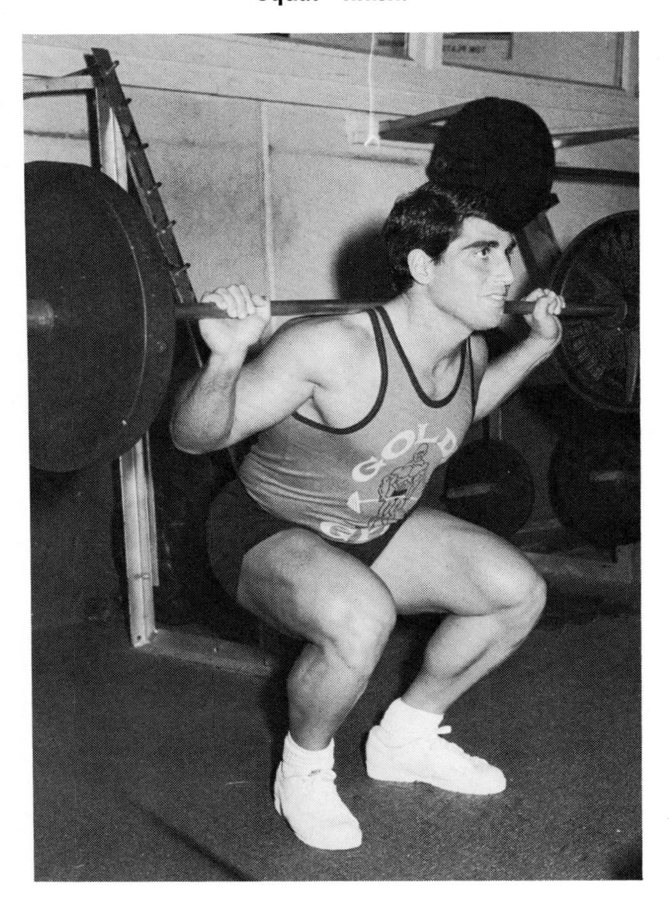

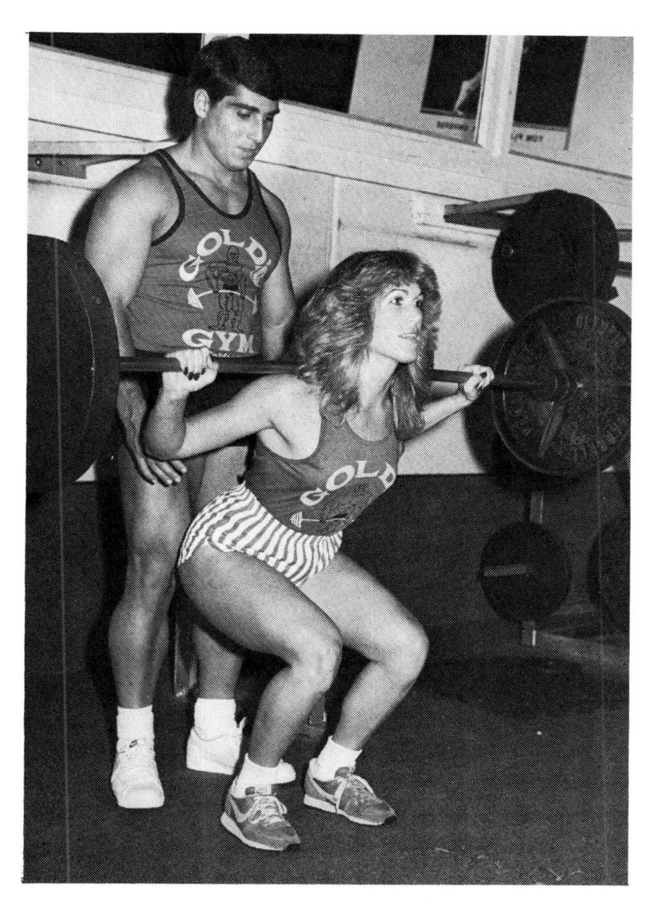

Proper position of spotter for squats.

throughout the movement. This will keep your head up and your back upright during the exercise.

Exercise Performance: Keeping your torso as upright as possible throughout the movement, slowly bend your legs and lower your body into a full squatting position. As you squat down, be sure that your knees travel out over your feet (i.e., your legs will be spread so they form an approximate 90-degree angle with each other at their juncture with the body). Go down as far as you can before beginning to straighten your legs to return to the starting position. Do *not* bounce at the bottom of the movement, since this can injure your knees and/or lower back. Once you are fully erect, immediately begin another repetition.

Training Tips: If you have difficulty balancing at the bottom position of the movement, or if your heels have a tendency to come off the floor, rest your heels on a 2 × 4-inch board during the movement. Once you can use at least your own body weight on Squats (for women the appropriate figure would be 75% of body weight), you should always wear a weightlifting belt to protect your lower back and abdomen from injury.

Leg Press

General Comments: This movement is similar in effect to the Squat, but it does not stress the thigh muscles with as great a degree of intensity during each set. Leg Presses can be done on a freestanding machine, a 45-degree-angled machine, a Universal Gym machine, or a Nautilus machine. Of these four alternatives, most Gold's Gym members prefer the 45-degree-angled machine or the Nautilus machine.

Starting Position (freestanding machine): Lie on your back on the angled pad beneath the

Leg Press on freestanding machine—start.

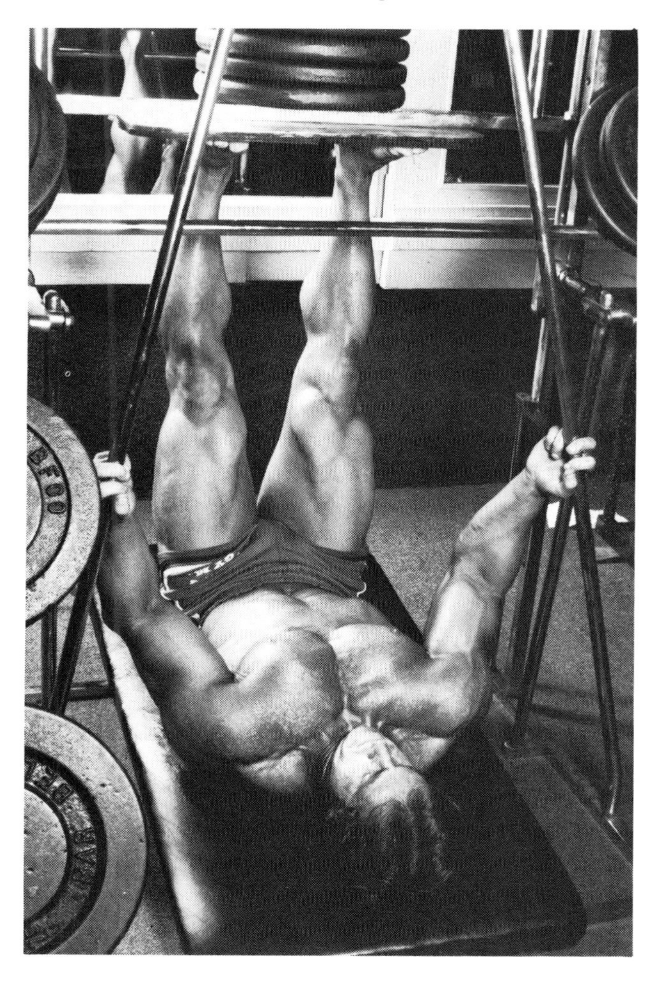

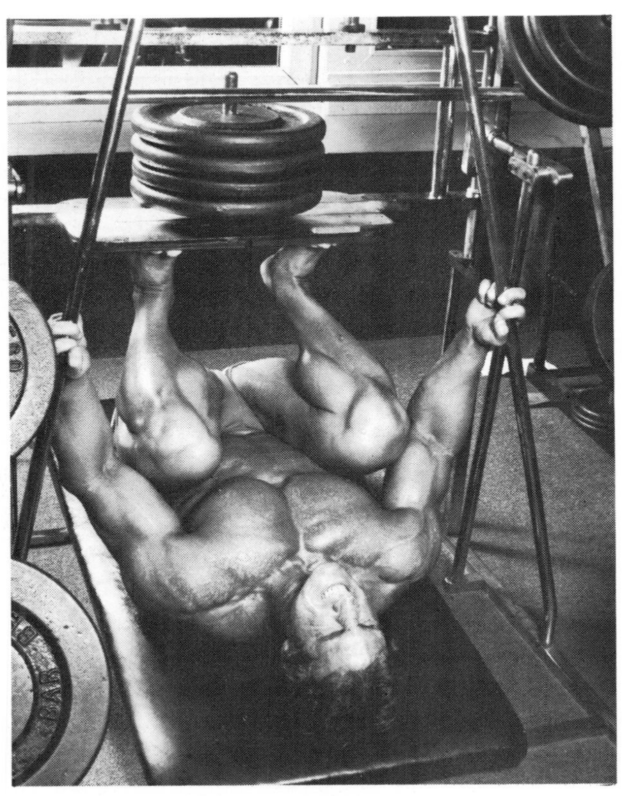

Leg Press on freestanding machine—finish.

weight platform. You should position your body so your hips are directly under the platform, at the upper end of the angled pad. Place your feet on the sliding platform at about shoulder width, your toes angled outward about 45 degrees on each side. Straighten your legs and rotate the stop bars at the sides of your hips to release the weight.

Starting Position (45-degree-angled machine): Sit in the machine so your back rests on the padded surface at the lower edge of the machine. There will be a corner where the back and seat pads join, and your hips should rest firmly in this corner. Place your feet on the sliding platform in the same position as for Leg Presses on a freestanding machine. Straighten your legs and release the stop catches at the sides of the machine to release the weight for your set.

Starting Position (Universal Gym machine): Sit on the seat of the machine. Place your feet on the lower set of pedals (if there are two sets). Grasp the handles at the sides of your seat and

Leg Press on 45-degree-angled machine—midpoint.

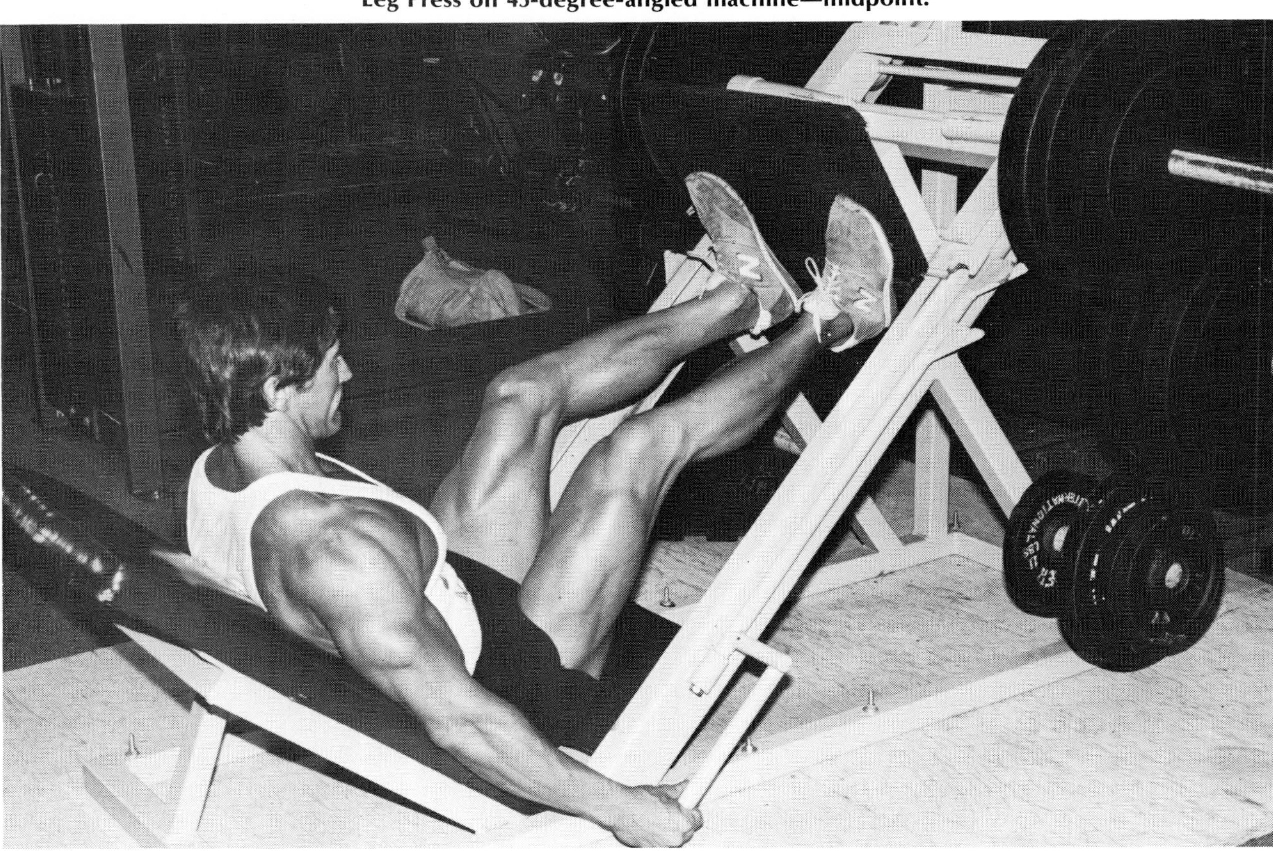

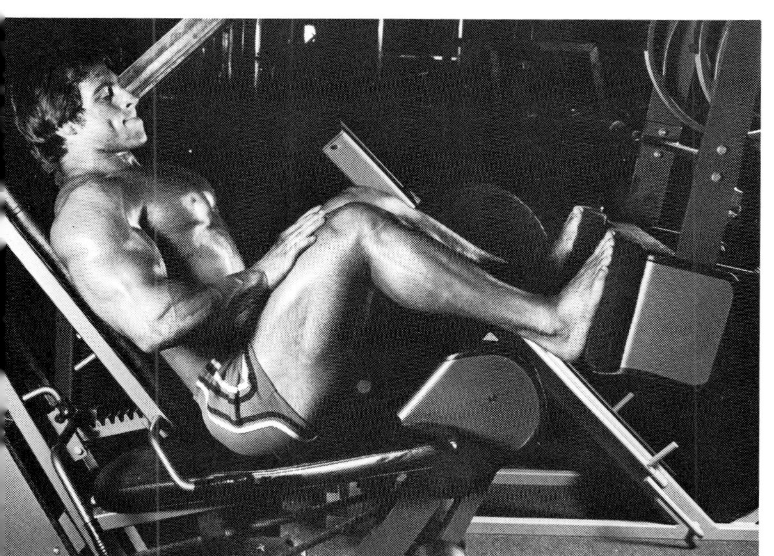
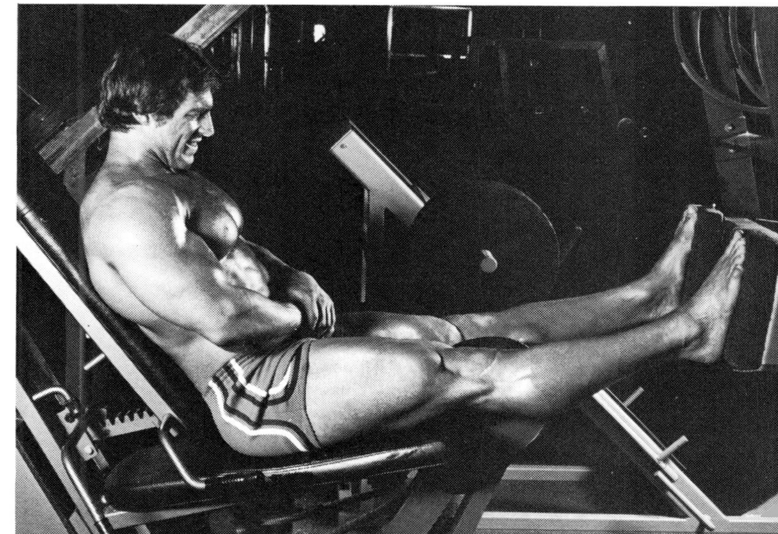

Leg Press on Nautilus machine—start, left; finish, right.

straighten your legs. The seat on the machine is adjustable both forward and backward. Simply pull up on the knob at the front of the seat and slide the seat to the position desired. Be sure the seat locks into the new position before you do your set. The closer you place the seat to the pedals, the longer the range of motion you will experience when doing the movement.

Starting Position (Nautilus machine): Assume the same starting position as for Leg Presses on a Universal Gym machine. On both machines you should angle your toes outward slightly on the pedals. The Nautilus machine seat is adjustable forward and backward in the same manner as the Universal Gym machine seat. The only difference is that on the Nautilus machine the seat is adjusted by moving a lever at the right side of the machine while you are sitting in the seat.

Exercise Performance: The exercise performance is identical for all four types of machines. Starting with your legs straight, bend your legs as fully as possible, being certain that your knees travel out over your toes as they did for the Squat. Straighten your legs to within five degrees of full lockout (when your knees can bend no further and seem locked) and repeat the movement for the required number of repetitions. At the completion of the set you must rotate the stop bars back to the locked position on the freestanding and 45-degree-angled machines before stepping out of the machine.

Training Tips: On the Universal Gym and Nautilus machines it is essential that you keep your back perfectly straight while you sit in the seat. Hunching your shoulders forward will eventually result in an injury to your middle or upper back. Generally speaking, the Universal Gym and Nautilus machines are safer than the other two types, since they obviate the possibility of becoming pinned under the weight if you fail to complete a repetition. When you are doing this movement on machines with a weight stack, be careful to avoid slapping the weights in the stack together very forcefully. The weights in the stack are made from cast metal, and they break rather easily if abused in this manner.

Leg Extension

General Comments: This exercise allows you to train the quadriceps muscles at the fronts of your thighs with direct stress and in relative isolation from the muscle groups of the rest of the body. You can do Leg Extensions on freestanding, Universal Gym, and Nautilus machines.

Starting Position (for all three machines): Sit in the machine with the backs of your knees at

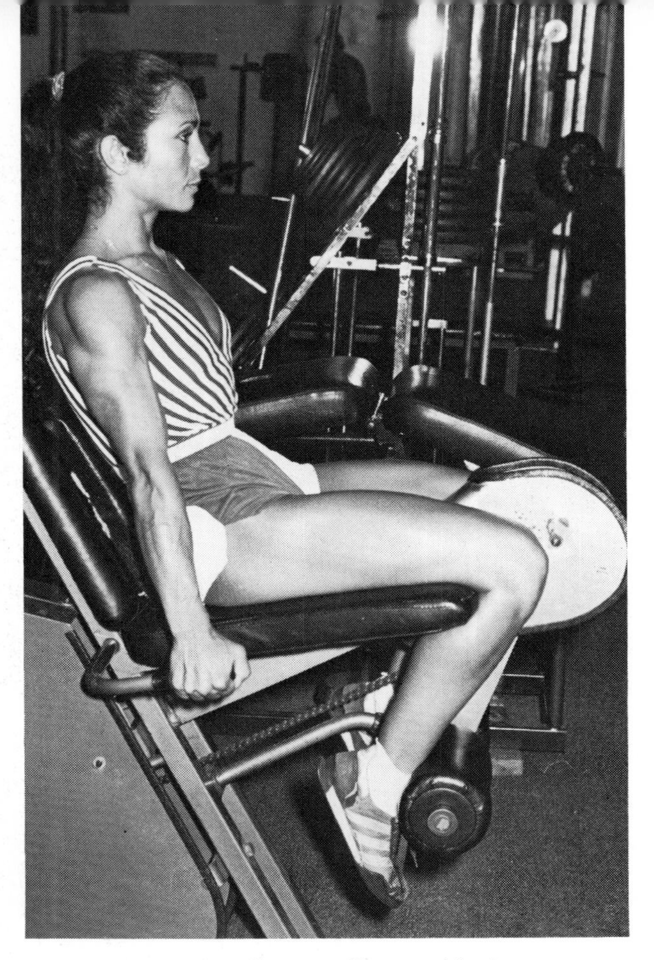

Leg Extension (freestanding machine)—start.

the edge of the padded surface and your legs facing the movement arm of the machine. Place the insteps of your feet under the lower set of roller pads (there will be only one set on the Nautilus machine). To steady your body as you perform the movement, grasp either the handles provided at the sides of the machine or the edges of the padded surface. The seat back on some Nautilus machines is adjustable forward and backward for added comfort when doing the exercise. As with the Leg Press machine, this adjustment is accomplished by moving a lever at the right side of the seat as you are sitting in it.

Exercise Performance: From this basic starting position, simply straighten your legs slowly. In the top position of the movement you should hold your legs straight for a count of two before lowering the weight back to the starting position. Repeat the movement for the desired number of repetitions.

Training Tips: Many bodybuilders, most notably 14-time World Champion Boyer Coe, do

Leg Extension (freestanding machine)—finish.

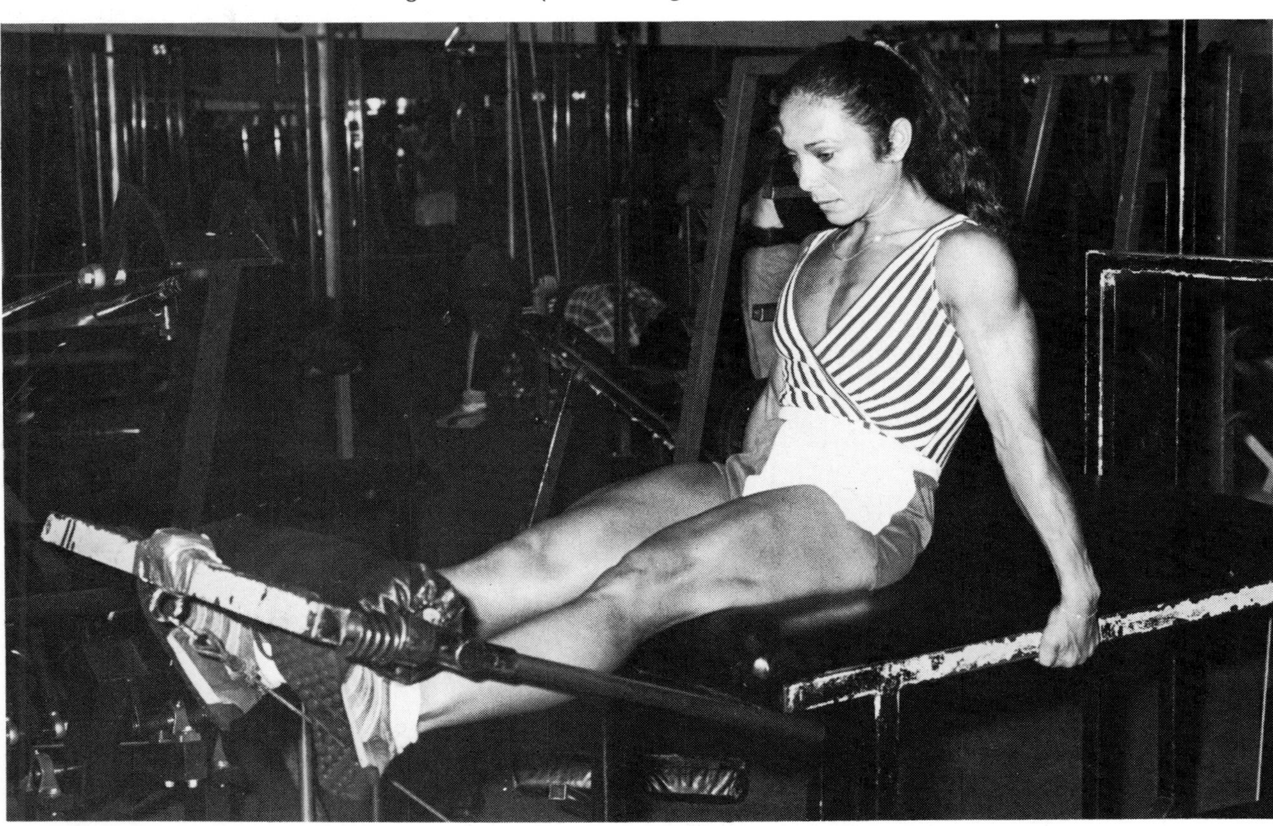

this exercise one leg at a time. When you do any movement one leg or one arm at a time, you will receive a better quality of stress than when using both arms or legs. This is because your concentration can be focused on one working muscle group rather than split between two. By holding the weight briefly in the fully contracted position (i.e., at the top of the movement), you will receive a "peak contraction" effect on your muscles (peak contraction is discussed in detail in Chapter 8).

Leg Curl

General Comments: This exercise allows you to train the biceps femoris (hamstrings) muscles at the backs of your thighs with direct stress and in relative isolation from other muscle groups. You can do Leg Curls on freestanding, Universal Gym, and Nautilus machines.

Starting Position (for all three machines): Lie face down on the padded surface of the machine with your knees at the edge of the pad, facing the lever arm of the machine. Place your heels under the upper set of roller pads (there will be

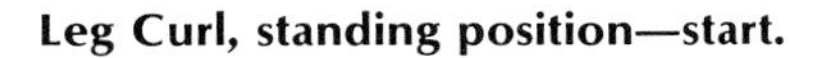

Leg Curl, standing position—start.

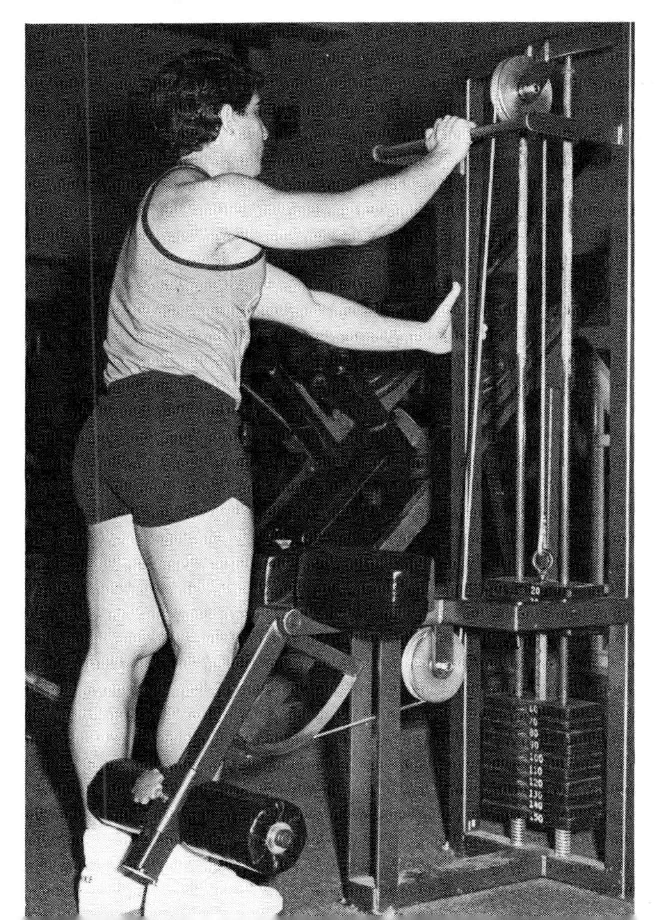

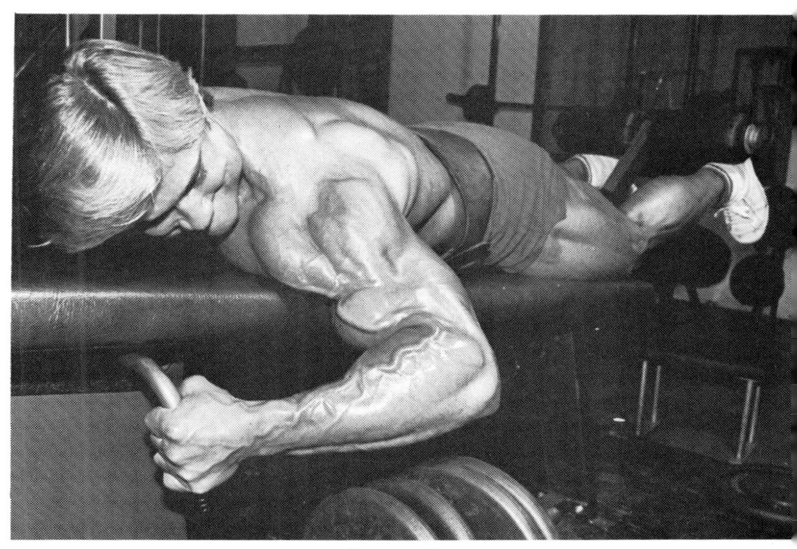

Leg Curl (Nautilus)—start.

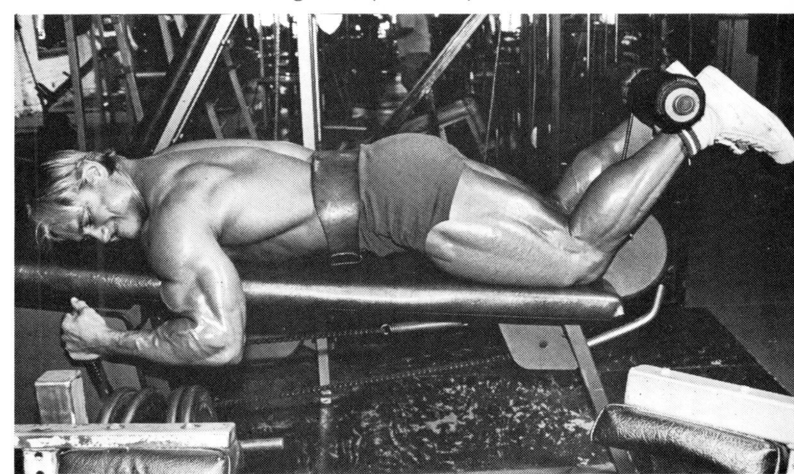

Leg Curl (Nautilus)—midpoint.

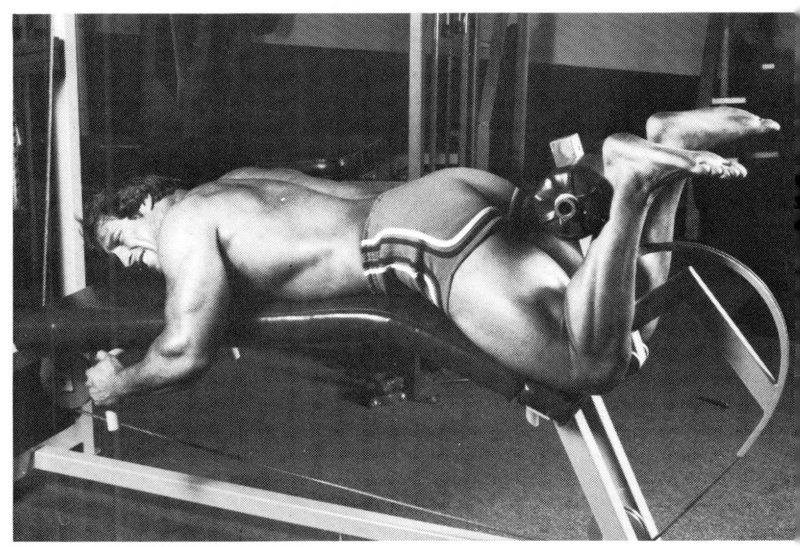

Leg Curl (freestanding)—finish.

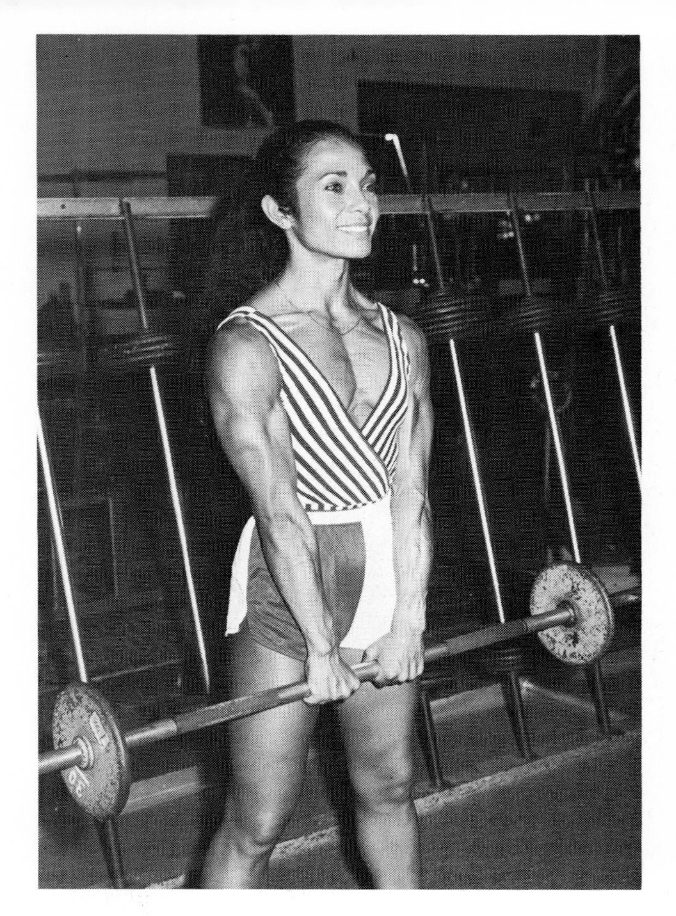

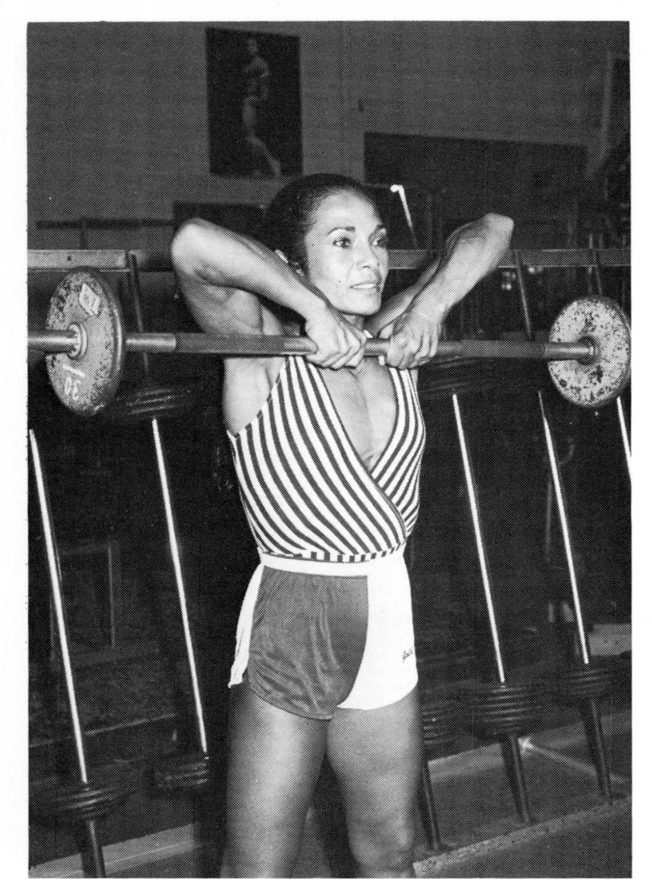

Upright Rowing—start, left; finish, right.

only one set on the Nautilus machine). Grasp either the handles provided or the sides of the padded surface to steady your body in position while you do the movement.

Exercise Performance: From this basic starting position, slowly bend your legs as fully as possible. Hold the fully bent position for a count of two before slowly lowering the weight back to the starting position.

Training Tips: As with Leg Extensions, you can do Leg Curls one leg at a time if you desire a more concentrated stimulation of your hamstrings. And holding the contracted position of the movement for two or three seconds will apply a peak contraction effect to your biceps femoris muscles.

Back Exercises

Upright Rowing

General Comments: This is an excellent exercise for building all the muscles of your shoulder girdle (the deltoid and trapezius muscles) at once. Secondary stress is placed on the muscles of the forearms and the biceps. This exercise can be done with a barbell, two dumbbells, or the floor pulley of a Universal Gym machine or other apparatus.

Starting Position (barbell): Take a narrow grip (about six inches between your index fingers) in the middle of a barbell so that your palms are toward your body when you stand erect and hang your arms down at your sides. When you stand erect, the barbell in your hands should be across your upper thighs.

Starting Position (dumbbells): Start in exactly the same position as with a barbell, except that you will be holding two dumbbells in your hands. As the dumbbells rest across your upper thighs, your palms should be toward your body, and the plates of one dumbbell will rest against the plates of the other.

Starting Position (floor pulley): Stand about 12 inches back from a floor pulley and take the same grip on a straight-bar handle attached to the pulley as you would take on a barbell for this movement. Since you are standing back from the pulley, your hands will be one or two inches from your thighs in the starting position.

Exercise Performance: From the basic starting position, slowly pull the weight, weights, or handle upward, close to your body, until it touches the underside of your chin. As you pull upward on the apparatus, keep your elbows above the level of your hands at all times. At the top of the movement you should especially emphasize this elbows-up position. Pause for a moment at the top of the movement and slowly lower the apparatus back to the starting position. Repeat the movement for the required number of repetitions.

Training Tips: You should experiment with various grip widths on the bar. You can move your hands inward until they are touching in the middle of the bar or outward until they are at approximately shoulder width on the bar. A few bodybuilders have noted that it is best to do this movement with dumbbells whenever you have a shoulder injury, since the dumbbells allow you to vary your grip width as you are pulling the weights upward. This allows you to avoid hand and arm position that might aggravate the injury.

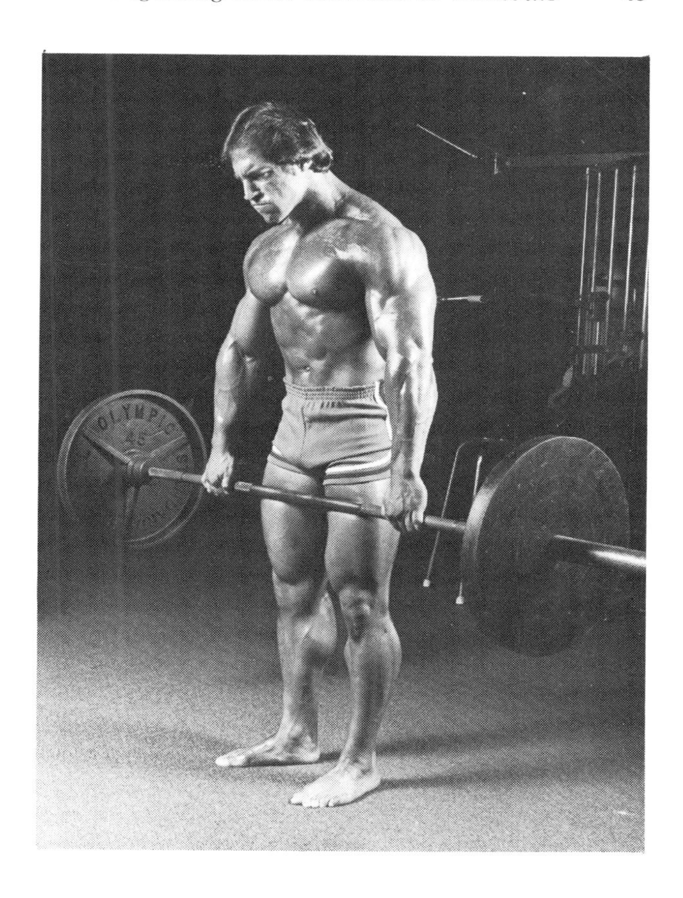

Barbell Shrug—start, above (*photo by Bill Dobbins*); **finish, below.**

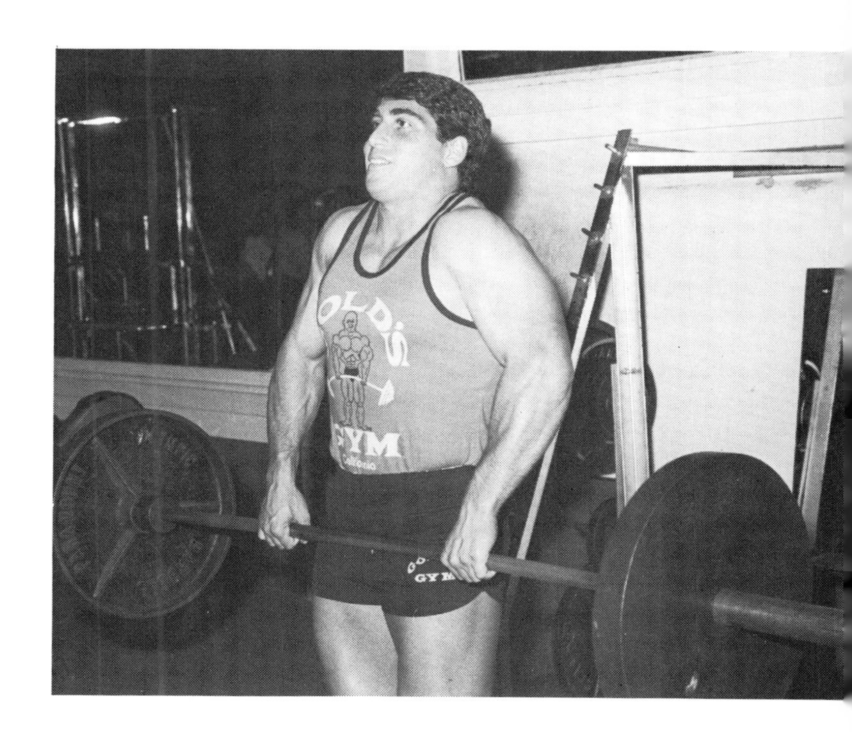

Barbell Shrug

General Comments: This is a very direct and intense type of movement for developing the trapezius muscles of your upper back. Secondary emphasis is placed on the gripping muscles of your forearms.

Starting Position: Take a shoulder-width grip on a barbell so your palms are toward your body as you stand erect and rest the barbell with straight arms across your upper thighs. Be sure to stand perfectly erect throughout the movement. Your arms should not bend at all during the exercise, since to bend them when you are using an exceedingly heavy weight could result in a torn biceps. Instead, think of your arms merely as cables with hooks (your hands) at the ends. These cables are the means by which you can hang a heavy barbell from your shoulders as you do Shrugs.

Exercise Performance: Sag your shoulders as far downward as possible. Then slowly shrug them upward and slightly backward to the full extent of the range of motion of your shoulder joints. Try to visualize yourself shrugging your shoulders high enough to touch them to your

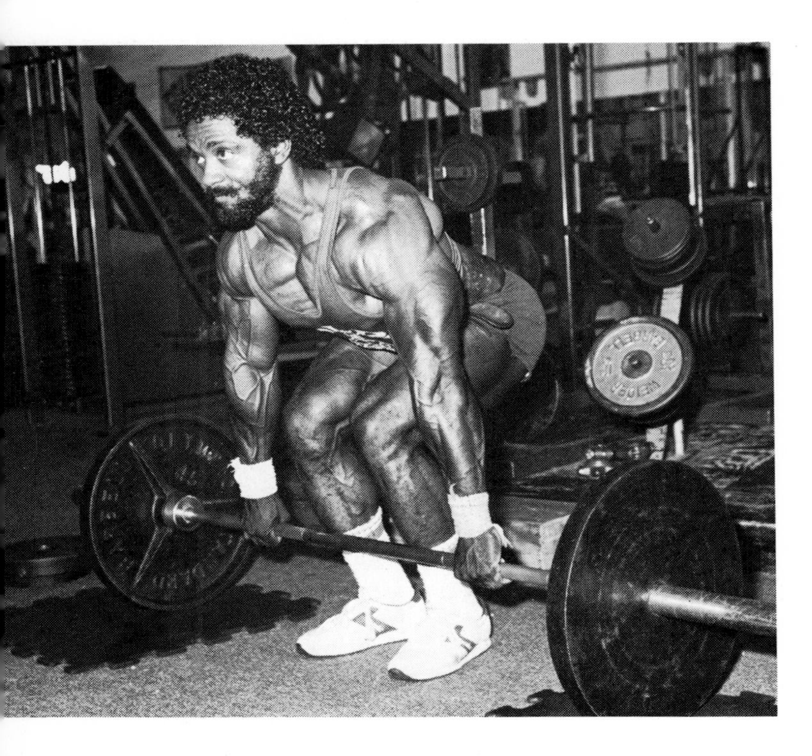

Deadlift—start, above; finish, below.

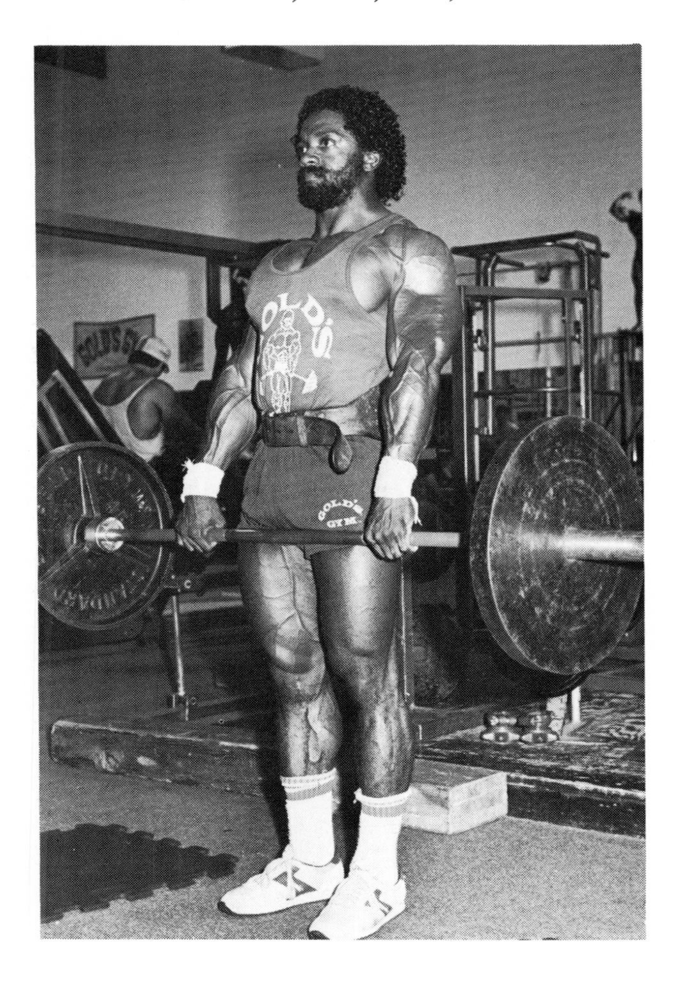

ears. Lower the weight back to the starting position and repeat the movement for the desired number of repetitions.

Training Tips: As with most barbell movements, you should experiment with different grip widths on the barbell. With very heavy weights you will find it a good practice to strap your hands to the barbell. There are various ways to use these straps, and any competitive powerlifter or weightlifter can show you how to use them. By the time you are using heavy enough poundages to require straps, you will be training in a large gym, where these competitive lifters should be accessible.

Deadlift

General Comments: This is a very important movement for beginning and intermediate bodybuilders. It develops muscle mass and a great deal of power in the large lower back, hip, thigh, and upper back muscles. It also places a great deal of stress on the gripping muscles of the forearms. Generally speaking, advanced bodybuilders shy away from using Deadlifts in their training. They are so strong that they must use exceedingly heavy weights on this movement to get any benefit from it. And when using such heavy poundages they run a magnified risk of injuring their lower backs. Andreas Cahling, Mr. International and one of the most enthusiastic Gold's Gym members, learned this lesson the hard way. While doing heavy Deadlifts a year before he won the International, Andreas injured his lower back badly enough to put him out of action for three months. Beginning and intermediate bodybuilders run very little risk of injuring their backs, however, as long as they use correct biomechanics (as outlined in this exercise description).

Starting Position: Load up a barbell that is resting on the floor. Bend over and grasp the bar with your hands set at shoulder width and your palms toward your feet. Place your feet a little narrower than shoulder width and close enough to the barbell for your shins to touch the bar. Dip your hips, straighten your arms fully (they must remain straight throughout the movement), and look straight ahead. When you are in the correct starting position, your shoulders should be above the level of your hips

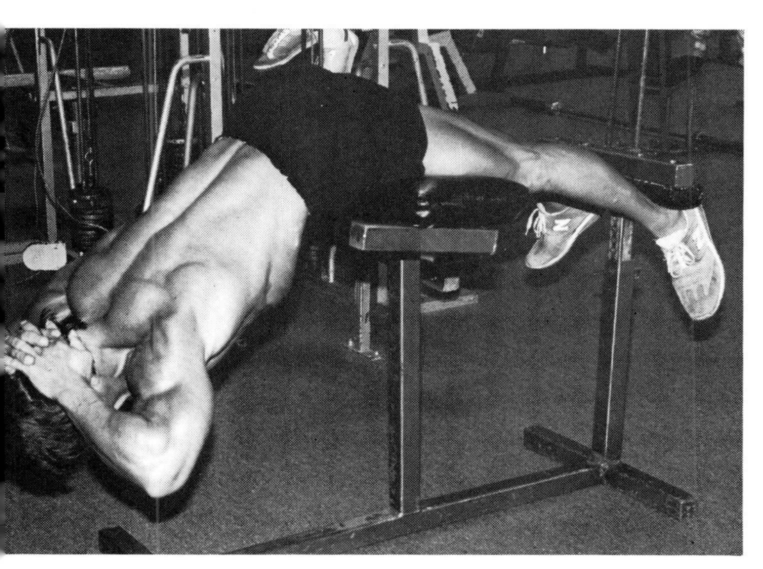

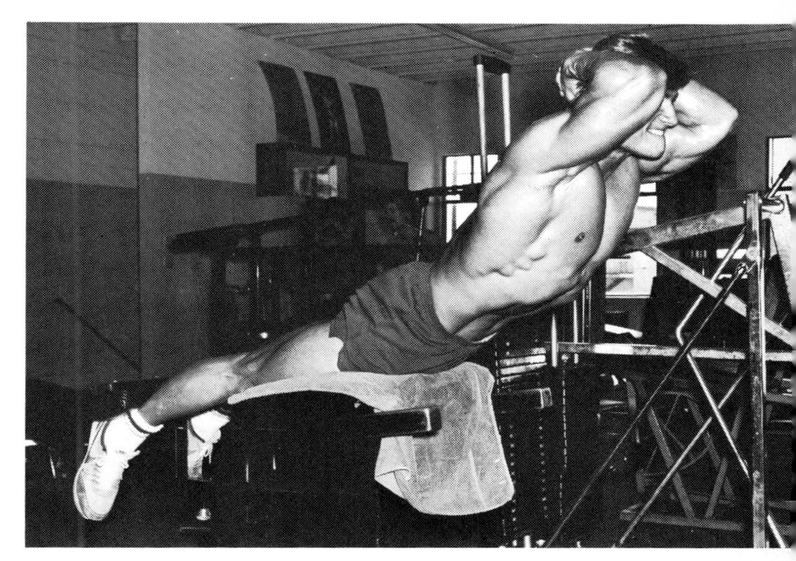

Hyperextension—midpoint, left; finish, right (*photo by Peter Brenner*).

and your hips should be above the level of your knees. Be sure to inspect carefully the photos included with this exercise. This starting position is the basic pulling position that you should assume whenever you are lifting a heavy weight from the floor. Such a position is biomechanically sound and will protect your lower back from injury.

Exercise Performance: Begin pulling the barbell from the floor by slowly straightening your legs. As your legs straighten, also begin to straighten your back. If you do this movement in a coordinated fashion, your legs and back should straighten simultaneously to bring your body fully erect with the weight resting at arms' length across your thighs. Lower the weight back to the floor by precisely reversing the procedure you used to raise it. Repeat the movement for the required number of reps.

Training Tips: When you are using very heavy weights, the barbell will have a tendency to roll from your fingers. When this is the case you should use a "reversed grip" in which the palm of one hand faces forward and the palm of the other faces backward. You will find this gripping method quite secure with even the heaviest poundages. There is also a type of Deadlift in which the legs are held straight throughout the movement. This is called a Stiff-Leg Deadlift, and it is explained in detail in Chapter 5.

Hyperextension

General Comments: This exercise allows you to place stress on the erector spinae muscles of your lower back without a compression pressure on your spinal vertebrae (as is the case with all forms of Deadlifting). Therefore, this movement is the only one that you can do for your lumbar muscles when you have a sore lower back. Hyperextensions place secondary stress on the hamstring muscles at the backs of your thighs.

Starting Position: Stand in a Hyperextension bench with your back toward the bar that is padded on its lower surface. You will be facing the larger of the machine's two pads. Lean forward on this larger pad so the top edge of your pelvis is at the front edge of the padded surface. As you lean forward, allow the backs of your ankles to come up against the rear pad. They will remain against this pad throughout the movement. Flex your body at the waist until your torso is perpendicular to the floor. Place your hands behind your neck and hold them in this position while you do the exercise.

Exercise Performance: From this starting position, slowly straighten your body until your torso reaches a position parallel to the floor. Do *not* arch your back, though you will frequently see male and female bodybuilders do this (cheating) in a gym. Arching your back compresses your lumbar vertebrae. Lower your torso back to the starting position and repeat the movement.

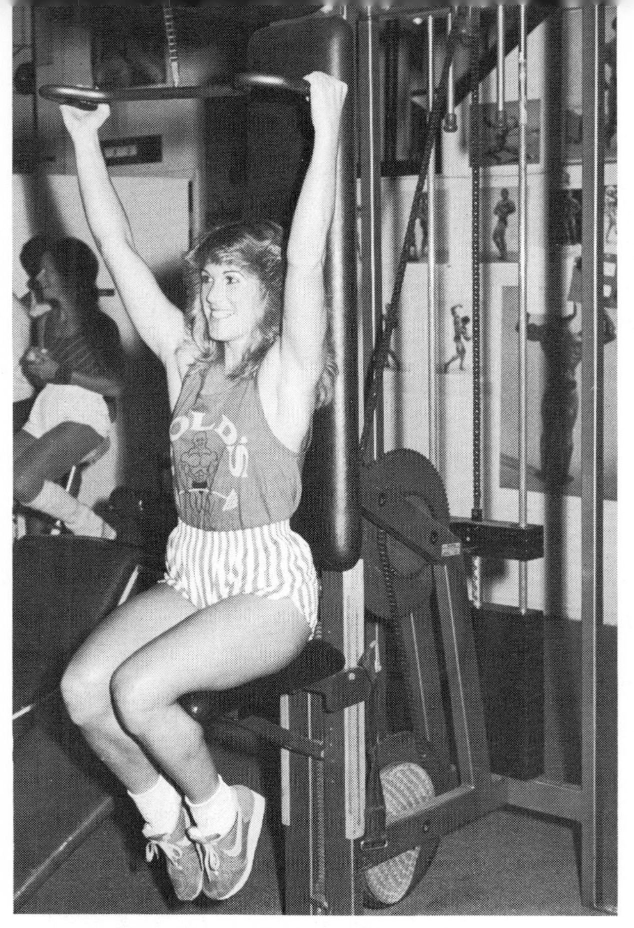

Lat Machine Pulldown on Nautilus—start.

Training Tips: Your back muscles will very quickly become strong enough for you easily to do several sets of 20–30 repetitions. At that point you will need to add resistance to the movement. This is best done by holding a loose barbell plate or two behind your head.

If a Hyperextension bench isn't available, you can do this movement lying with your legs on a high table or bench. A training partner can rest his torso across your calves or hold down your feet while you do the movement.

Lat Machine Pulldown

General Comments: This movement is similar to doing Chins. Instead of pulling your body up to a high bar, however, you pull a movable bar down to your body. Thus this is a good exercise to do when you are a little too weak to do a set of Chins. Lat Pulldowns develop the large latissimus dorsi muscles of your upper back. They place secondary emphasis on the gripping muscles of your forearms, your biceps, and your

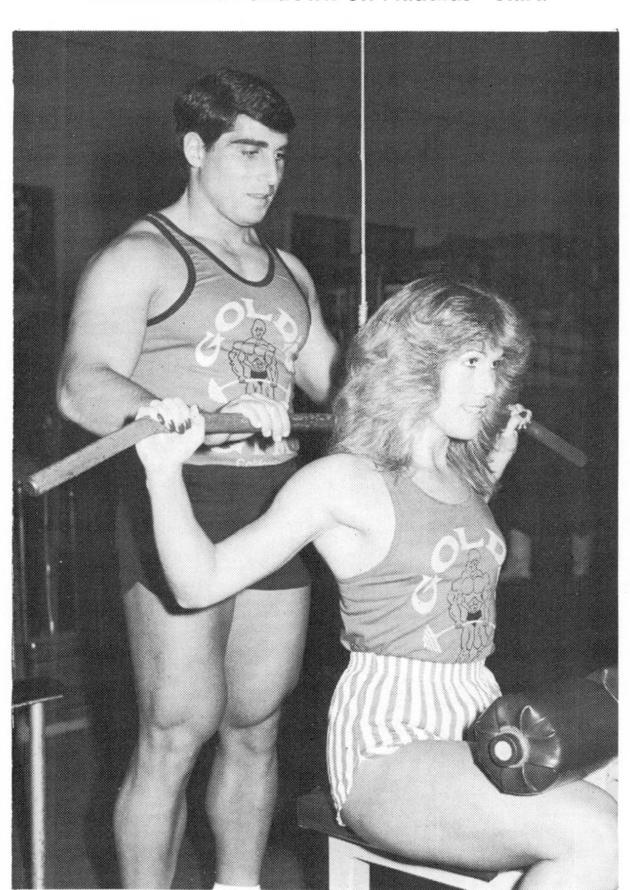

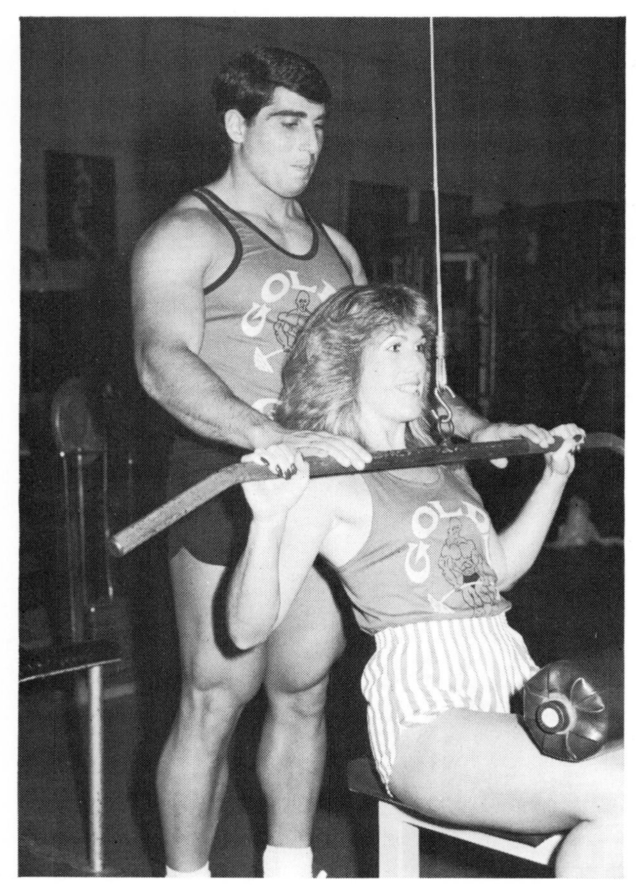

Lat Machine Pulldown on freestanding machine—finish behind neck, left; finish in front of neck, right. Note how partner is helping with forced reps.

trapezius muscles. Lat Pulldowns can be done on a freestanding lat machine, on the lat machine of a Universal Gym complex, or on a Nautilus machine.

Starting Position (Universal Gym and freestanding machine): Grasp a lat machine handle with a grip a little wider than your shoulders. Your palms will be facing forward—away from you—when you are in position to do the exercise. Slowly straighten your arms and either sit or kneel directly beneath the pulley. On some freestanding lat machines there will be a seat with a special knee-restraining bar attached to it. Simply sit in the seat and place your knees under this bar, and you will be able to do Lat Pulldowns with a very heavy weight, one heavy enough to pull your body from the floor under ordinary circumstances.

Starting Position (Nautilus machine): On this machine you sit in the seat that is provided and buckle the waist belt around your hips and waist to restrain your body in the machine while you do the exercise. Then reach up and grasp the handles of the machine with your palms facing inward. With your hands in this position (rather than with them facing forward during the movement), your biceps are put in a stronger mechanical position to assist the lats in pulling on the bar.

Exercise Performance: As you do this movement, visualize your elbows pulling downward and backward at the same time. The latissimus dorsi muscles' function is to pull the upper arm bones downward and backward, so this is the movement you should try to duplicate when doing all lat exercises. From the basic starting position, slowly pull the bar down until it touches your upper chest. Slowly allow your arms to straighten and repeat the movement.

Training Tips: You should experiment with various grip widths while you are doing Lat Pulldowns. You can also use a grip in which your palms are toward your body rather than away from it while you do the movement. Earlier, we mentioned Andreas Cahling and his lower back injury. His lower back was still weak from the injury when he was training to win the Mr. International competition. As a result, he was unable to do any Bent Rowing movements for his lats. Still, he was able to develop his upper back muscles fully by using six different types of grips on the bar of a lat machine. Generally speaking, bodybuilders do Chins and Lat Pulldowns to develop width in their latissimus dorsi muscles.

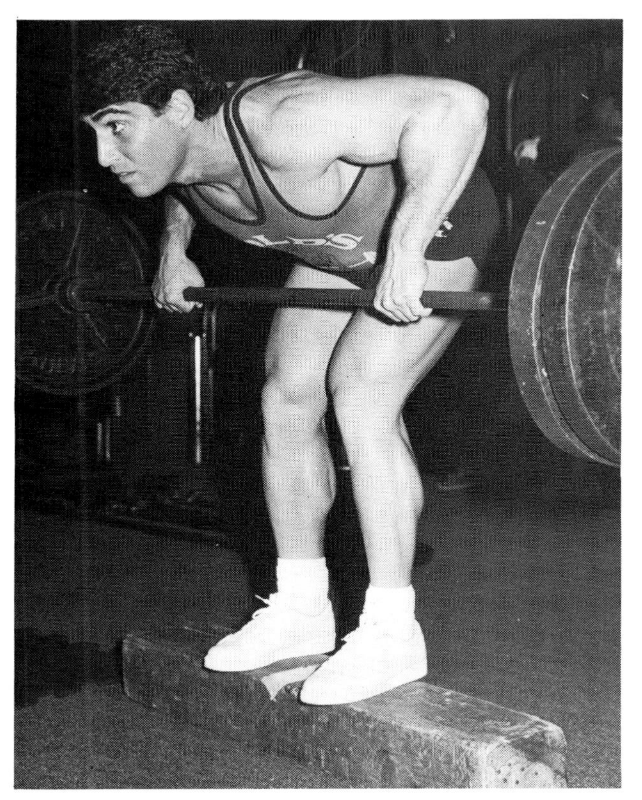

Barbell Bent Rowing: close to finish.

Barbell Bent Rowing

General Comments: This is an excellent upper back developer. In fact, it is one of the favorite lat movements of Lou Ferrigno, the two-time Mr. Universe winner who played the role of "The Incredible Hulk" for four seasons on television. Barbell Bent Rowing helps build thickness in the latissimus dorsi muscles. It places secondary emphasis on the upper and lower back muscles, the biceps, and the gripping muscles of the forearms.

Starting Position: Place a loaded barbell on the floor. Bend over and take a grip on the bar with your hands set a little wider than shoulder width and your palms facing your legs. Place your feet at about shoulder width about a foot back from the barbell. Bend your legs slightly and keep them bent throughout the movement in an effort to avoid unduly stressing your lower

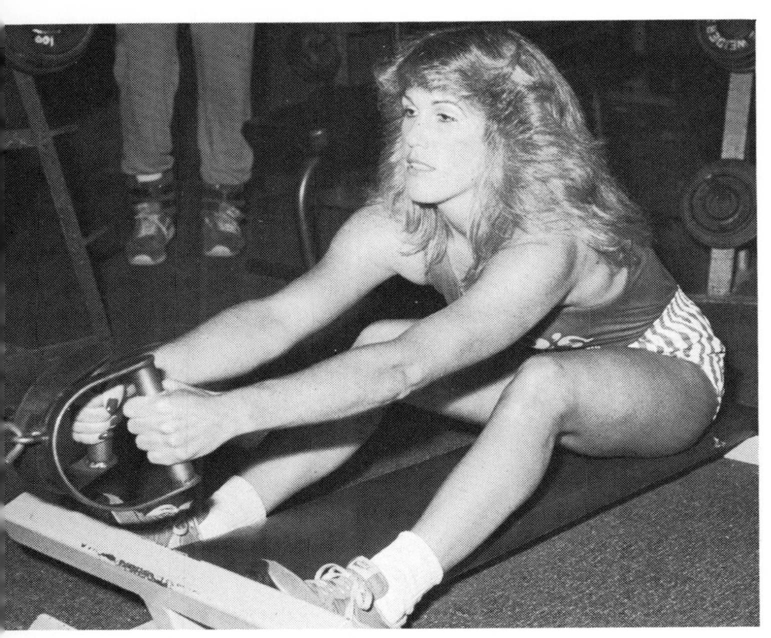

Seated Pulley Rowing—start.

back. Straighten your arms and pull your shoulders upward until your torso is parallel to the floor and the bar is hanging at arms' length below your shoulders. Your back should be either completely flat or, better yet, actually arched a bit during the movement.

Exercise Performance: From this basic starting position, bend your arms to pull the weight from arms' length to touch the lower part of your rib cage. As you pull the barbell upward, be sure that your elbows travel both upward and backward. Lower the barbell slowly back to the starting position and repeat the movement for the desired number of repetitions.

Training Tips: You can experiment with various grip widths on the barbell handle. Some bodybuilders seem to like a rather narrow grip in which the index fingers are placed on the bar about 8–10 inches apart. Others like a very wide grip on the barbell. Very few bodybuilders use a grip in which the palms face away from the body during the movement. One notable exception to this rule is the legendary Serge Nubret, one of the greatest bodybuilders of all time and a man who defeated Lou Ferrigno in the 1975 Mr. Olympia show. Nubret often does Barbell Bent Rowing with his palms facing away from his body, and his latissimus development is superb. Give all grip variations a good trial in your own workouts to see which works best for your unique body structure.

Seated Pulley Rowing

General Comments: This is an excellent movement for building both thickness and width in the latissimus dorsi muscles of the upper back. Secondary emphasis is placed on the trapezius, erector spinae, biceps, and forearm muscles. Virtually all of the great bodybuilders who have trained at Gold's Gym over the years favored this movement for back development.

Starting Position: Grasp a parallel-grip handle on a floor pulley apparatus so your palms are facing each other during the movement. Place your feet on the foot bar at the end of the seat toward the pulley. Sit down on the seat so your legs are bent slightly throughout the movement. Straighten your arms fully and lean forward over your legs to stretch your lats fully.

Exercise Performance: Simultaneously bend your arms to pull the handle toward your chest and sit backward until your torso is erect. Pull the handle in to touch your upper abdomen just under your rib cage. As you pull the handle in to touch your torso, be sure that your upper

Seated Pulley Rowing—finish.

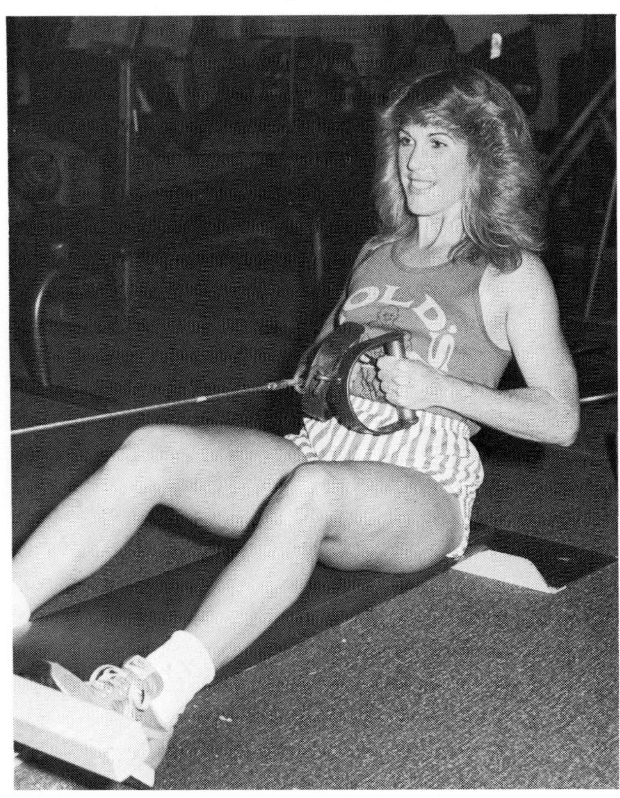

arms are held in close to your body. Reverse the pulling procedure to return to the starting position, again leaning forward over your legs. Repeat the movement for the desired number of repetitions.

Training Tips: You can experiment with several types of handles and hand grips when doing Seated Pulley Rowing. The first of these is a short straight bar handle, which is usually gripped with a narrow grip and the palms facing the floor. The bar can, however, also be gripped with the palms facing upward, a favorite grip used by the great French bodybuilder Serge Nubret. You can also use a long straight bar handle, on which you can take a wider grip with your palms facing downward. In addition, you can take a shoulder-width grip, with your palms facing inward toward each other, on a handle often used on lat machines. You can easily tell this handle from the others, because it will have rings of steel welded to the ends of the bar. Inside these rings are welded the handles that allow you to grip the bar with your palms facing inward.

Chest Exercises

Bench Press

General Comments: This excellent upper body movement has often been called "the Squat of upper body movements." Bench Presses can be done with free weights, on a Universal Gym machine, or on a Nautilus machine. Bench Presses strongly stress the pectorals, deltoids, and triceps. Secondary emphasis is placed on the latissimus dorsi muscles.

Starting Position (barbell): Take a grip on a barbell with your hands set four to six inches wider on each side than shoulder width. Your hands should be facing your feet when you have the bar supported at arms' length above your chest while lying on your back on a flat exercise bench. Viewed from the side, your arms will appeai to be perpendicular to the floor when the barbell is in the correct starting position. With heavier weights, you won't be able to get the barbell into the correct starting position unassisted. In such a case, you will need to use a bench press rack. Using such a rack, you load the barbell up while it is resting on the rack. Then you lie on the bench and lift the weight a couple of inches to the starting position. When finished with your set, simply place the barbell back on the rack.

Starting Position (Universal Gym machine): Lie on your back on a flat exercise bench so that your shoulders are positioned directly beneath the handles of the Bench Press station of a Universal Gym machine. Grasp the middle of

Bench Press on Universal Gyms machine—start.

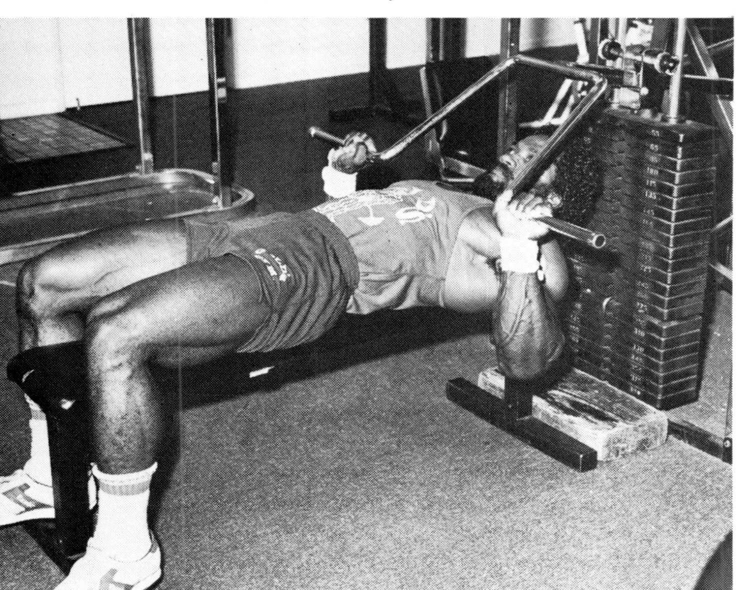

Bench Press with barbell—finish.

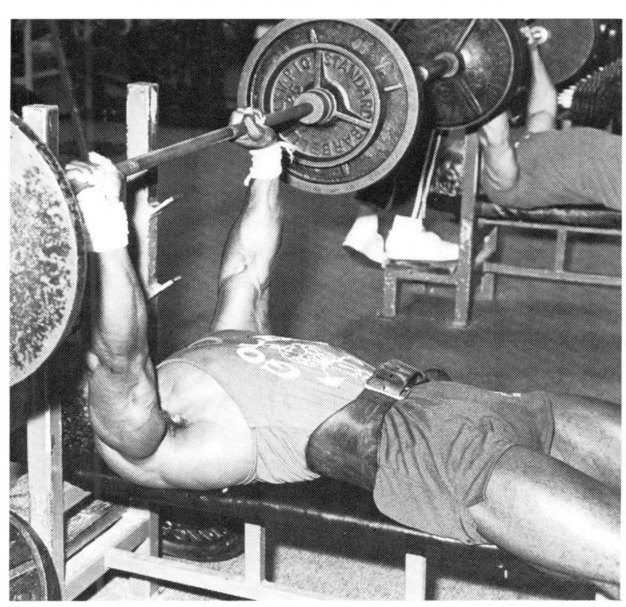

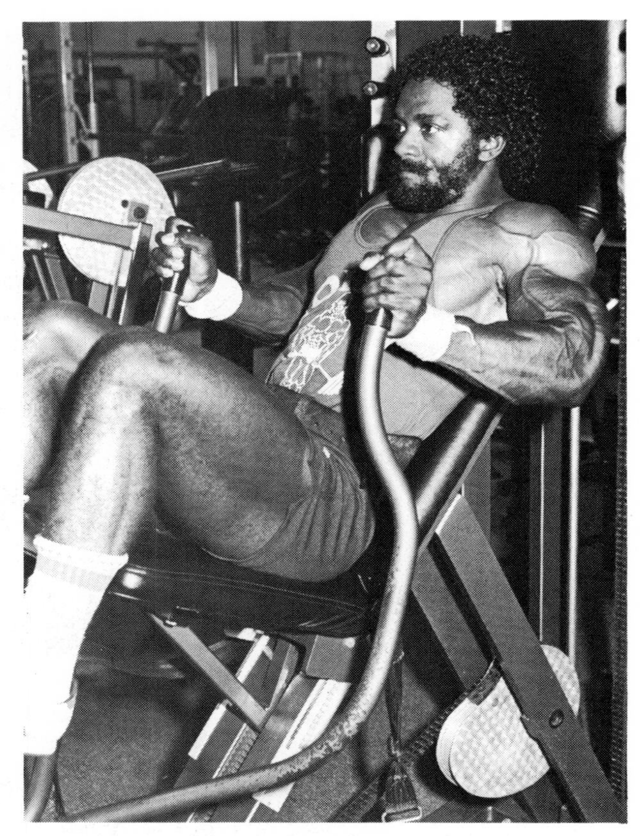

Bench Press on Nautilus machine—midpoint.

each handle with your palms facing your feet. Straighten your arms.

Starting Position (Nautilus machine): Sit in a Nautilus double chest machine and adjust the seat upward or downward so that the handles of the Bench Press apparatus are even with your pectoral muscles. Grasp the handles with your palms facing each other. You can push on the foot pedal to get the Bench Pressing handles into a position where you can grasp them. Using the foot pedal, push your arms straight.

Exercise Performance: The exercise performance is identical for all three types of apparatus. Lower the weight directly downward to the full extent of your range of motion or until the bar touches your chest. Then simply straighten your arms and return the weight to the starting position. Repeat the movement for the required number of repetitions.

Training Tips: The Nautilus and Universal Gym machines are quite safe to use, but using a barbell for Bench Presses can be dangerous in some contexts. Bodybuilders have been severely injured—and even killed—while Bench Pressing alone with a barbell. Never, under any circumstances, should you do limit-poundage (the heaviest weight you can handle) Bench Presses with a barbell alone. Always use a spotter at the head end of your bench under such circumstances. Additionally, never hold your breath while doing Bench Presses. You should always breathe outward as you are pressing up the weight. Holding your breath can cause you to faint while pressing out a weight. Then the barbell will fall swiftly downward where it can land across your neck or face.

Barbell Incline Press

General Comments: This movement is similar to the Bench Press, except that it is done lying back on a 30- to 45-degree incline bench. Pressing a barbell from this position places more stress on the front deltoids and upper part of the pectorals than on the deltoid group and the whole pectoral mass stressed by Bench Presses done on a flat bench.

Starting Position: Take a grip on a barbell similar to the one used for Bench Pressing. Again your palms will be facing forward during the movement. Lie back on an incline bench and press the barbell to arms' length above your shoulder joints. Viewed from the side, your upper arms will appear to be perpendicular to the floor when you have them in the correct starting position.

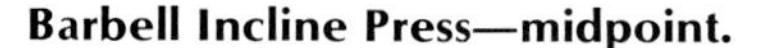

Barbell Incline Press—midpoint.

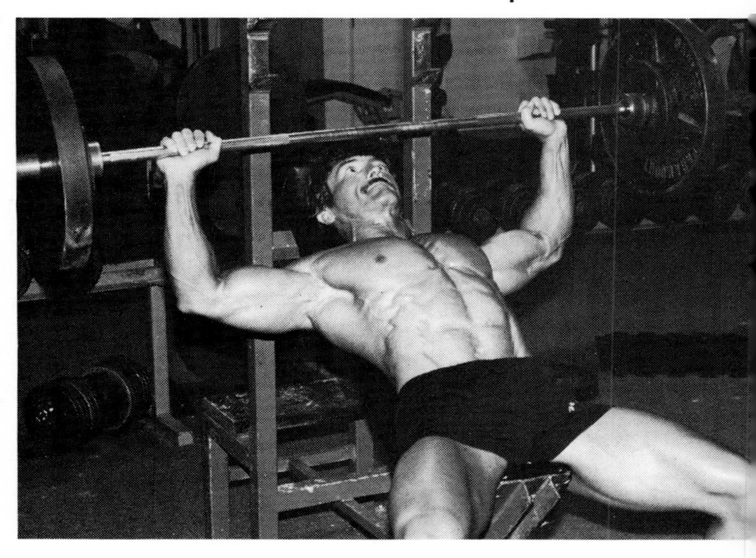

Exercise Performance: Slowly lower the barbell straight downward until it touches your upper chest, just at the base of your neck. As you lower the barbell, be sure your upper arms are held directly out to the sides. This arm position should also be maintained as you press the weight back to the starting position. Repeat the movement for the desired number of repetitions.

Training Tips: When this movement is done on an incline bench set at 30 degrees you will find that it places more stress on your upper pectorals and less on your deltoids, compared with doing the movement on a 45-degree bench. You can also improvise an Incline Press with an incline bench set at the Seated Press station of a Universal Gym machine. At Gold's Gym there is also a very low incline bench that can be placed beneath the Bench Press station of a Universal Gym machine. With this apparatus, you simply sit on the bench and press on the handles of the machine.

Flye

General Comments: This movement is used by most champion bodybuilders. It primarily stresses the pectoral muscles, and it secondarily stresses the front deltoid and latissimus dorsi muscles. Generally speaking, Flyes are considered more of a shaping movement than a mass-building exercise.

Starting Position: Grasp two light dumbbells and lie back on a flat exercise bench. Press the dumbbells to arms' length above your shoulder joints. Rotate your hands in this position so that your palms face each other and the plates of one dumbbell rest against the plates of the other directly above your chest. Bend your arms slightly and keep them bent throughout the movement.

Exercise Performance: Keeping your palms facing in and upward throughout the movement, lower the dumbbells in semicircles directly out to the sides until they are well below the level of your chest. As you raise and lower the dumbbells, be sure that your upper arms travel directly out to the sides. Raise the dumbbells back along the same arc to the starting point, and repeat the movement for the correct number of repetitions.

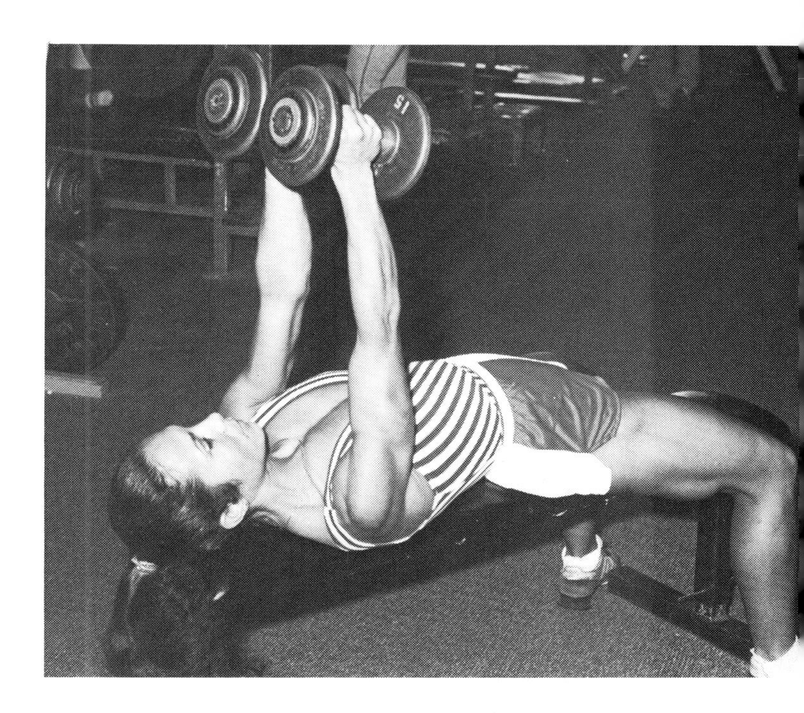

Flat-Bench Flyes—start, above; finish, below.

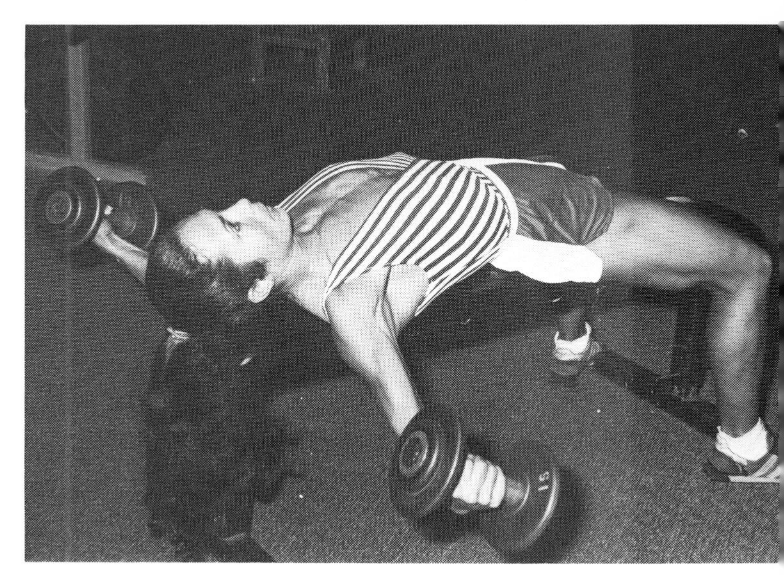

Training Tips: Be sure not to bend your elbows excessively as you do this movement. Bending your elbows too much allows you to use heavier weights as you do Flyes, but it places no more stress on your pectoral muscles. It merely is harder on your shoulder and elbow joints.

Deltoid Exercises

Military Press

General Comments: This is an excellent exer-

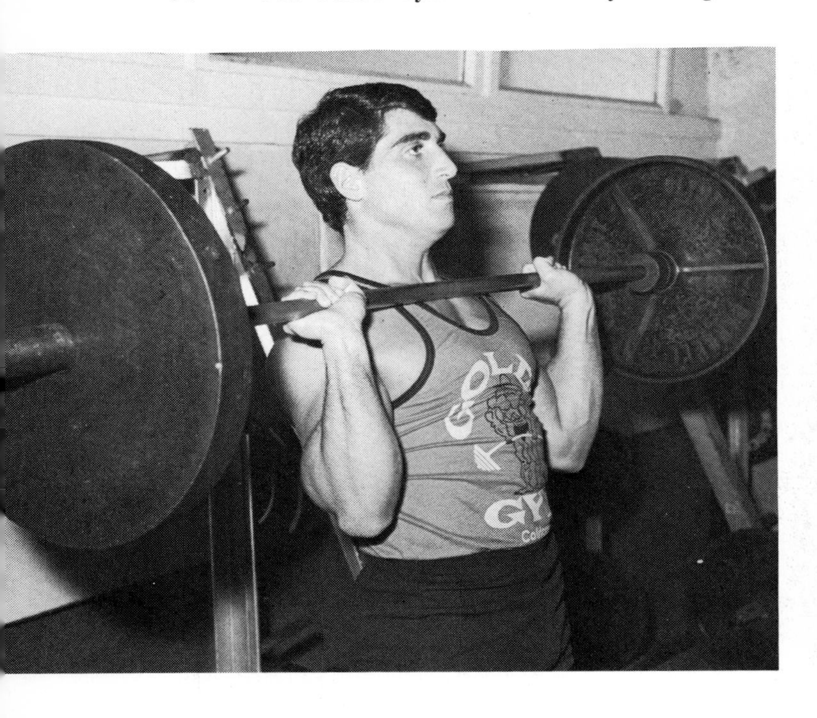

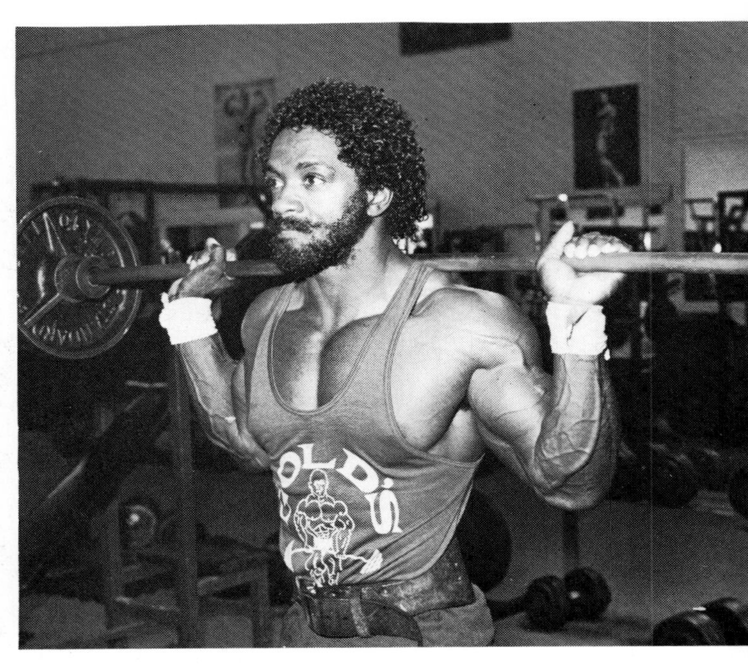

Military Press—start, above; finish, below.

Press Behind the Neck—start, above; finish, below.

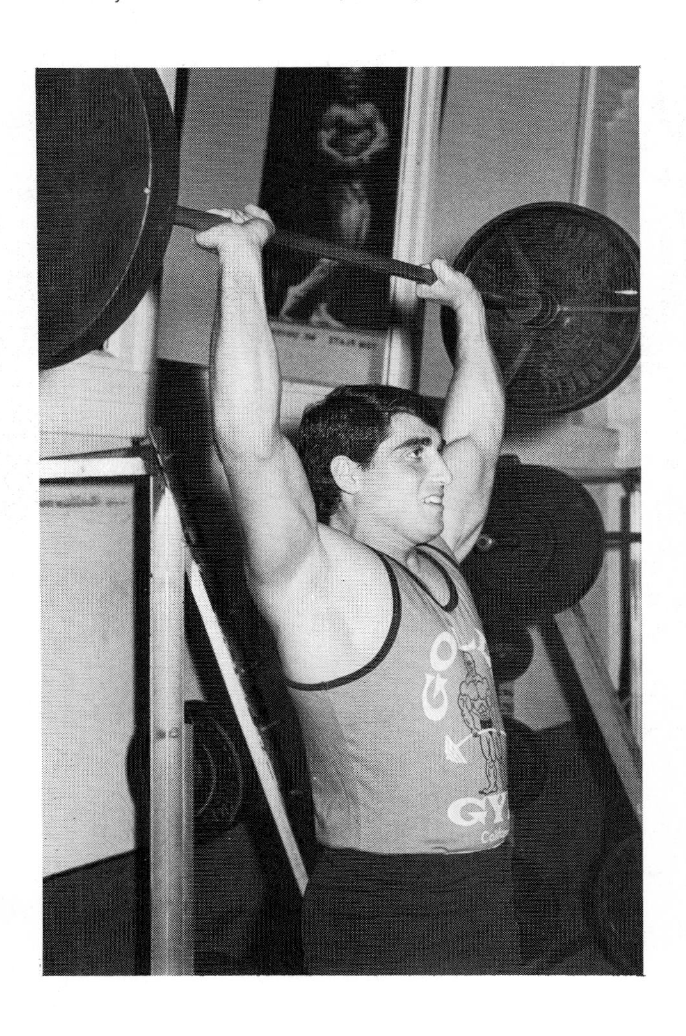

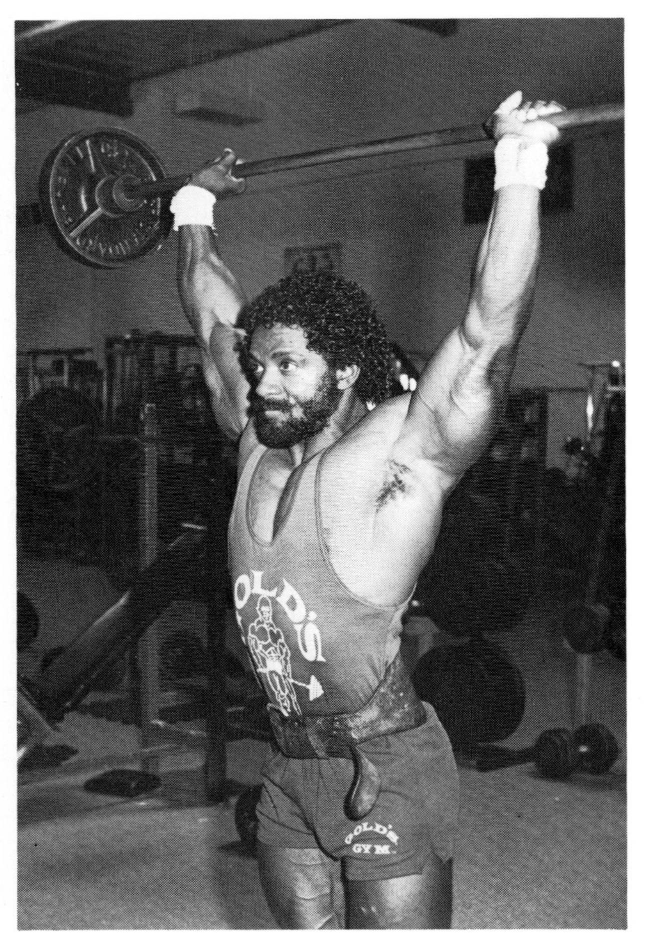

cise for developing the front deltoids and triceps. Secondary stress is placed on the trapezius muscles and upper pectoral muscles.

Starting Position: Take a grip on a barbell so that your hands are set slightly wider than shoulder width, your palms facing away from you at the starting position at the shoulder. Assume a correct pulling position—knees bent and back straight—and pull the barbell up to your shoulders, being sure to move your elbows under the barbell to hold it in this starting position.

Exercise Performance: Being sure not to lean backward as you push the weight upward, press the barbell directly upward until it reaches arms' length over your head. Be sure to keep the weight close to your face as you press the barbell up. Lower the barbell straight downward until it is again at the starting position. Repeat the movement for the desired number of repetitions.

Training Tips: On Military Presses and all other barbell movements you should periodically experiment with different grip widths. Using a wider grip, however, usually limits the range of motion on barbell exercises.

Press Behind the Neck

General Comments: This exercise is similar to Military Presses, except the barbell is pressed from a position across the shoulders and behind the neck rather than from in front of the neck. Presses Behind the Neck are a very direct front deltoid movement, more direct than Military Presses. There is also more stress on the trapezius muscles and less on the upper pectorals. Presses Behind the Neck still stress the triceps muscles rather hard.

Starting Position: Take a grip slightly wider than shoulder width on a barbell, so that your palms face forward during the movement. Pull the barbell up to your shoulders and move it to a position behind your neck. Stand erect and place your feet a comfortable distance apart.

Exercise Performance: Holding the barbell behind your neck, press it directly upward to arms' length above your head. Lower it slowly back to the starting position and repeat the movement for the required number of repetitions.

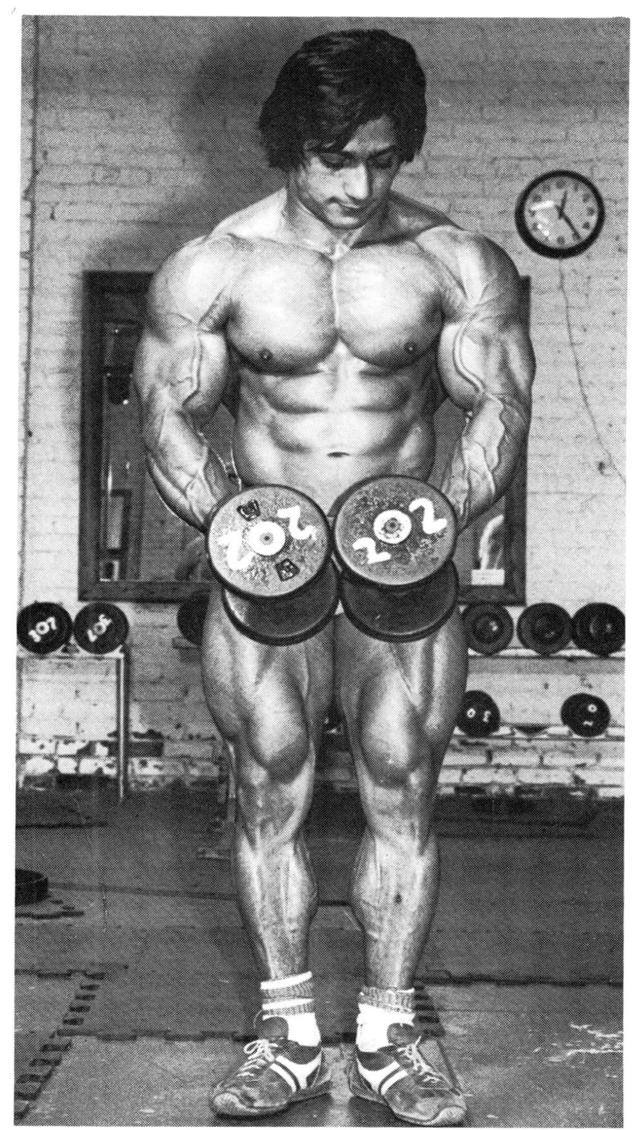

Side Lateral Raise—start.

Training Tips: You can do both Military Presses and Presses Behind the Neck standing at the Pressing station of a Universal Gym machine. For Military Presses, stand facing the weight stack. For Presses Behind the Neck, stand facing away from the weight stack.

Side Lateral Raise

General Comments: Also called a *Side Lateral,* this movement strongly stresses the front and side heads of the deltoids. Secondary stress is placed on the trapezius muscles of the upper back.

Starting Position: Grasp two light dumbbells.

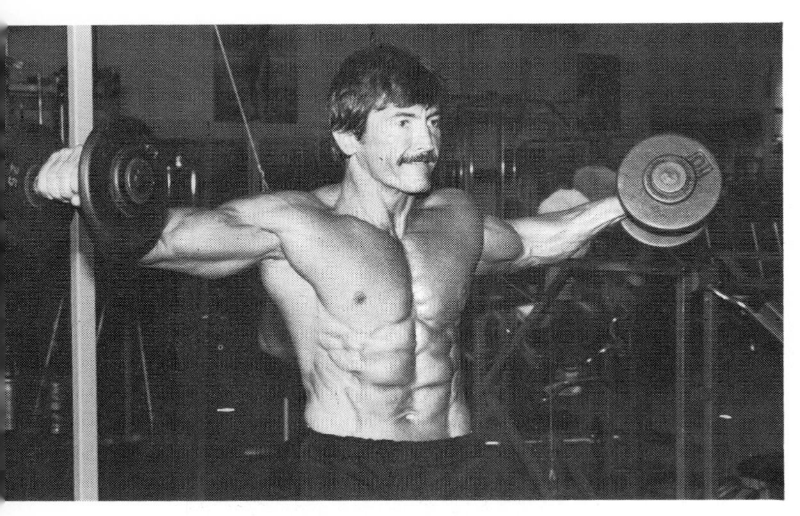

Side Lateral Raise—finish.

Stand erect with the dumbbells touching each other just in front of your hips, your palms facing inward. Bend your arms slightly and hold them in this bent position throughout the movement. Lean slightly forward at your waist, and hold this position throughout the movement.

Exercise Performance: From this basic starting position, slowly raise the dumbbells in semicircles directly out to the sides until they reach the level of your shoulders. Hold this top position for a moment and rotate the front end of the dumbbells forward and downward so that the front plates are slightly below the level of the back plates. Lower the dumbbells slowly downward along the same arc to the starting point and repeat the movement for the desired number of repetitions.

Training Tips: Robby Robinson used to do this exercise with very heavy weights, performing only the first quarter or third of the movement. Some bodybuilders also do this exercise occasionally with their palms facing upward rather than downward. Done in this manner, Side Laterals stress the front deltoids far more strongly than the medial heads of your deltoid muscles.

Arm Exercises

Barbell Curl

General Comments: This is the basic biceps movement, and it has been favored over the years by most champion male and female bodybuilders. Arnold Schwarzenegger had phenomenal biceps development during his career, and he almost always did Barbell Curls while he was a member of Gold's Gym. Barbell Curls also secondarily stress the muscles on the insides of the forearms.

Starting Position: Take a shoulder-width grip on a barbell so that your palms are facing forward at the start of the movement. Stand erect and rest the barbell across your upper

Barbell Curl—start.

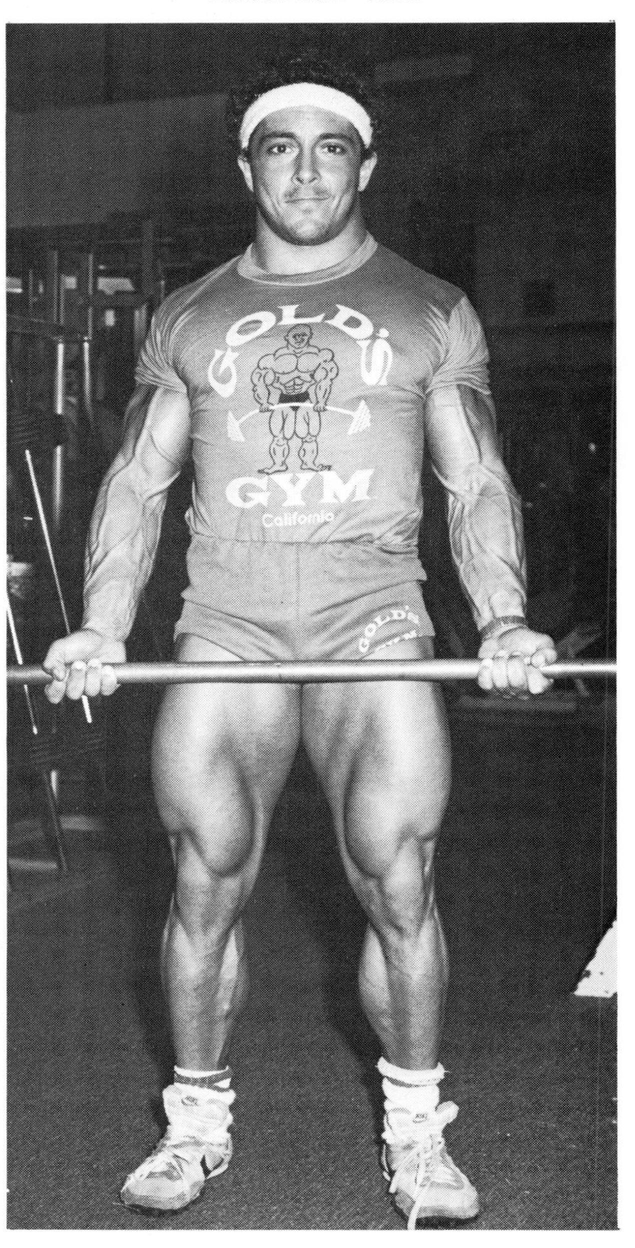

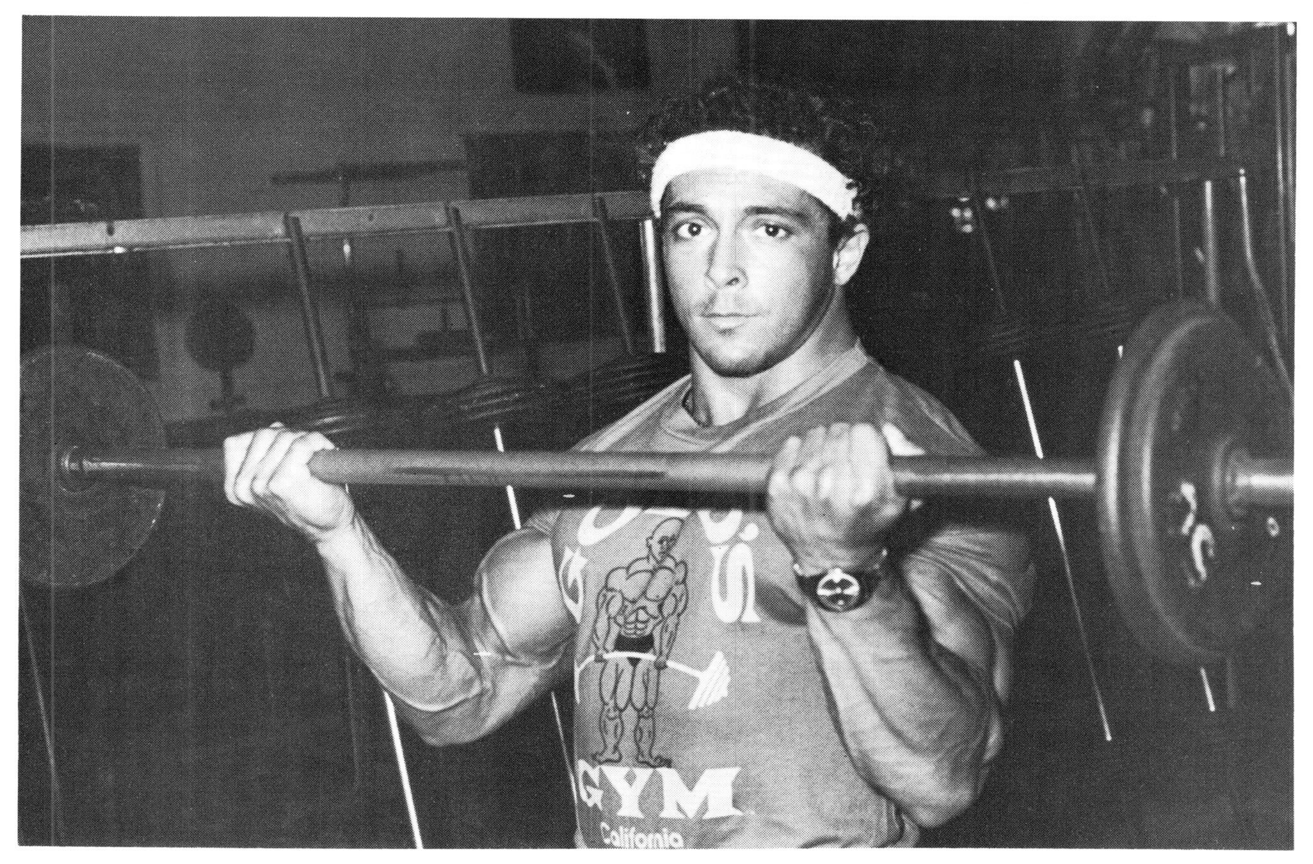

Barbell Curl—finish.

thighs. Press your upper arms tightly against the sides of your torso and fully straighten your arms.

Exercise Performance: Standing perfectly erect, slowly move the barbell in a semicircle from your thighs to your chin, using only the strength of your biceps muscles to move the barbell. Pause for a moment in the top position, then slowly lower the barbell back along the same arc to the starting position. Repeat the movement for the correct number of repetitions.

Training Tips: If you tend to cheat on this movement by swinging your upper body back and forth, try doing Barbell Curls with your back pressed against a wall. As with all barbell exercises, you should experiment with various grips on the barbell. You will find that you stress the inner head of your biceps more strongly if you use a very narrow grip on the barbell, while a wide grip will place more stress on the outer head of your biceps muscles. Generally speaking, Arnold Schwarzenegger used a grip four to six inches wider on each side than shoulder width.

Nautilus Curl

General Comments: This movement strongly stresses the biceps muscles over their full range of motion. Far less stress is placed on the forearm muscles using a Nautilus machine than when doing Barbell Curls.

Starting Position: Adjust the machine's seat upward or downward so that when you sit in it your shoulders are slightly below the level of the angled pad in front of your body. Run your upper arms across the pad, placing the outsides of your upper arms against the vertical pads at the edges of the angled pad. Place your wrists under the movable pads of the machine and sit down on the seat. Straighten your arms.

Exercise Performance: Slowly bend your arms as fully as possible. Hold this fully contracted position for a count of two and then

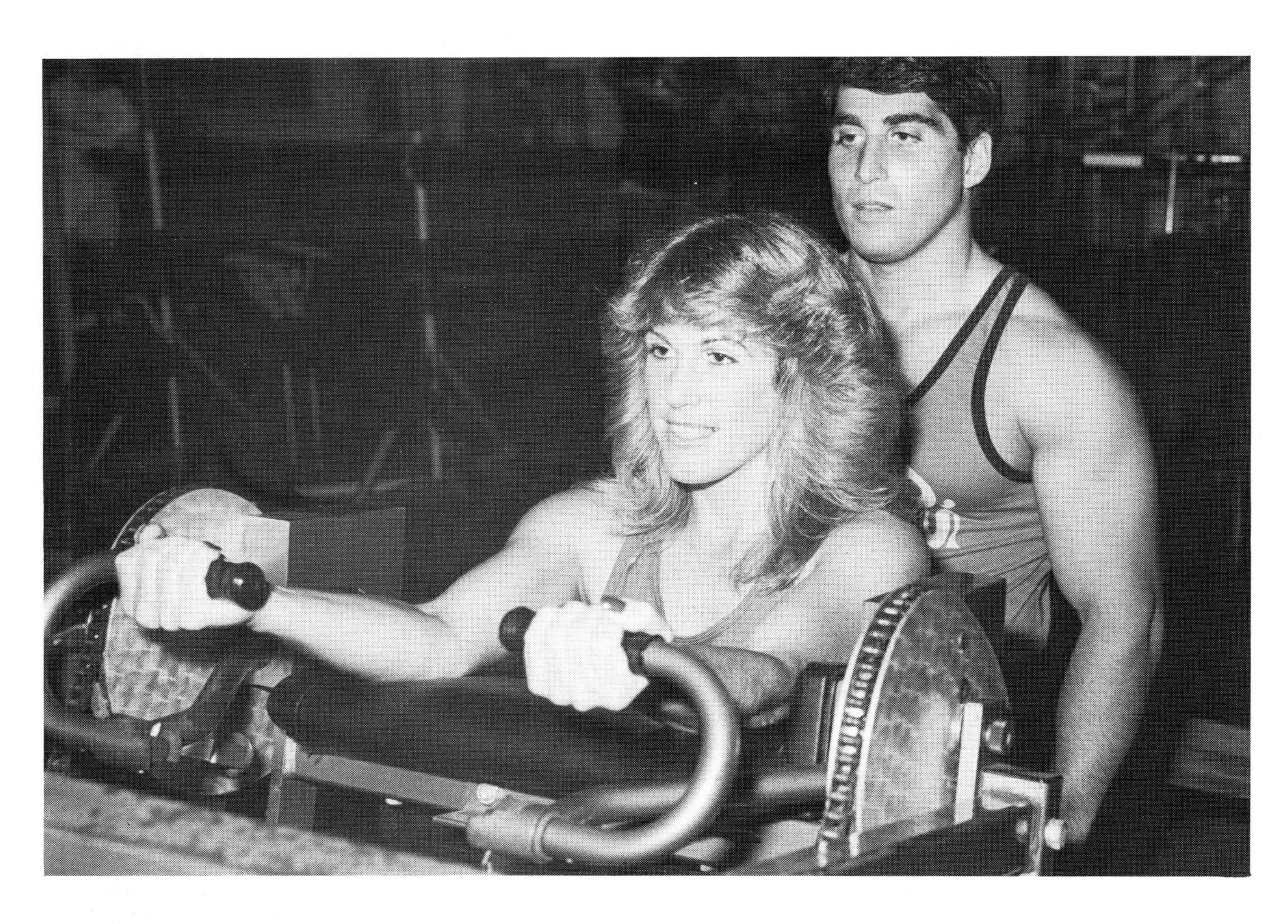

Nautilus Curl—start, above; finish, below.

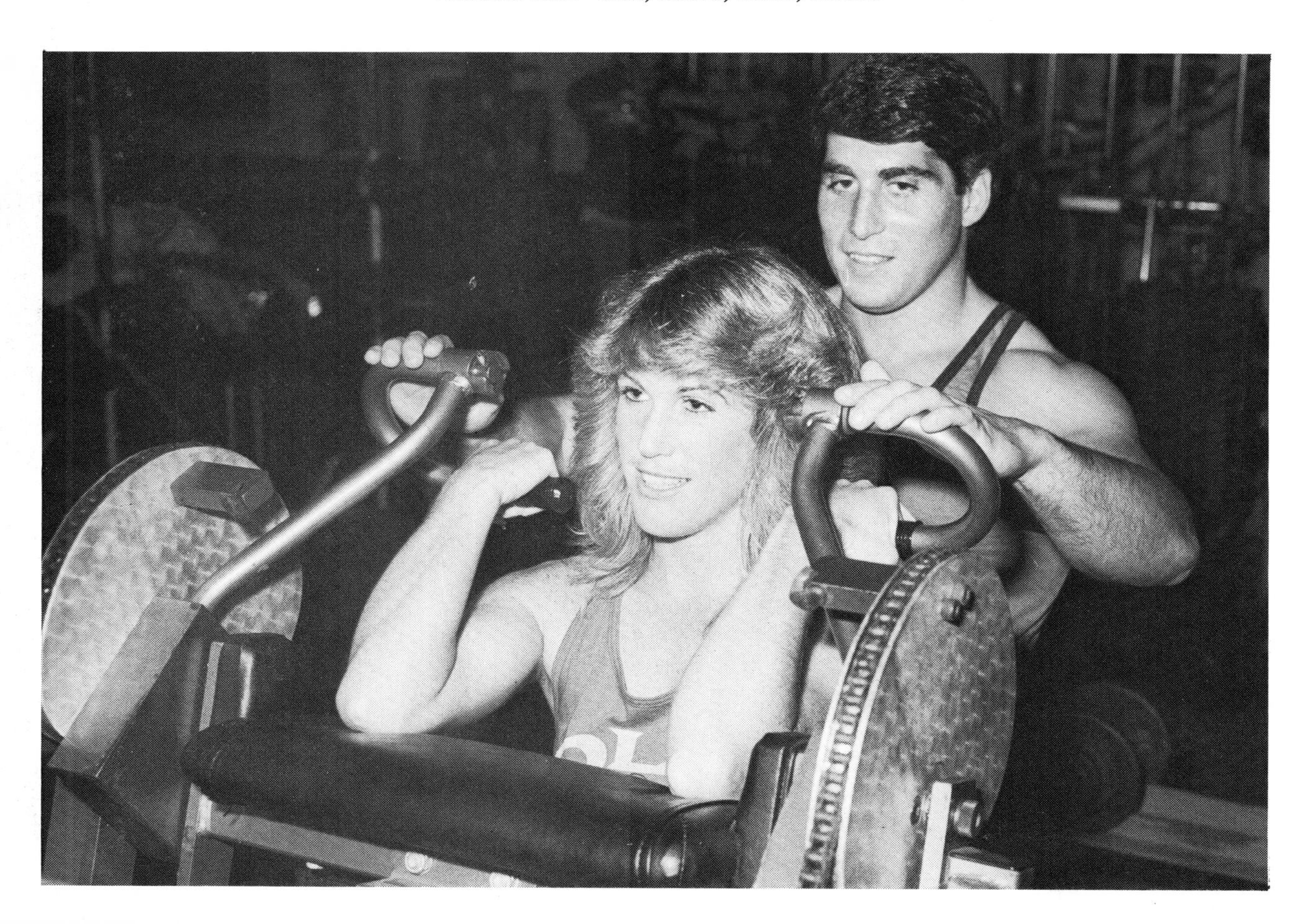

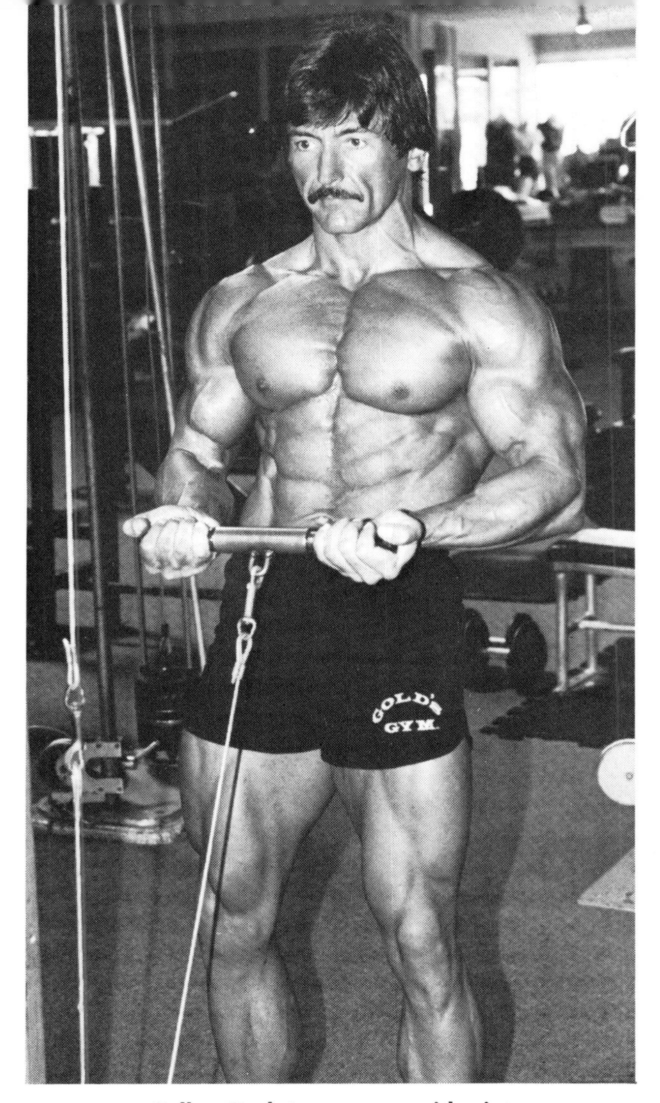

Pulley Curl, two arms—midpoint.

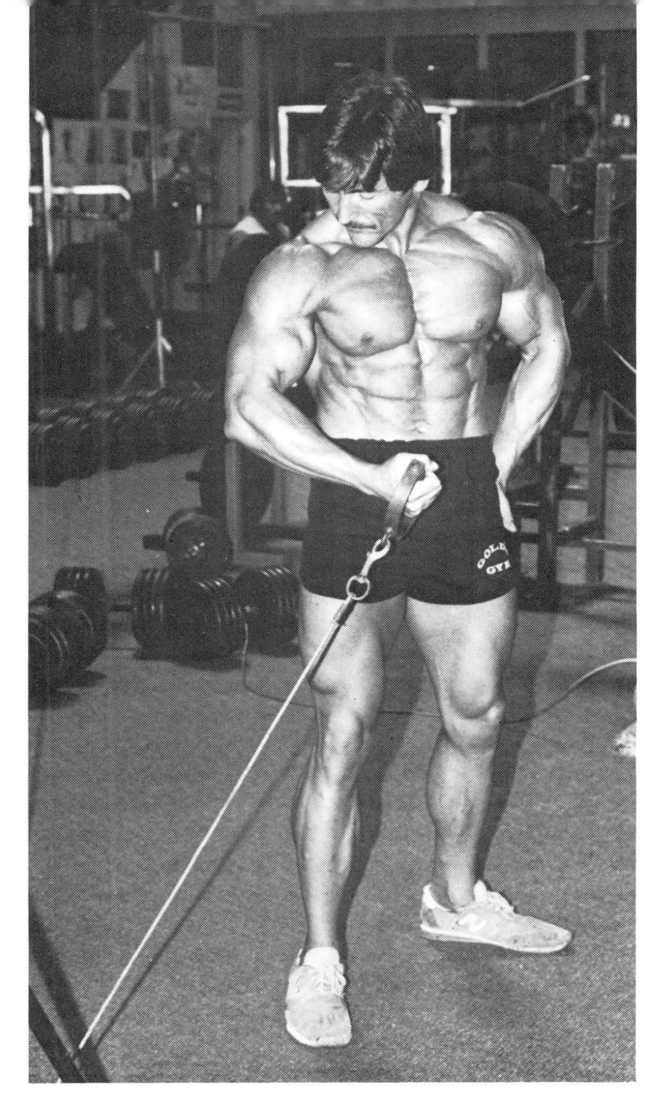

Pulley Curl, one-arm variation.

slowly straighten your arms. Repeat this movement for the required number of repetitions.

Training Tips: You can also do this movement with one arm at a time. Doing an exercise with one arm allows you to put more mental intensity into the movement than when you do it with both arms simultaneously. You can also use your free hand to assist your working hand in completing the movement when you are doing the exercise to failure.

Pulley Curl, one-arm variation, in supported position.

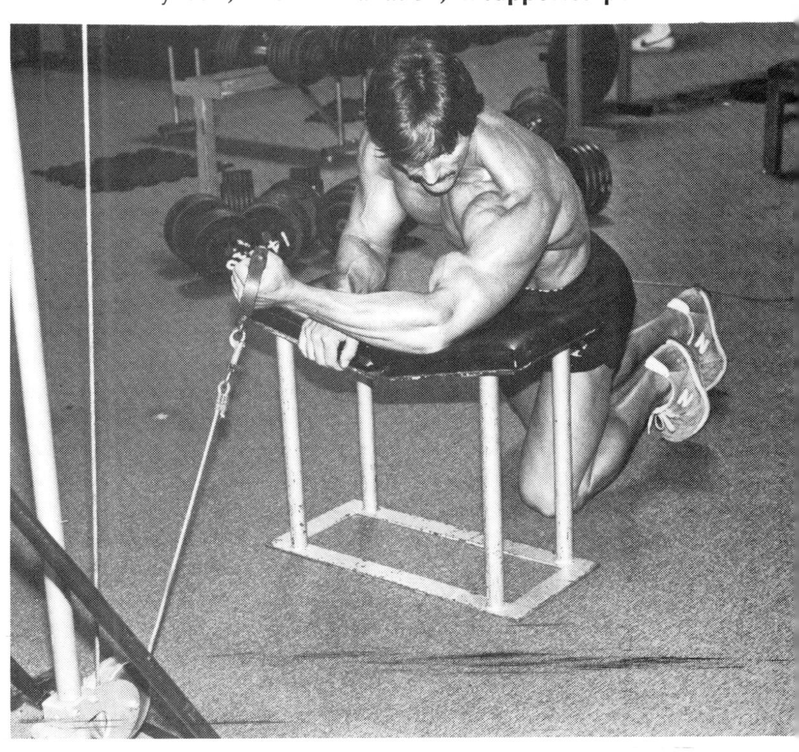

Pulley Curl

General Comments: This exercise is very similar, in both performance and effect, to Barbell Curls.

Starting Position: Grasp a straight bar handle attached to the floor pulley of a Universal Gym machine or a free-apparatus floor pulley so your palms are facing forward throughout the move-

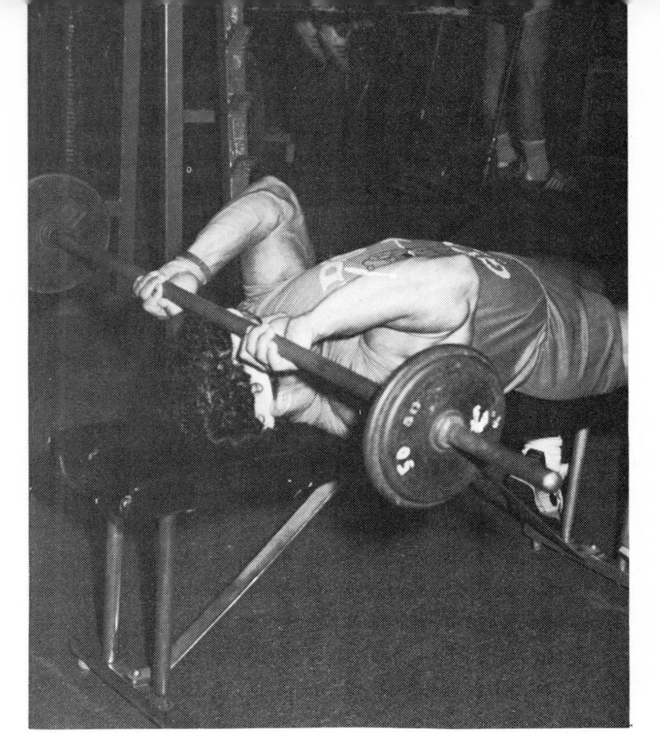
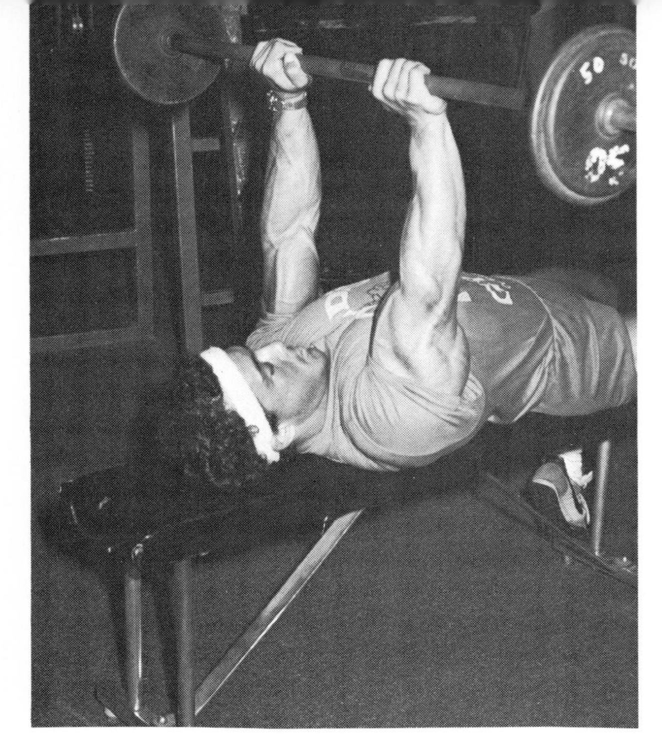

Lying Triceps Extension—start, left; finish, right.

ment. Stand erect and press your upper arms against the sides of your torso. Fully straighten your arms.

Exercise Performance: From this basic starting position, slowly curl the handle up in a semicircle until your hands are directly below your chin. Slowly straighten your arms and repeat the movement for the desired number of repetitions.

Training Tips: You can also do this movement with one arm at a time. Simply attach a loop handle to the cable that runs through the floor pulley that you are using. You can also do this exercise with two arms at a time while lying face up on the floor with your feet toward the pulley.

Nautilus Triceps Extension—start, left; finish, right.

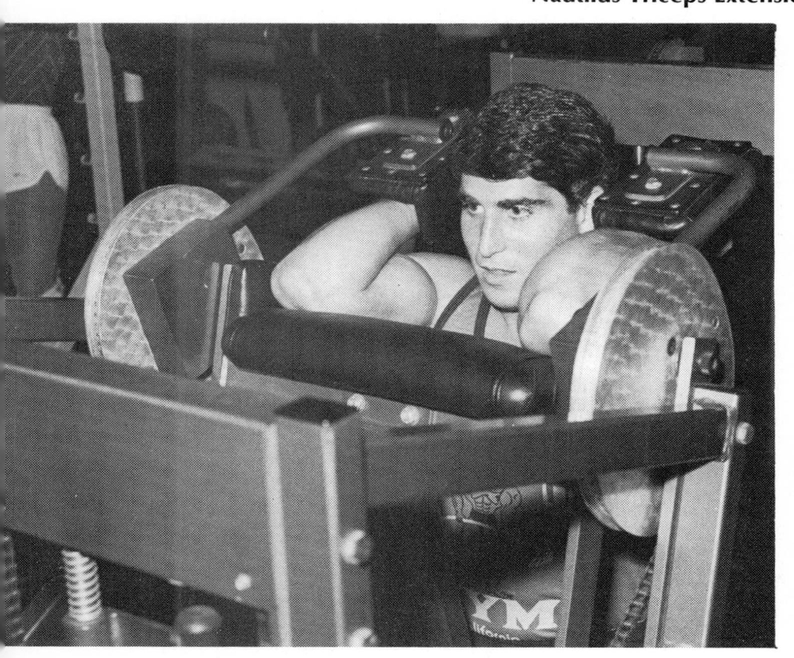
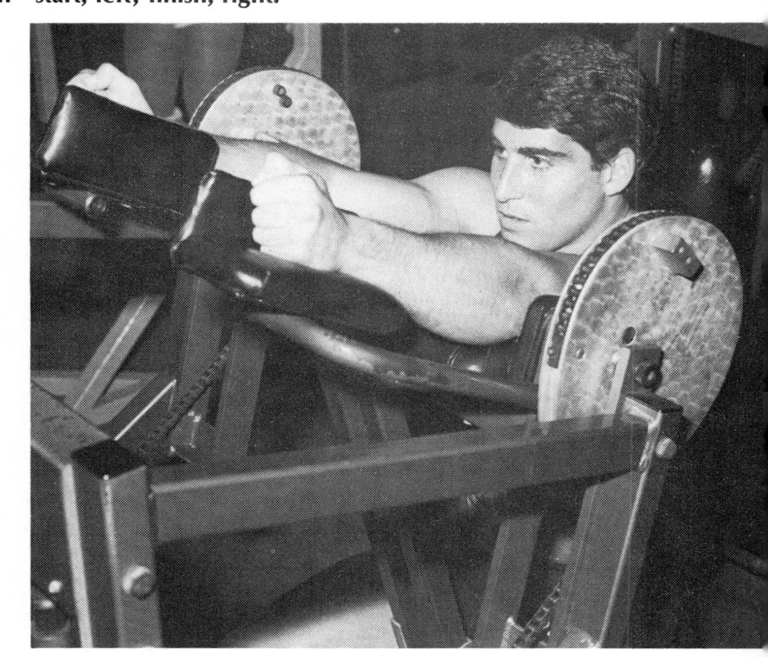

Lying Triceps Extension

General Comments: This is the most basic of all triceps exercises. It strongly stresses the full complex of your triceps muscles, but particularly the inner head of the triceps.

Starting Position: Grasp a barbell with a narrow grip (six inches or less between your index fingers) in the middle of the bar. Your palms should face your feet when you are in the correct starting position. Lie back on a flat exercise bench and place your feet flat on the floor to balance yourself in position. Extend your arms to hold the barbell directly above your shoulder joints.

Exercise Performance: Holding your upper arms in the same position throughout the movement, bend your elbows and lower the barbell in a semicircle from the starting point until it lightly touches your forehead. Then slowly return the barbell along the same arc to the starting position. Repeat the movement for a full set of the required number of repetitions.

Training Tips: You will find that your triceps muscles are usually stressed most strongly when you use the recommended grip. Still, you will find it valuable to experiment with a wider or narrower grip. Each change of grip will stress your triceps muscles a little differently.

Nautilus Triceps Extension

General Comments: This exercise strongly stresses the triceps muscles over their full range of movement.

Starting Position: Adjust the seat of the machine so that when you sit in it your shoulders are slightly below the level of the angled pad in front of your body. Bend your arms and put your wrists under the movable pads of the machine. Then run your upper arms down the pad with the outer parts of your upper arms resting against the vertical pads attached to the edges of the angled pad. Sit down on the machine's seat and bend your arms fully.

Exercise Performance: From this basic starting position, slowly straighten your arms fully. Hold this position for a count of two, then

Pulley Pushdown—start, left, finish, right.

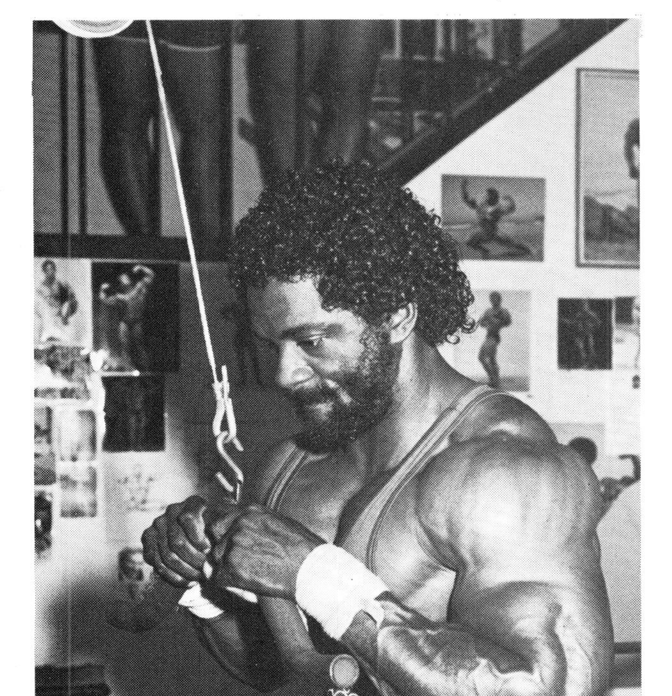

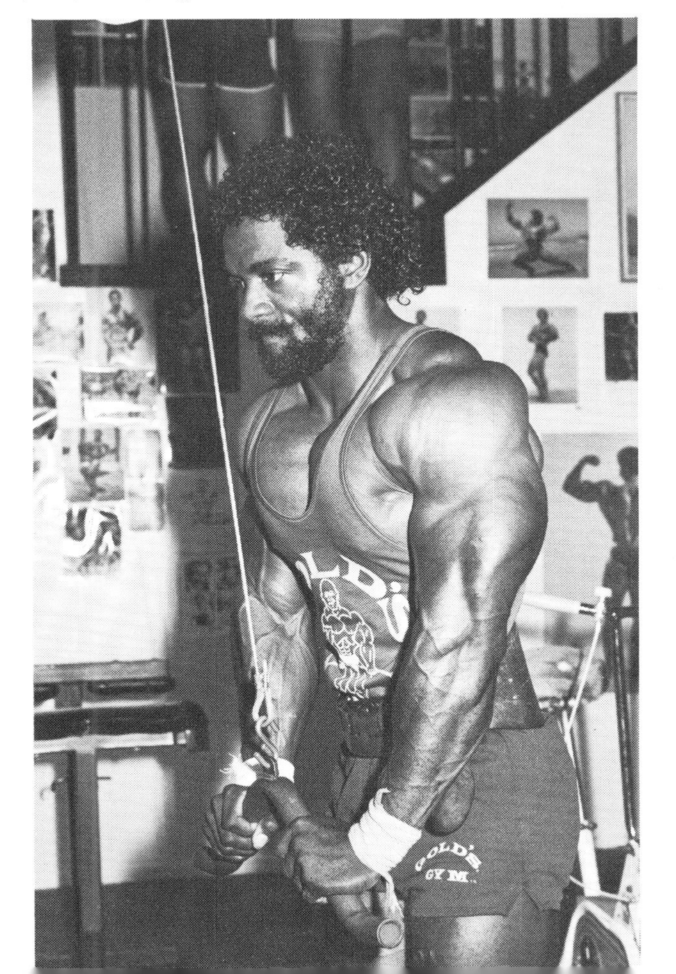

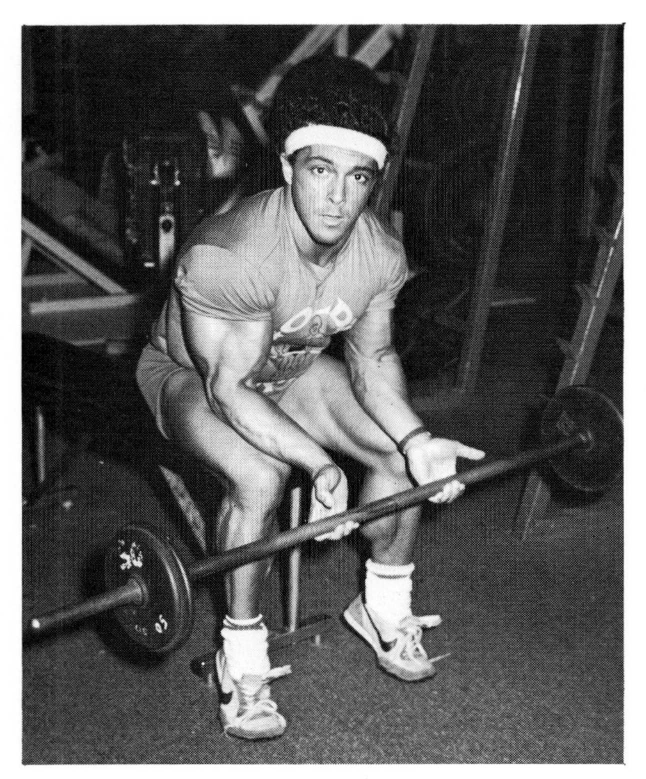

Barbell Wrist Curl—start.

slowly return your arms to the fully bent position. Repeat the movement for the required number of repetitions.

Training Tips: You can do this movement one arm at a time rather than with both arms simultaneously.

Pulley Pushdown

General Comments: This excellent movement can be done at the lat machine station of a Universal Gym machine or on a free-apparatus lat machine. Pushdowns work the entire triceps muscle, but particularly the outer head of the triceps.

Starting Position: Take a narrow grip in the middle of a lat machine handle so that your palms are facing away from your body when you are in the correct starting position. Stand about six inches back from the pulley and pin your upper arms against the sides of your torso during the movement. Bend your arms fully. Lean slightly forward.

Exercise Performance: From this basic starting position, slowly straighten your arms. Hold your arms in this position for a count of two, then slowly bend your arms fully. Repeat the movement for the desired number of repetitions.

Training Tips: You can do this movement with your palms facing in the opposite direction for a little different stress effect on your triceps. This exercise can also be done one arm at a time with a loop handle. Many bodybuilders also do Pushdowns with either a rope handle, which allows you to use a parallel grip, or a short-angled handle.

Barbell Wrist Curl

General Comments: When done with your palms facing upward, this movement stresses all of the muscles on the insides of your forearms. When done with your palms facing downward, it stresses all of the muscles on the outsides of your forearms.

Starting Position: Take a shoulder-width grip on a barbell so that your palms face upward

Barbell Wrist Curl—finish.

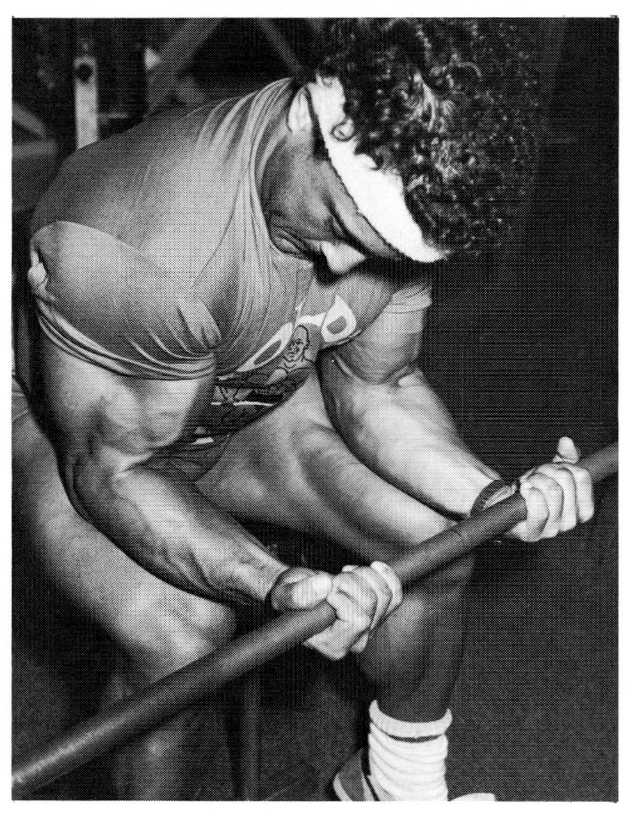

during the movement. Sit at the end of a flat exercise bench and run your forearms down your thighs so that your wrists and hands hang off the edge of your knees. Sag your fists downward as far as possible.

Exercise Performance: Slowly curl your fists upward in small semicircles by flexing your wrists. Lower the weight back to the starting position and repeat the movement for the required number of repetitions. Do an equal number of sets and reps with your palms facing downward.

Training Tips: You will find that you can use approximately half as much weight with your palms down as you can with your palms up. To make this movement more strict, you can run your forearms along the top of your exercise bench instead of along your thighs.

Pulley Wrist Curl

General Comments: This exercise can be done with either the floor pulley on a Universal Gym machine or a free-apparatus floor pulley. It is very similar in both performance and effect to the Barbell Wrist Curl.

Starting Position: Grasp a straight bar handle attached to a floor pulley with your palms facing either downward or upward. Sit at the end of a flat exercise bench placed close enough to the pulley so that the cable runs as near to straight up and down as possible. Run your forearms either along your thighs or along the top of the bench.

Exercise Performance: Slowly sag your wrists downward as far as possible, then curl the weight upward in small semicircles by flexing your wrists. Lower the weight back to the starting position and repeat the movement for the required number of repetitions. Do an equal number of sets and reps with your palms facing downward and upward.

Training Tips: You can do Pulley Wrist Curls with one arm at a time by attaching a loop handle to the floor pulley.

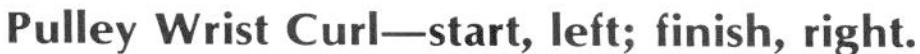

Pulley Wrist Curl—start, left; finish, right.

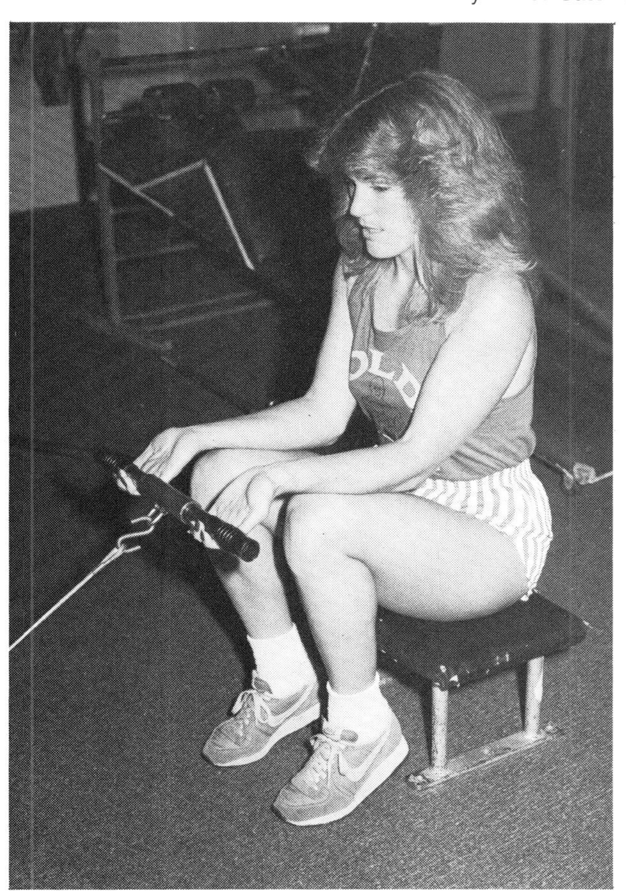

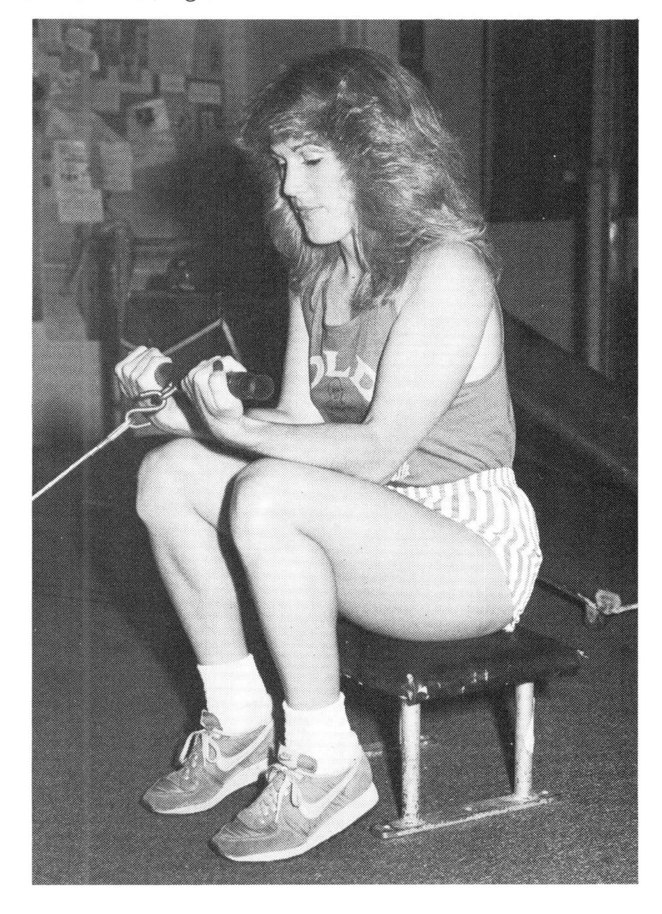

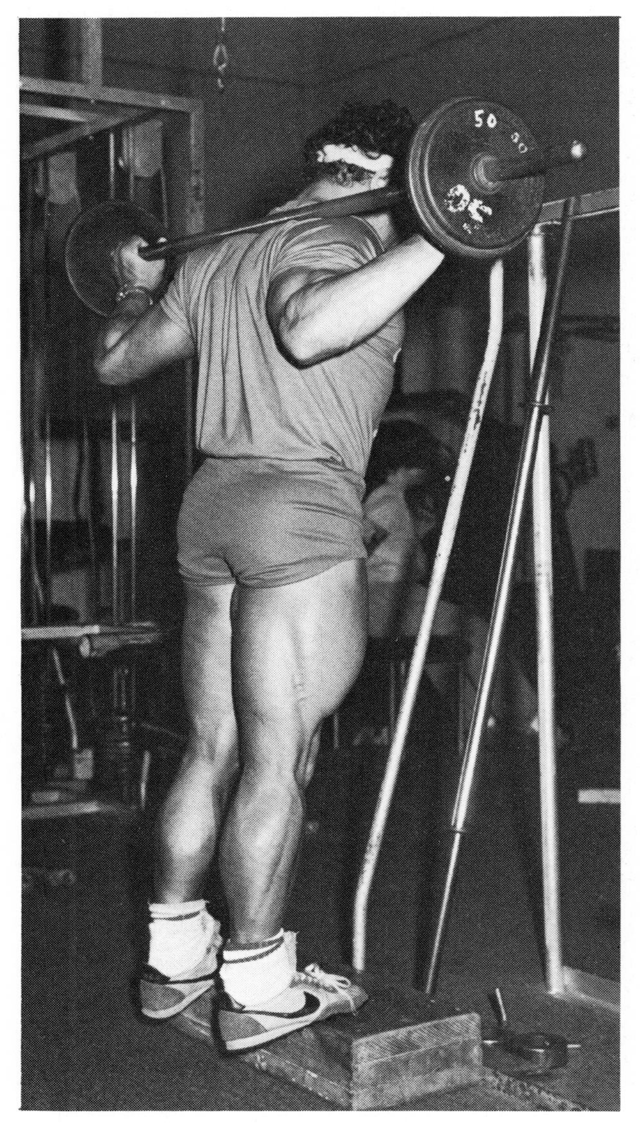

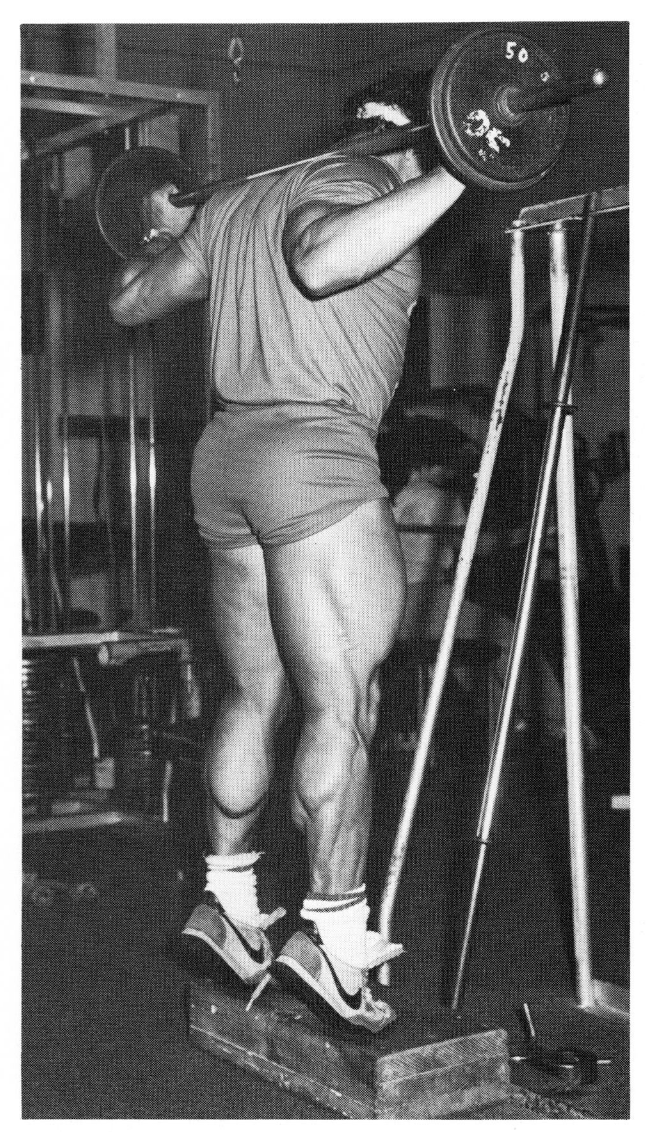

Standing Barbell Toe Raise—start, left; finish, right.

Calf Exercises

Standing Barbell Toe Raise (Calf Raise)

General Comments: This exercise strongly stresses the calf muscles. It is similar to the Standing Calf Machine exercise, which is discussed next.

Starting Position: Place a barbell behind your neck and across your shoulders as when doing a Squat. Stand with your toes and the balls of your feet on a four-by-four inch wooden block. Stand erect and slowly sag your heels as far below the level of your toes as possible to stretch your calf muscles prior to doing the exercise.

Exercise Performance: From this starting position, slowly rise up on your toes as high as possible. Lower back to the starting position and repeat the movement for the required number of repetitions.

Training Tips: You should do your Calf Raises with your feet held in three basic positions. You can angle your toes outward at 45 degrees on each side, place your toes directly forward, or angle your toes inward at 45 degrees on each side. Each of these three toe positions will stress your calf muscles somewhat differ-

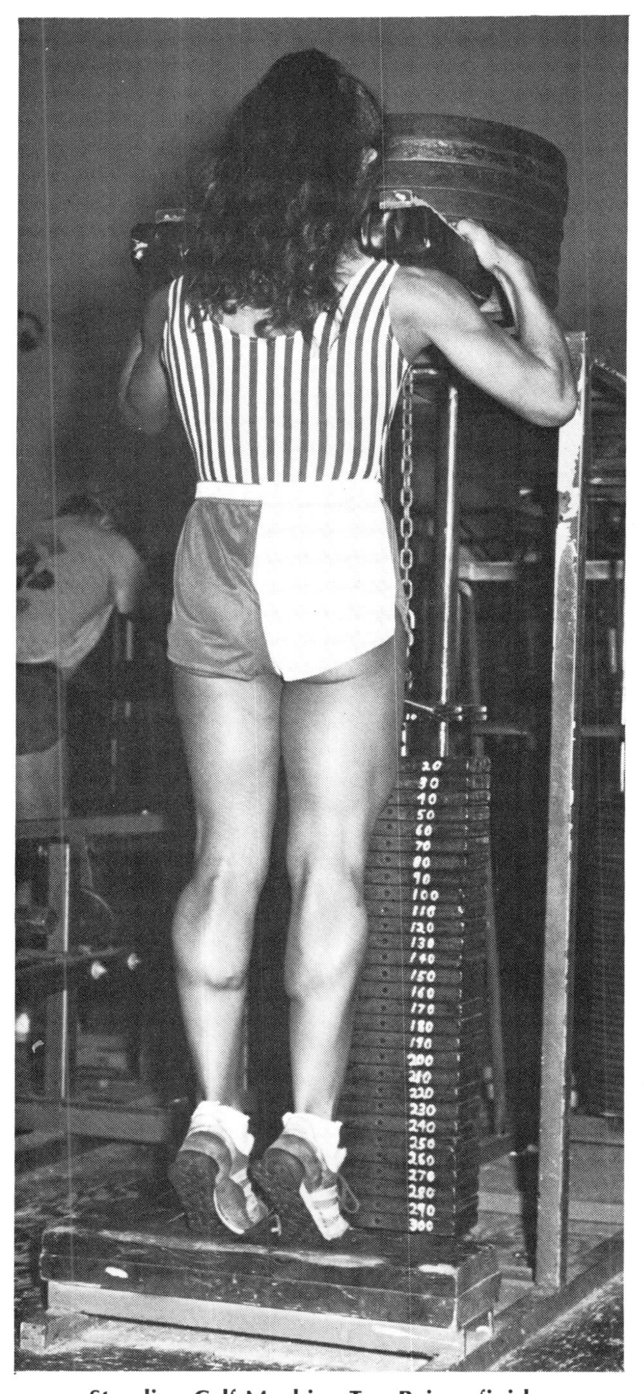

Standing Calf Machine Toe Raise—finish.

ently from the other two, giving them fuller shape and definition.

Standing Calf Machine Toe Raise

General Comments: You will probably find it somewhat difficult to balance your body when

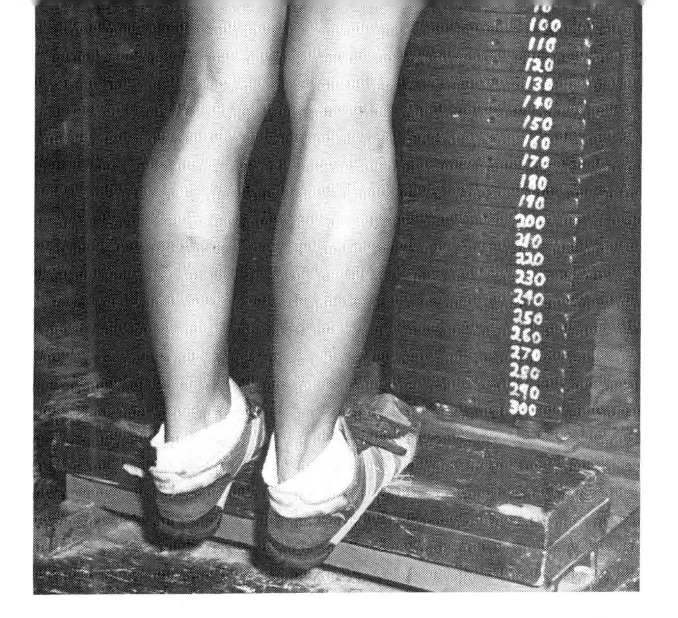

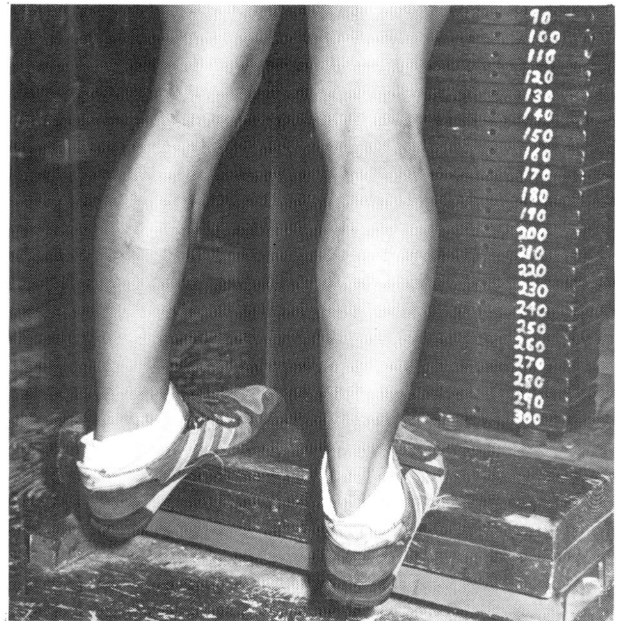

Toe Positions—forward, top; inward, middle; and outward, bottom.

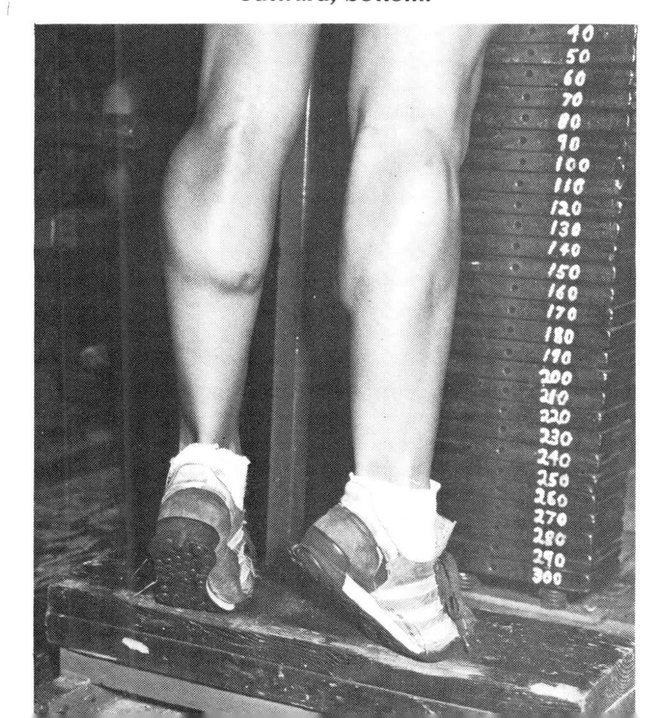

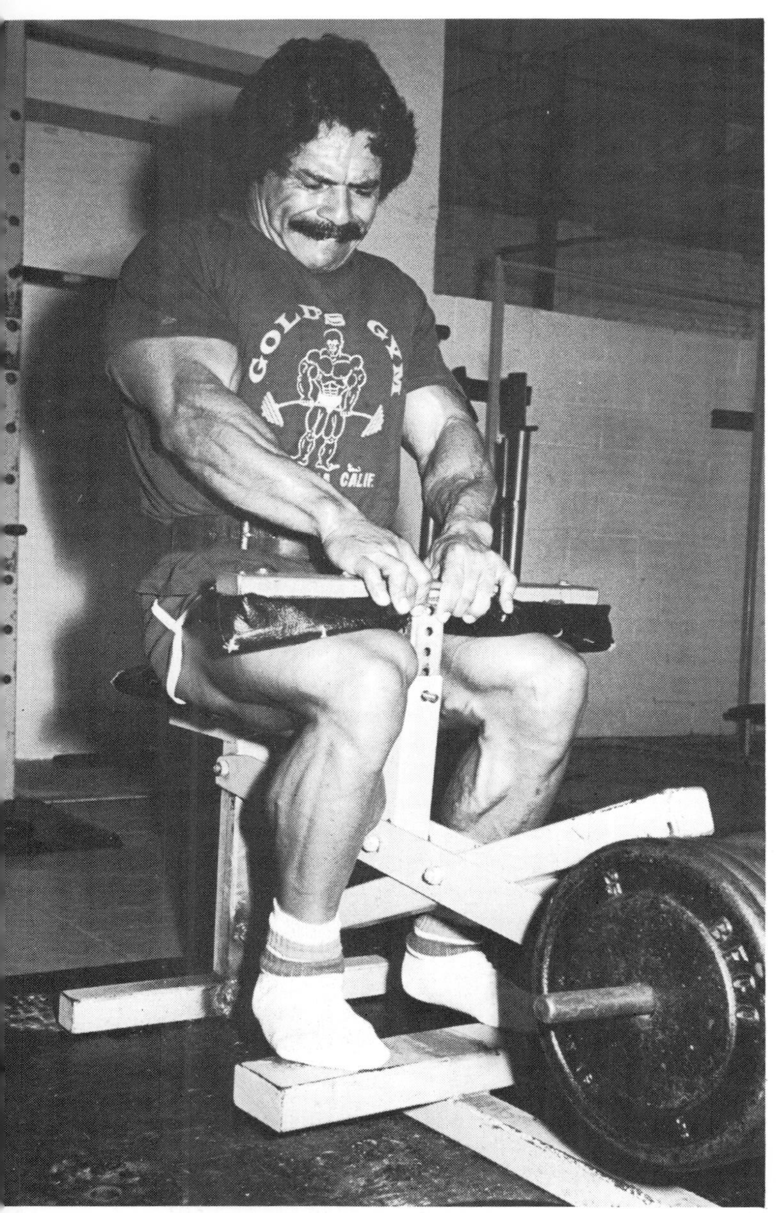

Seated Calf Machine Toe Raise—start.

you do Standing Barbell Toe Raises. If this is the case, you can do Toe Raises on a standing calf machine, which eliminates the balance problem.

Starting Position: Place your feet in the appropriate position on your toe block and bend your legs enough so that you can rest the yokes of the machine across your shoulders. Straighten your legs to take the weight of the machine across your shoulders. Sag your heels as far below your toes as possible.

Exercise Performance: Rise as high as you can on your toes and the balls of your feet. Then, lower your heels back down as far below your toes as possible. Repeat the movement for the required number of repetitions.

Training Tips: Experiment with all three toe positions noted in the description for Standing Barbell Toe Raises. You can also experiment with moving your feet closer together or wider apart. Spacing your feet differently also stresses your calves differently.

Seated Calf Machine Toe Raise

General Comments: To stress the soleus muscle lying beneath the gastrocnemius muscles of your calves, you must rise up on your toes with your legs bent at least 30 degrees. So the best type of soleus exercise you can do is Toe Raises on a seated calf machine.

Starting Position: Sit on the seat of a seated calf machine and place your toes and the balls of your feet on the foot bar. Then force your knees under the padded bar by sagging your heels below the level of your toes. The height of the padded bar can be adjusted by means of a movable pin within the column of metal attaching the pad to the machine. Move the stop bar of the machine forward to release the weight. Sag your heels below the level of your toes.

Exercise Performance: From this basic starting position, simply rise as high as you can on

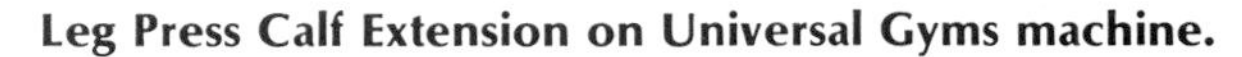

Leg Press Calf Extension on Universal Gyms machine.

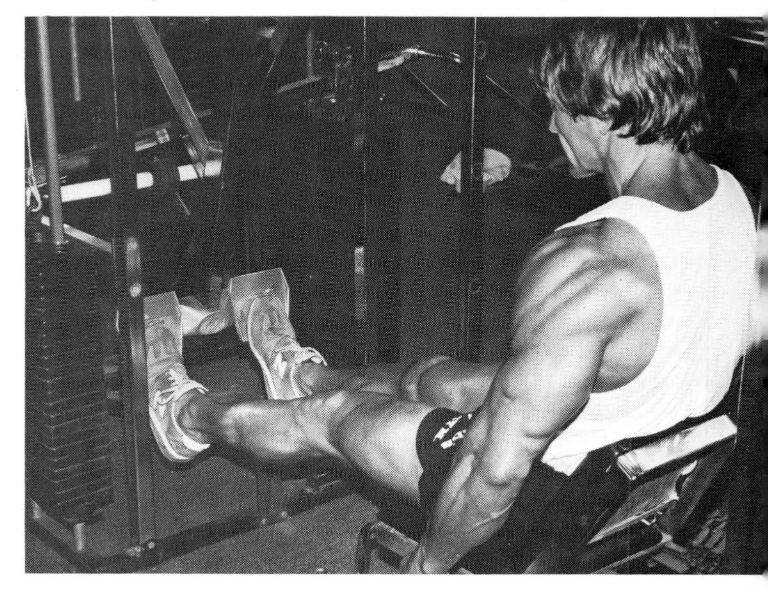

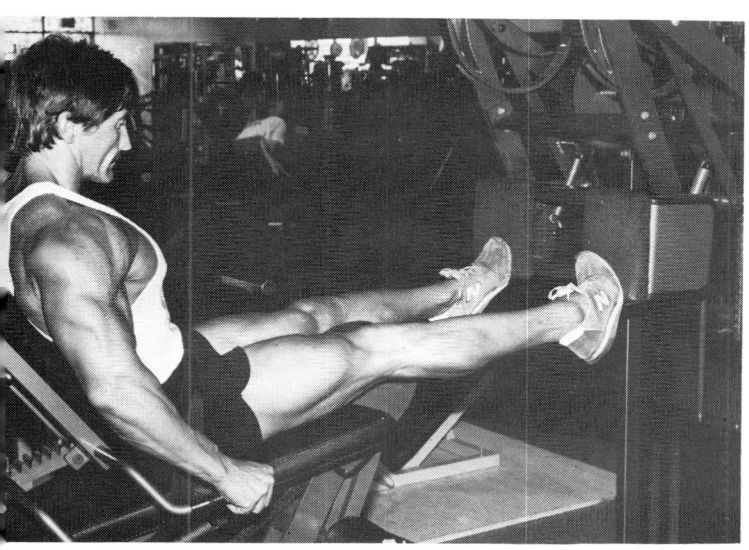

Leg Press Calf Extension on Nautilus machine.

your toes. Lower your feet back to the starting position and repeat the movement for the required number of repetitions. When you are finished with your set, return the stop bar to its locked position.

Training Tips: Use the three toe positions recommended for other calf exercises. You will probably find that the soleus muscles respond best to low repetitions (8–10), while the gastrocnemius muscles respond better to higher reps (15–20).

Leg Press Machine Calf Press

General Comments: You can do this excellent movement on either the Leg Press station of a Universal Gym machine or a Nautilus Leg Press machine. This movement strongly stresses the gastrocnemius muscles of your lower legs.

Starting Position: Sit in the seat of either type of Leg Press machine and place your toes and the balls of your feet on the pedals of the machine. Straighten your legs and sag your heels as far away from your body as possible.

Leg Press Calf Extension on vertical machine.

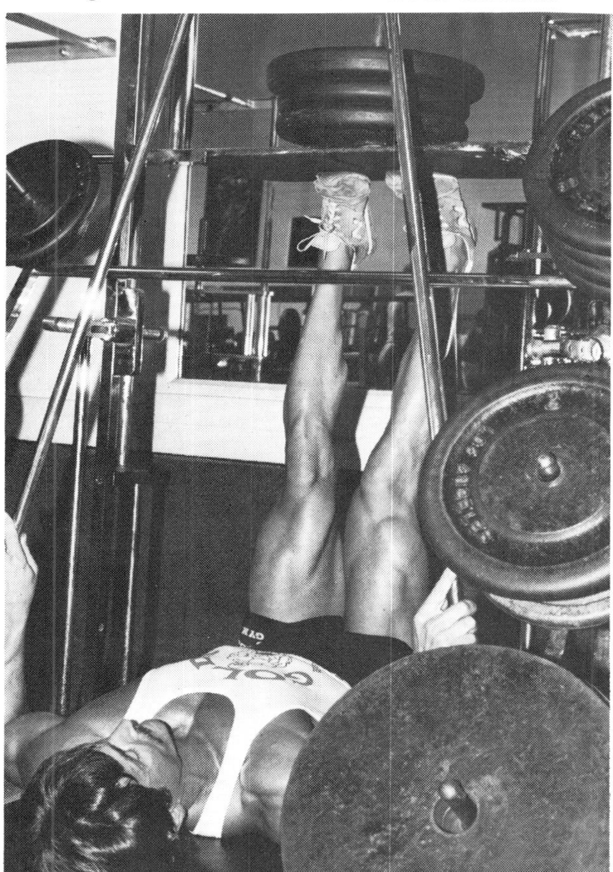

Leg Press Calf Extension on 45-degree-angled machine.

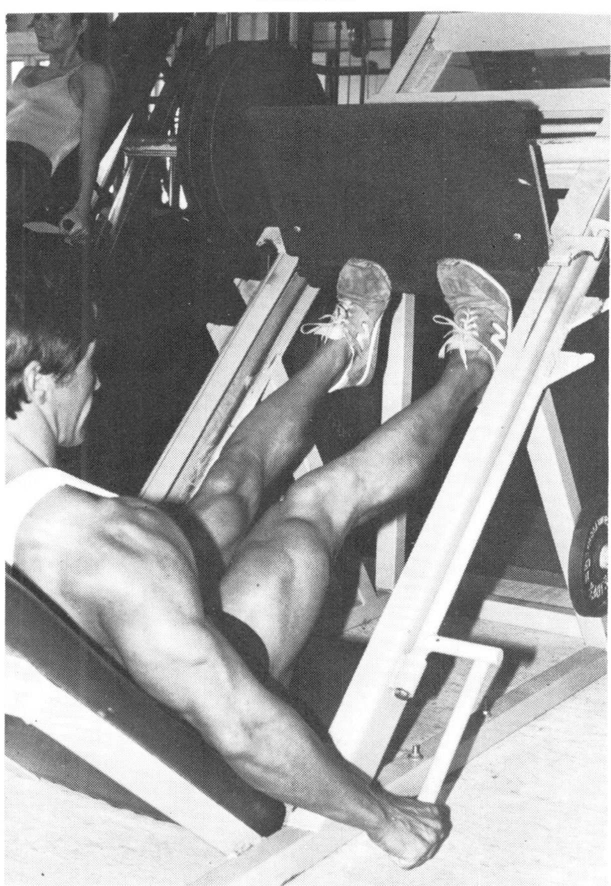

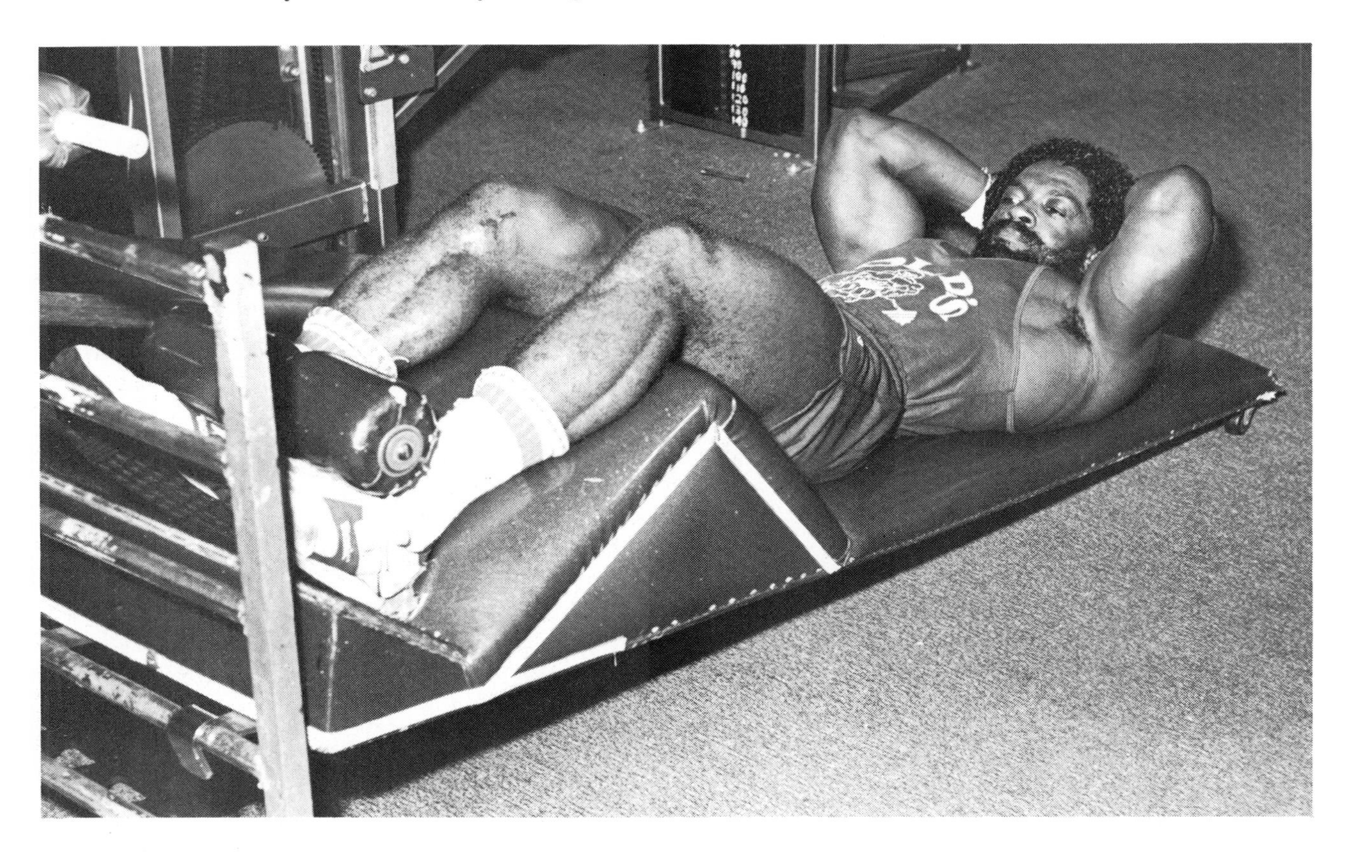

Sit-Ups—start, above; finish, below.

Exercise Performance: From this basic starting position, extend your feet as completely as possible. Return your feet to the starting position and repeat the movement for the required number of repetitions.

Training Tips: This movement is also done on a vertical Leg Press machine while lying on your back and placing your toes and the balls of your feet on the edge of the movable platform.

Abdominal Exercises

Sit-ups

General Comments: This movement stresses all the muscles on the front of your abdomen, particularly the upper half of this front abdominal muscle group.

Starting Position: Lie on your back on either the floor or an adjustable abdominal board. Hook your feet under a heavy piece of furniture or the strap or roller pads of the abdominal board. Bend your legs at approximately a 30-degree angle to take stress off your lower back during the movement. Place your hands behind

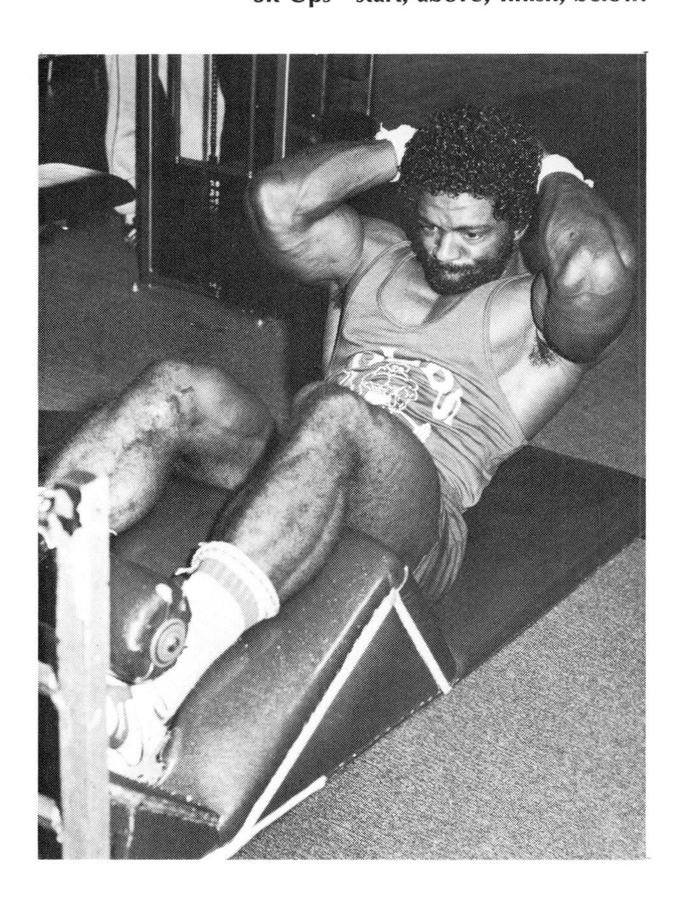

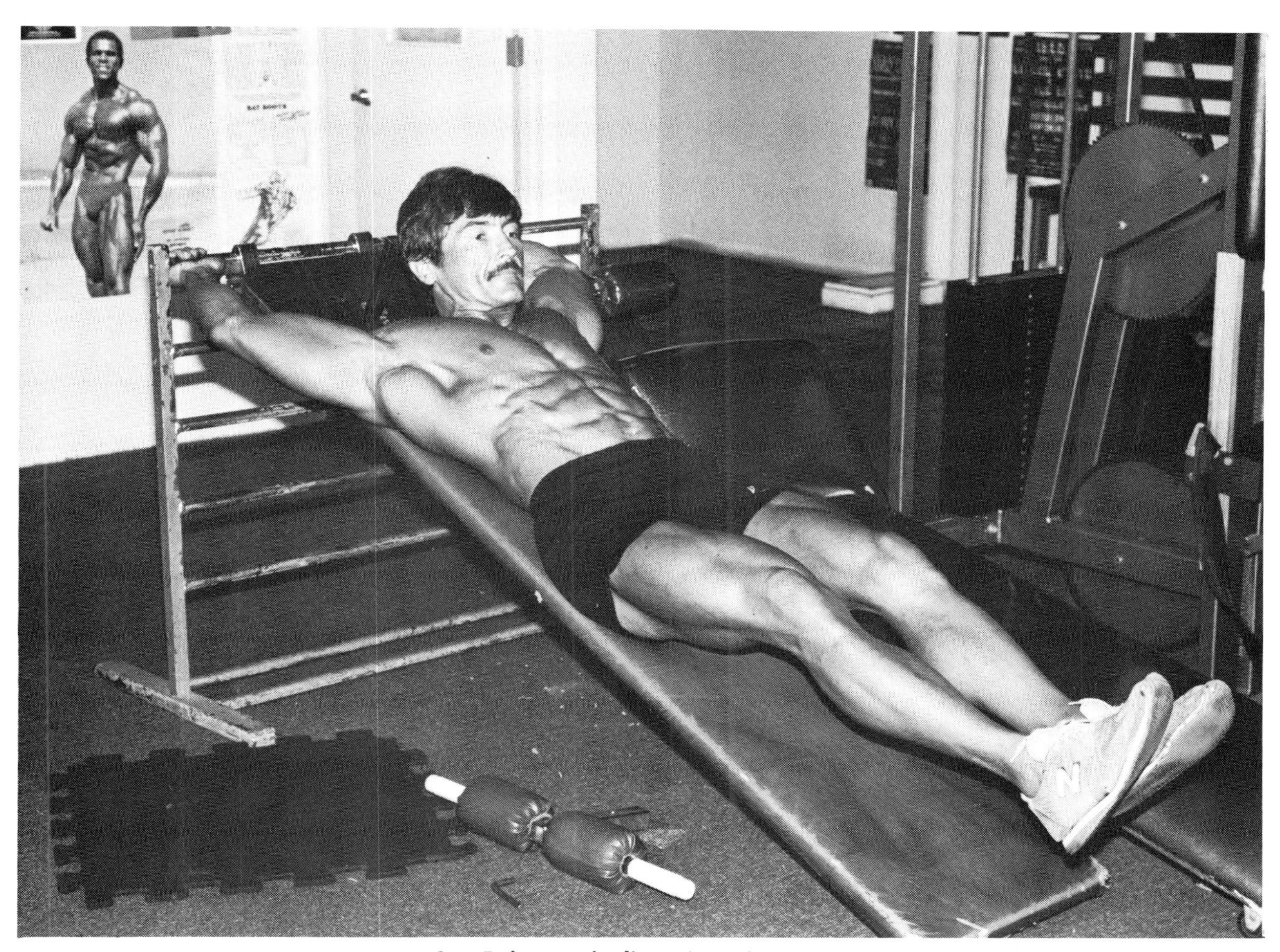

Leg Raises on incline—just after start.

your neck and interlace your fingers to hold them in this position throughout the movement.

Exercise Performance: From this position, curl your torso off the floor or board by lifting first your shoulders, then your middle back, and finally your lower back, until your torso is perpendicular to the floor. Return your torso to the starting position and repeat the movement for the required number of repetitions.

Training Tips: To add resistance to this movement you can either hold a barbell plate behind your head or raise the foot end of the abdominal board. You can shift stress in this movement more to your external obliques and intercostal muscles by twisting alternately to each side on succeeding repetitions.

Leg Raises

General Comments: This movement stresses all the muscles on the front of your abdomen, particularly the lower half of this front abdominal muscle group.

Starting Position: Lie on your back on either the floor or an adjustable abdominal board, but this time lie with your head toward the heavy piece of furniture or the strap or roller pads of the board. Grasp the piece of furniture or the restraint on the abdominal board to steady your body throughout the movement. Bend your legs slightly to take stress off your lower back and keep them bent throughout the movement.

Exercise Performance: Slowly raise your legs so that your feet travel in a semicircle from the floor or board to a position directly above your hips. Lower your legs back along the same arc to the starting position. Repeat the movement for the correct number of repetitions.

Training Tips: You can add resistance to this exercise by either wearing iron boots or raising

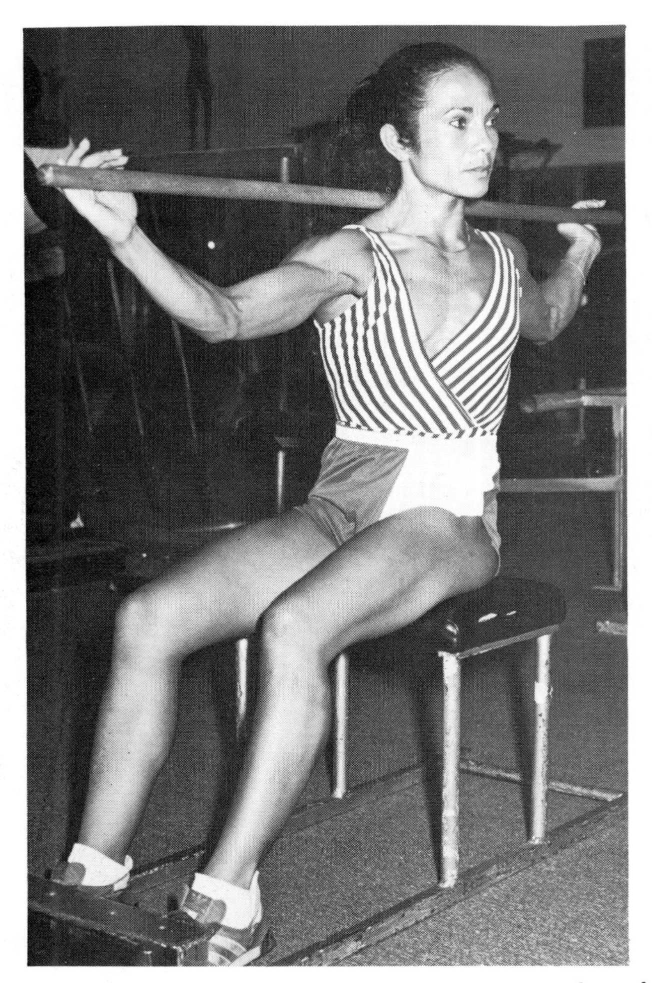
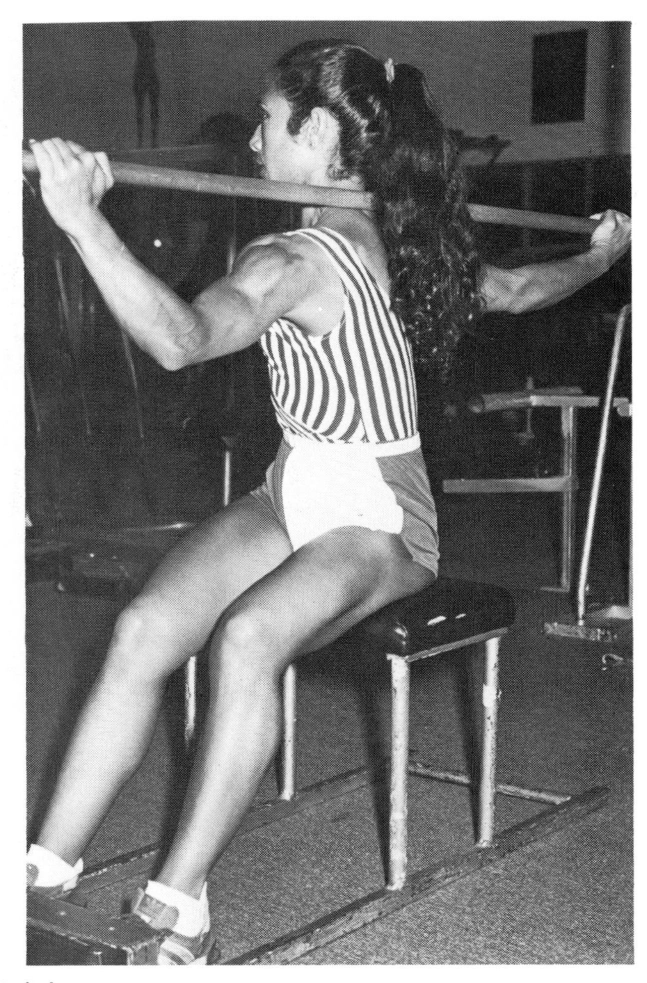

Seated Twisting.

the head end of the board progressively higher and higher.

Seated Twisting

General Comments: This movement tones the muscles at the sides of your waist. It also loosens your lower back prior to a training session.

Starting Position: Place an unloaded barbell bar or a broomstick across your shoulders behind your neck. Wrap your arms around the bar. Sit astride a flat exercise bench and wrap your legs around the upright legs of the bench to restrain your body during the movement.

Exercise Performance: Twist your torso briskly as far as you can to the right and left for the required number of repetitions, counting each full cycle from side to side as one repetition.

Training Tips: This movement is often done standing, but it's difficult to do the movement standing and still restrain hip movement. To solve this problem, many bodybuilders do Bent Twisting. In this exercise they bend over until their torso is parallel to the floor and then do the twisting movement in this position.

Side Bends

General Comments: This exercise stresses the muscles at the sides of your waist more strongly than does Seated Twisting.

Starting Positions: Several starting positions can be used when doing Side Bends. In the first one you place a light barbell behind your neck and hold it in this position during the movement. You can also hold two light dumbbells in your hands or one dumbbell in one hand with your free hand held behind your neck (in which case you switch the dumbbell to your free hand on each succeeding set). Regardless of the manner in which you add resistance to this movement, you should stand erect, with your feet set a little wider than shoulder width.

Exercise Performance: Bend directly to your left side as far as you can, being sure to keep your legs straight and your hips in the same position. Immediately bend as far to your right as possible. Alternately bend to each side with a brisk rhythm for the required number of repetitions. Count one full cycle of bending to each side as a single repetition.

Training Tips: Concentrate on doing high repetitions (at least 30 in each direction) with light weights on Side Bends. Doing this movement with heavy weights and low repetitions will build up the external oblique muscles, making your waist look unesthetically wide. It is better merely to tone the muscles with high reps than it is to build them up.

Beginning-Level Workouts

In this section we present four training routines of progressive difficulty. If you are a total beginner in bodybuilding, you should use the Level 1 workout for 4–6 weeks. Then you should progress through each succeeding rou-

Side Bends.

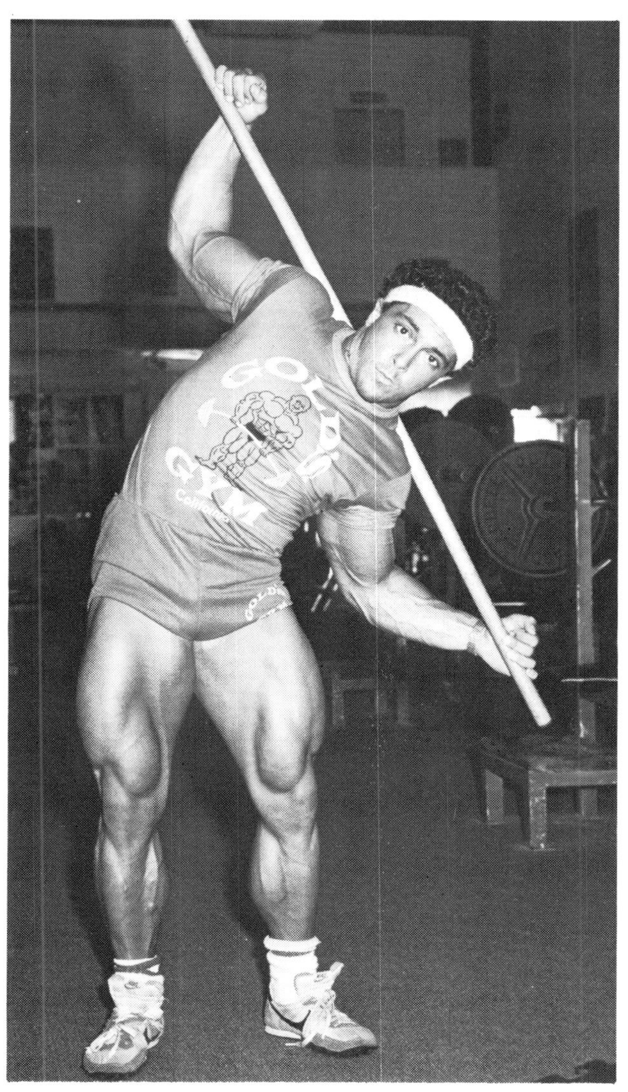

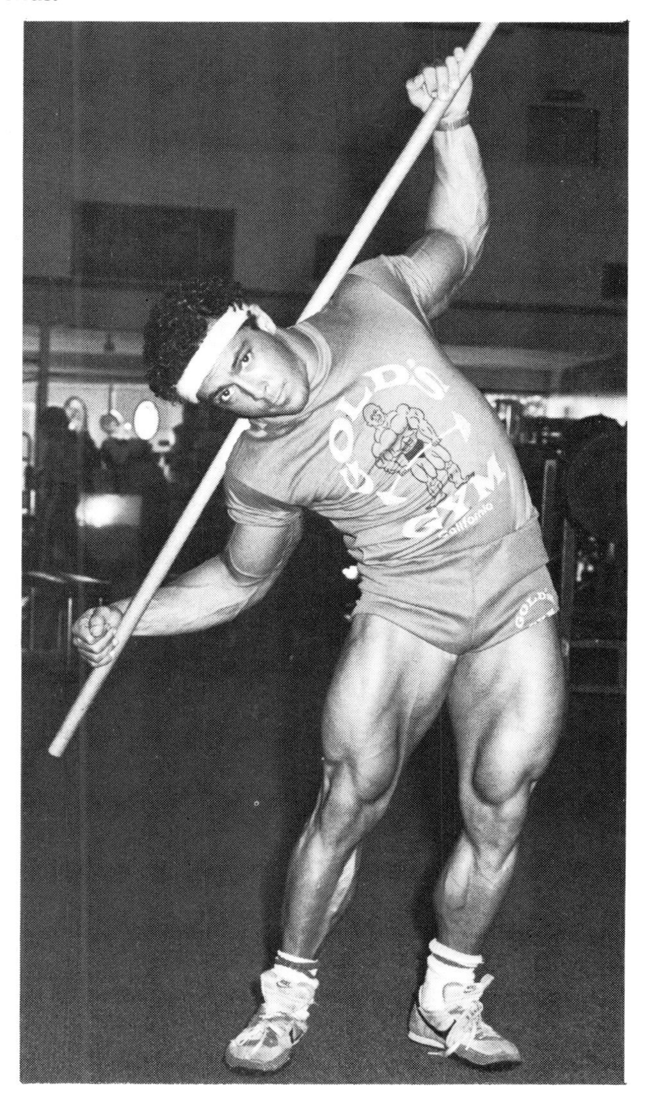

tine, spending 4–6 weeks with each new workout. By then, you will not need suggested percentages for poundage. When you have finished the Level 4 program you will have reached sufficient physical condition to be considered an intermediate bodybuilder. You will also be much more muscular-looking than when you first started training.

Now that you have survived the beginning level of bodybuilding training, you can look forward to even harder training at the intermediate level. To paraphrase Winston Churchill, the noted former British prime minister, bodybuilding offers you little but blood, sweat, tears, and toil. Truly, the strong survive in our sport. Do you have what it takes?

LEVEL 1

Exercise	Sets	Reps	% Men	% Women
1. Sit-Up	1	20–30	0	0
2. Squat	3	10–15	30	20
or Leg Press	3	10–15	40	30
3. Barbell Bent Rowing	3	8–12	25	15
or Lat Pulldown	3	8–12	25	15
4. Upright Rowing	2	8–12	20	10
or Barbell Shrug	2	10–15	30	20
5. Bench Press	3	8–12	25	15
6. Military Press	2	8–12	20	10
7. Barbell Curl	2	8–12	20	10
or Pulley Curl	2	8–12	20	10
8. Lying Triceps Extension	2	8–12	20	10
or Pulley Pushdown	2	8–12	15	7½
9. Barbell Wrist Curl	2	10–15	20	10
or Pulley Wrist Curl	2	10–15	20	10
10. Standing Calf Machine (Toe Raise)	3	15–20	35	25
or Leg Press Calf Extension	3	15–20	40	35

LEVEL 2

Exercise	Sets	Reps
1. Leg Raise	2	25–50
2. Seated Twisting	2	50–100
3. Squat	4	10–15
4. Leg Curl	3	10–15
5. Hyperextension	2	10–15
6. Barbell Shrug	3	10–15
7. Seated Pulley Rowing	3	8–12
8. Lat Pulldown	2	8–12
9. Barbell Incline Press	3	6–10
10. Flyes	2	8–12
11. Press behind the Neck	2	6–10
12. Side Lateral	2	8–12
13. Nautilus Curl	3	8–12
14. Nautilus Triceps Extension	3	8–12
15. Barbell Wrist Curl	3	10–15
16. Barbell Reverse Wrist Curl	3	10–15
17. Seated Calf Machine (Toe Raise)	2	8–12
18. Leg Press Calf Extension	2	15–20

LEVEL 3

Exercise	Sets	Reps
1. Sit-Up	3	25–50
2. Seated Twisting	3	50–100
3. Leg Press	3	10–15
4. Leg Extension	3	10–15
5. Leg Curl	3	10–15
6. Deadlift	2	8–12
7. Upright Rowing	3	8–12
8. Incline Press	3	6–10
9. Bench Press	3	8–12
10. Military Press	3	6–10
11. Side Lateral	3	8–12
12. Barbell Curl	4	8–12
13. Lying Triceps Extension	4	8–12
14. Cable Wrist Curl	4	10–15
14. Cable Reverse Wrist Curl	4	10–15
15. Standing Calf Machine (Toe Raise)	3	15–20
16. Seated Calf Machine (Toe Raise)	3	10–15

LEVEL 4

Day One (Monday-Thursday)

	Exercise	Sets	Reps
1.	Hyperextension	2-3	10-15
2.	Squat	4	10-15
3.	Leg Extension	4	10-15
4.	Leg Curl	4	10-15
5.	Barbell Shrug	3	10-15
6.	Seated Pulley Rowing	3	8-12
7.	Lat Pulldown	3	8-12
8.	Incline Press	4	6-10
9.	Flye	3	8-12
10.	Press behind the Neck	4	6-10
11.	Side Lateral	3	8-12
12.	Barbell Curl	3	8-12
13.	Pulley Curl	2	8-12
14.	Lying Triceps Extension	3	8-12
15.	Pulley Pushdown	2	8-12

Day Two (Tuesday-Friday)

	Exercise	Sets	Reps
1.	Sit-Up	3	25-50
2.	Leg Raise	3	25-50
3.	Side Bend	3	50-100
4.	Standing Calf Machine (Toe Raise)	4	15-20
5.	Seated Calf Machine (Toe Raise)	4	10-15
6.	Barbell Wrist Curl	4	10-15
7.	Reverse Wrist Curl	4	10-15

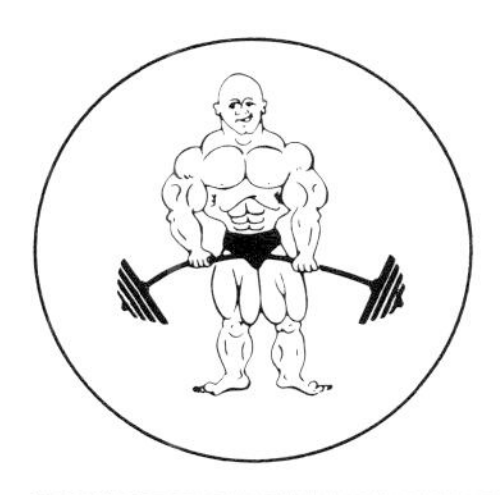

4 INTERMEDIATE BODYBUILDING

In this chapter we will discuss a number of bodybuilding concepts and training techniques that are far more advanced than the information presented in Chapter 2. Added to the knowledge that you gained in Chapter 2 and actually applied via the exercises and routines in Chapter 3, this new information will push you quickly through the intermediate level of bodybuilding training and on to the advanced level.

The rate at which each man and woman progresses through the various intensity levels of bodybuilding is highly individual. It depends on such factors as genetic bodybuilding potential (discussed in detail in the next section of this chapter), dedication to regular training, and mental drive to succeed as a bodybuilder.

Some exceptionally gifted and highly motivated male and female bodybuilders can progress through both beginning and intermediate levels of training intensity in as little as three months. And on the other side of the coin, a few men and women may never progress—or even care to progress—past the intermediate level of bodybuilding training.

You should place little importance on how quickly you move from one level to another, because in competitive bodybuilding the moral behind the tortoise-and-hare fable is particularly important. A methodical and consistently intense approach to training ultimately leads to success. We have seen literally hundreds of supertalented bodybuilders burn themselves out by attempting to progress too quickly, while most of the greatest bodybuilders of the present day are men in their late 30s and early 40s who have spent 15–20 years in consistently hard training!

Like fine wine, bodybuilders can slowly age to sublime physical perfection. A 20-year-old cabernet sauvignon is infinitely more satisfying to the palate than an immature year-old bottle of cabernet, just as a fully matured bodybuilder's physique is vastly superior to that of a younger and less experienced athlete. You should progress in your training at your own unique pace, but always strive to work out consistently and intensely. With this approach and sufficient time and patience, you can ultimately become a superb bodybuilder.

Looking ahead, we will discuss the following topics in this chapter: bodybuilding potential, muscle priority training, coping with sticking points, augmenting training enthusiasm, outdoor workouts, training partners, intermediate diet tips, mental approach to training, weight reduction, weight gain, power training, training to failure, changing workout programs, free weights versus machines, basic versus isolation exercises, heavy versus light movements, split routines, supination in biceps training, the use of weightlifting belts and body wraps, and a variety of factors unique to women bodybuilders (e.g., menstruation, birth control, amenorrhea, childbearing, and menopause).

Bodybuilding Potential

Over the past few years the topic of genetic potential for bodybuilding has been discussed widely. There *are* a wide variety of genetically determined factors that can influence your degree of success as a competitive bodybuilder, but few—if any—bodybuilders have even remotely approached their true genetic physical potential.

In most cases you should think of your bodybuilding potential not as a limiting factor but as a quality that makes your body unique among all others. All men and women have genetic pluses and minuses in their overall bodily makeup, and no bodybuilder has ever had "perfect" potential. Sergio Oliva and Arnold Schwarzenegger among the men and Laura Combes and Rachel McLish among the women have come close to having perfect bodybuilding potential, but each still had to work incredibly hard to bring up inherently weak points. And a critical eye can still easily pick out minor flaws in the physiques of each of these superstars, as well as in the physique of every other bodybuilder competing today.

The real trick to bodybuilding is being able to evaluate your potential correctly and then work hard and intelligently to maximize it. Among bodybuilding's elite athletes, the greatest degree of respect is accorded to those who have triumphed over great genetic obstacles.

Champion bodybuilders speak reverentially of how Larry Scott started with a skeletal structure in which his hips were actually wider than his shoulders, and yet he trained so diligently that he won two Mr. Olympia titles. They are in awe of how Arnold Schwarzenegger built his broomstick lower legs up to the level where his calves measured nearly 20 inches in circumference. And they speak admiringly of how naturally pudgy Laura Combes has been able to define her physique fully to become one of the world's truly great women bodybuilders.

So where should you begin in evaluating your bodybuilding potential? Dennis Tinerino, winner of the Mr. America, Mr. World, and Mr. Universe titles, has succinctly and authoritatively answered this question for all bodybuilders: "Before a person even starts to train, he or she should consider his or her skeletal structure and body metabolism. A potential superstar will almost always have a low degree of natural body fat, small knees and ankles, shoulders wider than his hips when in an untrained state (or for a woman, shoulders not too much narrower than her hips), and a relatively small and narrow hip and waist structure.

"After a year of training, a bodybuilder should ask several crucial questions: Do I genuinely love to train hard and consistently? Am I gaining muscle mass fast enough to maintain my enthusiasm for training? Do I have any exceptionally weak body parts? Am I willing to make the sacrifices necessary to become a champion? Do I sincerely believe I can become a champion bodybuilder? The bodybuilder's basic physical structure and answers to these questions will provide a good picture of his or her bodybuilding potential.

"Even if you have a poor skeletal structure, you can still develop a great physique if you are sincerely and completely devoted to achieving your goals. The classic example of a bodybuilder succeeding despite poor potential is, of course, Larry Scott. Burdened with narrow shoulders and the inability at first to make even modest muscle gains, he persevered for many years—even squeezing in his workouts while working full-time and attending night school—and built one of the most admired physiques in bodybuilding history. Even if your own potential is relatively poor, you can succeed as magnificently as did Larry Scott, *if* you have a burning desire to succeed!"

To Dennis Tinerino's advice we might add that the champion bodybuilders of the future will also invariably possess above average intelligence. To be successful, tomorrow's bodybuilder must have the intelligence to understand and apply to his or her training information

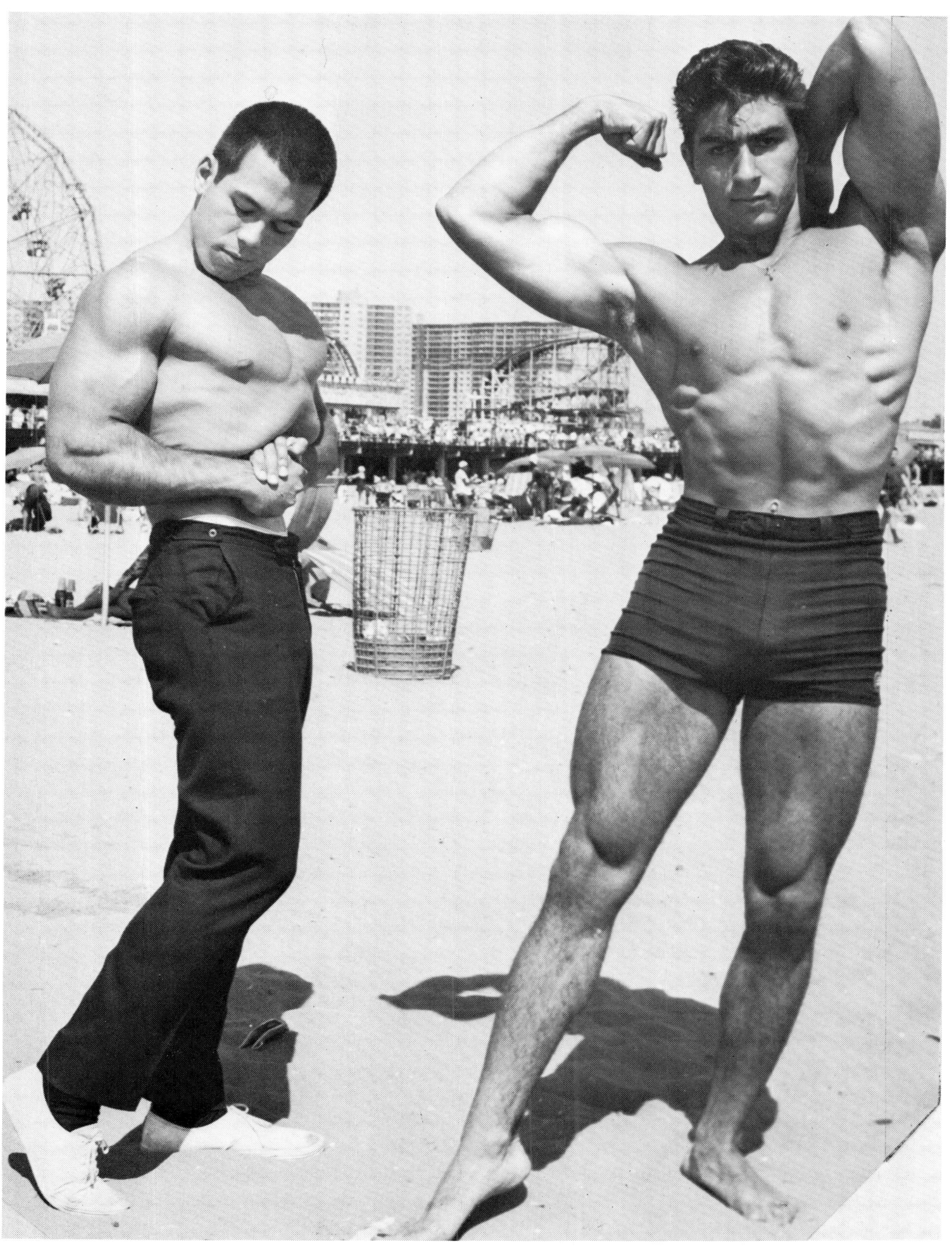

A great "before" photo of Dennis Tinerino (right) at the age of 17. He is posing at Coney Island with his friend Tommy Aybar. *(Photo courtesy of Dennis Tinerino)*

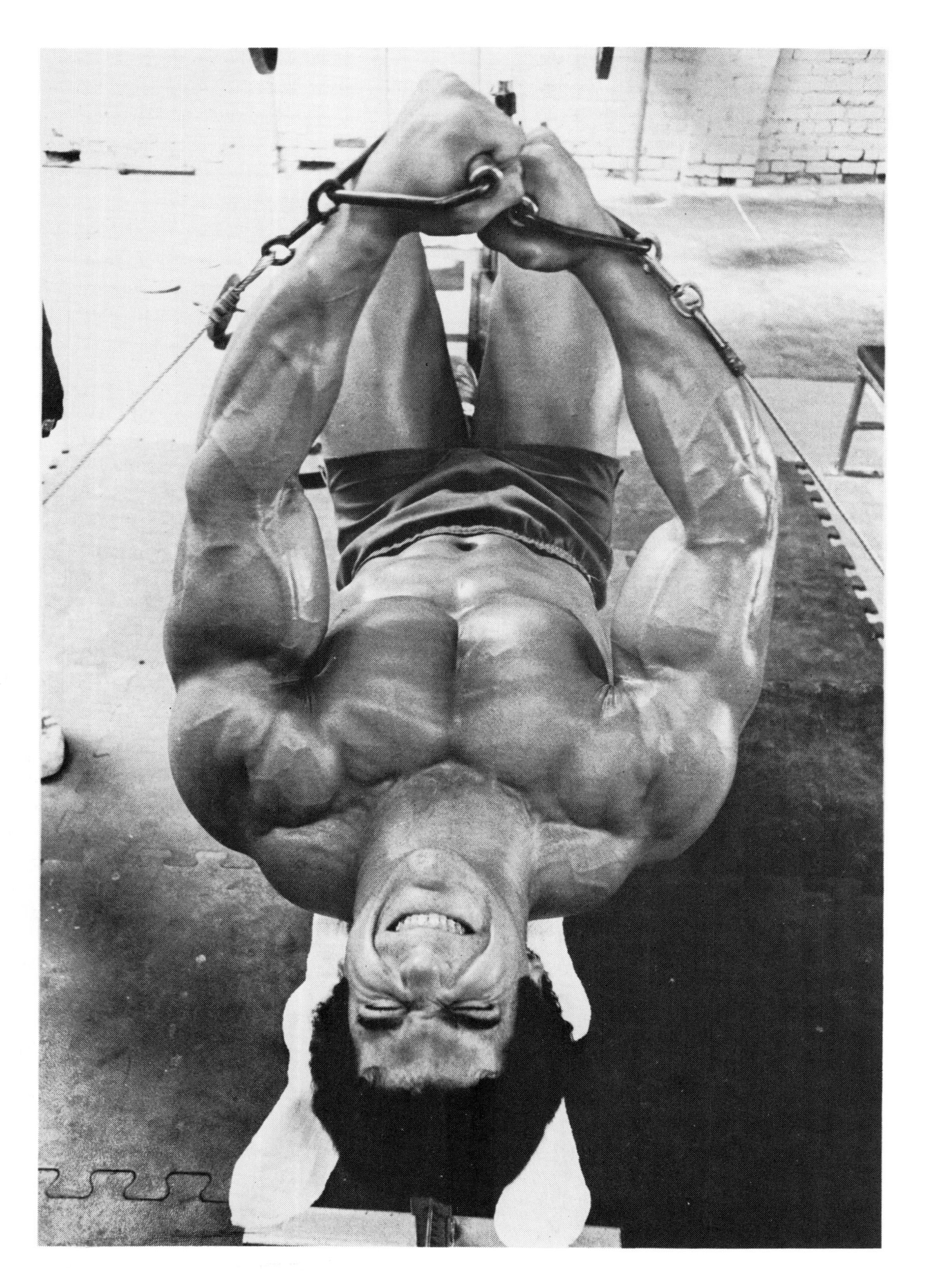

Few bodybuilders crashed through the pain barrier as consistently as hulking Lou Ferrigno. Here he carves extra striations across his pecs with Decline Cable Flyes. *(Photo by Craig Dietz)*

from such diverse scientific disciplines as exercise physiology, kinesiology, biomechanics, biochemistry, psychology, anatomy, and pharmacology.

Bodybuilding potential is truly what you make of it. Without hard and consistent training, a positive mental approach, and adherence to a healthy nutritional program, even a bodybuilder with the world's greatest potential will fail to win a regional bodybuilding title. By faithfully following a sound bodybuilding philosophy, however, scores of men and women with very poor genetic potential for bodybuilding have won state, regional, national, and even international titles!

Muscle Priority Training

After several months of steady training you will inevitably notice one or more muscle groups lagging a bit behind the rest of your body. Since the ultimate object of competitive bodybuilding is to develop a physique with each muscle group in perfect proportion with every other group, it is essential that you begin to deal with weak body parts as soon as they become evident.

The only way to improve a weak muscle group is to concentrate on it by training it longer, heavier, and more intensely. Such specialization involves training to failure, using forced reps, utilizing preexhaustion, working out with cheating movements, using negative reps, and employing a variety of other training intensification techniques that will be explained later in this chapter and in subsequent chapters.

Specializing in a weak muscle group demands a great energy expenditure, a much greater expenditure than will ever be required to train a body part that responds at a normal pace. Because specialization requires so much energy, it is best to train your lagging muscle group(s) at the beginning of your workouts, when your physical and mental energies are at their greatest level. If you waited until late in your workout to bomb your weaker body parts, your energy reserves would undoubtedly be too low to train a weak muscle group with sufficient intensity to jolt it into growth.

Training a weak body part first in your workout is a technique known as *muscle priority training*. Most champion bodybuilders either use or have used muscle priority training, and in combination with high-intensity workouts it is a very effective method of improving lagging muscle groups.

Sticking Points

The human body tends to gain muscle mass in cycles. For several weeks or months every body part grows a little in size and strength after each succeeding workout. But occasionally you will hit a sticking point during which you will make no progress whatsoever, even though you are dieting correctly and training both intensely and consistently.

Often your body encounters such a sticking point as it enters a short reconsolidation cycle prior to making good gains in muscle mass once again. In such a case, after two or three weeks of growth stagnation, your muscles will abruptly begin to add muscle mass and strength with each new workout.

At other times sticking points can linger for many weeks, even for several months. In such a case you must consciously attempt to explode past your sticking point and resume making acceptable muscle mass gains from your workouts. And how successfully you overcome such sticking points can influence your ultimate degree of success as a competitive bodybuilder.

Sticking points unrelated to your body's normal growth cycles are usually caused by the body becoming too accustomed to a particular type of training program. And these sticking points can be avoided by regularly changing training routines, as explained in detail later in this chapter.

To smash past a particularly persistent sticking point you should first take a complete layoff from training for a full week. Don't even go near a set of weights, but feel free to engage in other types of physical recreational activities, such as swimming, jogging, or participating in some type of vigorous team sport.

During your one-week layoff from working out, give serious consideration to your mental commitment to training. Are you consistently endeavoring to increase the resistance you use on each exercise in your routine? Is your level of training enthusiasm high? Do you really *want* to improve? If you discover any deficiencies in these areas of mental commitment, consciously rededicate yourself to your training.

Finally, at the end of your short layoff, resume your training on a totally different workout schedule than the one you had previously been following. It would be particularly beneficial to follow a shorter workout in which you use maximum training poundages in strict form for no more than five or six reps in each set.

This method will allow you to smash past even the most stubborn sticking points. Then, once you have begun to make acceptable muscle gains, be careful to avoid future sticking points by regularly changing your training programs and maintaining a high level of enthusiasm for your bodybuilding workouts.

Workout Enthusiasm

Most champion bodybuilders agree on the easiest way to keep their training enthusiasm at its maximum level. Lou Ferrigno explains: "Whenever I feel a little unenthusiastic about a workout that I have to do later in the day I turn to my collection of old muscle magazines. I've saved literally hundreds of these mags over the years, and just thumbing through them for an hour or so peaks my enthusiasm for the coming workout. I look at the photos of past and present champions, I think about how hard they trained to get where they are, and I then think about how hard I'll have to train myself to exceed the best standards of these champs. This procedure invariably sends me stomping into Gold's Gym with the momentum of a bull elephant in my eagerness to ferociously attack the weights!"

Dr. Lynne Pirie, a champion bodybuilder and physician, suggests another method of improving training enthusiasm: "As I was coming up through the ranks in bodybuilding I would get a tremendous boost in training drive from attending high-level bodybuilding competitions. I saw the best male and female bodybuilders going through their posing routines, and I vowed to eventually be up there myself, winning the big titles. Ultimately, I fulfilled these goals, because I was able to keep up my training enthusiasm by attending every possible bodybuilding show. I recommend this practice to any aspiring bodybuilder, man or woman."

Outdoor Workouts

Most bodybuilders train exclusively indoors—in a commercial bodybuilding gym like Gold's, at school, in a YMCA, at a health spa, or in a home gym. If you live in an area with a congenial climate, however, an occasional outdoor workout can be both an enjoyable change of pace and a chance to work on your tan.

Very few gyms have outdoor training facilities, such as that at the famed "Muscle Beach" weight pen on Venice Beach, California. Membership dues at the old weight pen, which is administered by the city parks and recreation department, are a mere $12 per year, and the weather usually allows for a good outdoor workout there all but a couple of weeks per year. Many regular Gold's Gym members pump a little iron from time to time at the Venice Beach weight pen, just as a change of pace.

The easiest way to train outdoors periodically is with a home gym. Simply lug your weights and benches out into the yard (the *backyard* if you have any respect for bodybuilding public relations), and take your workout in the sun.

Since no bodybuilder relishes training outdoors when it is either raining or excessively cold, there are two other environmental factors that should concern you when taking outdoor workouts. The first of these is excessive heat, which can—when coupled with a vigorous training session—lead to dehydration and possibly to heat prostration. It's not a good practice, then, to take prolonged workouts when the temperature is above 90 degrees Fahrenheit. And whenever it is warm enough to cause you to perspire profusely you should replenish your body fluids by drinking a little liquid every 10–15 minutes. Water is the most commonly used fluid replacement, though electrolyte replacement drinks are becoming increasingly popular with bodybuilders.

A second environmental consideration, particularly in large urban and/or highly industrialized areas, is air quality. There are numerous days each summer here in Los Angeles when the

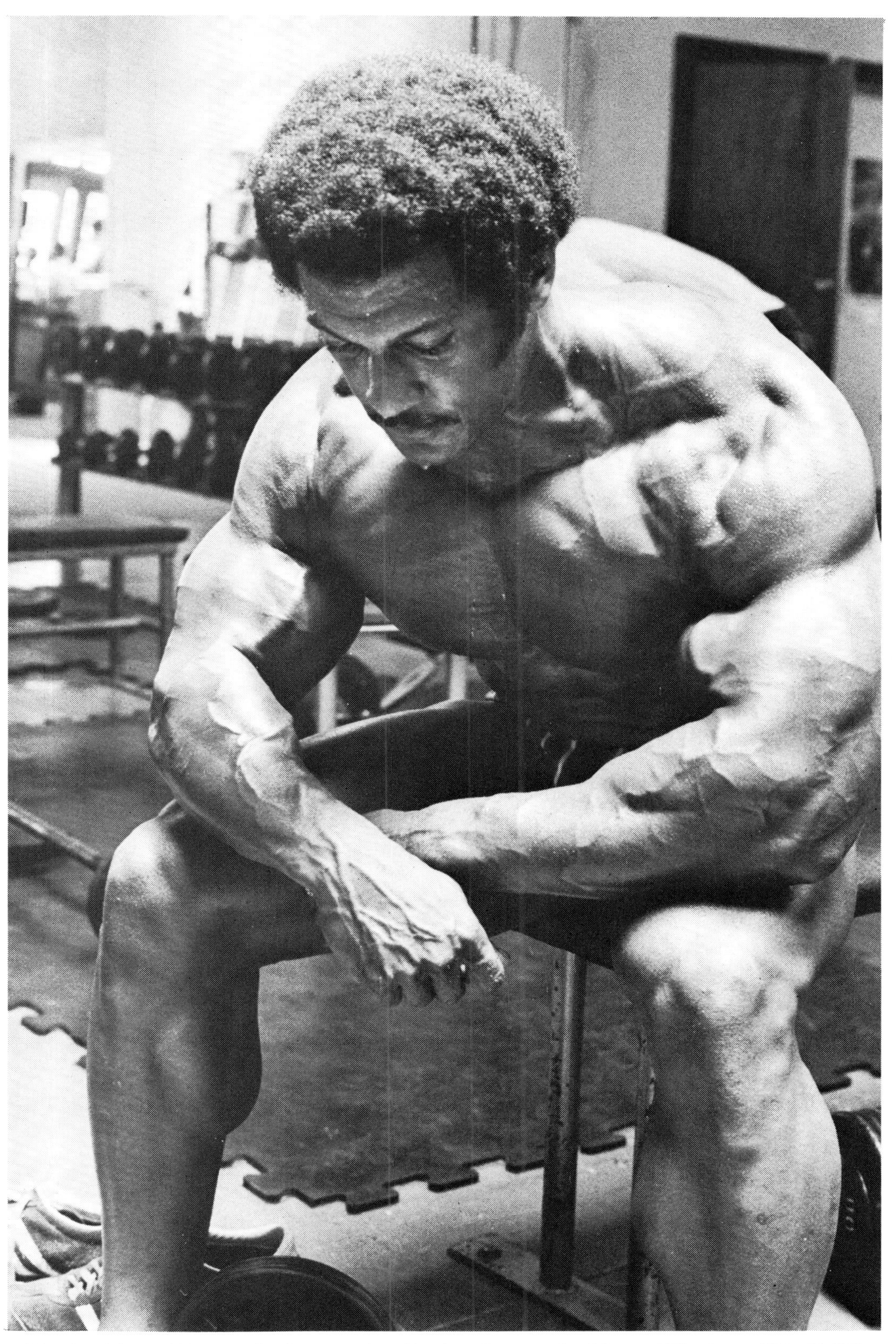

Massive Manuel Perry, who became Lou Ferrigno's stunt double on "The Incredible Hulk" television series, concentrates intensely before a heavy set of Bench Presses. Have you ever seen such upper body development!?! *(Photo by Craig Dietz)*

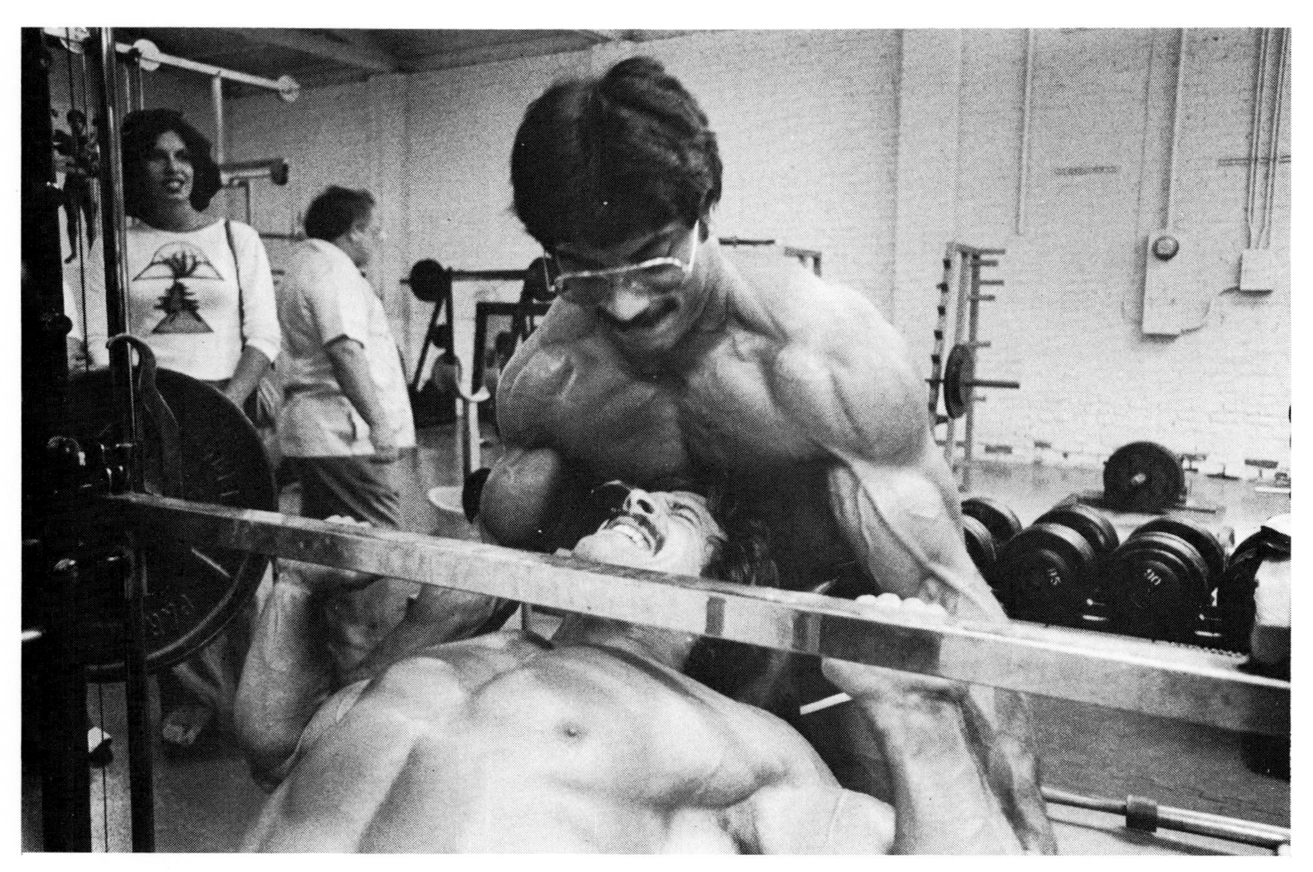

Ray Mentzer gives his brother, Mike, forced reps on Smith Machine Incline Presses. What a powerful duo for training together! Both have won Mr. America titles. *(Photo by Craig Dietz)*

smog is so dense that the local Air Quality Control Board issues warnings against strenuous outdoor exercise. If the air pollution where you live is sufficiently heavy to make normal outdoor training hazardous to your health, you might try your outdoor workouts early in the morning. Air pollution levels are normally much lower in the morning than they are later in the day, when vehicular exhaust emissions and industrial pollutants have had time to build up again after having been largely dissipated overnight.

If you follow these health precautions, you will find outdoor training a welcome change of pace from time to time. You'll still take the vast majority of your workouts indoors, but an occasional outdoor workout will be quite pleasurable.

Training Partners

To use a training partner or not to use one? That is the question invariably asked of serious bodybuilders. Certainly there are more competitive bodybuilders who use a training partner than there are athletes who prefer to train alone, but there are advantages and disadvantages to both methods.

From the standpoint of workout safety it is definitely best to train with a partner. As you will recall from our discussion of bodybuilding safety in Chapter 2, a training partner can act as a spotter whenever you are using near-maximum or maximum poundages in the Bench Press and Squat movements. A good partner can also assist you in using forced reps, a very advanced bodybuilding technique that will be explained in Chapter 6.

Alternating sets on each exercise with your workout partner, resting only long enough for him or her to complete a set before starting your own next set, guarantees a fast exercise pace. Resting excessively long between sets is

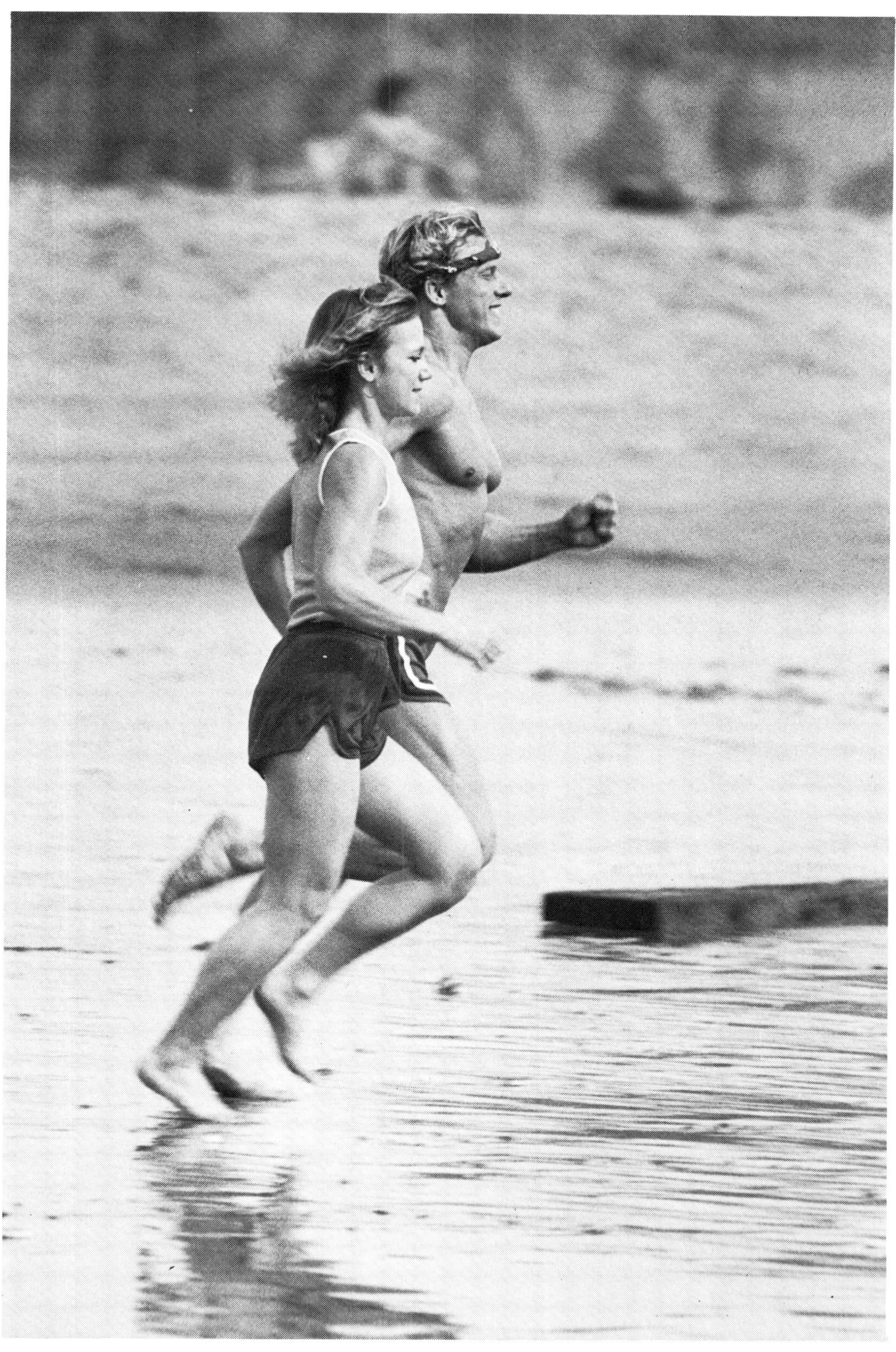

Stacey Bentley and Andreas Cahling pace each other during an aerobic workout on the beach.
(Photo by Mike Neveux)

disastrous during the weeks leading up to an actual competition, so many bodybuilders who normally train alone will use a workout partner when peaking for a competition.

There is also a measure of moral support that can be gained from having a workout partner. It's much more difficult for you to miss a workout when you know someone is waiting for you at the gym. And a well-chosen word of encouragement from your training partner can often spell the difference between getting and not getting a final result-producing rep in a hard set.

Unfortunately, however, when two bodybuilders form a partnership, either one or both of them will be forced to somewhat modify training philosophy. No two bodybuilders train identically, so adjustments must be made, and many bodybuilders feel that this disadvantage outweighs the advantages of having a training partner.

Many bodybuilders, who tend to be loners by nature, abhor training with someone else. Frank Zane, Chris Dickerson, and Deborah Diana are good examples of such bodybuilders. For these bodybuilders, training with a partner tends to detract from their degree of concentration on each set.

As a final thought on the subject of training partners, it's becoming increasingly popular to have male-female training partnerships. Andreas Cahling capsulizes the value of such an arrangement: "I often prefer to train with a woman. I'll always be much stronger than her, but women generally have higher thresholds of pain than do men. As a result, they can really push the pace of a workout, which is quite beneficial. In essence, I can encourage them to use heavier weights, while they encourage me to train longer and faster.

"I've also noticed a sort of show-off factor in cases where a man trains with a woman. The man seems to train even heavier and harder than he would with a male training partner, probably as a result of subconsciously trying to impress the woman. She, on the other hand, does the same thing, though probably more to show that she's not the 'weaker sex' after all. Either way, the training is heavier, faster, and harder, and you can't help but make good muscle gains while you work out in such a manner."

Intermediate Nutrition

In Chapter 2 we outlined several basic nutritional guidelines, as well as a sample daily menu that any beginning or intermediate bodybuilder can follow. In this section we will explain how to develop an individualized program of vitamin, mineral, and protein supplementation; how to diet to lose weight; and how to eat to gain muscular body weight.

Dietary Supplements

A huge and often bewildering array of vitamin, mineral, and protein supplements is available in health food stores as well as through advertisements in the various bodybuilding magazines. Undeniably, these supplements are of some value to an aspiring bodybuilder, though seldom of as great importance as the promoters of various brands of food supplements will claim.

Over the next few months you should gradually attempt to develop an individualized program of food supplementation that allows you to train with maximum vigor and energy production. To begin with, take two or three multipacks of vitamins, minerals, and trace elements per day, preferably with your meals, as recommended in Chapter 2. The manner in which you choose which brand of multipack to take, as discussed below, will later be repeated in choosing which individual vitamins and minerals you will use on a regular basis.

Multipacks provide insurance against progress-slowing nutritional deficiencies, but there are so many different brands on the market that you almost need to be a detective to decide which is the best value. To determine that, you must compare the nutritional values of each supplement packet and correlate each of these relative values with the price of each packet.

Reading the nutritional values of each packet can be a bit misleading, however. Some distributors of these multipacks list the values for two or three packets, noting that fact in exceedingly small type on the carton. Two packets of inferior-potency vitamins and minerals can look quite good in comparison to one high-potency packet if you fail—as many do—to note the fact that the posted nutritional data is for more than one packet.

The actual number of tablets and capsules in one packet has little bearing on the nutritional values of the entire packet. *More* doesn't necessarily mean *better,* because some packets have two small tablets of multiple minerals instead of a single larger, equal-potency tablet. Some have two B-complex tablets instead of one, and some have separate vitamin E and vitamin A and D capsules instead of one larger capsule or tablet incorporating all three vitamins.

The main places you can be ripped off with these packets are in the potencies of B-complex vitamins and the type of multiple minerals included. Compare the B-vitamin potencies carefully, because many supplement distributors cut corners with these nutrients, since they are relatively expensive. And all minerals included in the packets must be *chelated.* Chelation is a process by which protein molecules are chemically bonded to inorganic minerals, thereby making them much more assimilable in the human body than are unchelated minerals.

With multipack supplements—as well as all other vitamins, minerals, and protein supplements—you can save 30%–50% by banding together with friends in the gym where you train and ordering large quantities of supplements directly from distributors at wholesale prices. In effect, your group sets itself up as a health food store that sells supplements to each member, but without a retail markup.

Once you have chosen a multipack to use each day, you should experiment with various individual nutrients to see which help you make the best progress from your training. Introduce each supplement into your diet individually, taking careful note of its effect on your energy levels and muscle growth rate.

Experiment first with a powdered protein supplement. The best type of protein supplement is one formulated solely from milk and eggs. Nutritionists have evaluated the assimilability of various protein sources and established a Protein Efficiency Ratio (PER). The PER is based on egg albumen (egg white), the most assimilable source of protein available for human consumption. The protein in fish is second and milk is third in biological quality to that of eggs, in that it is about 80% as assimilable as egg albumen.

Egg albumen is very expensive, so most milk-and-egg protein powders have very little actual egg content. The milk protein content usually comes from calcium caseinate, which is approximately 95% protein. A lot of so-called milk-and-egg protein powders contain a significant percentage of yeast- or soya-based protein, both of which are very inexpensive in comparison to egg albumen and calcium caseinate. Such "milk-and-egg" protein powders are attractively priced but are of considerably lesser value to a bodybuilder. In effect, they're a rip-off.

Meat-based proteins are highly touted by some bodybuilders, but these preparations are exceedingly expensive and have a markedly lower PER than either milk- or egg-based protein. And soya-based protein powder supplements—as well as all others made from vegetable sources—have very low PERs and are of little value to a serious bodybuilder.

Protein supplements should be used as *supplements,* not as substitutes for regular food. They are best taken between regular meals, since the body can only assimilate approximately 30 grams of protein per feeding. A protein supplement can also be valuable as a substitute for a meal that might ordinarily have been missed if you are on more than a three-meal-a-day schedule. A protein shake can be whipped up and consumed in only three or four minutes, so if you're too rushed to eat a normal meal, use a protein supplement in its place.

Most serious bodybuilders have invested in heavy-duty, variable-speed blenders with which to mix up their protein shakes. It's a good investment because you will use it often and will undoubtedly experiment with difficult-to-blend vegetables or fruits. You can mix the protein powder with milk, fruit juice, or vegetable juice, though milk is preferred by most bodybuilders. Here is a good recipe for a blended protein drink (yields one large shake with approximately 40 grams of protein content).

- 8–10 oz. milk (raw milk is preferable)
- 2 tablespoons of milk-and-egg protein
- ½ piece soft fruit (such as a banana or peach) for flavor

Blend these ingredients for 45–60 seconds and

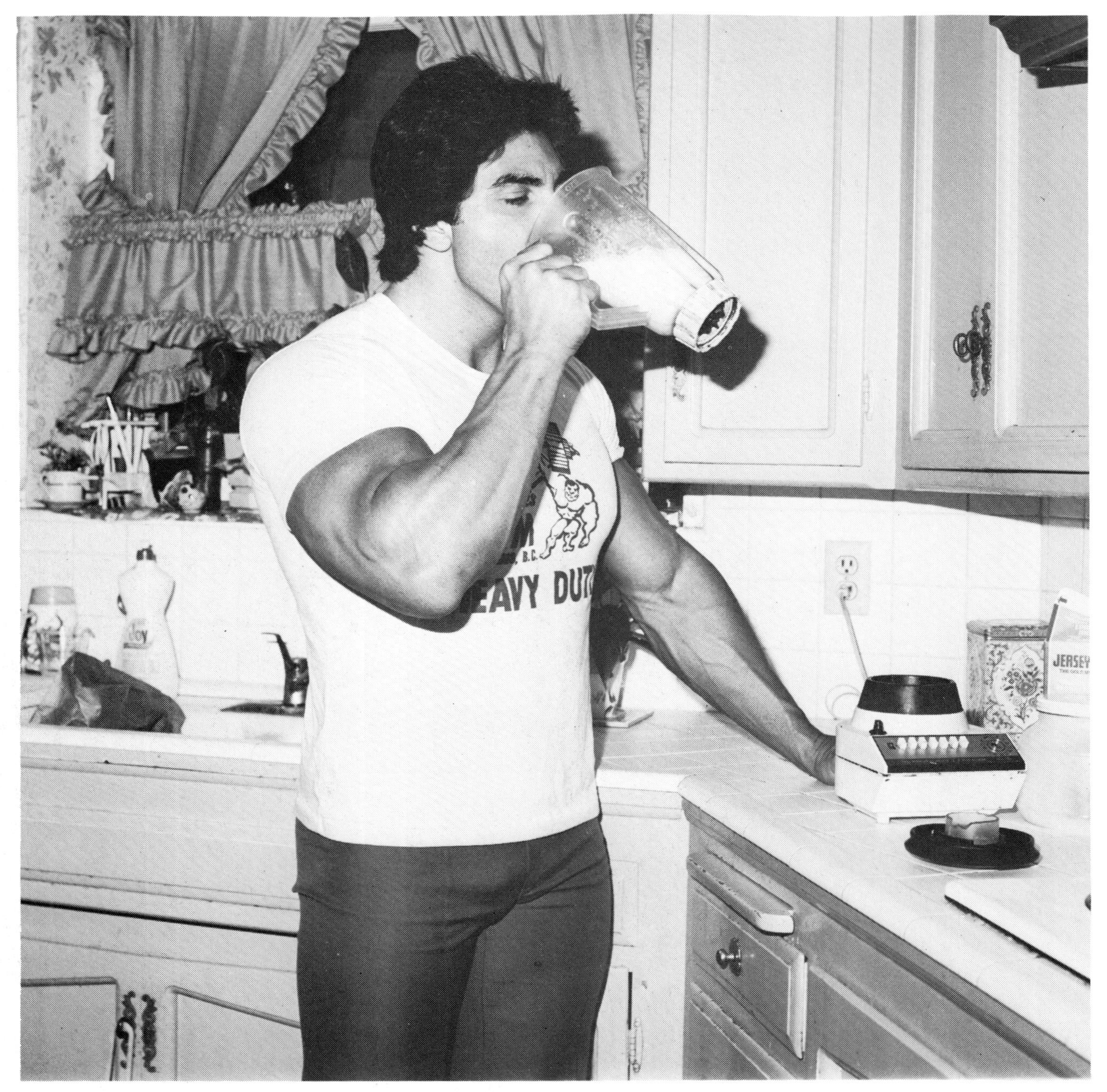

Even superstar bodybuilders like Dennis Tinerino drink protein shakes between meals to increase total protein assimilation and speed up muscle growth. *(Photo by Bill Reynolds)*

you will have a frothy and delicious drink. Raw (unpasteurized) milk can be purchased in most health food stores and in some supermarkets. For even greater protein content, many bodybuilders blend one or two raw or lightly poached eggs into this drink. Cooking the eggs lightly before blending destroys the avidin in the eggs, a substance that combines with biotin, a valuable B vitamin to make the biotin inactive.

Protein supplements are also available in liquid form and as tablets. Liquid protein has a very low PER, since it is made from animal byproducts that would normally be considered unfit for human consumption. These protein concoctions also taste terrible. A lot of bodybuilders use these "liquid amino acids" (which, incidentally contain negligible quantities of tryptophane, one of the eight essential amino acids), but they are essentially of little value nutritionally.

Protein tablets used to be very popular, but few bodybuilders use them today. On a per-gram basis, they are far more expensive than protein powders, and few types of tablets are manufactured from milk and/or egg proteins. They can, however, be conveniently carried and munched on throughout the day instead of eating a junk food snack.

Once you have thoroughly investigated protein supplements you should gradually experiment with individual vitamins and minerals, plus a few other types of food supplements. In descending order of importance (based on a combined experience of 40 years), you should try vitamin B-complex capsules, vitamin C (with bioflavonoids), chelated potassium, vitamin E, chelated calcium-magnesium, vitamin B-6, vitamin B-12, vitamin B-15, zinc, iron, pantothenic acid, and vitamins A and D.

Most bodybuilders use large quantities of dessicated liver tablets, particularly before competitions (Tim Belknap, Mr. America, uses up to 200 per day). Dessicated liver is approximately 70% protein and 30% carbohydrate. It also contains significant quantities of B vitamins and iron. Bodybuilders generally believe that dessicated liver helps build workout endurance, though this may be an individual matter. There is, however, some scientific evidence to support this claim.

In a classic experiment scientists fed three groups of laboratory rats various diets for a month. Group I was fed the normal lab rat diet, Group II the regular diet plus synthetic B vitamins, and Group III the regular diet plus all of the dessicated liver they wanted to consume. Then each group of rats was placed in its own drum of water, from which escape was impossible. The rats literally were forced to swim or drown, a definitive test of physical endurance.

The rats in Groups I and II swam an average of approximately 15 minutes before drowning. The Group III rats, however, swam approximately three times as long before drowning, and several were still swimming vigorously when the experiment was concluded two hours later! Many researchers, as a result of this experiment, have concluded that dessicated liver greatly augments energy and endurance levels.

The problem with this experiment—and the conclusions drawn from it—is one of isolating experimental variables from all other possible variables that can weigh on the result of an experiment. In this case many researchers have questioned whether the liver itself was responsible for the increase in endurance rather than the increase in dietary protein that it provided. This question has still not been resolved, so tread lightly as you experiment with dessicated liver in your own diet.

Dieting to Lose Weight

Forget about following fad diets. Eating nothing but pineapple for a week, cutting carbohydrate consumption nearly to zero, and eating five pounds of rice per day will all result in a loss of body weight, some of it water, some fatty tissue, and some muscle mass. But such nutritionally unbalanced diets are very unhealthy to follow. While you're shedding pounds on one of them, you may also be seriously damaging your health.

Low-carbohydrate diets, for example, have been widely popular in recent years, but they can result in low blood sugar, depression, and binge eating. And much of the body weight lost on a low-carbohydrate diet results from dehydration. One gram of carbohydrate in your body normally retains four times its weight in water. As a result, when you severely restrict dietary carbohydrate intake, your body will flush out water that it normally holds. Such a water loss can also be unhealthy, since it can disturb the normal functioning of your heart and other internal organs.

A low-carb regimen used to be *the* bodybuilding precontest muscle definition diet, and some bodybuilders still follow it to achieve a cut-up appearance. It is a fairly effective diet for these purposes, though many champion bodybuilders have experienced a loss of muscle mass on a low-carb diet. And, more crucially, following a low-carbohydrate diet prior to competition is very uncomfortable, both physically and mentally. Every bodybuilder we've observed on this diet prior to competition has been highly nervous and irritable, has had a very low degree of training energy, and has been prone to significant mood swings.

The most sensible and healthy type of weight-loss regimen—for both bodybuilders and the average person—is a nutritionally balanced diet in which caloric consumption is restricted. For a competing bodybuilder, or a bodybuilder who is chronically overweight, this type of diet results in a safe and gradual loss of body fat accompanied by a minimal loss of muscle tissue.

In a human body that maintains a steady weight there is an equilibrium, or a dynamic balance, between energy intake and outflow in terms of calories. A calorie is merely a unit of energy measurement. More precisely it is a measure of the energy stored in the body as fat (potential energy), consumed in the foods we eat, or expended through physical movement or to keep the body's metabolism and vital processes functioning at a healthy level.

When dieting, we think of calories primarily in terms of stored body fat and food intake. There are 3,500 calories in one pound of fat, so to lose one pound of body fat while following a low-calorie diet, you must restrict your dietary intake by 3,500 calories over the period of a few days. On a severely restricted diet, you might be able to lose one pound of fat in two or three days, but it's much more healthy to think in terms of losing approximately one pound per week (7 × 500 calories per day in a caloric deficit). Such a slow loss of body weight, in addition, allows you to maintain a diet that is relatively easy to follow, especially when compared to diets of 1,000 calories or less per day.

You *cannot* be scientifically accurate in calculating your exact caloric expenditure each day for both metabolic maintenance and physical activities such as bodybuilding training and aerobic workouts. But you can fairly accurately calculate your maintenance caloric intake level by using this formula:

Body Weight (in pounds) × Sex Factor × Exercise Activity Factor × Age Factor = Daily Caloric Maintenance Level

The sex factor for women is 1.0, while for men it is 1.2, since men are generally more physically active in their work environment. And scientific data indicate that men have a somewhat higher BMR (Basal Metabolic Rate) than women, burning up proportionately more calories each day simply to stay alive.

You must also estimate your exercise activity factor. If you hardly exercise at all, rate yourself below 7; if you exercise infrequently but fairly hard when you do, rate yourself between 7 and 15. If you feel that you exercise only moderately hard each day, assign yourself a factor of 15. If you work out very hard and for a relatively long period of time each day, however, you can use a factor of 20. You might also assign yourself any other factor between 15 and 20 to reflect your relative level of intensity and duration of exercise.

General physical activity and metabolic caloric consumption decline with age, so if you are over 35, you should consider the age factor:

- Up to age 35, your age factor will be 1.0.
- From 36–40 years of age, assign yourself an age factor of 0.95.
- From 41–45 years of age, assign yourself an age factor of 0.90.
- From 46–50, assign yourself an age factor of 0.85.
- At any age over 50, assign yourself an age factor of 0.80.

Using this formula, a 25-year-old male bodybuilder who weighs 200 pounds and trains very hard two hours a day, six days per week, would require approximately 4,800 calories to maintain his body weight (200 × 1.2 × 20 × 1 = 4,800). An inactive woman over 50 and weighing 130 pounds would require only approximately 1,560 calories to maintain her weight (130 × 1.0 × 15 × 0.80 = 1,560).

By purchasing an inexpensive calorie counter booklet at a health food store and recording everything you eat in your training log, you can easily calculate your daily nutritional caloric intake. Then, by simply adjusting your food intake to 500–600 calories less than your maintenance level each day, you can lose about one pound of body fat per week.

What foods should you cut out of your diet? First, any type of junk food should go, because calories from these foods are of little nutritional value to an aspiring bodybuilder. Such foods include anything containing refined sugar or flour, plus alcoholic beverages.

Next, endeavor to avoid *drinking* your calories, since it's very easy to consume an excessive number of calories in this manner. As an example, you can easily prove to yourself that by drinking two or three glasses of orange juice (a very concentrated source of calories), you can consume 10 times the calories you would by eating a couple of oranges. Similarly, it's very easy to ingest a huge number of calories while drinking milk, particularly if it's full-fat milk.

Finally, and most importantly, you should reduce the consumption of fats in your diet. Fats are more than twice as concentrated a source of calories than are proteins or carbohydrates. More specifically, one gram of fat yields nine calories when metabolized for energy in the human body. In contrast, one gram of either protein or carbohydrate yields only four calories.

Based on the foregoing information, it seems logical enough that you can comfortably and significantly reduce your caloric intake simply by limiting your consumption of fats while perhaps eating more carbohydrates and/or proteins. In actual practice, this is indeed the case, and the vast majority of high-level competitive bodybuilders follow a low-fat/low-calorie diet prior to a contest. With this diet's relatively high carbohydrate intake allowance, bodybuilders are able to train much harder and more energetically, while still losing body fat at an acceptable rate of speed, than is possible on a low-carb regimen.

The following table lists foods that are very high or very low in fat content.

Do Eat	Do Not Eat
Egg whites	Egg yolks
Poultry white meats (skinless)	Pork and beef
Green vegetables	Full-fat milk products
Fresh fruits	Corn
Salad greens	Oils
Potatoes (no butter or sour cream)	Nuts, seeds, and some grains

To give you a clear idea of how you can eat while on a low-fat diet, here is a sample daily meal plan for someone dieting moderately strictly.

Meal 1 (8:00 a.m.)—six poached egg whites, one bran muffin, half a cantaloupe, hot tea, supplements.

Meal 2 (11:30 a.m.)—tuna salad (minimum of mayonnaise), an apple, iced tea with lemon, supplements.

Meal 3 (3:00 p.m.)—broiled chicken breast, rice, salad with vinegar, two green vegetables, iced tea with lemon, supplements.

Meal 4 (6:30 p.m.)—broiled fish, a baked potato, two green vegetables, iced tea with lemon, supplements.

Snacks—fresh fruit, fresh raw vegetables.

To more fully define the low-fat/low-calorie diet, here are 10 additional dietary rules suggested by the superb Boyer Coe:

1. In a hierarchy of fatty meats, pork is more fatty than beef, beef is more fatty than poultry with skin on it, poultry with skin is more fatty than skinned poultry, and skinned poultry is more fatty than fish. Furthermore, within the category of poultry, dark meat is somewhat higher in calories than is white meat.

2. Never fry foods. Cooking oil is pure fat, and fried food soaks up the oil it's cooked in. Your fish and poultry should be baked, boiled broiled, or grilled. Broiling meat over a charcoal fire provides a true taste treat.

3. Avoid full-fat milk products, particularly butter. Full-fat cheese and milk are much higher in calories than low-fat cheese (such as mozzarella and nonfat milk). Since an enzyme factor in milk products tends to promote water retention in the body, you should avoid milk products for approximately two weeks prior to competing. If you continue milk usage right up to the day of a contest, your skin can be bloated with water, which blurs your true muscular definition.

4. Avoid using oil or commercial dressings on your salads. Add parsley and other herbs to your salad and use lemon juice and/or vinegar as a dressing. As a bonus from this practice, many top bodybuilders believe that vinegar helps to metabolize body fat.

5. Dry baked potatoes (without butter or sour cream) are quite low in calories in proportion to their bulk. As with many other foods, the toppings traditionally put on potatoes provide the bulk of calories associated with the food. And dry baked potatoes taste just fine once you have become used to them. Along the same lines, dry popcorn is also a good low-calorie food.

6. Use a wide variety of herbs and spices in your cooking. Each herb and spice adds a distinctive flavoring to your meat, vegetables, and salads, and all herbs and spices have a negligible caloric content.

7. If you eat bread, use whole-grain bread and don't spread butter, peanut butter, jam, or jelly on it. Similarly, use only whole grains whenever you consume grain products. As with milk, avoid consuming grains for the final two weeks before a competition, because they can also cause your body to retain water.

8. Avoid boiling vegetables. Boiling leeches valuable vitamins and minerals from the foods. Avoid using butter or oil in cooking vegetables.

9. Avoid using all forms of sodium in your diet, since it retains 50 times its weight in water. The main offenders in your diet will be table salt and artificial sweeteners, which are based on sodium saccharide. Surprisingly, celery also is very high in sodium.

10. Everyone on a diet gets cravings now and then. You will particularly crave fats and refined sugar products. Avoid both. When a craving is particularly great, eat naturally sweet fruit, such as watermelon and peaches, until the craving abates.

Following these guidelines, you can adjust your caloric consumption upward and downward according to how slowly or quickly you are losing body fat. And you can also use a variation of this diet—but with a higher total caloric intake each day—to maintain your body fat level throughout the year.

Dieting to Gain Weight

In a way, dieting to gain weight involves eating a surplus—rather than a deficit—of calories. It's more important during the weight-gaining process, however, to increase your daily protein intake, since protein forms the skeletal muscles of your body. Combined with heavy exercise (described in detail later in this chapter), a high-protein diet will allow you to gain solid muscle mass at the fastest possible rate of speed.

There are two primary ways in which to increase the amount of protein digested and assimilated by your body: (1) Eat smaller and more frequent meals; (2) Consume digestive aids, such as hydrochloric acid and digestive enzymes. By combining these two methods, you can achieve optimum protein digestion and assimilation. And by melding optimum protein assimilation with heavy, high-intensity bodybuilding training, you can most efficiently add muscular body weight to your frame.

Under normal circumstances, your digestive system can process only 25–30 grams of protein at each meal. Any protein in excess of these figures will simply pass from the body as waste in the feces. Additionally, heavy-protein meals can actually make the digestive process more sluggish and result in even less protein assimilation.

By eating smaller meals more frequently, however, you can augment the total daily amount of protein that your body digests and ultimately assimilates as muscle tissue. You can eat 4–6 smallish meals, each with 20–30 grams of protein content, every day rather than the customary two or three gigantic daily repasts that most North Americans and Europeans consume.

Assuming that you will eat six protein-rich meals in one day, here is a sample daily menu for weight gaining.

Meal 1 (8:00 a.m.)—five-egg cheese omelet, a piece of fruit, a glass of milk, supplements.
Meal 2 (10:15 a.m.)—protein shake, supplements.
Meal 3 (12:30 p.m.)—tuna salad, a glass of milk, supplements.
Meal 4 (2:45 p.m.)—protein shake, supplements.
Meal 5 (5:00 p.m.)—roast beef, baked potato, salad (blue cheese dressing), glass of milk, supplements.
Meal 6 (7:30 p.m.)—fruit-flavored yogurt, boiled eggs, glass of milk, supplements.

Notice the heavy reliance on milk in this diet. Although a few athletes are unable to consume milk, most bodybuilders consider it an ideal weight-gaining food. And certified raw milk, which hasn't been heated in the pasteurization process, is the best type of milk to drink. This milk comes from cows regularly inspected and certified to be free from disease. In addition to presenting it as a beverage, many certified dairies manufacture a variety of other raw-milk products, such as cottage cheese, hard cheese, and yogurt. These products can often be obtained from health food stores and health food departments of progressive supermarkets.

Some individuals are unable to digest milk properly due to a deficiency of lactase in their digestive systems. Lactase is the enzyme that digests lactose, the sugar found in milk. This condition is called galactose intolerance, and if you have it, you can still eat hard cheeses from which the lactose has been removed in the manufacturing process.

Galactose intolerance becomes more common as an athlete gets older. Men are more prone to having this malady than are women. And Blacks and Orientals are more likely to suffer from galactose intolerance than are Caucasians.

Your family physician can tell you if you suffer from galactose intolerance, or you can self-diagnose this digestive enzyme deficiency. The most common symptoms of galactose intolerance are bloating of the stomach and drowsiness and/or lethargy soon after consuming milk products.

To fortify the natural digestive acids and enzymes in your digestive tract you can purchase a variety of supplements at a health food store. The best of these is a formula of hydrochloric acid and pepsin, the primary digestive media of the human stomach. You can also take other commercially produced digestive enzyme preparations, particularly papain, the digestive enzyme found in pineapple. All digestive aid supplements should be taken with your meals.

There are other food supplements that you can take to optimize your weight-gaining nutritional program. Vitamin B-complex, for example, stimulates the appetite, and several of the B vitamins are essential for the formation of enzymes and coenzymes in the human body.

Even more important, supplementing the diet with a wide spectrum of high-potency vitamins and minerals ensures that the body will remain in optimum health. And if your body is not completely healthy, you will find it difficult to gain solid body weight very quickly.

Mental Approach

The essence of a champion bodybuilder's mental approach to the sport can be expressed in a single word—*positive.* It is difficult under any circumstances to succeed as a bodybuilder, and it's totally impossible if the mind has not been locked into a consistently positive mode.

Tom Platz, a Gold's Gym member and one of the sport's leading proponents of positive mental programming, has crystallized this frame of mind: "From the time I was 17, when I had already been training for about two years, I have *known* that I would become a great champion. And even though I have suffered several defeats in bodybuilding competition, I have never allowed the intensity of my self-belief and positive mental attitude to waver.

"A bodybuilder who always expects success, and who can clearly visualize himself or herself achieving this success, will surely succeed. The inverse of this statement is also true, however—whoever expects failure will surely fail. It is axiomatic in bodybuilding that the man or woman with the strongest mind will ultimately triumph."

Platz himself is an excellent illustration of the veracity of his argument. Through hard training, intelligent dietary practices, and consistent application of his theories on mental approach, he has become the most massively muscular bodybuilder in history.

Concentration

Oriental philosophers have written that any person who can concentrate 100% of his or her mental awareness on a single entity for five minutes can rule the world. The kicker, of course, is that even highly trained masters of concentration are unable to achieve this goal. And few untrained individuals are able to concentrate on one topic or concept for more than 15–20 seconds.

During every set of every bodybuilding workout you do you should concentrate as fully as possible on the working muscles. "To get the most out of a heavy set," notes Tom Platz, "you must have a very strong link between your mind and the working muscles. Over a period of years you can make this link stronger and stronger, until it is totally unbreakable.

"You should begin to forge this mind link with your muscles by thinking hard about the

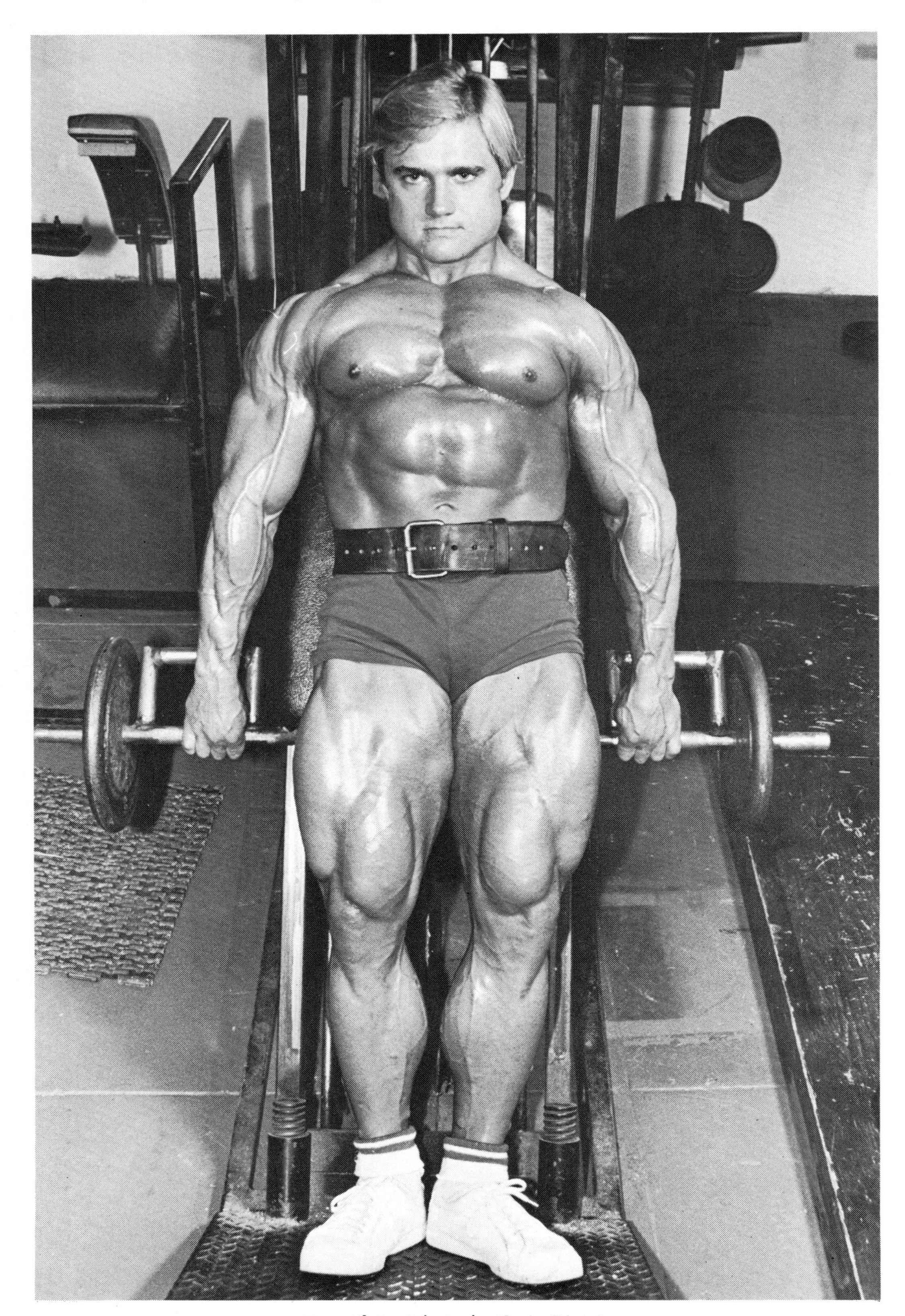

Tom Platz. *(Photo by Craig Dietz)*

muscles being worked as you perform an exercise. When doing Dumbbell Concentration Curls, for example, focus your mind on your biceps. Visualize the muscle group shortening and peaking into a miniature Mount Everest as you curl up the dumbbell. Visualize it flattening and extending as you lower the weight back to the starting position.

"By constantly focusing your mind on the working muscles, you will gradually strengthen the mind link I have mentioned. It's somewhat like a spider going back and forth along one thread of silk, laying a new thread each trip, until it has fabricated a thick cable of silk. Once you are able to concentrate effectively, a jumbo jet could crash on the roof of the gym during your set and you wouldn't notice anything but your working muscles!"

We can suggest a nonbodybuilding concentration exercise that will help improve your ability to focus your concentration during a workout. Lie on your back in a comfortable position. Choose a number and try to concentrate solely on it for longer and longer periods of time.

At first, other thoughts will intrude on your ability to focus only on the number you have chosen. Each time you notice your mind wandering from its focus point, force it back on the point. Practice this exercise for about 10 minutes once or twice per day, and you'll soon notice that you can focus your concentration without interruption for a longer and longer period. And as your focusing ability becomes more and more acute, your workouts will become better.

Transcendental Meditation classes can effectively improve your concentration as well. Several champion bodybuilders, among them three-time Mr. Olympia winner Frank Zane, have gained greater powers of concentration via classes in TM and other forms of meditation. Give it a try!

Goal Setting

Goal setting is one of the most effective tools that a bodybuilder can have in his or her kit. By effectively using goal setting, you can maintain a consistently high level of enthusiasm for your workouts and diet, which in turn will allow you to make continued fast gains in both muscle mass and quality.

One problem with bodybuilding is that it's quite difficult to conceive of actually being as huge and muscular—and as powerful—as a champion bodybuilder is. If your upper arm is 14 inches in circumference, it's extremely difficult to visualize yourself with a 20-inch upper arm measurement. It's equally difficult to imagine yourself Bench Pressing 200 pounds more than you are currently handling.

The secret to coping with this problem is to go ahead and establish such mind-boggling long-range goals, then break these into numerous smaller and more manageable short-range goals. For example you could set a long-range goal of using 50 additional pounds in the Bench Press within a year, which would greatly augment your chest, shoulder, and arm development. You might feel put off at the prospect of repping out with 50 more pounds in the movement, but five additional pounds doesn't sound like that much. Yet 12 months of adding five pounds to the bar each month will result in a yearly increase of 60 pounds, not merely 50!

All goals should be set high enough to be challenging but not so high as to become unrealistic. Set your long-range goals at intervals of one year and record them in your training diary for periodic review. Set short-range goals at intervals of one week or one month and be certain to work as hard as possible to achieve each of these smaller goals. If you are unable to reach your short-range goals, you certainly won't reach your long-range goals.

Once you have achieved a goal, set a newer and higher target at which to shoot. Very quickly you will discover that the proper use of goal setting allows you to make faster progress and enjoy your training more. And this is a winning combination for any aspiring bodybuilder.

Exercise and Weight Reduction

Earlier in this chapter, when we discussed dieting for weight reduction, we stated that it was necessary to establish a caloric deficit in order to lose fat weight. It's easiest to do this through dietary means, but you should also be conscious of an exercise-oriented approach to weight reduction. By combining a sensible diet with vigorous exercise, you will be able to lose fatty body weight easily and efficiently.

Bodybuilders generally attempt to burn off fat by upping the total number of sets they do in a workout, plus occasionally doing a greater number of sets within a constant period of time. Training faster like this is called *quality training,* and it is discussed in detail in Chapter 8. For now, however, let's concentrate solely on increasing the amount of training you do.

Longer workouts necessitate the use of lighter training poundages. Most bodybuilders have also concluded that they receive greater weight-loss benefit from their bodybuilding workouts if they consistently do higher reps in each set.

Taking all of this into consideration, here is a good weight-loss workout that you can follow on three nonconsecutive days per week.

Exercise	Sets	Reps
1. Sit-Up	2–3	25–50
2. Leg Raise	2–3	25–50
3. Side Bend	2–3	50–100
4. Squat	4	10–20
5. Leg Extension	3	10–15
6. Leg Curl	3	10–15
7. Hyperextension	2	10–15
8. Upright Rowing	2	10–15
9. Seated Pulley Rowing	3	10–15
10. Lat Pulldown	2	10–15
11. Bench Press	3	10–15
12. Incline Press	2	10–15
13. Press behind the Neck	2	10–15
14. Side Lateral	2	10–15
15. Barbell Curl	3	10–15
16. Lying Triceps Extension	3	10–15
17. Barbell Wrist Curl	2	15–20
18. Barbell Reverse Wrist Curl	2	15–20
19. Standing Calf Machine (Toe Raise)	3–4	15–20
20. Seated Calf Machine (Toe Raise)	3–4	15–20

Resting 30–45 seconds between sets, you should be able to complete this workout comfortably in less than 90 minutes.

Aerobic Activities

We will discuss the relationship between aerobic activity and competitive bodybuilding in detail in Chapter 6. For now, however, you can use aerobic exercise on your nonworkout days to burn off extra calories.

Aerobic literally means *with air.* Aerobic exercise, then, is physical activity of low intensity that is carried on for extended periods of time within the body's ability to supply oxygen to the working muscles in amounts equal to or greater than those being burned up while exercising. Typical forms of aerobic exercise include running, cycling, swimming, fast walking, roller skating, and dancing.

Assuming that you do your bodybuilding workouts on Mondays, Wednesdays, and Fridays, you can do aerobic sessions on Tuesdays, Thursdays, Saturdays, and perhaps Sundays. To get any effect from your aerobic workouts you must exercise continuously for at least 20 minutes. Ideally, your aerobic workouts should last between 30 and 40 minutes.

There is a tendency to stick with one type of aerobic activity for all workouts, but you'll find it easier to stick to a program when you constantly vary the type of aerobic exercise you perform. Variety is, indeed, the spice of life, and variety in aerobic workouts makes them much more interesting over the long haul.

Exercise for Weight Gain

As a bodybuilder, you have no doubt already concluded that there is a definite relationship between the amount of weight you use in all of your exercises and the size of your muscles. Very simply put, the heavier you train, the larger will be your muscles.

It is possible to gain fatty body weight simply by pigging out on junk foods several time a day, but such a weight gain is obviously detrimental in bodybuilding. Instead, you should gain weight by increasing muscle mass, which means that you must train with heavy weights and low reps on basic exercises.

Basic exercises are discussed in detail later in this chapter. For now, you should understand that basic exercises are movements that work large muscle groups of the body—e.g., the thigh, chest, and back muscles—in concert with smaller muscles such as the biceps and triceps. On movements such as the Squat and the Bench Press you can use very heavy weights, and these are easily the best exercises for building exceptional muscle mass.

In order to use maximum poundages for low reps without the fear of incurring an injury, you must thoroughly warm up the muscles called into play in each movement. The best way to do this is to use a technique called *pyramidding* in which you begin each exercise using a light weight for relatively high reps, then increase the poundage and decrease the reps on each succeeding set.

To be sure that you understand specifically how pyramidding works, here is a typical pyramid of sets, reps, and poundages for the Squat.

Set Number	Reps	Weight (in pounds)
1	12	135
2	10	205
3	8	255
4	6	285
5	4	315
6	2	335

Based on the foregoing advice, here is a good three-day-per-week weight-gaining routine.

Exercise	Sets	Reps
1. Sit-Ups	2–3	25–50
2. Squat	5	12/10/8/6/4*
3. Barbell Bent Rowing	4	12/10/8/6/5*
4. Deadlift	3	8/6/4*
5. Barbell Shrug	3	12/10/8*
6. Bench Press	5	12/10/8/6/4*
7. Military Press	3	8/6/4*
8. Barbell Curl	3	8/6/4*
9. Lying Triceps Extension	3	10/8/6*
10. Seated Calf Machine (Toe Raise)	4	12/10/8/6*

* These exercises should be pyramidded.

A little later in this chapter we will explain a method of splitting your routine in half and doing each half twice per week on a four-day split routine. Using a split routine, here is a good four-day-per-week workout that you can use in conjunction with a protein-enriched diet for weight gain.

Monday and Thursday

Exercise	Sets	Reps
1. Incline Sit-Up	2–3	20–30
2. Hyperextension	2–3	10–15
3. Squat	6	12/10/8/6/4/2*
4. Barbell Bent Rowing	5	12/10/8/6/4*
5. Barbell Shrug	3	12/10/8*
6. Deadlifts	4	8/6/4/2*
7. Barbell Wrist Curl	3	12/10/8*
8. Barbell Reverse Wrist Curl	3	12/10/8*
9. Standing Calf Raise (Toe Raise)	5	15/12/10/8/6*

Tuesday and Friday

Exercise	Sets	Reps
1. Incline Leg Raise	2–3	20–30
2. Bench Press	5	10/8/6/4/2*
3. Incline Press	3	8/6/4*
4. Military Press	4	8/6/4/2*
5. Barbell Curl	4	10/8/6/4*
6. Lying Triceps Extension	4	12/10/8/6*
7. Seated Calf Raise (Toe Raise)	5	15/12/10/8/6*

* These exercises should be pyramidded.

In conjunction with the weight-gaining diet presented earlier and the recuperative procedures outline next, these weight-gaining routines will allow a man to gain one or two pounds of solid muscle mass each month and a woman up to one pound of new muscle tissue per month.

Recuperation

The most common cause of insufficient gains in muscle mass is the failure to recuperate fully between workouts. Your muscles will not grow in mass and strength until your body has recuperated fully from the previous workout. If you train again before your muscles have recuperated and gained in mass, you will fail to make good muscle gains. It is even possible to lose muscle mass if you do not allow yourself to recuperate fully between workouts, because your body will metabolize the protein in muscle tissue to meet unfulfilled energy needs.

You will most likely fail to recuperate fully if you train too frequently or take workouts that are too long. For this reason, you should never train more than four times per week when you are concentrating on gaining muscle mass. It also is important never to do more than 8–10 total sets for each major muscle group (6–8 total sets for smaller muscle groups like the arms) when gaining muscle mass, since doing an excessive number of sets can disrupt the recuperative process.

As described in Chapter 2, you must also be certain to sleep and rest sufficiently each day to allow your body to recuperate fully. You should also avoid energy leaks during the day. Avoid excessive aerobic training and attempt to maintain a tranquil mind at all times. Emotional energy leaks can be disastrous to the recuperative cycle.

Power Training

As when gaining muscle mass, you will train with low reps and heavy weights on basic exercises when you are training especially for added strength. But when training for power, your pyramid will consist of a lower range of repetitions than you used to gain muscle mass. Typically, your rep range will be 6–1, 5–1, or 4–1, decreasing the reps by one on succeeding sets.

Great strength is less a function of huge muscles than of tendon/ligament strength and the ability to will the contraction of a great number of muscle fibers on command. These abilities are best developed by doing 1–3 reps with very heavy weights. It is counterproductive, however, to do a maximum-weight single repetition on any exercise more frequently than once every two or three weeks, since going for a max single too often can quickly lead to overtraining.

Taking the foregoing suggestions into consideration, here is a good four-day-per-week split routine that you can use to augment your power.

Monday and Thursday

Exercise	Sets	Reps
1. Incline Sit-Up	2–3	20–30
2. Hyperextension	2–3	10–15
3. Squat	6	6/5/4/3/2/1*
4. Deadlift	5	5/4/3/2/1*
5. Barbell Bent Rowing	5	8/6/5/4/4*
6. Barbell Curl	4	6/5/4/3*
7. Standing Calf Raise (Toe Raise)	5	12/10/8/6/5*

Tuesday and Friday

Exercise	Sets	Reps
1. Incline Leg Raise	2–3	20–30
2. Bench Press	5	5/4/3/2/1*
3. Incline Press	3	4/3/2*
4. Military Press	4	5/4/3/2*
5. Lying Triceps Extension	4	8/6/5/4*
6. Barbell Wrist Curl	4	12/10/8/6*
7. Seated Calf Raise (Toe Raise)	5	12/10/8/6/5*

* These exercises should be pyramidded.

You should follow such a training routine for six to eight weeks once or twice per year. This will allow you to greatly increase your ability to handle heavier exercise poundages, which in turn dramatically increases your muscle mass.

Training to Failure

Any experienced bodybuilder will tell you that pushing a set to the limit will give you maximum response in terms of muscle mass and strength gain. Therefore, once you have warmed up thoroughly, you should go to failure on each remaining set of a movement. This means continuing a set in strict form until you literally can no longer do a full repetition. Training like this will give you a great response from each set.

There are two techniques through which you can actually push a fatigued muscle group past the point of failure, thereby receiving even more muscle-building benefits from a set. These techniques are *cheating* and *forced reps,* which will be discussed in detail in Chapter 6.

Changing Routines

If you stay on the same training program for an excessively long period of time, you may become bored with it and cease to make fast gains when following it. Therefore, you should periodically change to a new routine—the main

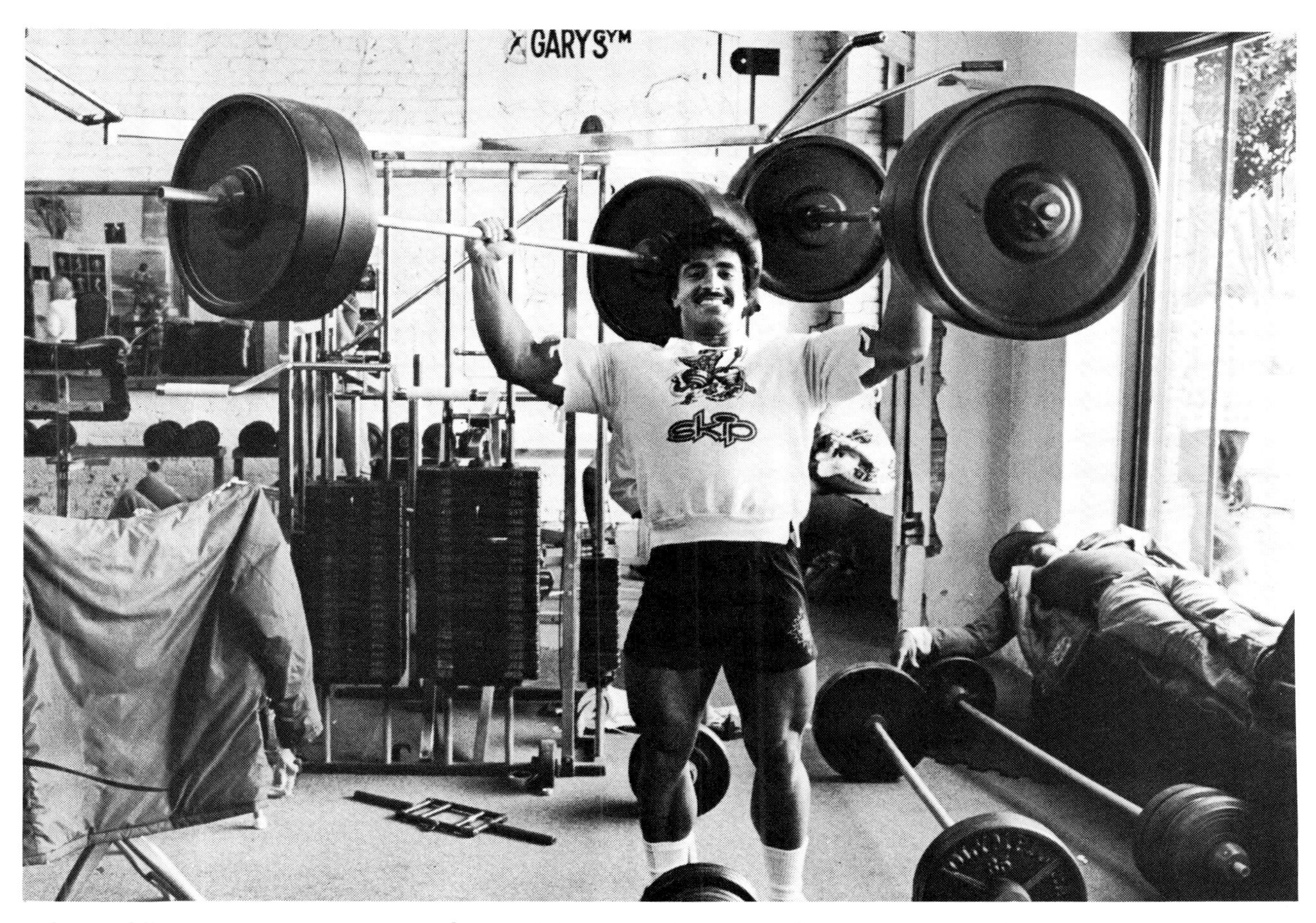

The world's strongest man? No, merely Mr. Universe Samir Bannout horsing around with prop weights at one of the many film productions shot at Gold's Gym. *(Photo by John Balik)*

reason why we have presented several workouts at the ends of chapters 3, 5, and 7.

There are three schools of thought on how frequently you should change routines. The two extremes of thought are represented by two of the sport's most noted actors, Lou Ferrigno *(The Incredible Hulk, Hercules)* and Arnold Schwarzenegger *(Conan the Barbarian).*

Ferrigno prefers to change his workouts from day to day, following a sort of "nonroutine routine." He has written, "This is the only way I can maintain peak interest in my training and hence make optimal progress. If I stay on a set routine, I very quickly become bored with my workouts."

Schwarzenegger, in contrast, seldom alters his training program appreciably. He believes that there are only a limited number of exercises and combinations of exercises that work for each bodybuilder. And once a bodybuilder finds these exercises and combinations, he or she should stick with them. "I've used basically the same biceps routine for virtually the entire time I have been bodybuilding," Arnold notes.

A majority of bodybuilders—typified by champs such as Boyer Coe, Ed Corney, Laura Combes, Danny Padilla, and Valerie Mayers—stick to the middle ground and change their training programs every 4–6 weeks. As you gradually develop your own unique training philosophy, it would doubtless be most sensible to start out by changing your workouts each 4–6 weeks.

Free Weights vs. Machines

In recent years there has been considerable controversy over the pros and cons of free weights compared to exercise machines. As discussed in Chapter 2, both types of apparatus have advantages, and a bodybuilder would profit most from using both types of equipment in his or her workouts. That's why Gold's Gym has made it a point to equip the gym with free weights and a variety of exercise machines.

The primary advantage of free weights and related benches, pulleys, and other apparatus lies in the huge number of possible exercises that can be done for each body part using them. Each type of machine allows only one to three exercises for each muscle group, while literally hundreds of movements can be done for each body part when using free weights and related apparatus.

Most exercise machines, however, are biomechanically constructed to stress a working muscle group more directly than free weight. This is because they offer such features as variable resistance and rotary resistance. You will, though, pay dearly for these features. Most types of exercise machines are far too expensive for the average person to purchase. And that's the reason why you'll seldom see such machines outside of a large commercial bodybuilding gym like Gold's.

Virtually all of the champions who train at Gold's Gym use the widest possible variety of free weights and exercise machines in their workouts. As a result, they achieve a much better quality of muscular development than those men and women who train exclusively with weights or exclusively with exercise machines.

Basic vs. Isolation Exercises

Earlier we defined basic exercises as those movements that work the body's large muscles with heavy weights in conjunction with other smaller body parts. Here is a list of the best basic exercises for each of the four major muscle groups.

Thighs—Squat, Partial Squat, Front Squat, Leg Press
Back—Upright Rowing, Deadlift, Barbell/Dumbbell Bent Rowing, Seated Pulley Rowing
Chest—Barbell/Dumbbell Bench Press (at all angles), Parallel Bar Dip
Shoulder—Barbell/Dumbbell Standing Press, Press Behind the Neck, Upright Rowing

Isolation exercises, in contrast, are done with lighter weights and provide direct stress to a single muscle group or a segment of a muscle group in relative isolation from the rest of the body. Here is a list of the best basic exercises for each body part.

Abdominals—Crunch, Side Bend
Calves—Seated/Standing Calf Raise
Thighs—Leg Extension, Leg Curl
Back—Pullover
Chest—Flye (at all angles), Cable Crossovers, Pec Deck Flye
Shoulders—Dumbbell/Cable Side Lateral, Dumbbell/Cable/Barbell Front Raise, Dumbbell/Cable Bent Lateral
Biceps—Barbell/Dumbbell Concentration Curl
Triceps—Pulley Pushdown
Forearms—Barbell/Dumbbell Wrist Curl, Barbell/Dumbbell Reverse Wrist Curl

Generally speaking, basic exercises are best for building general muscle mass and power, while isolation movements are useful for shaping and defining the various body parts, particularly just prior to a competition. Basic exercises are used year-round, but more heavily in the off-season than prior to competing. Isolation movements are also performed year-round, but far more heavily during the final few weeks before a bodybuilding contest.

Heavy vs. Light Training

Some bodybuilders, such as two-time Mr. Olympia Franco Columbu, train with very heavy weights at all times. In a way, this is a good practice, because—as we have mentioned—there is a direct relationship between the weights you use and the size of your muscles. And in a way it's a bad practice, because it is far easier to incur an injury when using maximum training weights. Even if you avoid a traumatic injury when using heavy poundages, the constant wear and tear that they put on your joints can cause long-term degenerative problems.

A few pumpers use almost exclusively light weights in all of their training sessions. They generally avoid injury, but they don't build large muscles or very much muscle quality.

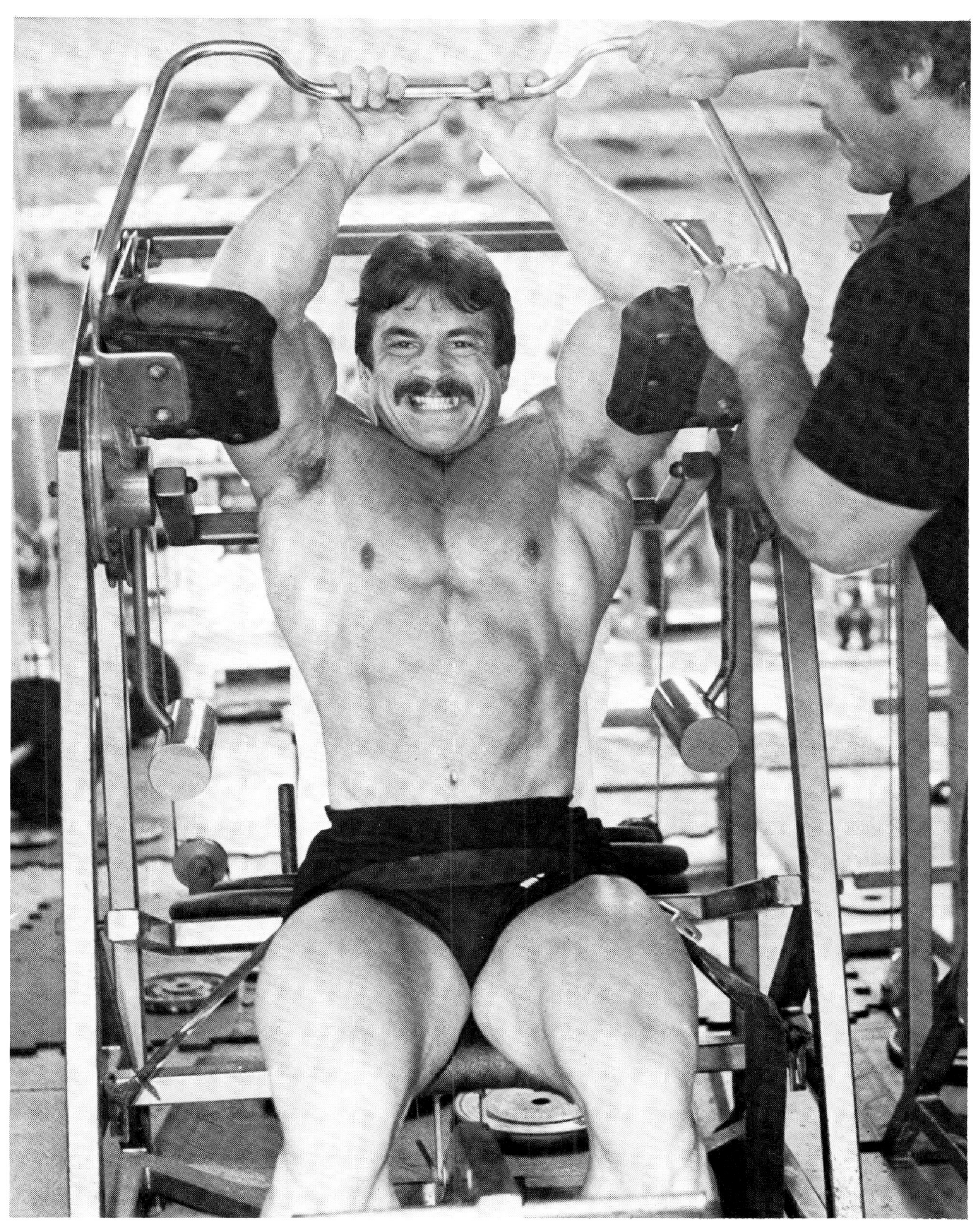

"Mr. Heavy Duty," Mike Mentzer (Mr. America, Mr. North America, and Mr. Universe) receives forced reps from Kent Keuhn (Past-40 Mr. America and Past-40 Mr. Universe) on a heavy set of Nautilus Pullovers at Gold's II.
(Photo by Bill Reynolds)

Overall, it's best to use moderately heavy poundages following a good warm-up in your routines. Occasionally, when you feel particularly energetic, you can use maximum weights in a workout. Training in this manner is both safe and enjoyable, and such workouts will build impressive muscle mass and quality.

Ultimately, you may discover that heavy training is very appropriate for your temperament and unique physical makeup. If this is the case, be very careful to use strictly correct biomechanical positionings in all exercises. You should also use a slow and smooth movement on each rep rather than jerking the weight anywhere along an exercise's range of motion. If you follow these two suggestions, you should be able to avoid traumatic joint and muscle injuries. You can also lessen the severity of any possible joint degeneration.

Split Routines

During your first year of bodybuilding training you will gradually add to the total number of sets that you perform for each muscle group. Eventually, this practice will make it difficult to finish a full-body workout in one session, since your native energy reserves are insufficient to handle the large total number of sets you are required to do.

At this point you should switch to doing a split routine in which you divide your body into halves, doing each part twice per week on a four-day split routine. Here are three different methods of following this type of split routine.

ROUTINE A

Monday and Thursday	Tuesday and Friday
Chest	Thighs
Back	Upper Arms
Shoulders	Forearms
Calves-Abdominals	Calves-Abdominals

ROUTINE B

Monday and Thursday	Tuesday and Friday
Chest	Thighs
Shoulders	Back
Triceps	Biceps
Forearms	Calves-Abdominals
Calves-Abdominals	

ROUTINE C

Monday and Thursday	Tuesday and Friday
Thighs	Back
Chest	Shoulders
Biceps	Triceps
Forearms	Calves-Abdominals
Calves-Abdominals	

This is the type of split routine you will use for the first year or two of your training. Eventually, though, you will wish to progress to using a five-day split routine.

The most commonly used five-day split routine involves first splitting the body into halves, using one of the three splits outlined above. Then, during the first week, half of Routine A is done on Monday, Wednesday, and Friday; half of Routine B is done on Tuesday and Thursday. During Week 2, half of Routine B is done on Monday, Wednesday, and Friday; half of Routine A is done on Tuesday and Thursday. Week 3 is a repeat of Week 1 and so on. In all cases Saturday and Sunday are rest days.

There are two types of six-day split routines, one in which each major muscle group is trained twice per week and one in which each major muscle group is bombed three times per week. Few bodybuilders use the second type of six-day split for more than a few weeks just prior to a contest, when they are trying to harden up their physiques. To do it regularly would quickly lead to overtraining, fatigue and loss of muscle mass, and vulnerability to injury.

With the first alternative, the body is split into three parts and trained in this manner.

Monday and Thursday	Tuesday and Friday	Wednesday and Saturday
Chest	Shoulders	Thighs
Upper Back	Upper Arms	Lower Back
Calves-Abdominals	Forearms	Calves-Abdominals

Again, Sunday is a full day of rest. This type of split routine has been used successfully by numerous champion bodybuilders, most notably Lou Ferrigno, Lisa Elliott, Jusup Wilkosz, and Carla Dunlap.

The six-day split in which each muscle group

is trained three times per week again involves splitting the body into halves. Then one half is trained on Mondays, Wednesdays, and Fridays; the other half on Tuesdays, Thursdays, and Saturdays. As with the first six-day split routine, Sunday is a day of full rest from bodybuilding training.

Supination

To get the most out of your biceps training you must understand the kinesiology of your biceps. Your biceps muscles bend your arm fully from a straight position, as all bodybuilders know. They also supinate the hands, however, and many bodybuilders unwittingly ignore this function as they train their biceps.

Supination involves rotating your hand from a position with your palm downward to a position with your palm upward. This function can't be duplicated when using a barbell or curling machine to train your biceps, but it can be accomplished conveniently when using dumbbells for Curls.

Let's assume that you are doing Dumbbell Curls. Begin with both palms facing your thighs. As you curl the weights upward, rotate your thumbs outward, until your palms are facing upward at the conclusion of the movement. Reverse this supination movement, a motion called *pronation,* as you lower the weights. By utilizing supination in this manner, you can develop considerably higher-quality biceps muscles than if you merely did Barbell Curls with no supination.

Weightlifting Belts and Body Wraps

Weightlifters and powerlifters habitually wear weightlifting belts to add stability to the midbody and protect their lower back from injury. For the same reasons many bodybuilders wear a weightlifting belt while training. A lifting belt is particularly valuable when doing Squats, back exercises such as Deadlifts and Bent Rowing, and all forms of overhead pressing.

These thick leather belts come in four-inch and six-inch widths, as measured at the back of the belt. Only the four-inch belt can be worn in lifting competitions, but the six-inch belt gives more lower back support than the four-inch version. It would be best to wear the six-inch belt while training. Weightlifting belts range in price from about $30 to more than $50 for custom-made models.

Two basic types of body wraps are used to support and protect an injured joint or muscle group. Neoprene rubber body bands provide minimal actual support for an injured joint, but the rubber effectively retains body heat around the joint, and this has considerable therapeutic value. These rubber bands are most commonly used around the knees, the waist (for a lower back injury), or the belly of an injured muscle.

Elastic gauze bandages strongly support injured joints, such as the wrist or knee. Some bodybuilders use a combination of elastic bandages and rubber body bands over a particularly tender joint. Dennis Tinerino (Pro Mr. Universe) is one such bodybuilder. First he places the neoprene bands around his knees; then he slips on his sweat pants and wraps the elastic gauze around his knees over the sweats. Then he can do heavy Squats and other thigh work in complete comfort and safety.

Bodybuilding Facts for Women

Since the authors of this book are both men, we turned to eminently qualified Lynne Pirie, an orthopedic surgeon from Phoenix, Arizona, who has placed as high as third in the 1982 Women's World Bodybuilding Championships, for data on uniquely female factors in bodybuilding. Lynne is quite articulate and we are fortunate that she candidly discussed each factor in the type of layperson's terms that anyone can understand.

"As a physician and competitive bodybuilder, I have been quite interested in a variety of specifically female factors in bodybuilding and weight training," Dr. Pirie told us. "Among these factors are birth control and competitive bodybuilding, menstruation and amenorrhea, pregnancy and childbirth, menopause, and anorexia nervosa."

Birth Control

"Many sexually active women bodybuilders are on birth control pills," Lynne noted, "but because of their estrogen and progesterone con-

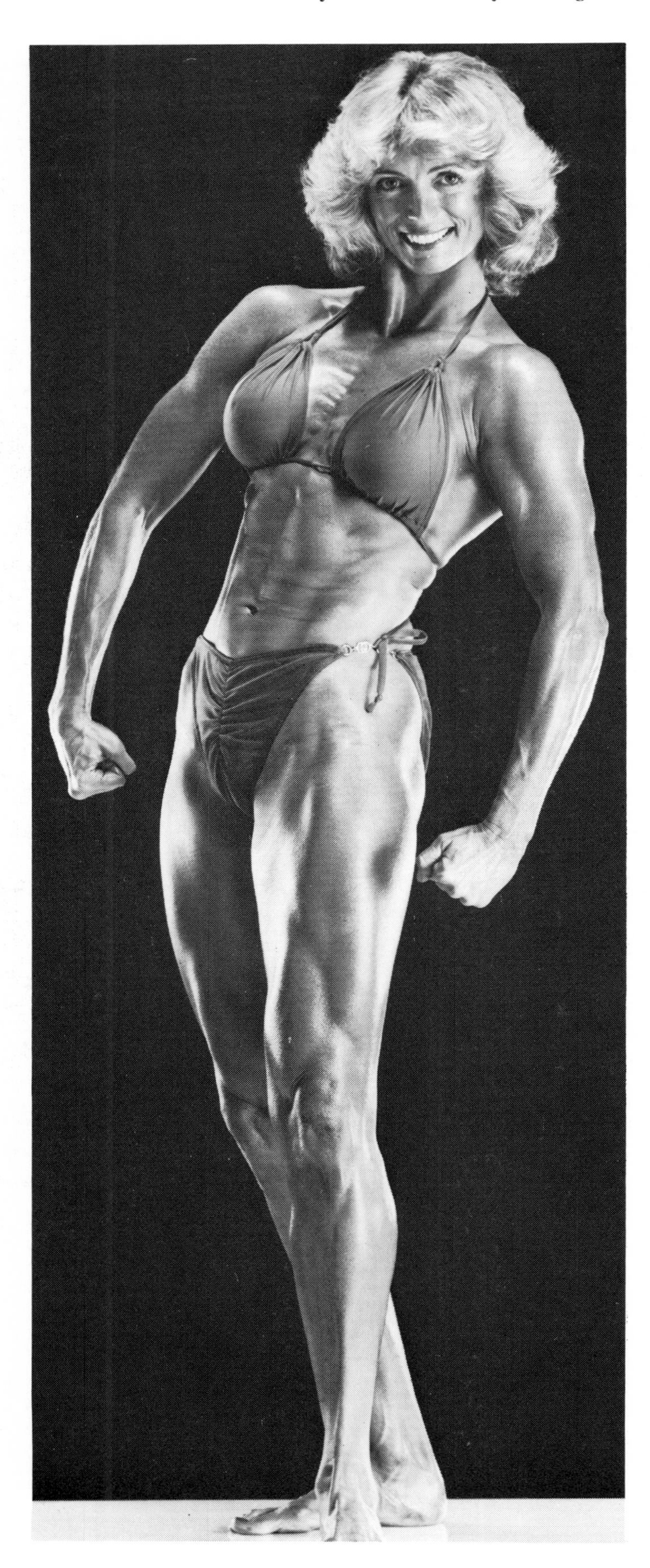

Dr. Lynne Pirie. *(Photo by John Balik)*

tent these pills can cause significant water retention. This is particularly true just before the menstrual cycle begins, and it can be a problem for many women bodybuilders. A woman doesn't know if the extra weight is body fat or retained water, and it's very hard to peak for a competition under such circumstances.

"Few women understand that progesterone has a protein catabolic effect. In other words, it breaks down muscle tissue, the exact opposite effect desired by a bodybuilder. So, the progesterone in oral contraceptives contraindicates the use of birth control pills by any serious woman bodybuilder.

"There also are other facts that contraindicate the use of birth control pills, and these are evident in a woman's medical history. One of these is the possibility of blood clotting. If you are dehydrating—and many women bodybuilders use a diuretic to bring out the maximum degree of muscular definition—you are going to increase thromboembolytic potential (that is, you will increase your body's potential to form blood clots).

"Blood clots are most likely to be very small, but they can occasionally be large as well. Small clots can damage various organs, such as the spleen, liver, kidneys, or any organ through which blood flows. Larger clots can cause strokes by blocking blood flow to part of the brain.

"If a woman is taking birth control pills and using anabolic steroids to increase muscle mass, she can do herself great damage. I don't know of any actual research that has been aimed specifically at this problem, but I can tell you that such a practice throws the whole endocrine system out of balance. It changes your entire hormonal environment. If you have a dormant tumor in your body and it responds to the new environment, it could grow with disastrous consequences. Steroids can also destroy your entire neural-hormonal axis, which can affect every organ system in your body. In short, it's much worse to take steroids if a woman is taking birth control pills than if she is not, and it's very bad for a woman to take steroids under any circumstances.

"So, what birth control method should a sexually active woman bodybuilder use? The use of an IUD was once considered quite safe, but with an IUD there is always a danger of perforation of the uterus or of the body outright rejecting the device. An IUD is made of metal and is foreign to the human body, so if the uterus doesn't want one, it'll try to reject it.

"Sometimes IUDs have actually gone through the wall of the uterus, and if the perforation is serious enough, it can force a hysterectomy. If a woman has never had children, that's a very high price to pay.

"I personally recommend the use of a diaphragm. It's a minor inconvenience at times, but it only takes a couple of minutes to insert one. Correctly used, a diaphragm is an effective birth control device. And, in a health sense, it is a safe one to use."

Menstruation and Amenorrhea

"There appears to be an optimum level of exercise that assists menstruation and relieves menstrual complications but still does not interfere with menstrual function," Dr. Pirie said. "The menstrual cramps that younger women often experience can definitely be eased by exercise, but excessive exercise can affect menstrual function.

"There are certain anti-inflammatory products, such as wine and tryptophane, that can relieve menstrual cramping to a small degree. Overall, however, exercise does a better job of relieving cramps.

"Bodybuilding, track, gymnastics, and other sports that require a low body weight and involve a high degree of stress can cause amenorrhea, or a cessation of menses. This is probably due to a very quick weight loss and/or general stress.

"Delayed menses are relatively common among girls who are serious bodybuilders, dancers, gymnasts, runners, or who participate in other strenuous sports and must maintain a low degree of body fat. There appears to be a height-weight ratio that must be achieved before such a young woman will menstruate.

"There is considerable speculation on whether or not an amenorrheic woman ovulates, but there is no scientific evidence to support either stand. Therefore, it would be foolish to assume that amenorrhea is an effective birth control system. Without relying on other forms of birth control, you could become pregnant.

"All of the investigations I have done on amenorrhea indicates that the condition is not dangerous. The menses simply seem to resume as soon as a woman's body weight goes back up to a 'normal' level.

"Unfortunately, many gynecologists are not experienced in treating amenorrhea, and they immediately prescribe hormonal therapy to induce menses. Such a procedure is both expensive and unnecessary. To resume your menses, simply gain body weight and perhaps reduce your physical activity level."

Pregnancy and Childbirth

"If a woman bodybuilder has been training regularly prior to becoming pregnant, she can profitably continue to work out," Dr. Pirie reported. "It's not a good idea, however, for an out-of-shape woman to commence hard training once she discovers she's pregnant. A pregnant woman shouldn't be doing anything physically that she's not used to. And it's important to avoid overtraining, which can cause anoxia (a deficiency of oxygen) to the fetus.

"Many women athletes have continued to train fairly vigorously up to and through the seventh and eighth months of their pregnancies. The better a woman's musculature, the better control she can have over her own delivery. This also takes into consideration such athletic-related abilities as self-control, self-discipline, and the ability to control pain. A woman who is in very good physical condition can push down harder and deliver more quickly. There's a lot of pain associated with childbirth, and a woman who is used to training in pain can handle it better.

"Nutritionally, a woman bodybuilder should make the same changes in her diet that any other pregnant woman should make, including an increased intake of folic acid and other vitamins. A pregnant woman bodybuilder should not be dieting—or training—for a contest. This should be obvious, but it must be said nonetheless, considering the competitive nature of most bodybuilders.

"After giving birth, all women are concerned with regaining their prepregnancy appearance and physical condition. Any woman who remained in excellent physical condition during her pregnancy will have a full and rapid recovery following childbirth. As a footnote, numerous champion women bodybuilders have had children and yet regained such superb condition that they have been consistent winners in bodybuilding competition."

Menopause

Dr. Pirie revealed, "There has been little research on the relationship between exercise and menopause, and none on the relationship between bodybuilding and menopause. I can only give you an informed opinion on it.

"Menopause is a time of general deterioration of the body as a consequence of the natural aging process. The effects of bodybuilding are in the reverse direction; that is bodybuilding promotes tissue growth rather than atrophy. Thus, regular bodybuilding and weight training will probably help minimize the negative effects of menopause."

Anorexia Nervosa

"Anorexia nervosa, a mental-physical disorder that affects primarily women (and more women from the upper middle class than from any other socioeconomic group), has gained considerable publicity in recent years," Dr. Pirie stated. "It is characterized by prolonged fasting or subsistence on a bare minimum of calories, as well as by frequent endurance-type exercise, all aimed at making an anorexic 'fashionably thin.' As the disorder becomes progressively more serious, it can be life-threatening.

"Anorexia nervosa is often difficult for a family member to identify, because anorexics become very devious about disguising their symptoms. They will even begin to pad their clothing to hide the fact that they are losing weight.

"While I personally know of no anorexic women bodybuilders, the requirements of the sport (strict dieting and copious exercise) can lead to anorexia nervosa. If a woman becomes anorexic, it's not something that should be handled by a friend in the gym or even by the family general practitioner. In my opinion, anorexia nervosa is a psychiatric emergency that should be treated only by a psychiatrist specifically experienced in handling the disorder. An anorexic should also be hospitalized in many cases.

"Bulemia is a related disease that also should be treated psychiatrically. Bulemics will gorge themselves with food and then purge themselves with a finger down the throat. As with anorexia nervosa, this is a potentially serious disorder that could occur to women in competitive bodybuilding, as well as in a variety of other sports."

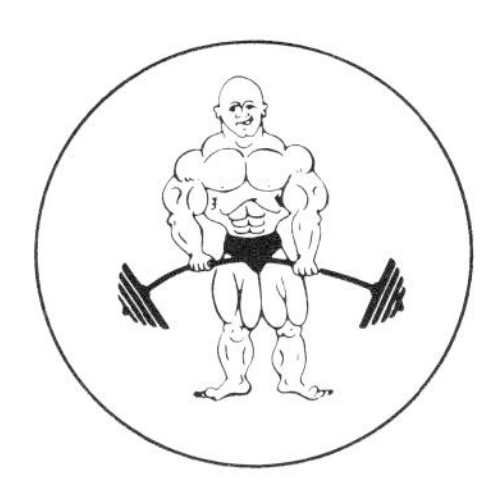

5 INTERMEDIATE-LEVEL EXERCISES & WORKOUTS

In Chapter 3 we began to develop a pool of bodybuilding exercises that you will use at various times for as long as you continue to train. In this chapter we will enlarge on that basic pool by fully describing and illustrating 35 additional movements.

At the end of the chapter we have also included several training routines suitable for use by an intermediate-level male or female bodybuilder. Using these programs sequentially, you can quickly work through the intermediate phase and go on to become an advanced bodybuilder.

Thigh Exercises

Hack Squat

General Comments: Most champion competitive bodybuilders consider the Hack Squat one of the best movements for developing front thigh cuts (definition) and adding mass to the area of the thighs just above the knees.

Starting Position: Place your feet flat on the angled foot platform at the bottom edge of the machine. Your heels should be placed six to eight inches apart, and your toes should be angled outward 30–45 degrees on each side. Bend your legs fully and place your back flat against the sliding platform of the machine. Grasp the handles at the sides of your hips and fully straighten your legs.

Exercise Performance: From this basic starting position, slowly bend your legs and lower your body downward under resistance until your legs are fully bent. As you lower your torso and the sliding platform, your knees should travel directly out over your feet. This means that your legs will spread apart as you bend your knees.

Once you reach the bottom position of the movement, slowly straighten your legs and return to the starting position. As you straighten your legs, be careful not to change your upper leg angle. You must also be careful not to bounce at the bottom of this or any other squatting movement.

Training Tips: Another version of the Hack Squat is used frequently by the champions at Gold's/Venice. In this variation two yokes are attached to the machine in such a way that you can rest them over your shoulders to bear the resistance provided by the machine. Two handles at the side of the machine act as "stops" to

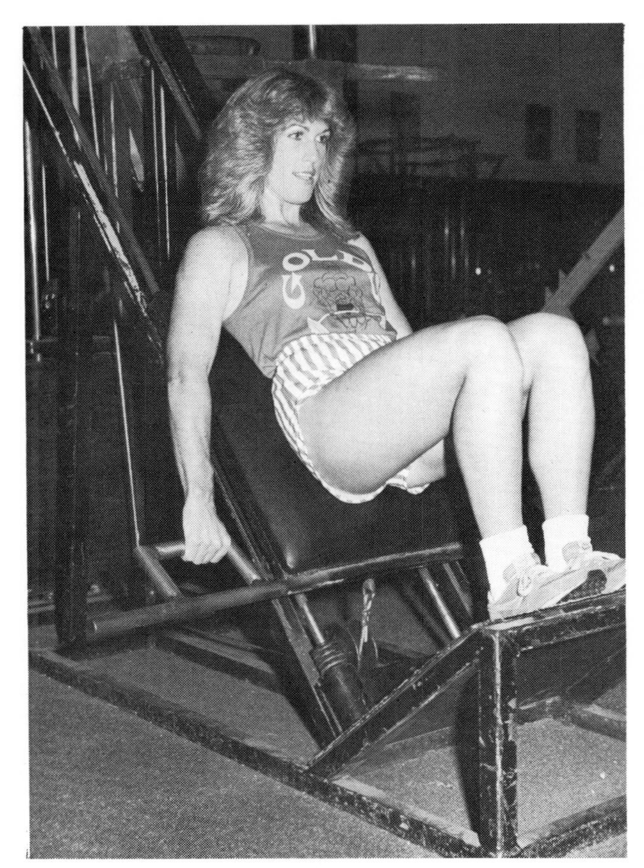
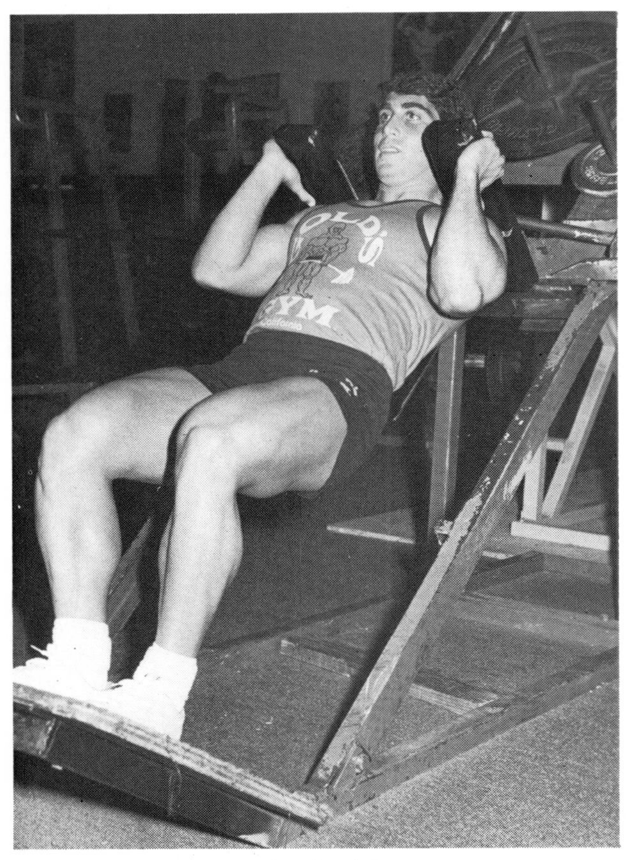

Hack Squat—platform machine finish, left; yoke variation near finish, right.

keep the machine in the finish position between sets. By rotating these stop handles outward you can release the machine for your set of Hack Squats. From there you will perform this variation of the Hack Squat the same as you do the original version.

Lunge

General Comments: This is an excellent movement for enhancing the cuts along the front thigh muscles, particularly at the upper edges of the muscle mass where the quadriceps tie into your hip structure. Lunges also tighten the buttock muscles.

Starting Position: Rest a barbell across your shoulders in the same manner as for the start of a Squat. Place your feet about shoulder width apart and point your toes directly forward. Stand erect.

Exercise Performance: Step forward 2½–3 feet with your left foot and place it flat on the floor. Keeping your back leg relatively straight, bend your left leg as fully as possible. Your torso should be held upright during this movement. At the bottom position your right leg will still be relatively straight and your knee will be between three and five inches from the floor. Your left knee will be bent fully and positioned several inches ahead of your left ankle. In the bottom position you will feel a strong stretching sensation in the thigh muscles of your back leg.

From the low position, slowly straighten your left leg and push yourself back to the starting position. Do the next repetition with your right foot forward. Alternate the foot that you put forward with every succeeding rep. Count one complete cycle with each foot forward as a full repetition.

Training Tips: You can do this movement while holding two dumbbells down at your sides with your arms straight. Some bodybuilders also do this exercise lunging upward onto a flat exercise bench with their forward foot. This variation tends to put more stress on the muscles of the back leg's thigh.

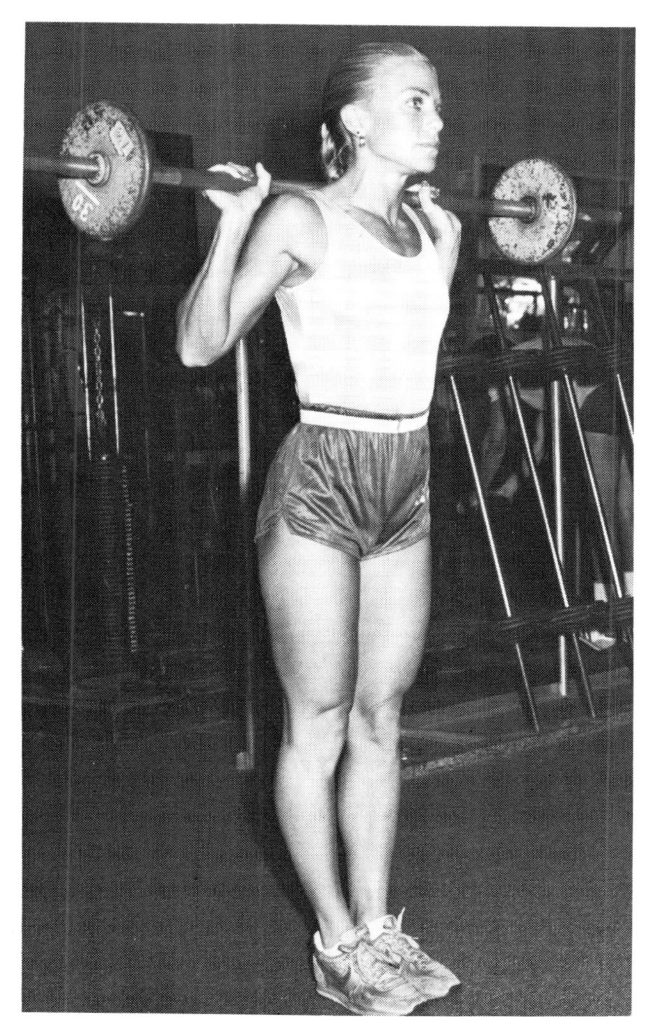

Front Squat

General Comments: This movement affects the same muscles as a Squat done with a barbell held across your shoulders behind your neck. Front Squats do stress the muscles just above the knees somewhat more than regular Squats.

Starting Position: Load up a barbell and place it on a Squat rack. Dip under it with your arms extended straight out from your shoulders. Rest the barbell across the base of your neck and your deltoids. Keeping your elbows up, fold your arms across the barbell. As long as your elbows are up as you do the movement, you can comfortably do Squats with the barbell held in this position. Once you have the barbell held securely in front of your neck, place your feet at about shoulder width, your toes pointed slightly outward.

Exercise Performance: Keeping your back as erect as possible, fully bend your legs, being sure that your knees travel directly outward over your feet. Pause for a second in the bottom position of the Squat, then recover to the starting point by straightening your legs. Repeat the movement for the required number of repetitions.

Lunge—start.

Lunge—finish.

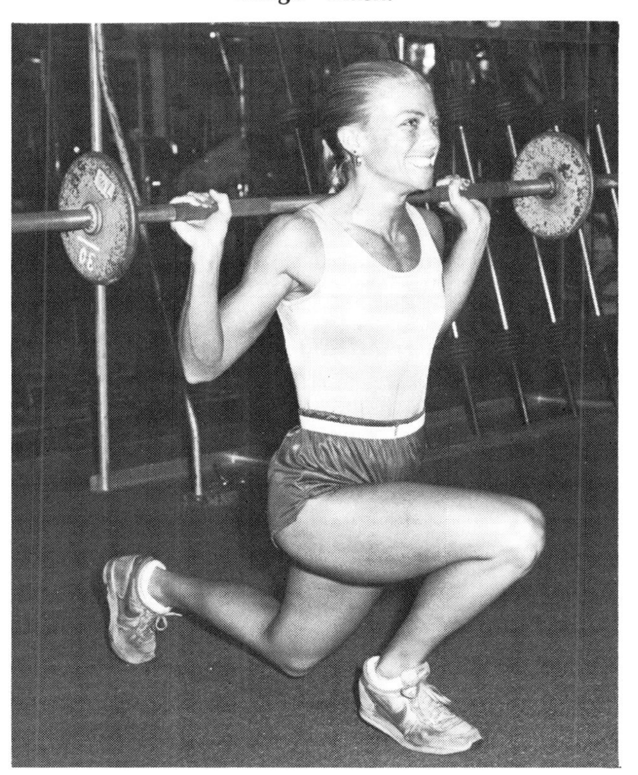

Front Squat—midpoint.

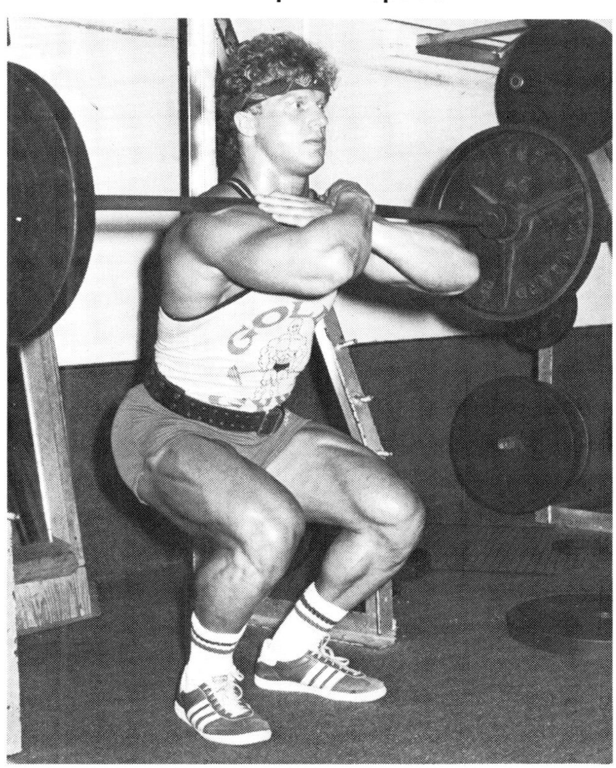

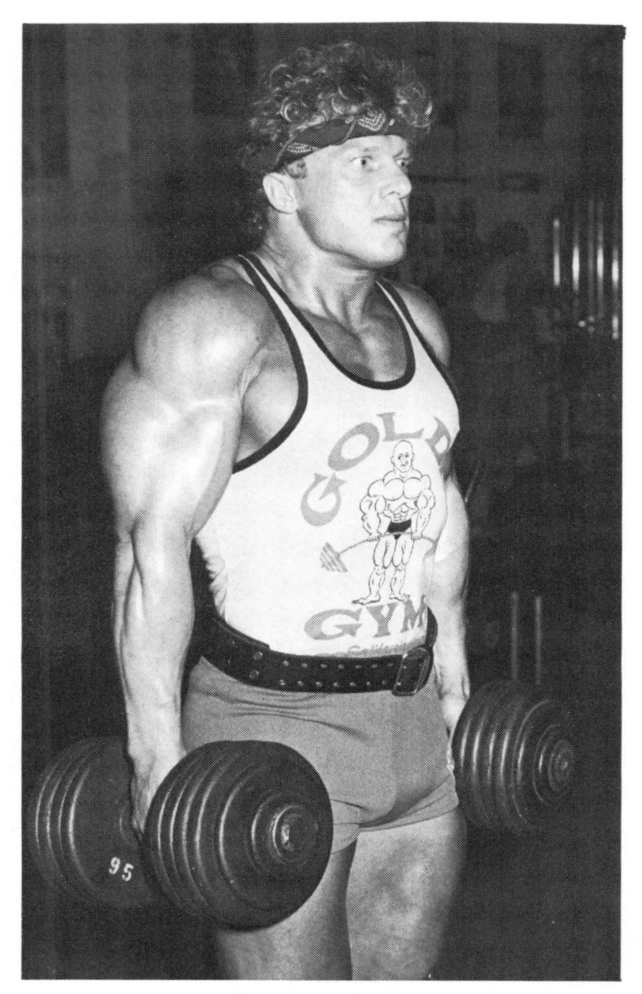

Dumbbell Shrug—finish.

Training Tips: Most bodybuilders find that they are forced to stand with their heels on a board to maintain good balance while doing Front Squats, even though they needn't use this board while doing regular Squats. You will probably also discover that you need to use a lifting belt more for Front Squats than for regular Squats.

Back Exercises

Dumbbell Shrug

General Comments: This exercise is somewhat better than a Barbell Shrug movement for developing the trapezius muscles, because it allows greater freedom of movement.

Starting Position: Grasp two heavy dumbbells and hang them down at your sides with your palms toward each other. Your arms should be held perfectly straight throughout the movement. Think of your arms merely as cables that attach your shoulder joints to the dumbbells.

Exercise Performance: Sag your shoulders downward and forward as far as possible. Then shrug your shoulders upward and backward as far as possible. You should actually touch the points of your shoulders to your ears at the top of the movement. Lower the dumbbells back to the starting position and repeat the movement for the desired number of repetitions.

Training Tips: Some bodybuilders actually use a rotating motion with the shoulders when they do Dumbbell Shrugs. You can rotate your shoulders both forward and backward for a good trapezius-building effect.

Stiff-Leg Deadlift

General Comments: This is a good exercise for adding strength and muscle mass to the lower back and hamstring muscles. Secondary

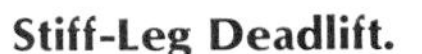
Stiff-Leg Deadlift.

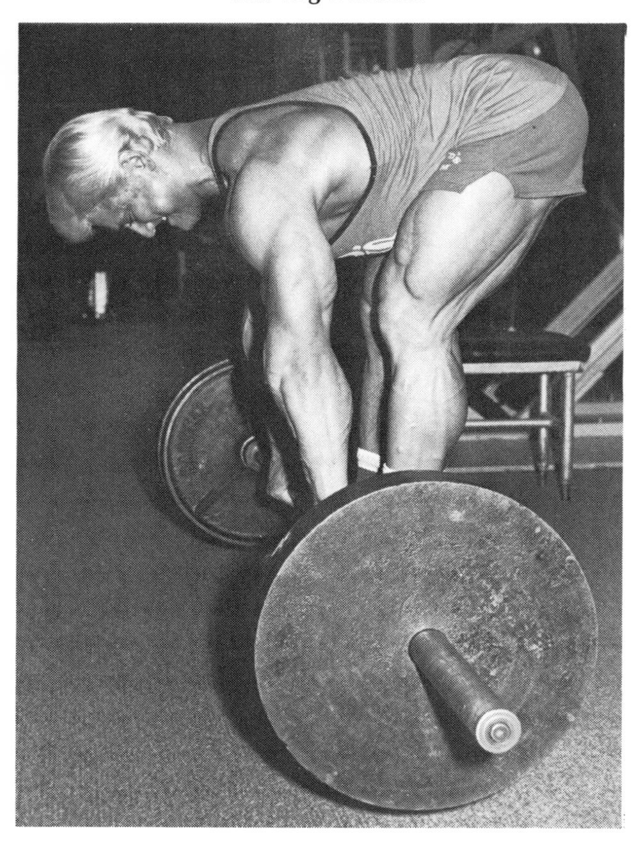

emphasis is placed on the gripping muscles of the forearms.

Starting Position: Grasp a barbell with a shoulder-width grip so that your palms are toward your body in the starting position of the movement. Stand on the padded surface of a flat exercise bench or on a high block of wood so that your feet are set at about shoulder width and your toes point directly ahead. Stand erect and hold your arms straight so that the barbell rests across your upper thighs.

Exercise Performance: Keeping your arms and legs held straight, slowly bend forward as far as you can. You will notice that by standing on an exercise bench or high block of wood you can lower the barbell much farther than if you were standing on the floor, since the plates of the barbell won't touch the floor prematurely. As soon as you have reached the bottom position, slowly return to the starting point of the movement. Repeat the movement for the required number of repetitions.

Training Tips: This exercise places your lower back in a weak mechanical position. It's essential, therefore, to warm up thoroughly before going heavy on it. You should also be careful to do the movement slowly and with no jerks.

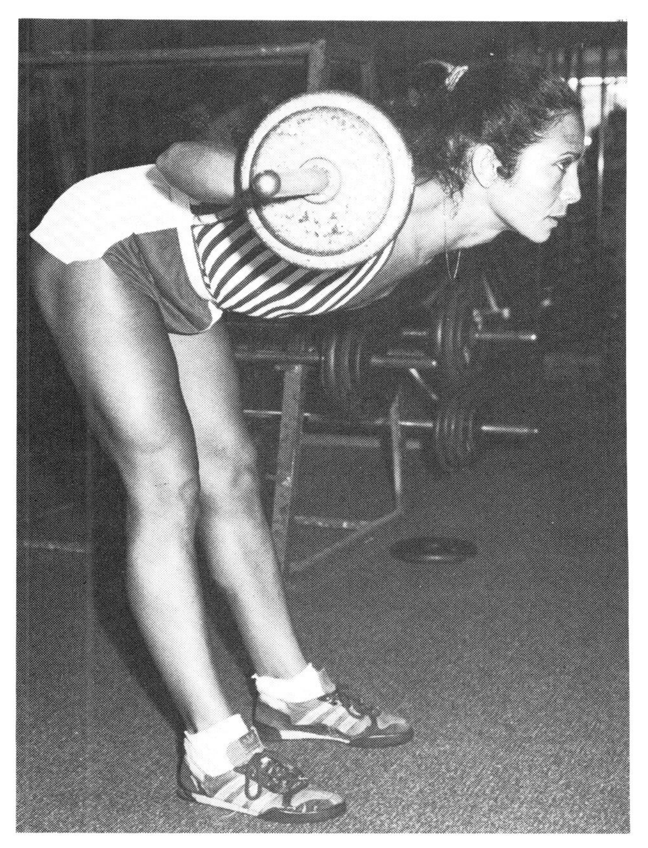

Good Morning—finish.

Good Mornings

General Comments: This exercise is similar in effect to Stiff-Leg Deadlifts. It develops the muscles of the lower back and hamstrings quite efficiently.

Starting Position: Pad the handle of a light barbell and place the barbell across your shoulders and behind your neck as for the start of a Squat. Place your feet approximately at shoulder width and point your toes directly forward. Grasp the handle of the barbell out toward the plates on each side. Straighten your legs.

Exercise Performance: Keeping your legs straight, slowly bend forward at the waist until your torso is parallel to the floor. Once you are warmed up you can actually go well below the parallel position with this movement. Return slowly to the starting position and repeat the movement.

Training Tips: If your lower back is at all sore, you should avoid this exercise. Again, be sure that you are thoroughly warmed up before going very heavy on the Good Morning movement.

Chin

General Comments: There are many variations of the Chin, and most bodybuilders use several of them to develop the flaring latissimus dorsi muscles of the upper back. Secondary stress is placed on the biceps and forearm muscles.

Starting Position: Jump up and grasp a chinning bar with your palms pointed forward and your hands set a little wider than shoulder width. Bend your legs anywhere from 45–70 degrees and cross your ankles. Hang motionless at arm's length below the bar.

Exercise Performance: Being sure that your elbows move downward and backward, bend your arms and pull your body up to the bar until your upper chest touches the bar. As you

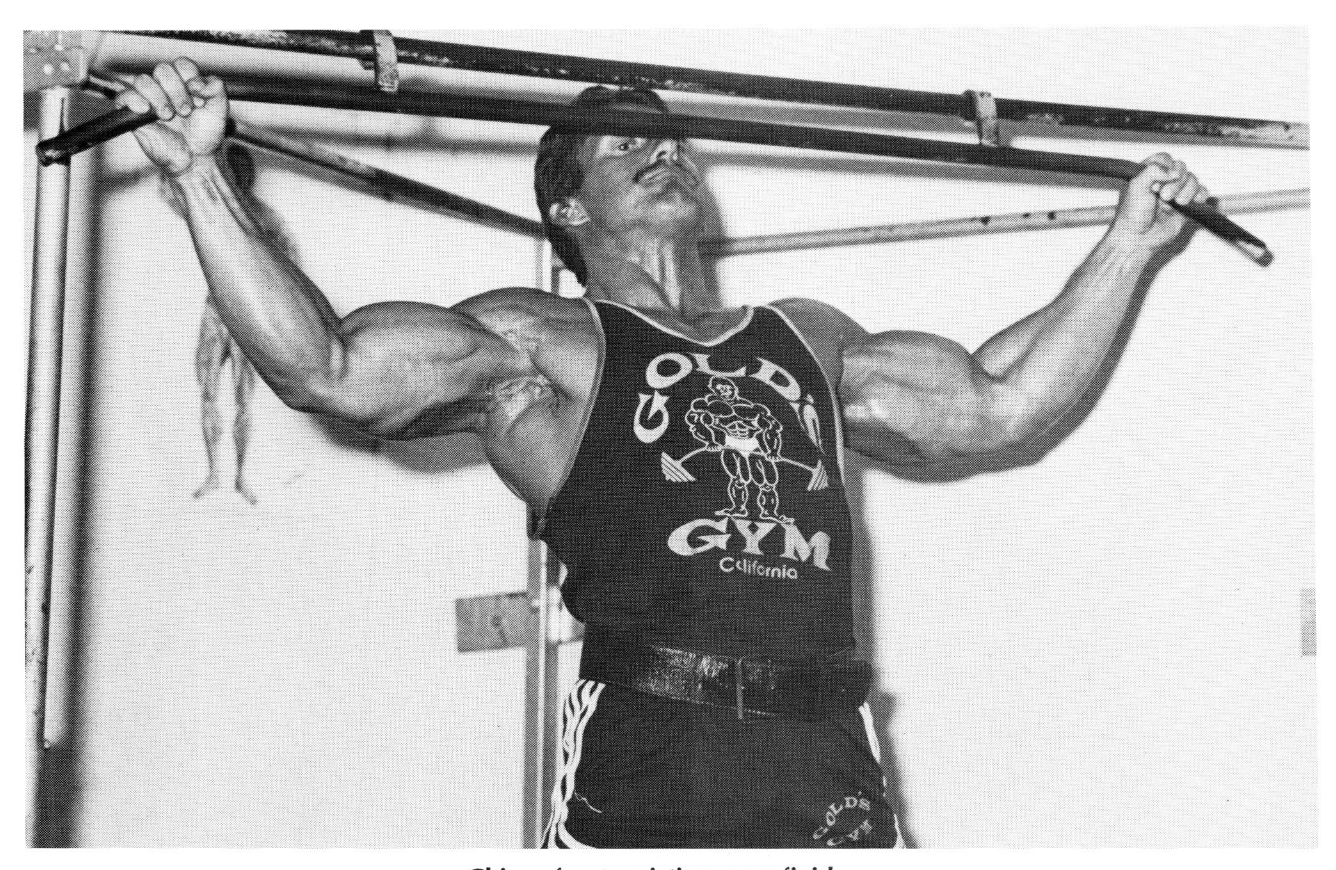

Chins—front variation, near finish.

pull your body up to the bar, you should arch your back, since your lats can't be contracted fully unless your back is arched. Slowly lower your body back to the starting point and repeat the movement for the required number of repetitions.

Training Tips: Many bodybuilders do Chins behind the neck by starting in an identical position to the Front Chins just described but pulling the torso up so the chinning bar touches the trapezius muscles at the back of the neck. You can do a number of other variations of the Front Chin and Chin behind the neck simply by varying the width of your grip. There is also a triangle-shaped chinning bar attachment that fits over the bar and allows a bodybuilder to do Narrow-Grip Chins with the hands set in a parallel grip.

Dumbbell Bent Rowing with one dumbbell, near finish.

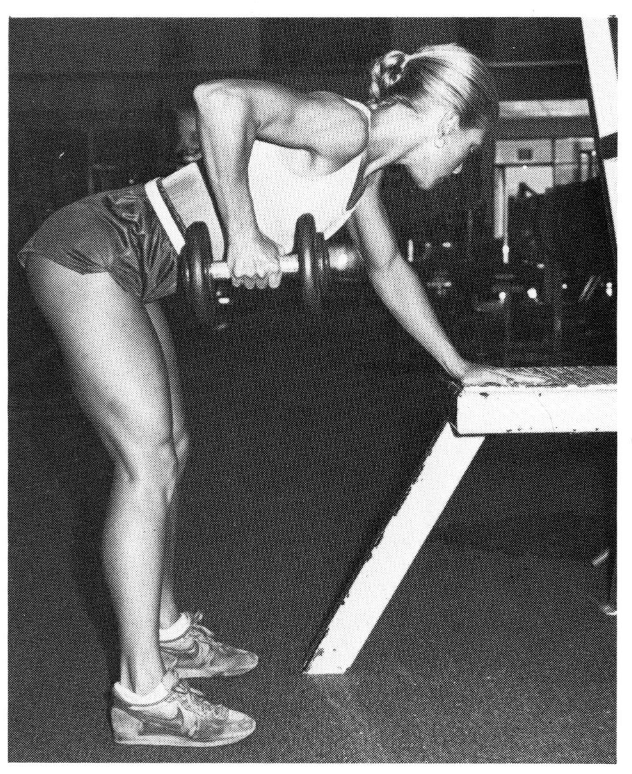

Dumbbell Bent Rowing

General Comments: This exercise is excellent for adding both width and thickness to the lats.

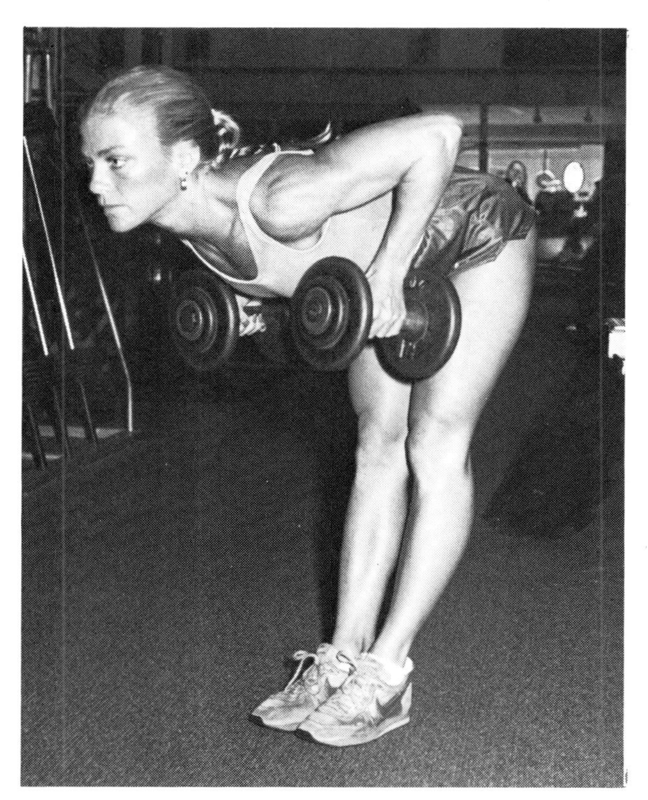

Dumbbell Bent Rowing with two dumbbells, finish.

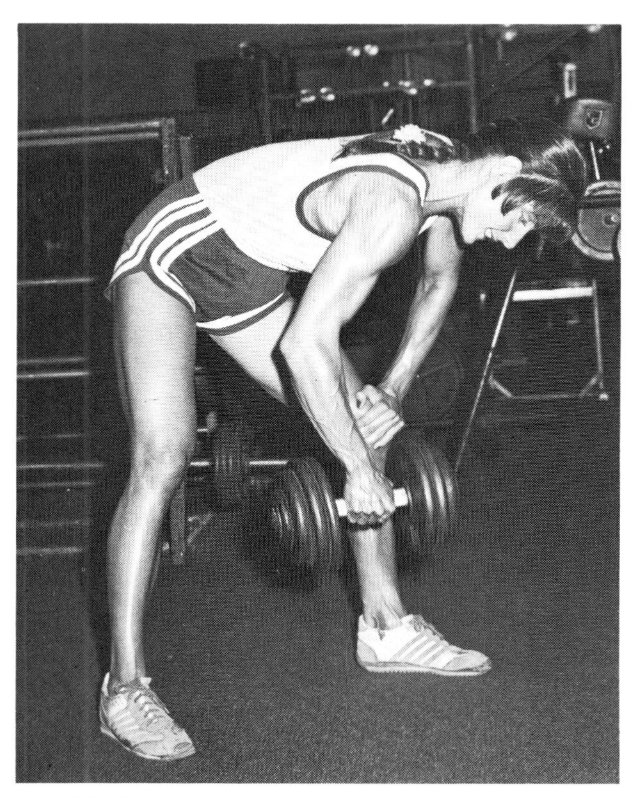

Dumbbell Bent Rowing with one dumbbell using knee for support, near start.

It is particularly good for bombing the lower lat insertions. Secondary stress is placed on the biceps, forearms, and posterior deltoid muscles.

Starting Position: Position yourself next to a flat exercise bench. As a support for your torso during the movement, place your left hand on the bench with your left arm straight. Extend your left leg forward about 1½ feet and bend it at a 45-degree angle. Extend your right leg to the rear about 2½ feet and hold it fairly straight. Grasp a relatively heavy dumbbell in your right hand and extend your right arm straight below your shoulder joint. Rotate your torso slightly toward the right to stretch the right lat.

Exercise Performance: Slowly pull the dumbbell directly upward until it touches the side of your torso. As you pull the dumbbell upward, rotate your torso slightly away from the exercising arm. Slowly lower the weight back to the starting point and repeat the movement for the required number of repetitions. Reverse your body position and perform an equal number of sets and reps with your right arm.

Training Tips: In recent years many bodybuilders have been doing this movement with the front leg fully bent and the knee resting on the padded surface of the flat exercise bench. You can also do this movement standing up, using two dumbbells simultaneously. A third variation, done with one arm at a time or both arms, is performed with the forehead resting on a padded surface at approximately waist level.

Chest Exercises

Parallel Bar Dips

General Comments: When done as a chest movement, this exercise is one of the favorite pectoral exercises of most bodybuilders. It strongly stresses the lower and outer areas of the pectoral muscles. Secondary stress is placed on the front deltoids and triceps.

Starting Position: Grasp a pair of parallel bars with your palms facing each other and jump up to support yourself above the bars on straight arms as illustrated. Tilt your head for-

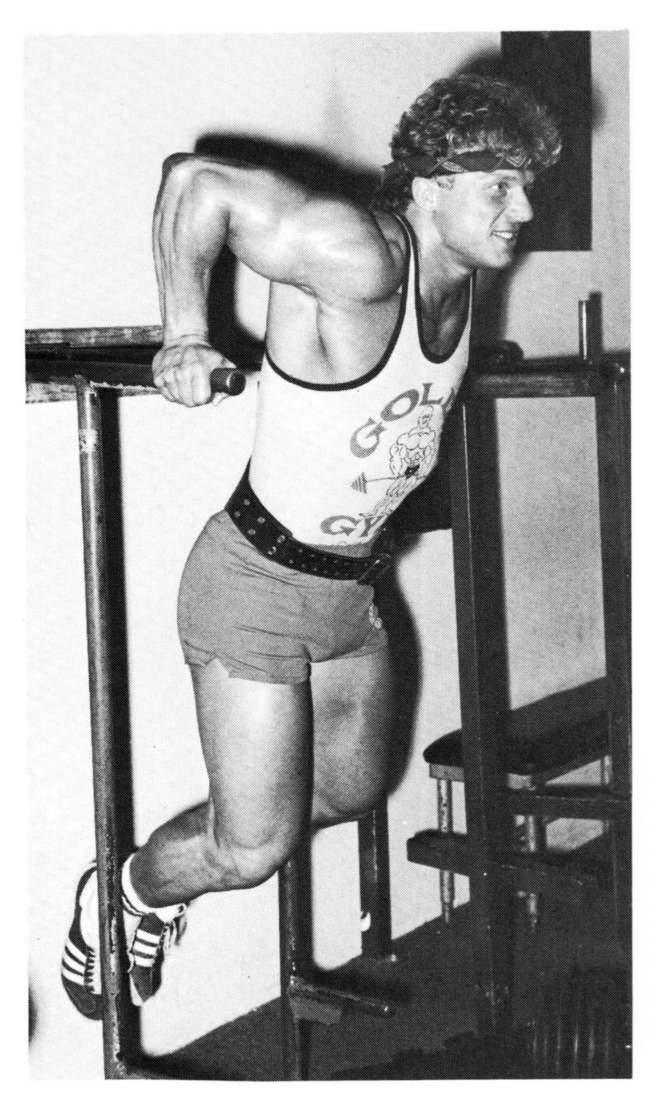

Parallel Bar Dip.

ward and bend your legs. This will help you lean into the movement as you do it.

Exercise Performance: Slowly bend your arms as fully as possible to lower your body down between the bars. You should try to bend your arms well past the point where they make a 90-degree angle between the upper arm and forearm. Push back up to the starting position by straightening your arms and repeat the movement for the desired number of repetitions.

Training Tips: By keeping your torso upright as you do Parallel Bar Dips, you can stress your triceps much more strongly than you do in the movement just described.

Some gyms, including Gold's/Venice, have bars that are about 32 inches wide on one end and angle inward on the other. These bars allow you to use a variety of grip widths when doing Dips. On the angled bars you will sometimes see a bodybuilder doing dips with his or her hands reversed, that is, with the palms facing away from each other.

Regardless of the variation of Parallel Bar Dips that you use, you will soon find that you can do the exercise relatively easily. At that point you can add resistance by tying a dumbbell or a barbell plate around your waist. This can easily be accomplished by tying a five-foot piece of rope in a loop. Step into the loop and position it around your waist. Then hang a dumbbell in the rope and wrap your legs around the dumbbell. If you hold the weight in this position, it will be very secure while you do your Dips.

Incline Dumbbell Press—midpoint.

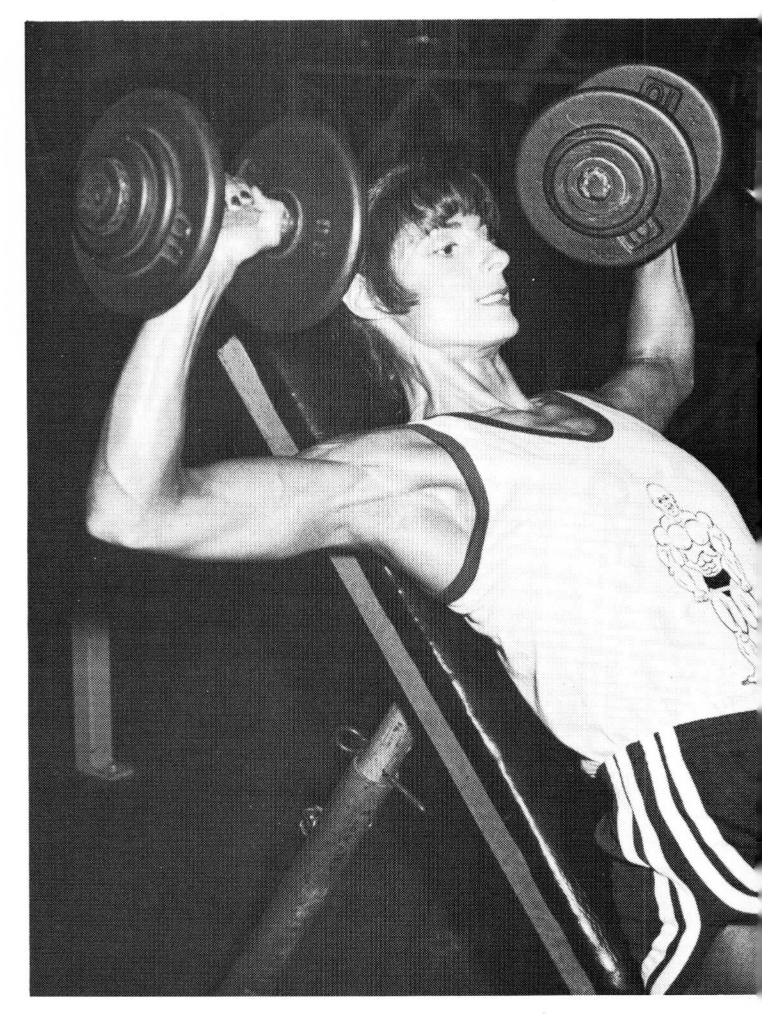

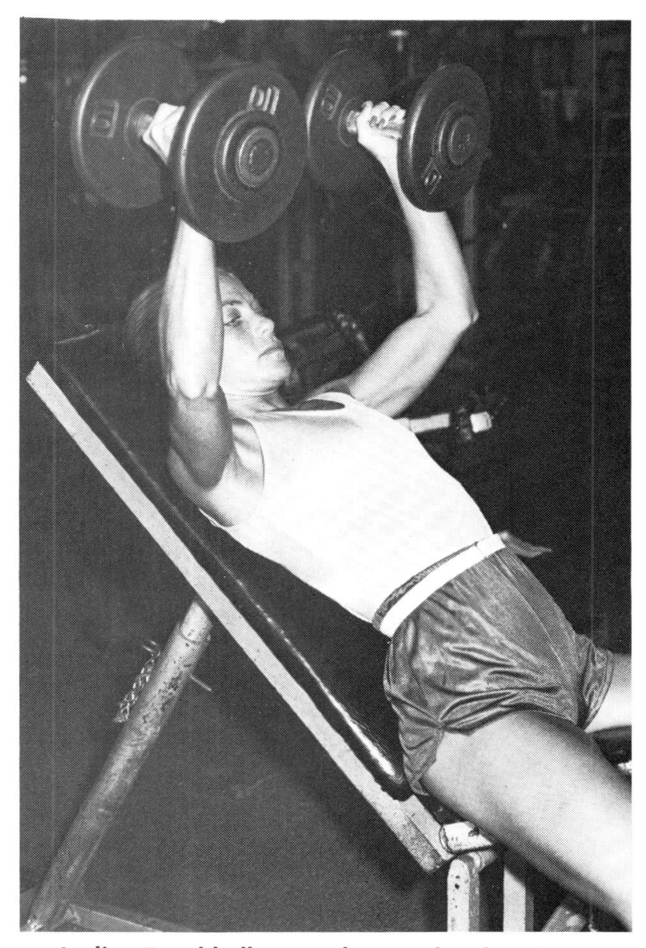

Incline Dumbbell Press, alternate hand position.

Dumbbell Incline Press

General Comments: This is an excellent upper pectoral and front deltoid movement. Secondary stress is placed on the triceps muscles. Generally speaking, doing Bench Presses at various angles with dumbbells is superior to doing the same movements with a barbell. Since the bar of a barbell touches your chest, it limits the range of motion you can achieve with your hands as you do the exercise. With dumbbells, however, you can lower your hands quite a bit farther, achieving a greater stretch in your pectorals at the bottom point of the movement.

Starting Position: Grasp two moderately heavy dumbbells and lie back on a 45-degree incline bench. Push the dumbbells to arms' length directly above your shoulder joints. Keep your hands facing forward and touch the inner plates of one dumbbell against those of the other.

Exercise Performance: Being careful to keep your elbows back throughout the movement, slowly lower the dumbbells as far as possible. Then press them back to the starting position and repeat the movement for the required number of repetitions.

Training Tips: While most bodybuilders do a majority of their Incline Presses on a 45-degree-angled bench, you will undoubtedly find that a 30-degree bench, or even one angled lower than that, will stress the upper pectorals more directly. Some bodybuilders do Incline Presses on a flat bench that simply has a four-by-four-inch block of wood placed under the legs at the head of the bench. This is a very low incline, but it is still effective in stressing the upper pectorals.

Dumbbell Bench Press

General Comments: As in the Barbell Bench Press, this movement stresses the pectorals, deltoids, and triceps fairly strongly. With dumbbells, however, you will achieve a much greater range of motion than when using a barbell.

Starting Position: Grasp two moderately heavy dumbbells and lie back on a flat exercise bench. Push the dumbbells to arms' length directly above your shoulder joints. Keep your hands facing forward and touch the inner plates of one dumbbell against those of the other.

Exercise Performance: Being careful to keep your elbows back during the movement, slowly lower the dumbbells as far as possible. Press them back to the starting position and repeat the movement for the desired number of repetitions.

Training Tips: With very heavy dumbbells you will find it somewhat difficult to get the weights into position to start the movement. There are two methods you can use to accomplish this. In the first you use a pair of training partners to hand you the weights. If you are training alone, however, you can get them into position by first resting the dumbbells on end on your knees while grasping the dumbbell handles. Keeping your legs flexed at the waist, roll backward onto your back. If you keep your arms straight and the dumbbells on your knees, you will find that they are now in the correct starting position. To lower them back to the

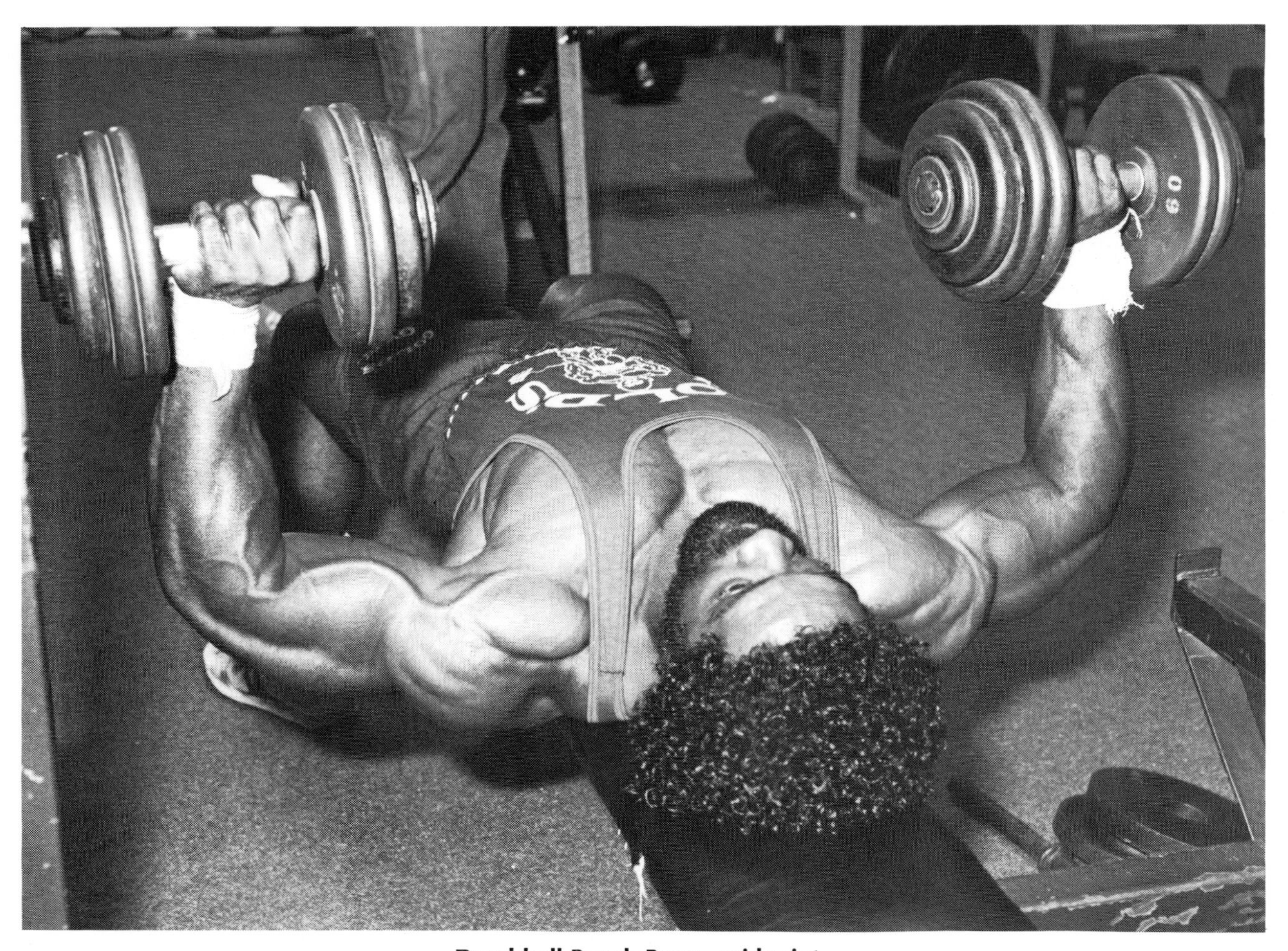

Dumbbell Bench Press—midpoint.

floor after completing your set, simply bend your legs and place the dumbbells against your knees. Tilt the dumbbells a little toward your feet and you will find that you can roll easily into a seated position at the end of the bench.

Decline Press

General Comments: All types of Decline Presses strongly stress the lower and outer edges of the pectorals. Secondary stress is placed on the deltoids and triceps.

Starting Position: Lie on your back on a 30-degree decline bench and take a grip a little wider than shoulder width on the barbell so that your palms are pointed toward your feet when you are in the starting position. Have a training partner help you move the barbell into the starting position, which is with it supported at arms' length directly above your shoulder joints.

Decline Press with dumbbells, near start.

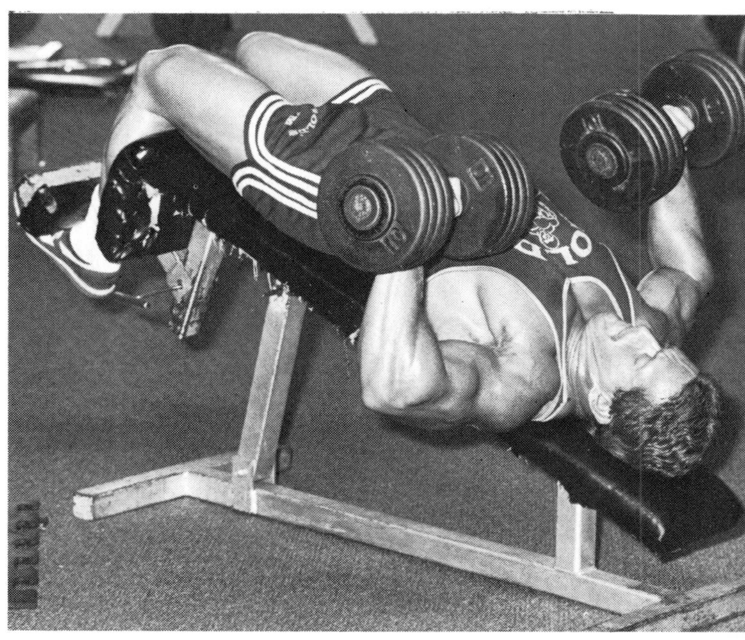

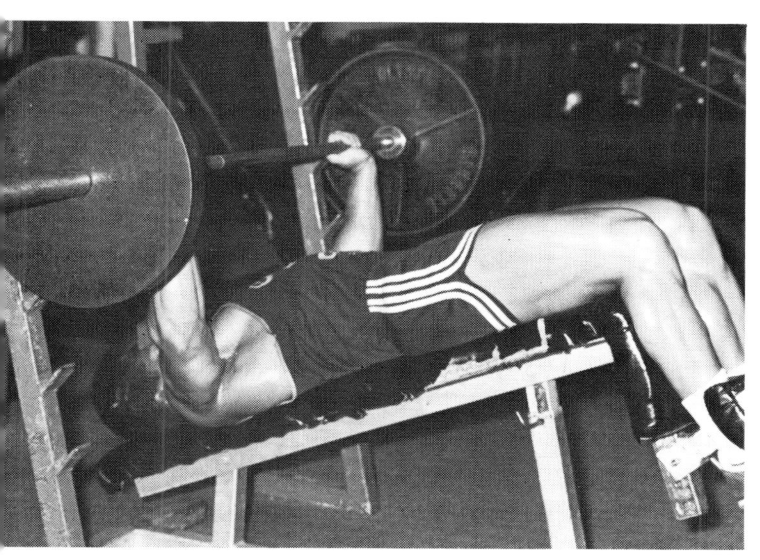

Decline Press with barbell, near finish.

Exercise Performance: Being careful to keep your elbows back, slowly lower the barbell directly downward until it touches your upper chest at the base of your neck. Then press it steadily back to arms' length and repeat the movement for the required number of repetitions.

Training Tips: As with Incline Presses, you can also do this movement quite profitably with dumbbells. A lot of top bodybuilders at Gold's/Venice do Decline Presses and Incline Presses on a bench set under the Bench Press station of a Universal Gym machine.

With a barbell or two dumbbells your training partner can easily help you get the weight(s) into position if you keep your arms straight and he or she simply pulls upward on your hands to move them in a semicircular arc from the floor to the starting position. Then, at the end of your set, you can simply reverse this procedure to place the weight(s) back on the floor.

Incline/Decline Flye

General Comments: As on a flat bench, you can also do Flyes on a decline or incline bench. Decline Flyes stress primarily the lower and outer sections of the pectorals, while Incline Flyes stress the upper pectorals and front deltoids.

Starting Position: Grasp two moderately weighted dumbbells in your hands and lie back on an incline or decline bench. Move the dumbbells so that they are supported at arms' length directly above your shoulder joints. Your palms should be facing inward throughout the movement. At the start of either version of the Flye the dumbbells should be touching each other above your chest. Keep your arms bent slightly at all times.

Exercise Performance: Slowly lower the dumbbells outward and downward in semicircular arcs on each side to as low a position as is

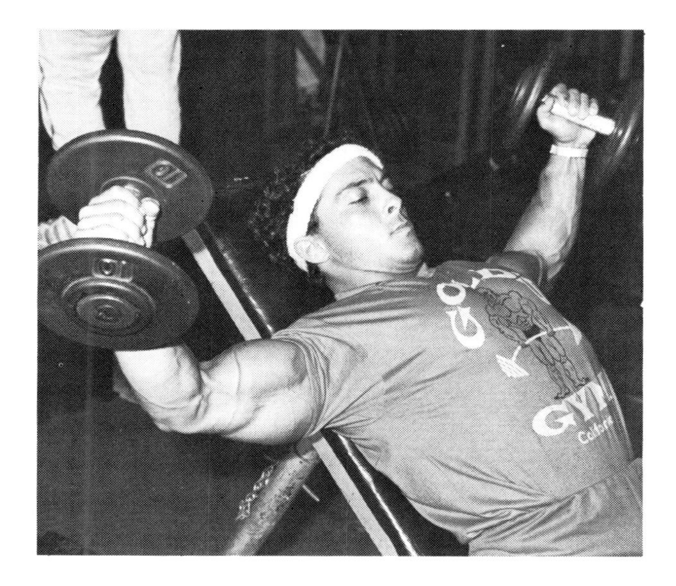

Incline Flye, above; Decline Flye, below.

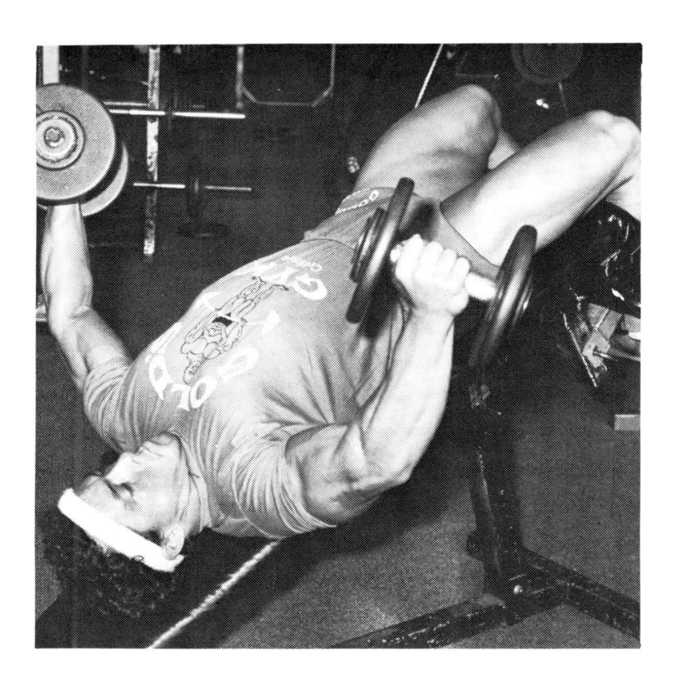

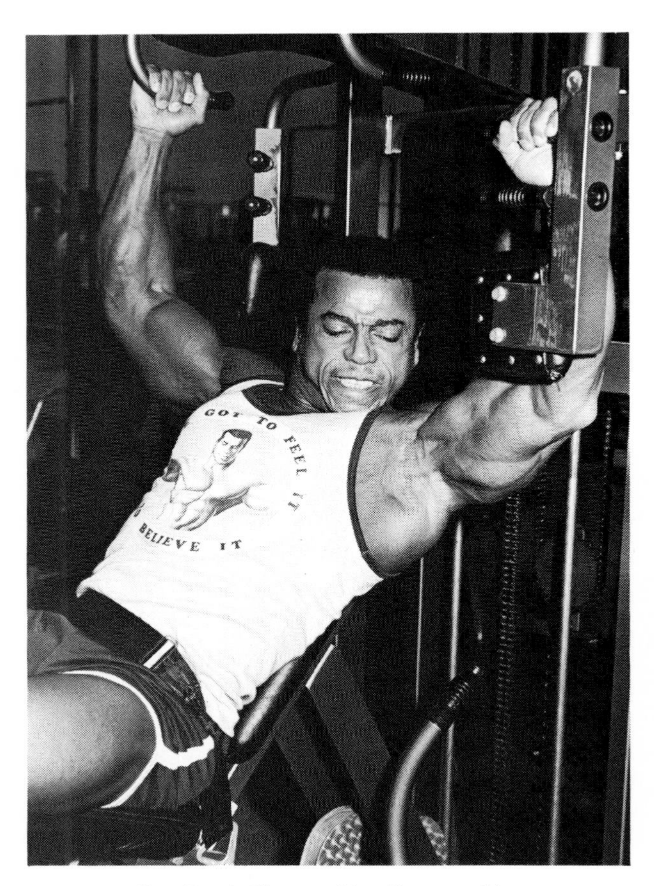

Pec Deck Flye on Nautilus machine.

comfortable. Raise them back along the same arcs to the starting point. Repeat the movement until you have done a full set.

Training Tips: On all incline and decline chest movements you should experiment with a variety of bench angles. Each new angle will stress your pectoral muscles somewhat differently.

Pec Deck Flye

General Comments: This is a relatively new movement, since the pec deck apparatus was invented during the mid-1970s. Flyes done on this machine stress the whole pectoral, but particularly the inner edges of the muscle. Since the machine has a cam (rotary pulley), you can keep tension on your pectorals throughout the range of motion of the exercise. This exercise can be done on either a Nautilus machine or a freestanding pec deck machine.

Starting Position (Nautilus machine): Adjust the seat to a height at which your upper arms will be parallel to the floor during the movement. Place your forearms against the movable pads of the machine and grasp one or the other set of handles. Allow the movable pads to travel backward as far as possible.

Starting Position (freestanding apparatus): Adjust the seat by revolving it until it is high enough so that your upper arms are parallel to the floor during the movement. Sit on the seat and force your forearms inside the pads so that they run along the pads and your hands can rest over the top edges of the pads. Allow the movable pads to travel backward as far as possible.

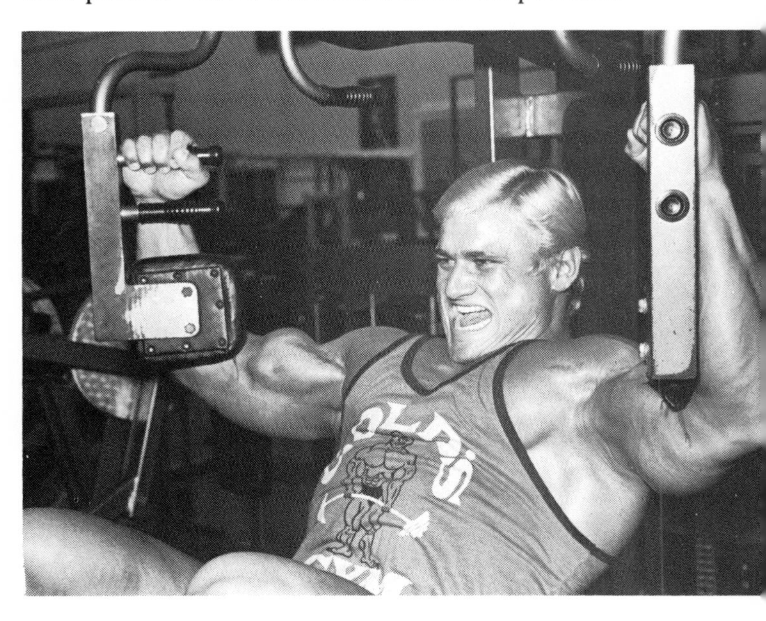

Pec Deck Flye—near start (on Nautilus machine), above; near finish (on freestanding machine), below.

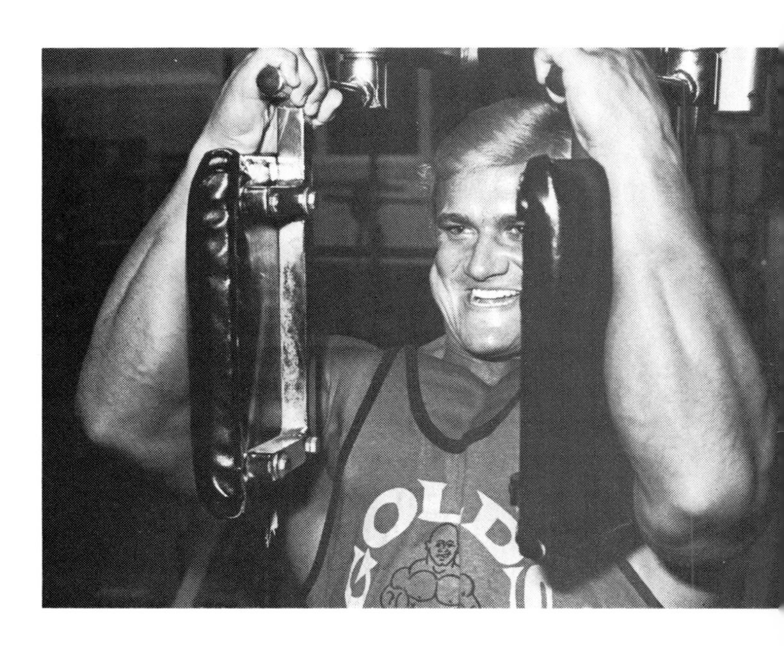

Exercise Performance: On both types of apparatus, move your elbows forward in semicircular arcs until the movable pads touch each other in the middle directly in front of your chest. Slowly return the pads to the starting position and repeat the movement for the desired number of repetitions.

Training Tips: You can vary the height of the seat on both types of apparatus for a somewhat different feel in your pectorals as you do the movement. On the Nautilus machine you will see two handles on the top edge of the machine, just above your chest as you are lying in the apparatus. Grasp the left handle in your left hand to do the movement just with your right arm (be sure, however, to do an equal number of sets and reps for each side). Doing the movement one arm at a time allows you to concentrate more fully on the muscle action.

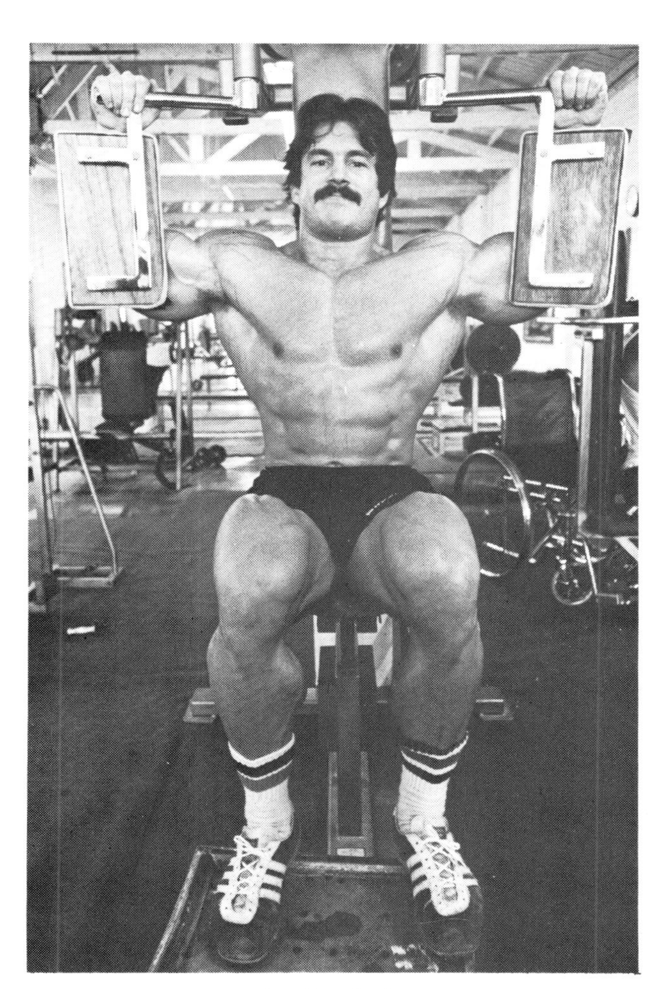

Pec Deck Flye.

Deltoid Exercises

Dumbbell Press

General Comments: Dumbbell Presses of all sorts are excellent movements for stressing the front deltoids and triceps. Secondary stress is placed on the upper back muscles.

Starting Position: Place your feet a comfortable distance apart and clean two dumbbells to your shoulders. Stand erect and be sure that your palms are pointed away from your body.

Exercise Performance: Slowly push the dumbbells directly upward to arms' length above your head. At the top of the movement the dumbbells can actually touch each other in the middle. Return the dumbbells slowly to your shoulders and repeat the movement for the desired number of repetitions.

Training Tips: Numerous variations of the Dumbbell Press exist. Instead of pointing your palms forward, you can face them toward each other. You can also do Alternate Dumbbell Presses in which one dumbbell is pressed upward as the other one is lowered. Most commonly, Alternate Dumbbell Presses are done with the palms facing each other. Both of these variations can be done seated on a flat bench, which isolates your legs from the movement.

Some bodybuilders do Dumbbell Presses one

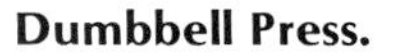

Dumbbell Press.

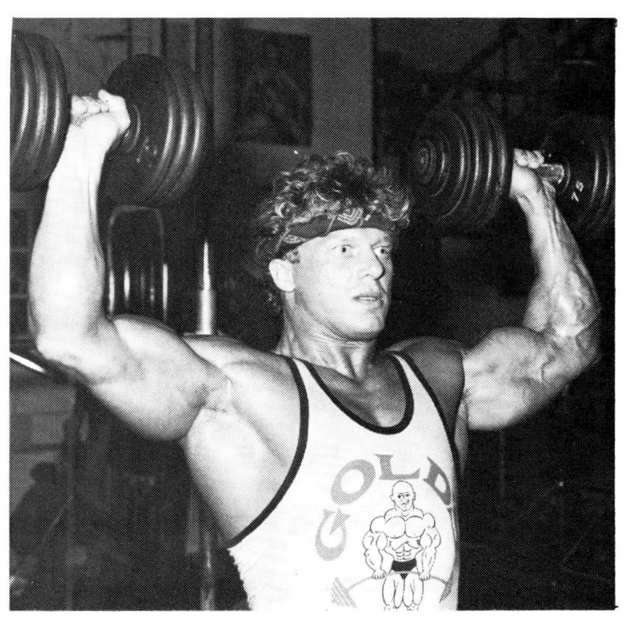

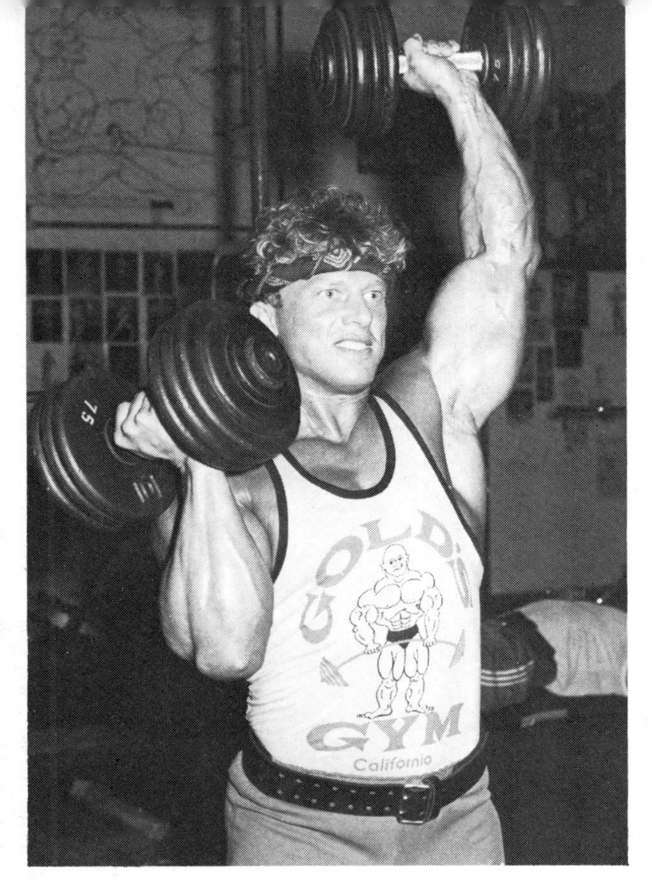

Dumbbell Press alternating arms.

arm at a time, usually holding onto something with the free hand to steady themselves.

Arnold Schwarzenegger did a unique Rotating Dumbbell Press quite often in his shoulder workouts. This movement started with the palms facing the body as at the finish of a Dumbbell Curl movement. Arnold would actually force his hands toward the floor in this position to stretch his deltoid muscles maximally. From there he would press the weights upward while rotating his thumbs inward until his palms were facing forward. He would not actually lock his elbows at the finish of the movement, because that would keep continuous tension on his deltoids. Arnold would simply reverse the movement to return the dumbbells to his shoulders for another repetition.

Seated Press

General Comments: As mentioned in the de-

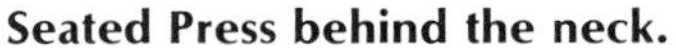

Seated Press behind the neck.

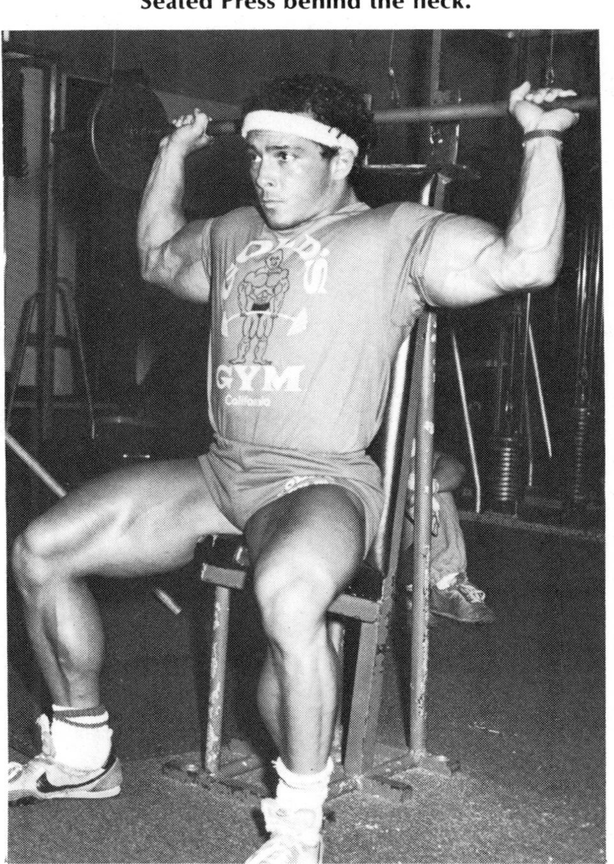

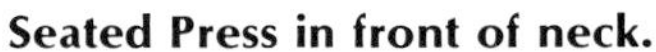

Seated Press in front of neck.

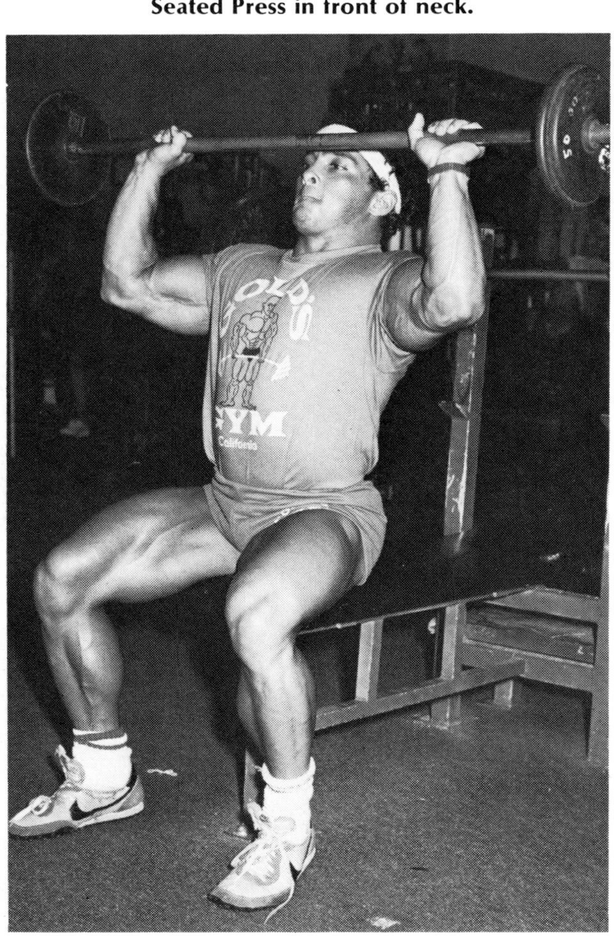

scription of Dumbbell Presses, all types of overhead pressing can be done while seated at the end of a flat exercise bench. Doing Seated Presses isolates the legs from the movement and prevents you from leaning backward to cheat up a heavier weight. Therefore, doing Seated Presses will prevent you from using as heavy a poundage as doing Presses when standing erect.

Machine Press

General Comments: Machine Presses strongly stress the front deltoids and triceps. Secondary stress is placed on the upper back muscles. Machine Presses can be done on a Smith machine, a Universal Gym machine, or on a Nautilus double shoulder machine.

Starting Position (Smith machine): Place a bench between the uprights of the machine and sit on it so that you can rest the movable bar of the machine either across the base of your neck in front of your neck or across your trapezius behind your neck. Grasp the bar with a grip a little wider than shoulder width, your palms pointed forward. Sit erect.

Starting Position (Universal Gym machine): Sit on the stool provided with a Universal Gym machine either facing toward or facing away from the weight stack at the shoulder press station. Grasp the handles of the machine with your palms pointed away from your body. Sit erect.

Starting Position (Nautilus machine): Adjust the seat height so that when you are sitting in the machine your shoulders are at the same level as the pressing handles. Sit in the seat and fasten the lap belt. Grasp the pressing handles with your palms facing each other.

Exercise Performance: Slowly straighten your arms by pushing upward against the apparatus. As soon as your arms are straight, slowly lower the apparatus back to the starting position. Repeat the movement for the desired number of repetitions.

Training Tips: Machine Presses are a good alternative to all types of free-weight Overhead Presses. Generally speaking, machines allow for a greater use of continuous tension on most shoulder exercises.

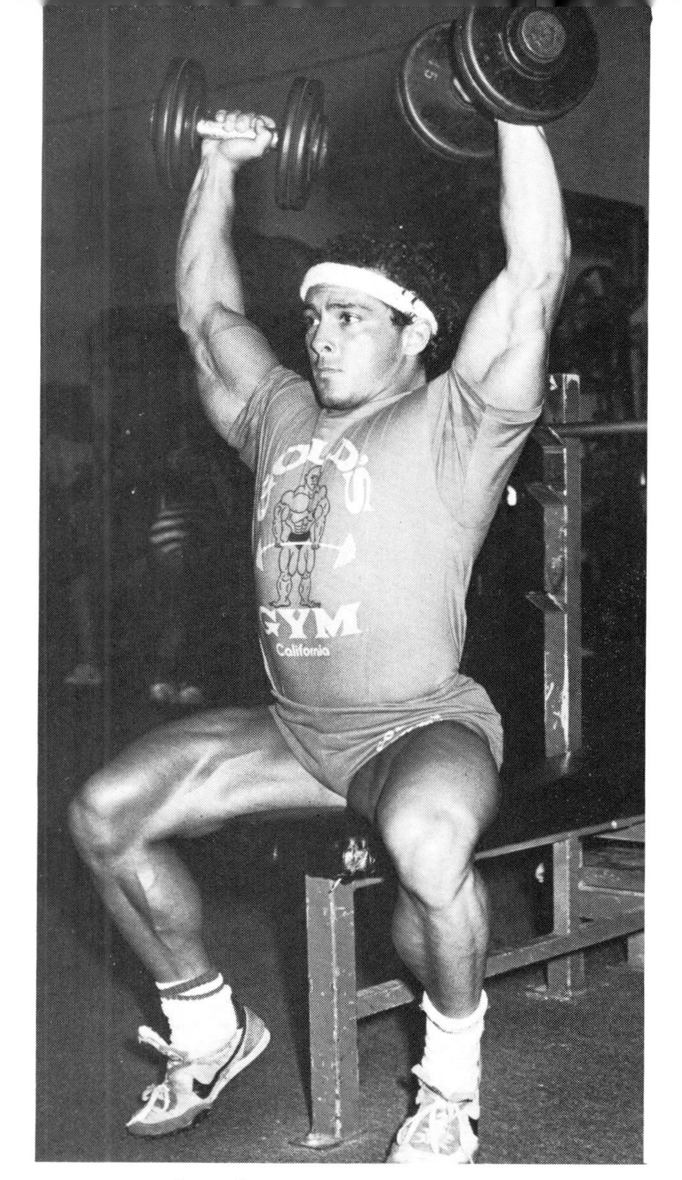

Seated Press using dumbbells.

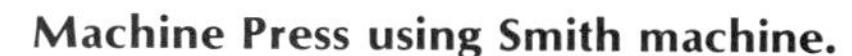

Machine Press using Smith machine.

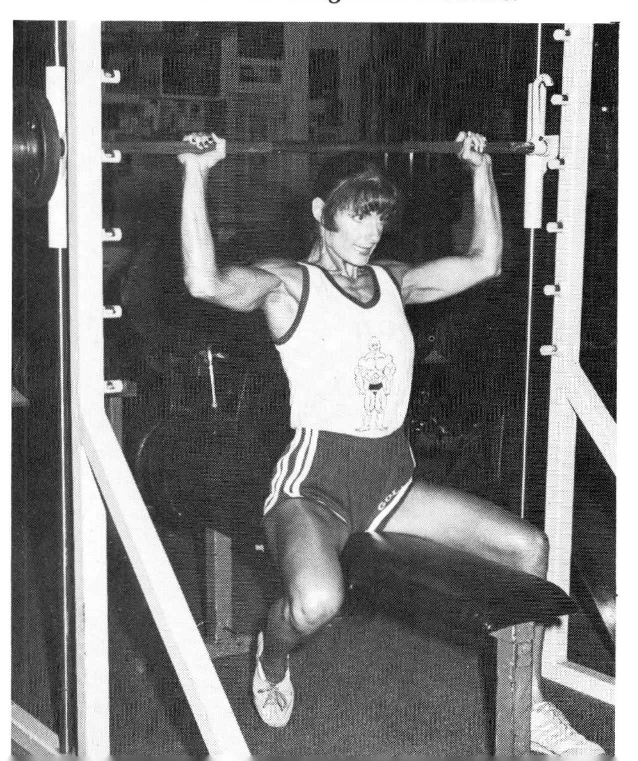

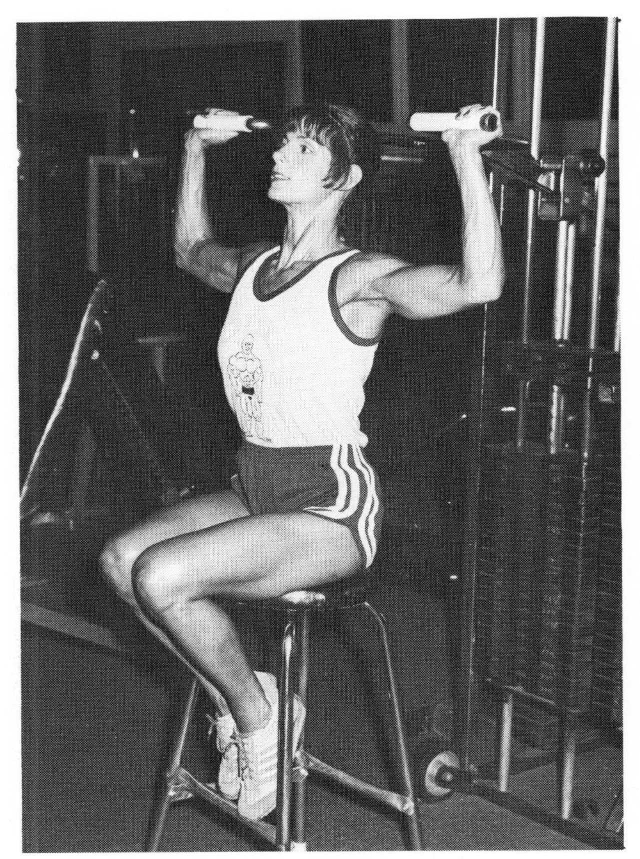
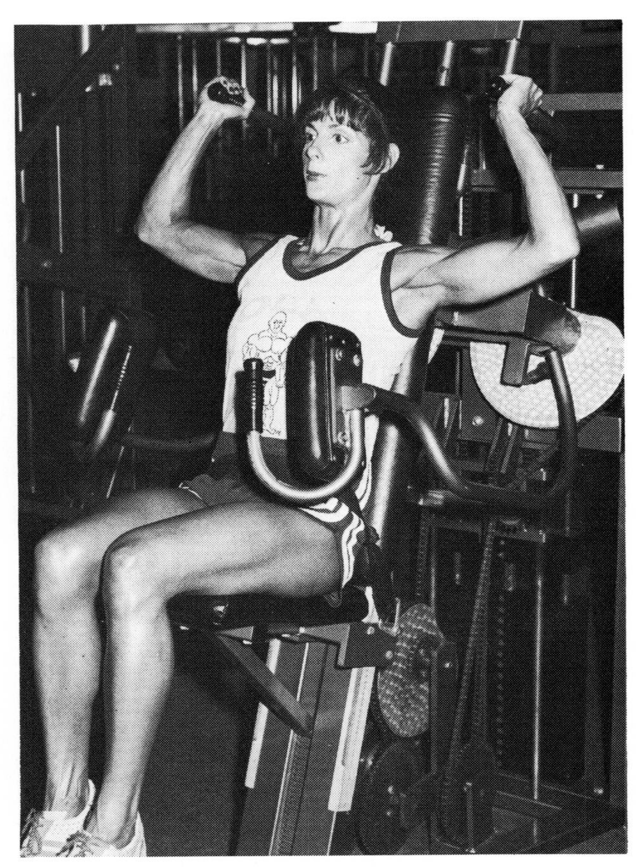

Machine Press using Universal Gyms machine, left, and Nautilus machine, right.

Bent Lateral

General Comments: This movement strongly stresses the posterior deltoid muscles, plus the muscles of the upper back.

Starting Position: Grasp two light dumbbells in your hands and place your feet a comfortable distance apart. Bend over at the waist until your torso is parallel to the floor. Hang your arms directly downward from your shoulder joints and bend them slightly. Maintain this slight arm bend throughout the movement.

Exercise Performance: From this basic starting position, use your posterior deltoid strength to move the dumbbells in semicircular arcs directly out to the sides and upward until they reach a line drawn parallel to the floor and through your shoulder joints. Slowly lower the weights back to the starting position and repeat the movement for the desired number of repetitions.

Training Tips: The most common mistake when doing this movement is to raise the dumbbells somewhat to the rear, rather than directly out to the sides. Try to watch yourself in the mirror to prevent this. You can also do this movement seated at the end of a flat exercise bench, an exercise that is fully described in Chapter 7.

Front Lateral

General Comments: This movement can be done with a barbell, two dumbbells, or a single dumbbell held in both hands. It strongly stresses the anterior head of each deltoid muscle.

Starting Position: Grasp a barbell with a shoulder-width grip. Stand erect with the barbell resting across your thighs, your palms toward your body. Straighten your arms and keep them straight throughout the movement.

Exercise Performance: Slowly move the barbell with deltoid strength in a semicircular arc forward and upward until it reaches shoulder

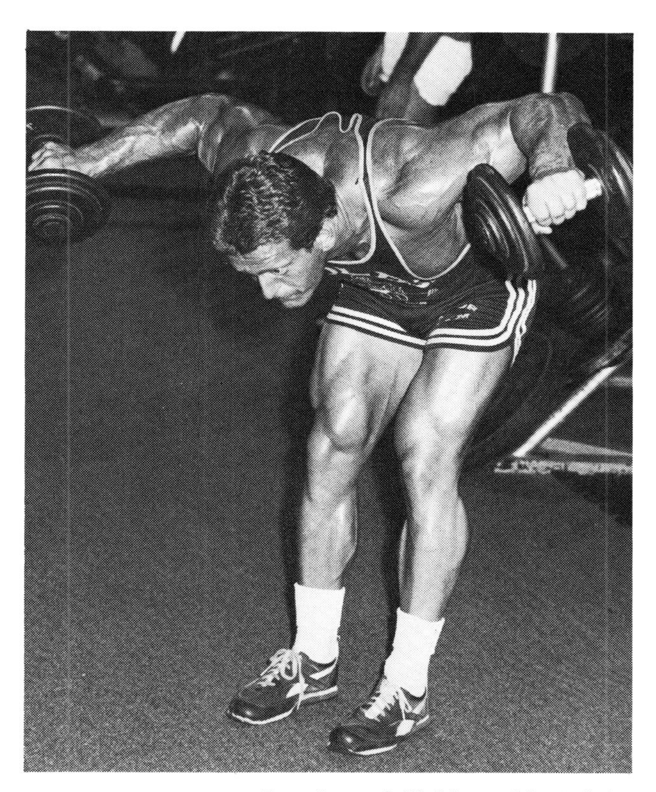

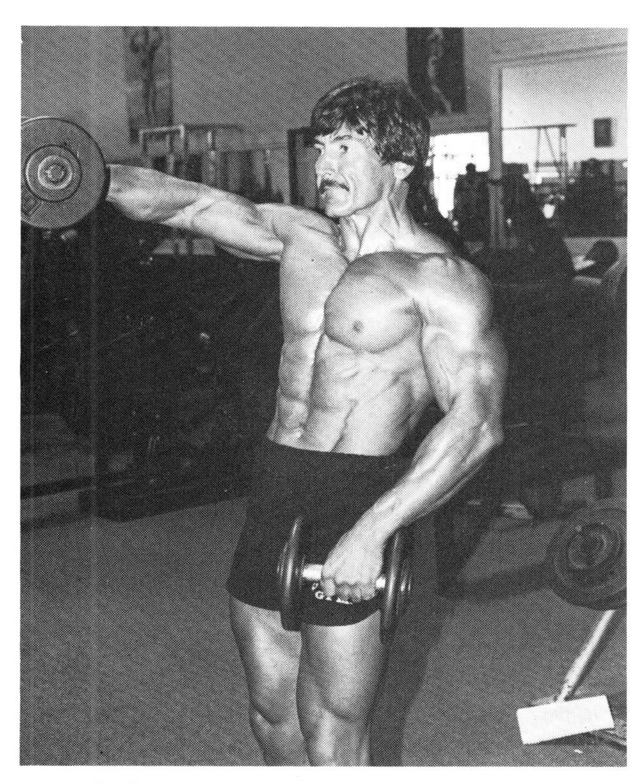

Bent Lateral (finish position), left; Front Lateral (alternating arms), right.

level. Slowly lower it back to the starting point and repeat the movement.

Training Tips: By holding a dumbbell in both hands you can do a similar movement. Or you can hold two dumbbells and raise them either together or alternately, one going up as the other comes down. If you do Alternate Front Raises, take a tip from Lou Ferrigno and move the dumbbells upward along the centerline of your body, rather than up along independent lines on a plane with your shoulder joints.

Arm Exercises

Dumbbell Curl

General Comments: Many bodybuilders feel that Dumbbell Curls are superior to Barbell Curls, because they allow bodybuilders to supinate each hand as they curl the weights upward. The function of the biceps muscle is not only to bend the arm, but also to supinate the hand.

Starting Position: Grasp two dumbbells and stand erect with your arms hanging down at

Dumbbell Curl, standing.

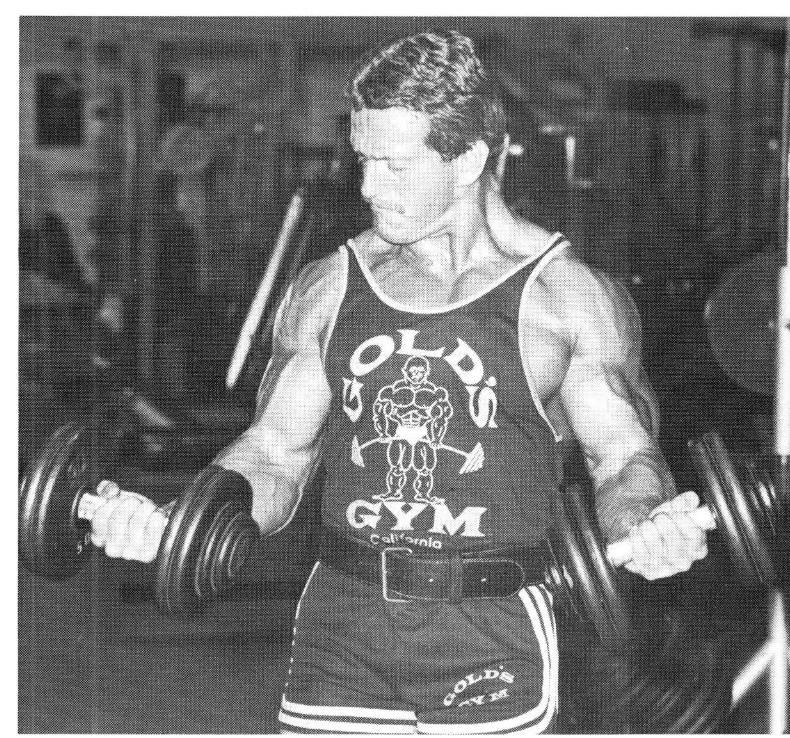

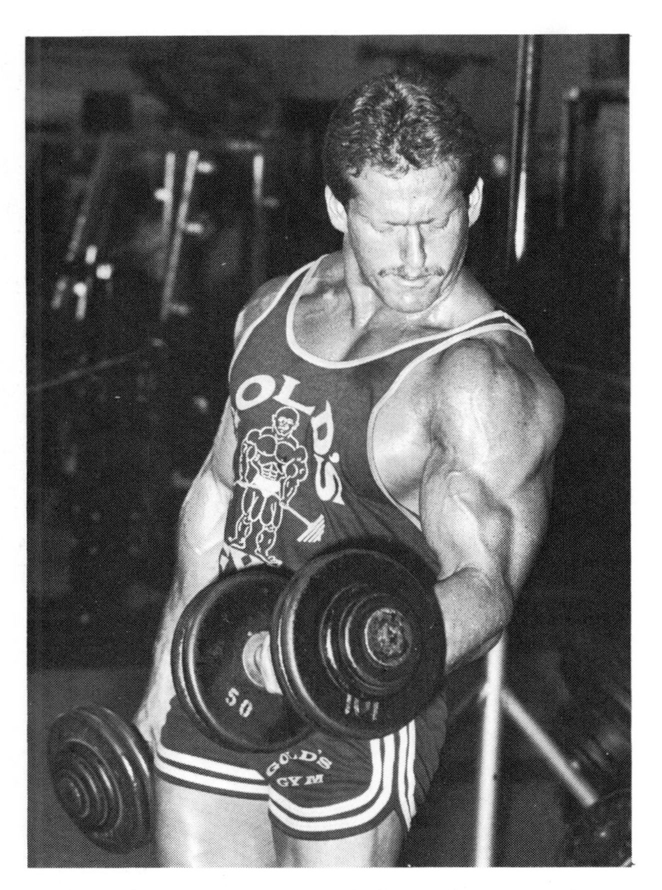

Dumbbell Curl—standing and alternating arms, above; seated using both arms, below.

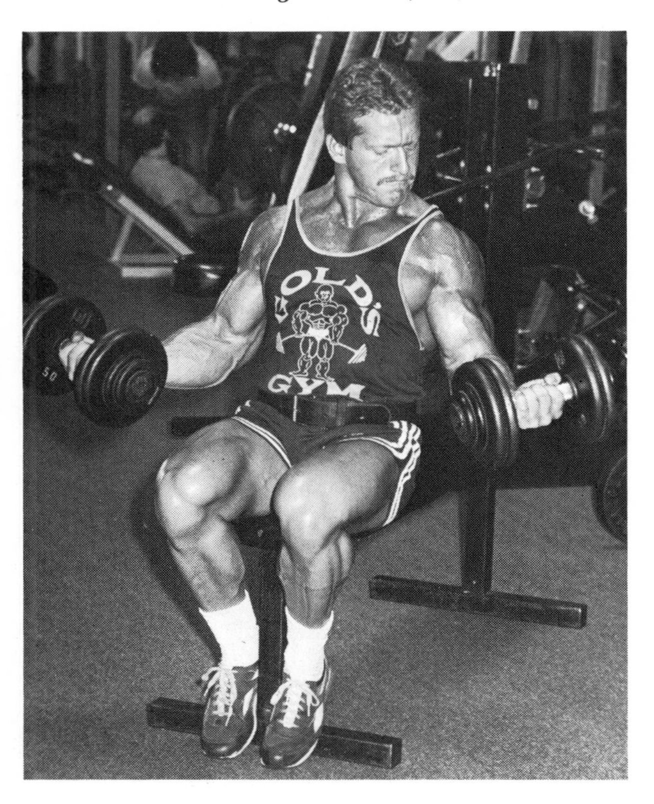

your sides. Your palms should be facing your body. Pin your upper arms to the sides of your torso and keep them in that position throughout the movement.

Exercise Performance: Slowly move the dumbbells in semicircular arcs upward from the sides of your body until they reach shoulder height. As you curl the dumbbells upward, rotate your wrists on each side to bring your palms into a position in which they are facing directly upward during the movement. Reverse the curling and supination procedure to return the dumbbells to the starting point. Repeat the movement for the required number of repetitions.

Training Tips: Two variations of the Dumbbell Curl are commonly used in bodybuilding gyms. In the first you curl the dumbbells alternately, one hand going up as the other comes down. In the second variation you sit on the end of a flat exercise bench and curl both dumbbells simultaneously. This variation isolates the legs from the movement and makes it more strict.

Preacher Curl

General Comments: This exercise strongly stresses the lower insertions of the biceps muscles. It also builds a thick, football-like biceps such as that exhibited by Larry Scott, the bodybuilder who popularized the movement. Preacher Curls can be done with a barbell, two dumbbells, or one dumbbell at a time.

Starting Position: Grasp a barbell with an undergrip, your hands set two or three inches wider than your shoulders on each side. Lean over a preacher bench so that the top edge of the bench is wedged under your armpits. Your upper arms should run parallel to each other down the angled surface of the bench, and your elbows should be set a little narrower than the width of your grip. Completely straighten your arms.

Exercise Performance: From this starting position, use your biceps strength to bend your arms fully, pulling the barbell in a semicircular arc up to rest against your neck under your chin. Slowly allow your arms to straighten fully, then repeat the movement for the required number of repetitions.

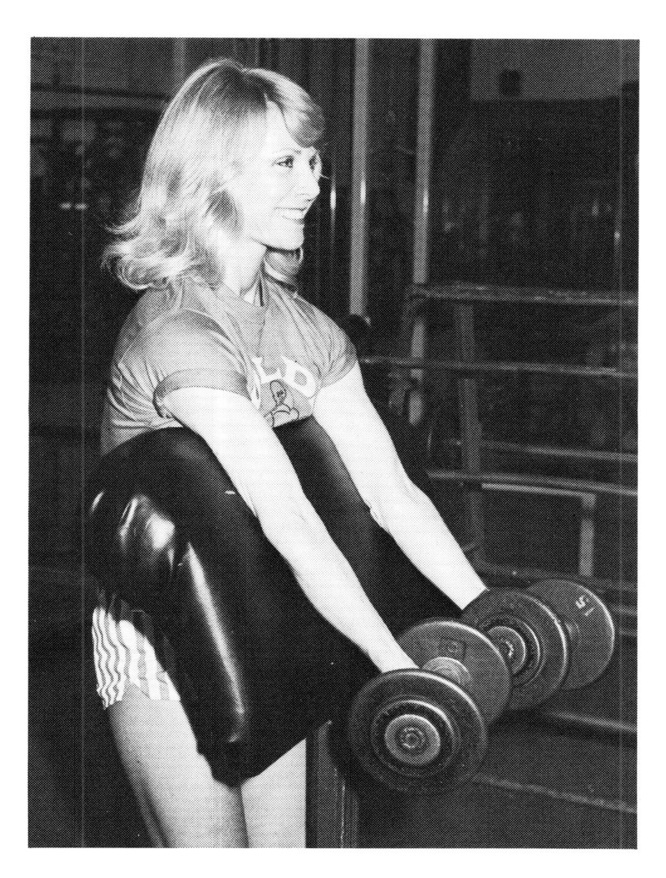

Preacher Curl starting positions—with dumbbells, above; with barbell, below.

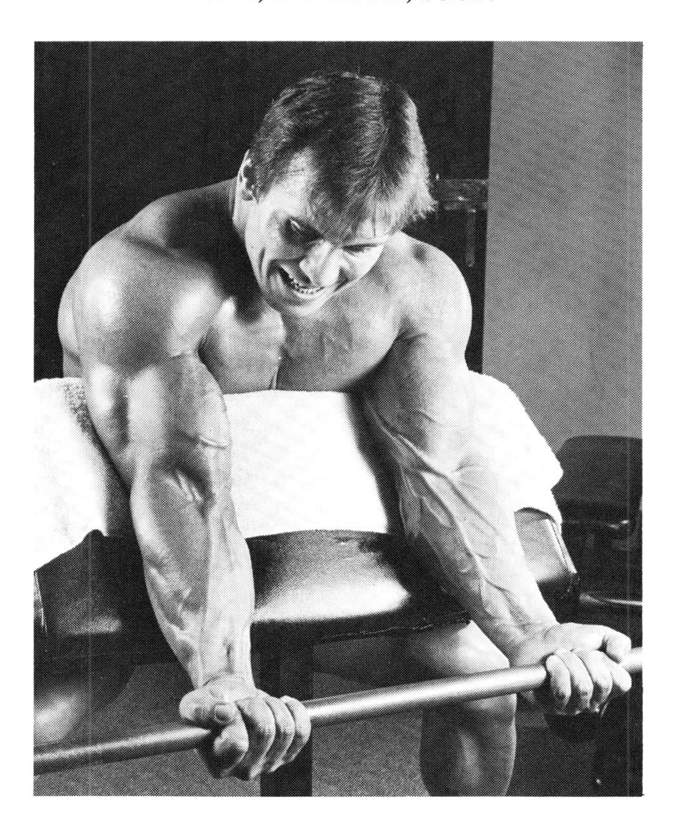

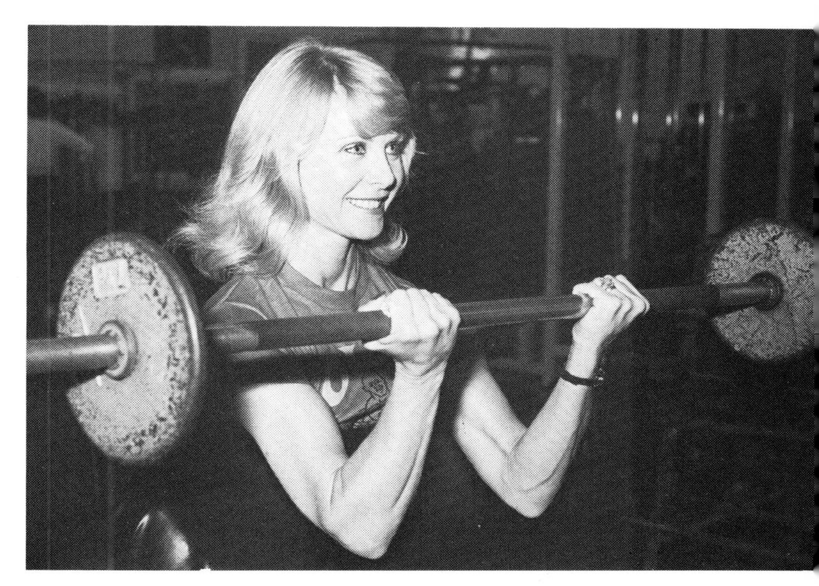

Preacher Curl with barbell—finish.

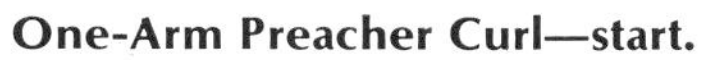

One-Arm Preacher Curl—start.

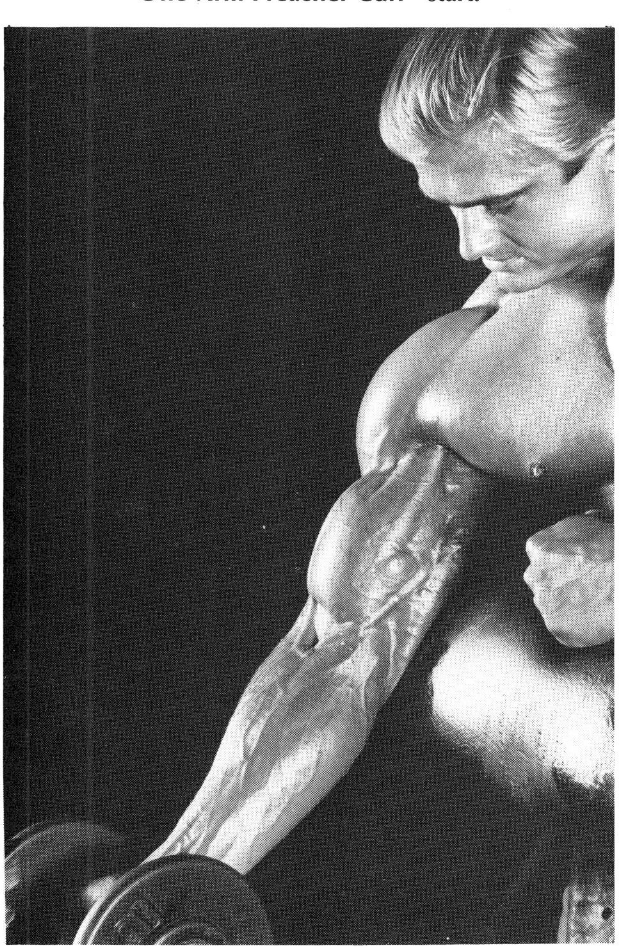

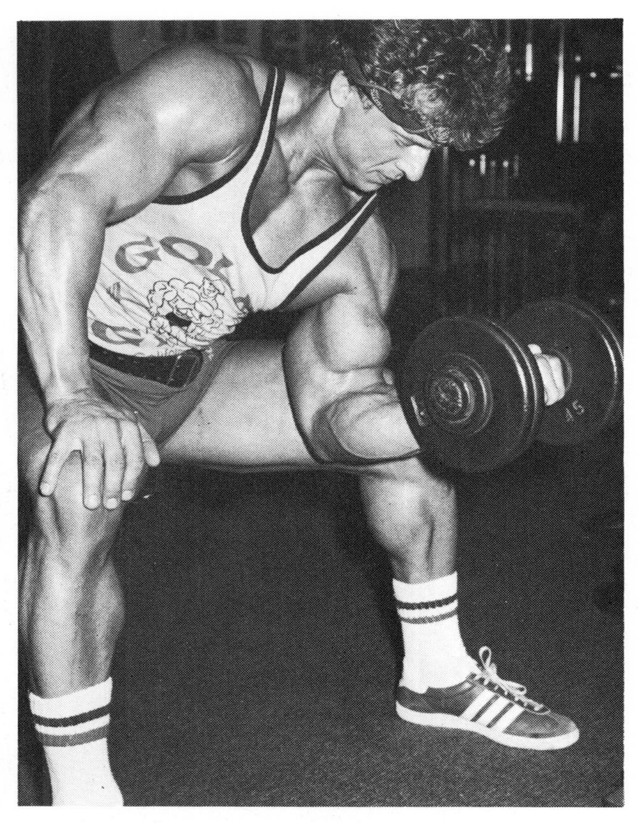

Concentration Curl with dumbbell.

Training Tips: Many bodybuilders, including Larry Scott, do this movement with two dumbbells. In such a case the method of performing the exercise is identical to that of Barbell Preacher Curls. As you curl up the dumbbells, however, you should be conscious of keeping the dumbbells a little outside of your elbows.

Some bodybuilders—most notably Boyer Coe—prefer to do Dumbbell Preacher Curls with one arm at a time. In this case you can usually concentrate harder on the movement than when using both arms simultaneously. Be sure to do an equal number of sets and reps with each arm.

Concentration Curl

General Comments: This is a good movement for accentuating the peak on your biceps. Some bodybuilders don't have good potential for biceps peak, and nothing will bring it out in such a case. Still, if you do have the potential to develop a high-peaked biceps, you should take every advantage of Concentration Curls.

Starting Position: Sit at the end of a flat exercise bench and place your feet flat on the floor with about 2½ feet of space between them. Grasp a moderately weighted dumbbell in your right hand. Bend over at the waist enough so that you can place the elbow of your right arm solidly against the inside of your right leg a few inches away from your knee. Maintain this arm position throughout the movement. You can rest your left hand on your left thigh. Fully straighten your right arm.

Exercise Performance: From this basic starting position, slowly curl the weight upward to your chin. As you curl the dumbbell upward, be sure to supinate your hand fully. Hold the peak contracted position at the top of the movement for a couple of seconds and then slowly lower the weight back to the starting point. Repeat the exercise for the desired number of repetitions.

Training Tips: Robby Robinson usually preferred to do this movement with a barbell held in both hands. He would take a narrow undergrip in the middle of the barbell handle, bend over until his torso was parallel to the floor and hang his upper arms directly downward throughout the movement. By doing Concentration Curls in this position, he was able to exert a very powerful peak contraction effect on the biceps muscles of both arms.

Standing Triceps Extension

General Comments: This movement strongly stresses the whole triceps muscle mass, but particularly the large inner head of the muscle. Standing Triceps Extensions can be done with a barbell, two dumbbells simultaneously, one dumbbell held in one hand at a time, or a single dumbbell held in both hands.

Starting Position: Take a narrow overgrip in the middle of a barbell handle (there should be about six inches of space between your index fingers). Stand erect and extend your arms fully above your head. In this position your upper arms will be placed against the sides of your head. They should be maintained in this position throughout the movement.

Exercise Performance: Slowly unlock your elbows and let the barbell travel in a semicircle from the starting position downward until it

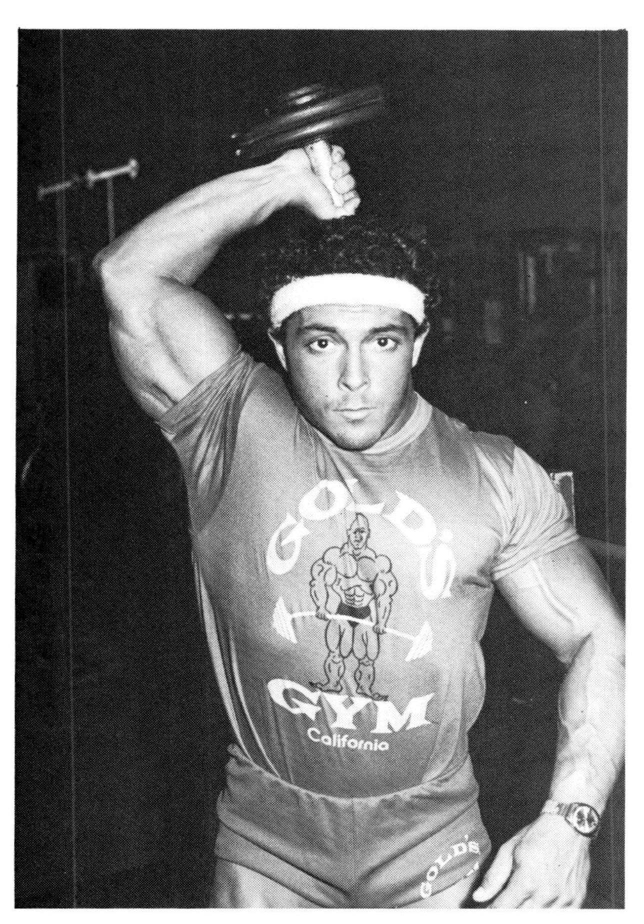

Standing Triceps Extension using one arm and dumbbell.

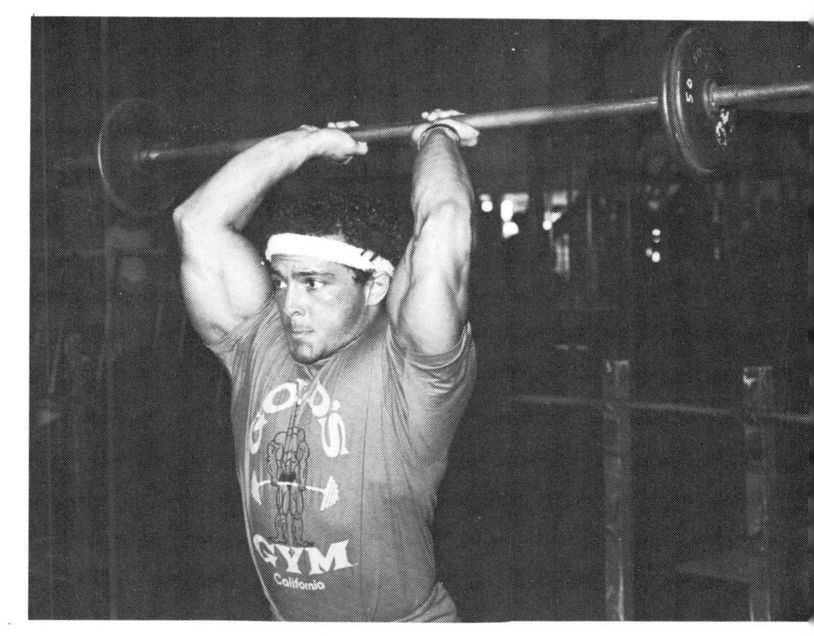

Standing Triceps Extension using barbell.

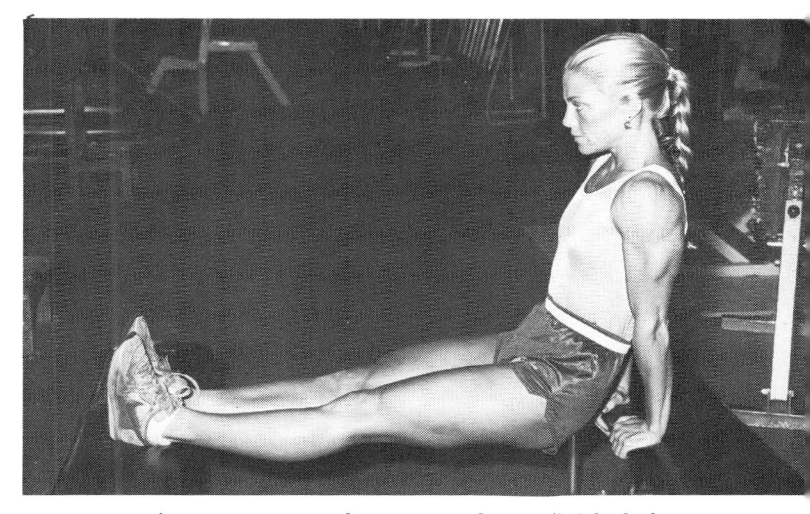

Dip Between Benches—start, above; finish, below.

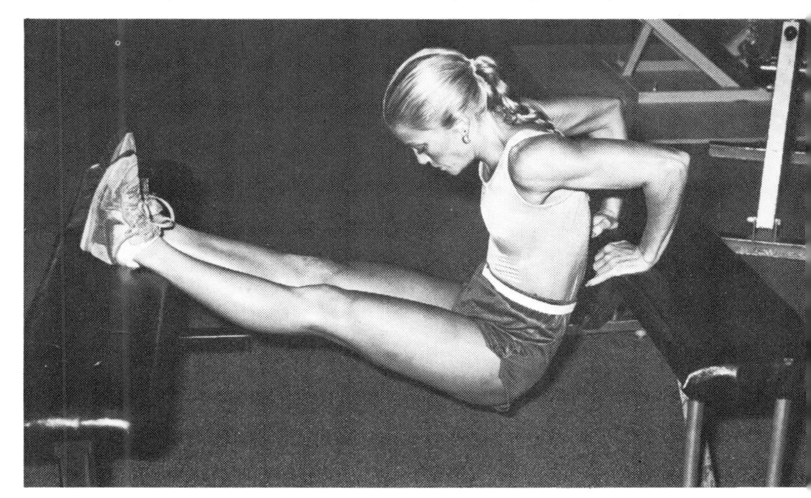

touches the back of your neck. Be careful when doing this exercise that you keep your elbows pointed directly upward and close to your head at all times. As soon as the barbell touches your neck, reverse the direction of travel and return it to the starting point with triceps strength. Repeat the movement for the required number of repetitions.

Training Tips: Using one arm at a time, you can move the dumbbell in a similar arc, or you can move two dumbbells simultaneously in the same arcs. By placing the palms of your hands against the inside plates at one end of a dumbbell, you can hang the dumbbell handle vertically and do Triceps Extensions with both arms at once.

Dips Between Benches

General Comments: Many bodybuilders do this exercise as a finishing-off movement to give

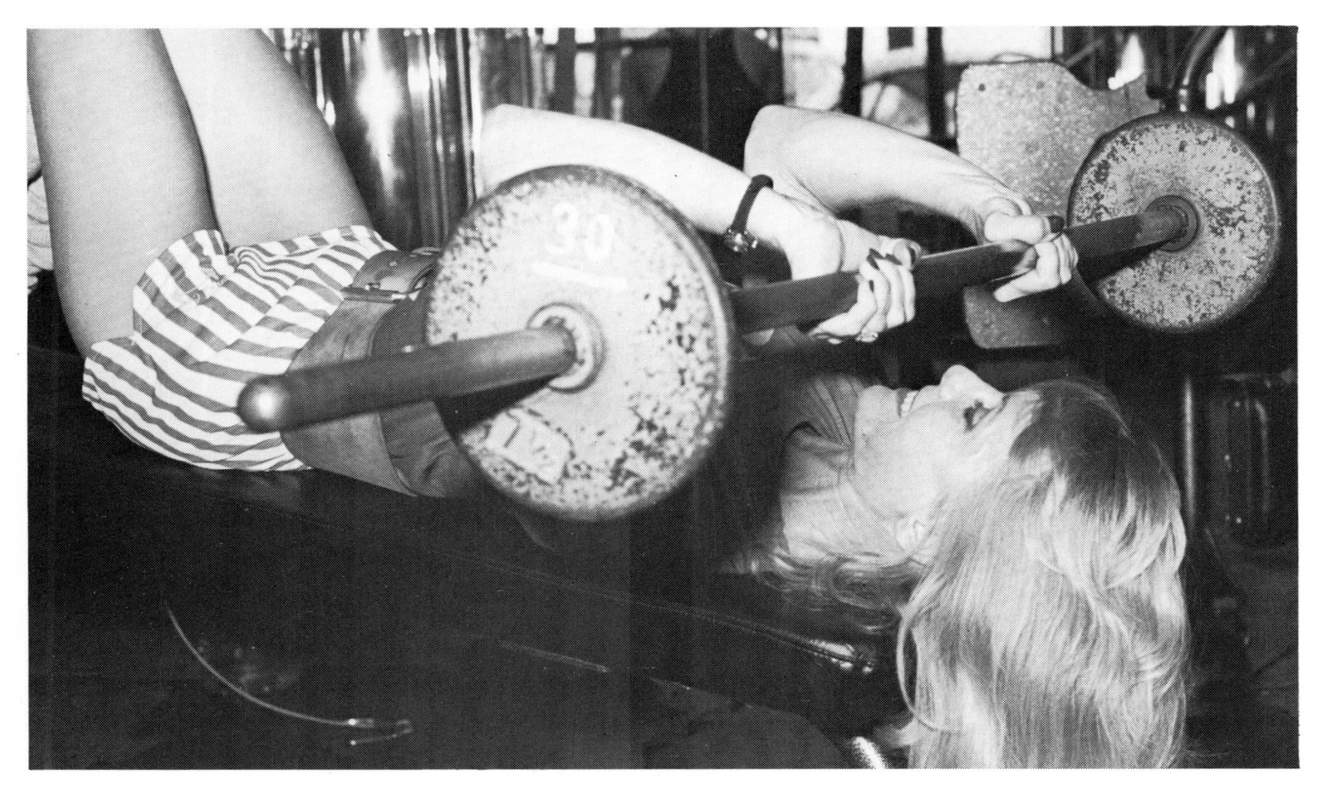

Decline Triceps Extension—start.

the final pump their triceps need for optimum response from training.

Starting Position: Place two flat exercise benches parallel to each other and about 2½–3 feet apart. Place your heels on one bench and your hand on another, fingers toward your feet. Your hands should be set fairly close together or should even touch each other behind your back. Straighten your arms fully.

Exercise Performance: Slowly lower your upper body between the benches by bending your arms as fully as possible. Once you reach the low position of this movement, reverse the direction of movement by slowly straightening your arms. Repeat the exercise for the required number of repetitions.

Training Tips: Some gyms have a special apparatus on which you can do this movement. When Dips Between Benches become easy to perform, you can add resistance by holding a dumbbell, or a barbell plate, in your lap.

Incline/Decline Triceps Extension

General Comments: These movements di-

Incline Triceps Extension—finish.

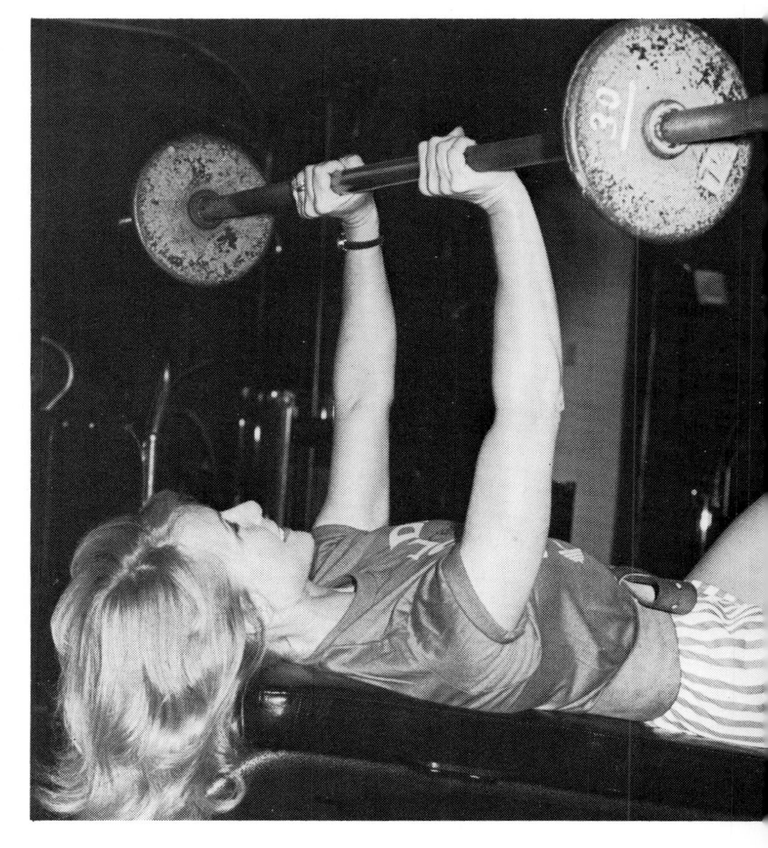

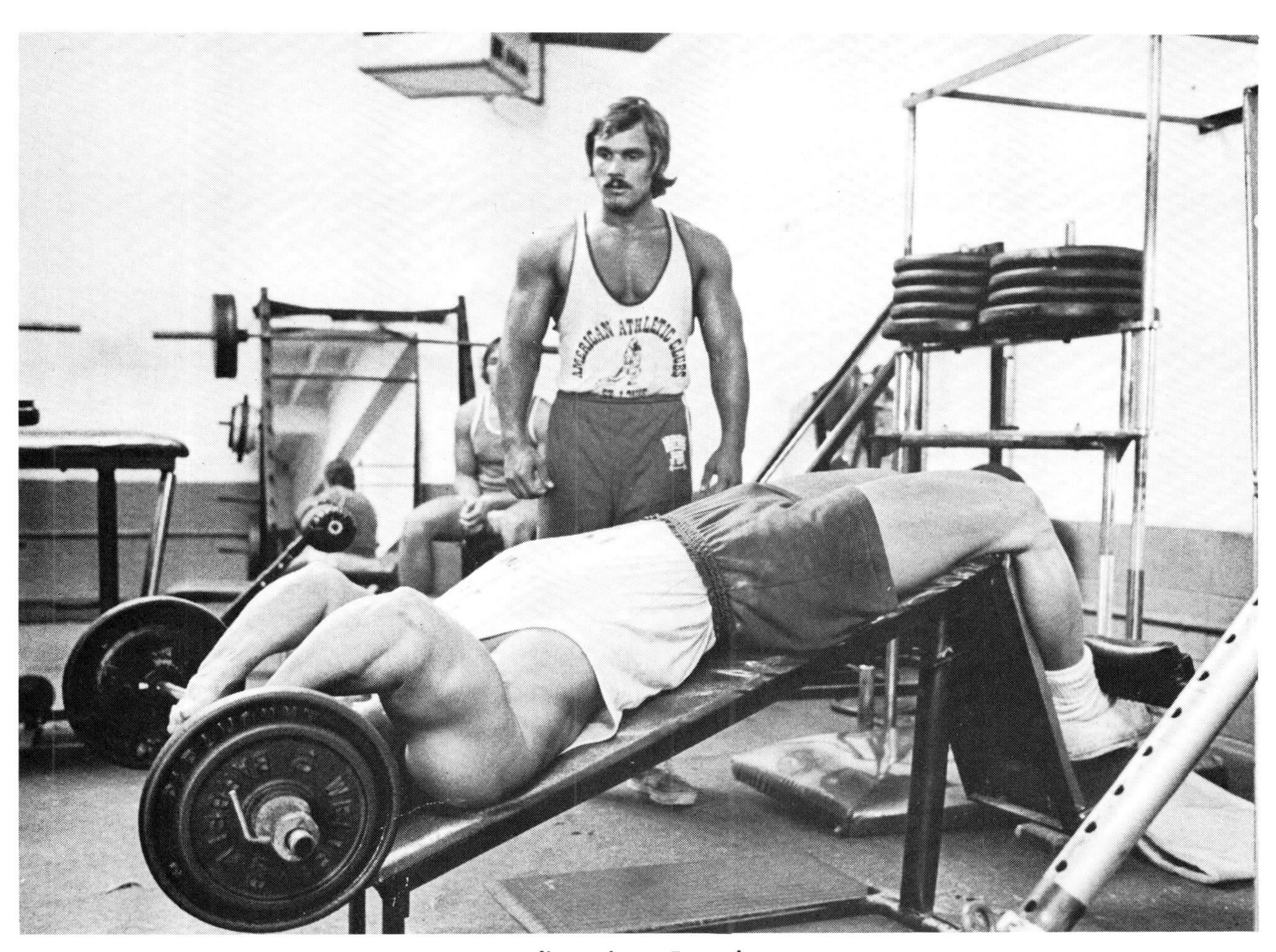

Decline Triceps Extension.

rectly stress the triceps muscles at the back of your upper arms. They are merely variations of the Lying Triceps Extension described in Chapter 3. The different angles, however, stress the triceps uniquely.

Starting Position: Lie back on an incline or decline bench and grasp a barbell with a narrow grip (about six inches between your index fingers) and your palms toward your feet when the barbell is in the correct starting position. Extend your arms perpendicular to the floor, as illustrated.

Exercise Performance: Keeping your upper arms motionless and your elbows pointed directly at the ceiling, slowly bend your elbows and lower the barbell in a semicircle from the starting point until it touches your forehead. Return the barbell along the same arc to the starting position and repeat the movement for the required number of repetitions.

Training Tips: You can vary the width of your grip on this movement and even occasionally use a reversed grip.

Reverse Barbell Curl

General Comments: Reverse Curls strongly stimulate the brachialis muscles lying under the biceps. These muscles are visible as an extra band of muscle between the biceps and triceps when a well-defined bodybuilder does a back double biceps pose. Reverse Curls also strongly stimulate the muscles on the outer forearm, particularly where the forearms tie into the upper arms.

Starting Position: Take a shoulder-width reverse grip on a barbell and stand erect with your arms hanging down the sides of your torso. The barbell will be resting across the tops of your thighs. Press your upper arms against the sides

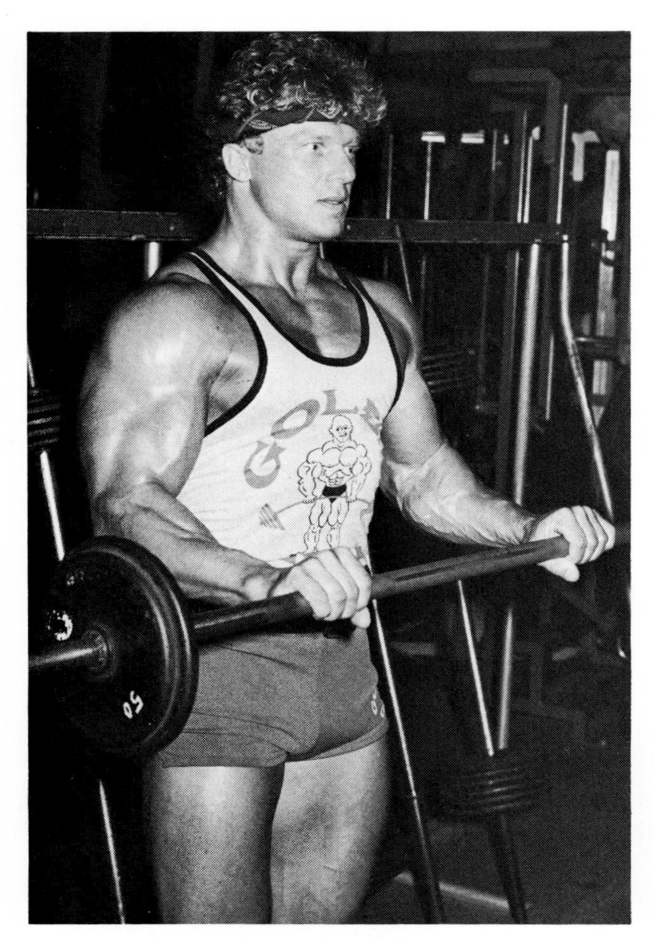

Reverse Barbell Curl.

of your torso and keep them in this position throughout the movement.

Exercise Performance: Without allowing your upper body to move, slowly bend your elbows and move the barbell in a semicircular arc from your thighs to your chin. Return the barbell along the same arc to the starting point and repeat the movement for the required number of repetitions.

Training Tips: You might find that a narrow grip gives your arms a good workout as well. You won't be able to use as much weight when your hands are set with your index fingers about six inches apart, but you'll still receive superior brachialis and forearm muscle stimulation.

Dumbbell Wrist Curl

General Comments: Dumbbell Wrist Curls are similar to Barbell Wrist Curls in that they stimulate all of the muscles of your forearms. You can do Dumbbell Wrist Curls with your palms up or palms down, and you can perform them with both arms simultaneously or with one arm at a time.

Starting Position: Sit at the end of a flat exercise bench and place your feet flat on the floor about shoulder width apart. Grasp two moderately weighted dumbbells and run your forearms down your thighs so that your wrists and hands, with the dumbbells, hang off the edge of your knees. You can hold your palms either up or down.

Exercise Performance: Sag your fists as far toward the floor as possible. Then curl your fists upward in small semicircular arcs as high as possible. Slowly return to the starting posi-

Dumbbell Wrist Curl with two dumbbells.

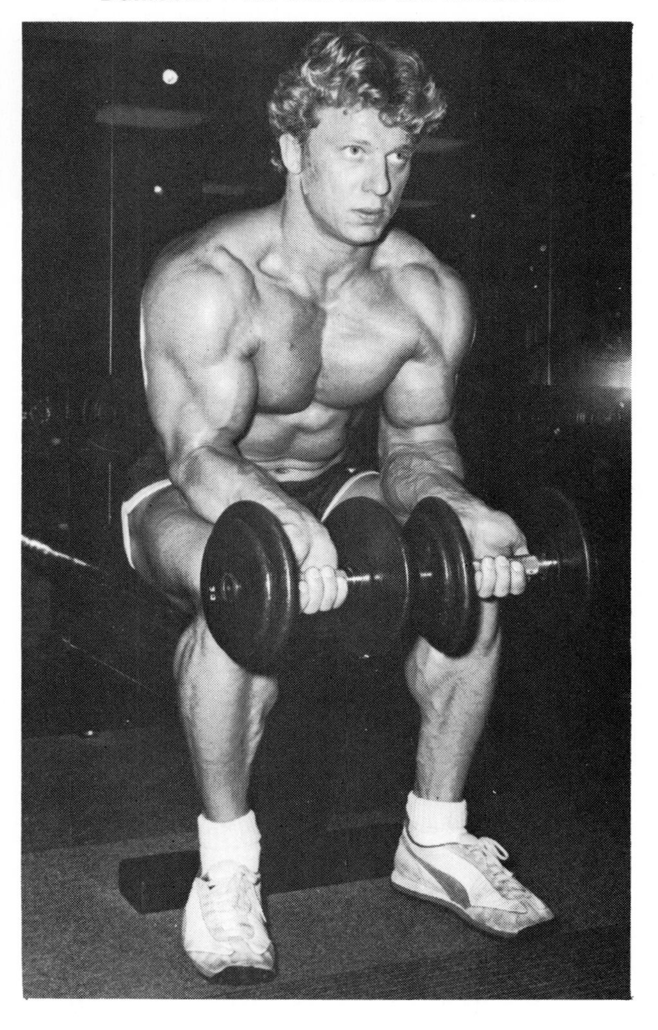

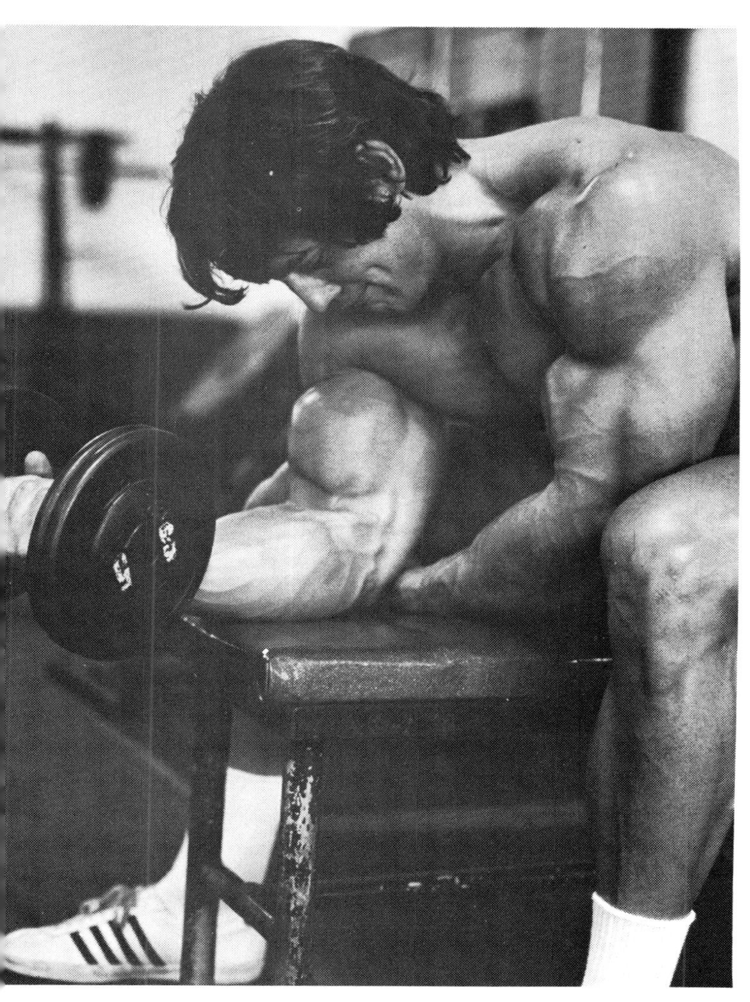

Dumbbell Wrist Curl with one dumbbell.

tion and repeat the movement for the desired number of repetitions.

Training Tips: Many bodybuilders prefer to do this exercise with a single dumbbell held in one hand. In such a case they usually run their working forearm along the padded surface of a flat exercise bench in such a position that their wrist and hand hang off the edge of the bench.

Wrist Roller

General Comments: This movement strongly stresses all the muscles of the forearms. It can be done with either a simple stick and piece of clothesline or on the wall-mounted apparatus found in some gyms.

Starting Position: Grasp a wrist roller with your palms down and hold it out at arms' length directly in front of your shoulders.

Exercise Performance: Slowly roll the rope up in one direction or another, then slowly lower it back to the starting point. Then roll it up in the opposite direction. Reverse directions for several repetitions until the forearms muscles are fully fatigued.

Training Tips: On the wall-mounted apparatus you can simply roll it up in each direction. You needn't worry about balancing the stick out in front of your shoulders when using this piece of equipment, however.

Calf Exercises

Donkey Calf Raise

General Comments: Some individuals in pub-

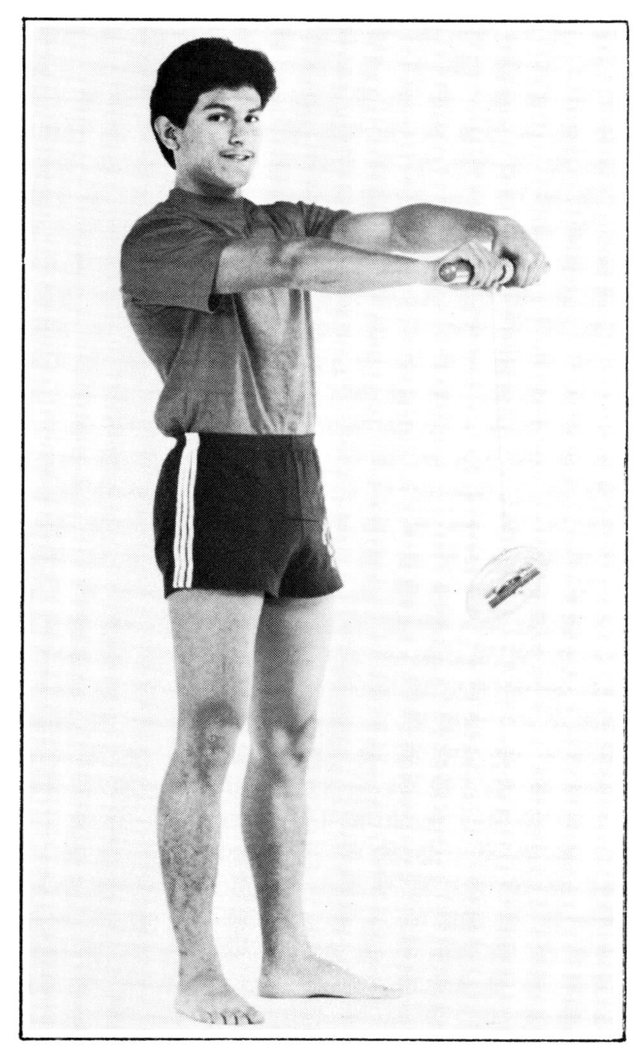

Wrist Roller.

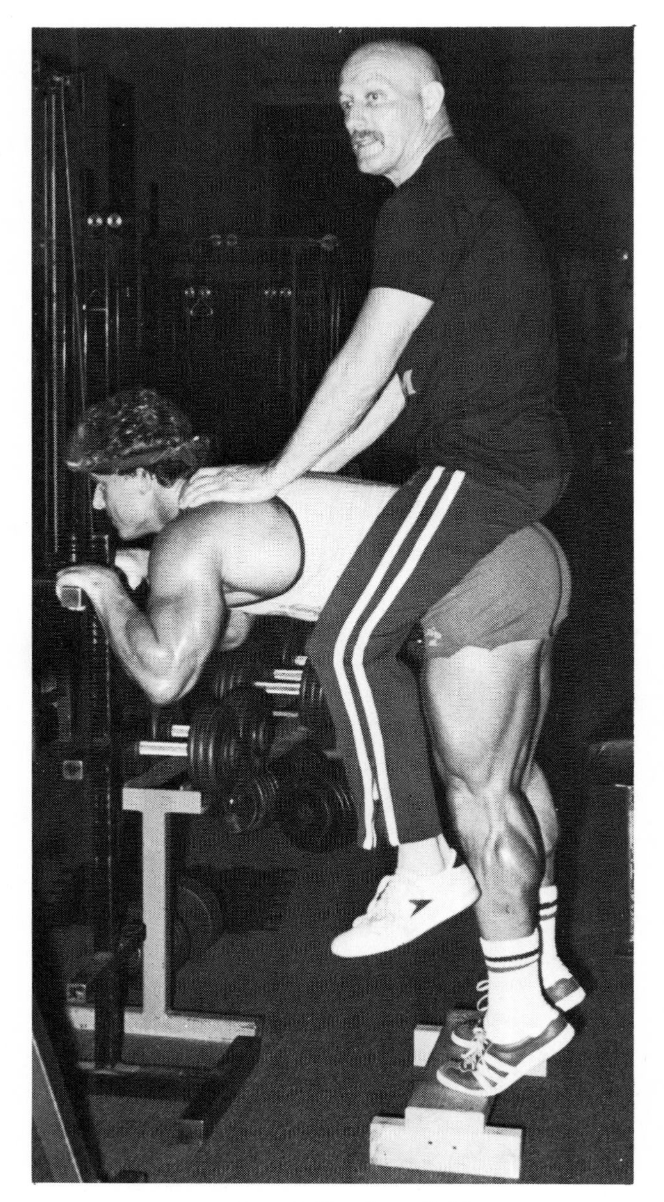

Donkey Calf Raise—finish.

lic gyms seem to feel that this exercise looks funny, but it is a very effective way to muscle up your calves.

Starting Position: Place your toes and the balls of your feet on a thick block of wood. Bend over at the waist so that your torso is parallel to the floor and place your hands on a flat exercise bench to keep your torso in this position. Have a heavy training partner hop up astride your hips as if he or she were riding a horse.

Exercise Performance: Sag your heels well below the level of your toes. Then rise up as high on your toes as possible. Lower slowly back to the starting point and repeat the movement.

Training Tips: Be sure to do some sets with your toes pointed outward at 45 degrees on each side, some with your toes angled inward at 45 degrees, and some with your toes pointed directly ahead.

Your training partner must be sure to sit as far back on your hips as possible. Sitting too far forward lessens the stress you put on your calves. Once your partner becomes too light for you, have him or her hold a barbell plate or a dumbbell in position on your lower back.

One-Leg Toe Raise—start.

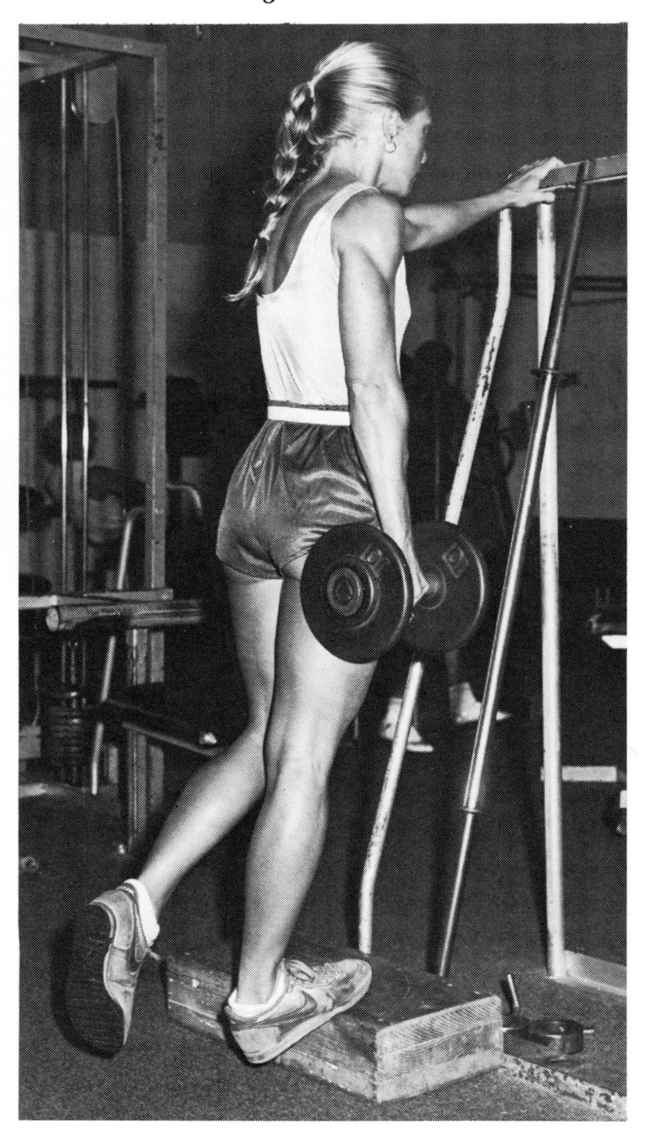

One-Leg Toe Raise

General Comments: As stated before, you can usually concentrate better on a movement that is done with one leg or one arm at a time. This exercise strongly stresses the calf muscles without requiring any apparatus other than a dumbbell and a calf block.

Starting Position: Stand with the toes and ball of one foot on a calf block and raise the other leg out of the way of the movement. Hold a dumbbell at arms' length down the side of your body in the hand on the same side as your exercising leg. With your other hand, grasp a solid object to steady your body throughout the movement.

Exercise Performance: Sag your heel as far below the level of your toes as possible. Then rise as high as possible before returning to the starting point. Repeat the movement for the desired number of reps.

Training Tips: You will find it a little difficult to use the suggested three toe positions on this movement, but you should attempt to do so nonetheless. If you have a staircase handy, you'll find it easy to do this exercise on one of the steps while holding the stair railing.

Abdominal Exercises

Hanging Leg Raises

General Comments: This exercise strongly stresses all the muscles of the front abdomen, particularly those of the lower abdomen.

Starting Position: Jump up and grasp a chinning bar with a shoulder-width grip, your palms facing forward. Hang your body straight down below the bar and bend your knees slightly to take pressure off your lower back as you do the movement.

Exercise Performance: Slowly raise your feet in semicircles to a position at which they are at the same height as your hips. Lower slowly back to the starting point and repeat the movement.

Training Tips: You will probably find that your body swings below the bar as you do this exercise. In such a case you should have a training partner press against your lower back to keep your body from swinging.

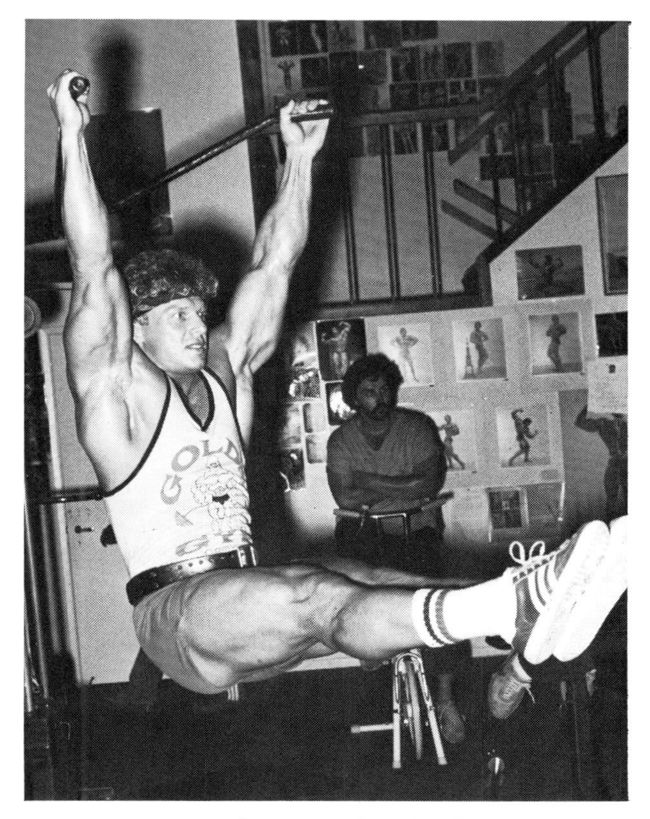

Hanging Leg Raise—finish.

Crunch

General Comments: This is a popular short-range movement for developing the front abdominal muscles, particularly those of the upper abdomen.

Starting Position: Lie on your back on the floor and drape your calves over a flat exercise bench as illustrated. Clasp your hands behind your neck and maintain this arm position throughout the movement.

Exercise Performance: You must do three things simultaneously to do this movement properly. First, use your lower abdominal strength to lift your hips from the floor. Second, attempt to force your shoulders toward your hips, which will result in your shoulders coming off the floor. And third, strongly blow your breath out. If you do all three of these things optimally, you will feel a very strong contraction in your front abdominal muscles. Lower back to the starting point and repeat the movement for the desired number of repetitions.

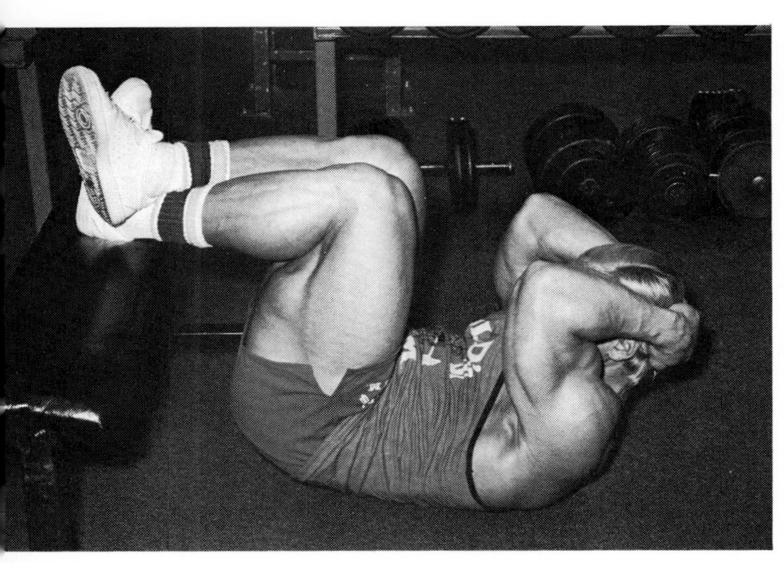

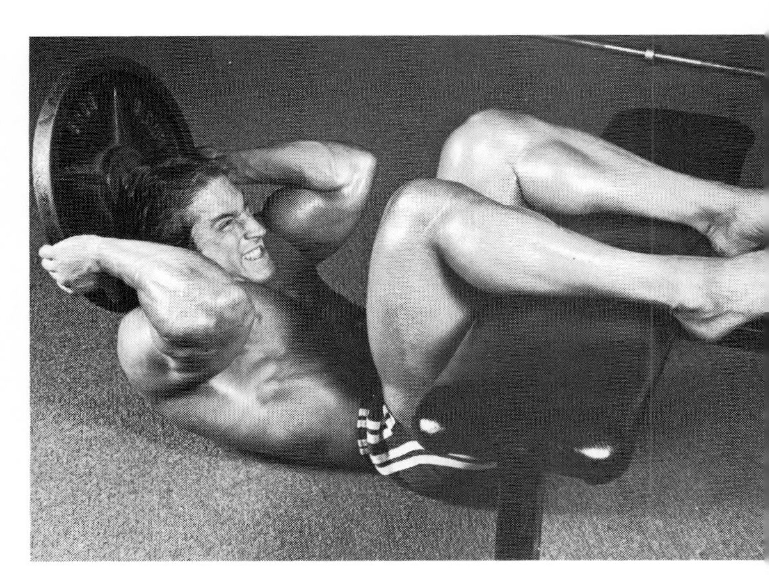

Crunches—top position, left; top position with extra weight, right (*photo by Bill Dobbins*).

Training Tips: Alternative foot positions include sitting with your hips in the *L* formed by a wall and the floor and running your legs up the wall, as well as merely placing your feet on the wall rather than having your lower legs resting on an exercise bench.

Bench Leg Raise

General Comments: This is a more stressful variation of the standard Leg Raise described in Chapter 3. It strongly stresses all the front abdominal muscles, but particularly those of the lower abdomen.

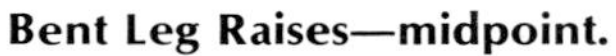

Bent Leg Raises—midpoint.

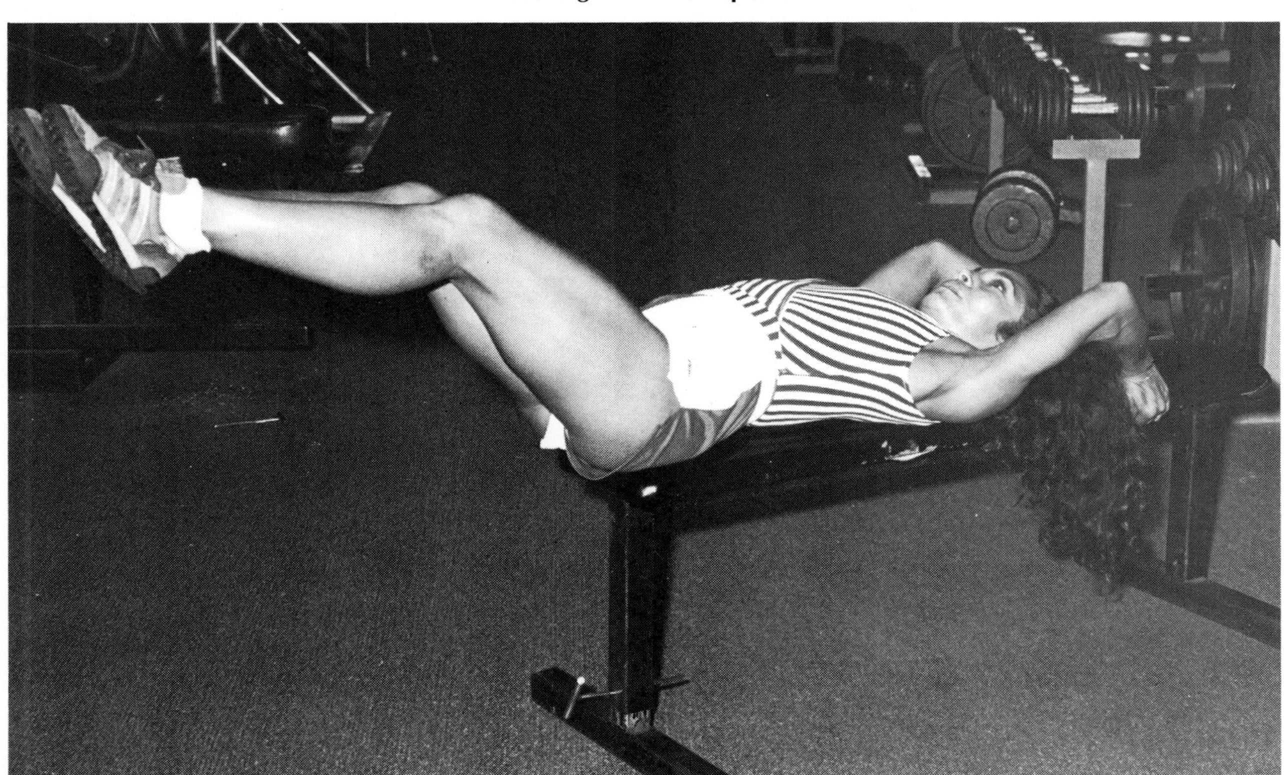

Starting Position: Lie on your back on a flat exercise bench so that your hips are at the end of the bench and your legs are hanging off. Bend your legs slightly to take undue stress off your lower back as you do the movement. Grasp the bench behind your head with your hands to steady your body on the bench during the movement.

Exercise Performance: Begin with your feet as close to the floor as comfortably possible. Then raise your feet in semicircular arcs until they are directly above your hips. Lower them slowly back down along the same arcs to the starting point. Repeat the movement for the desired number of counts.

Training Tips: To add stress to the muscles once this exercise becomes easy to do you can wear iron boots on your feet. You can also elevate the head end of your bench a little by placing a block of wood under the legs.

Roman Chair Sit-Ups.

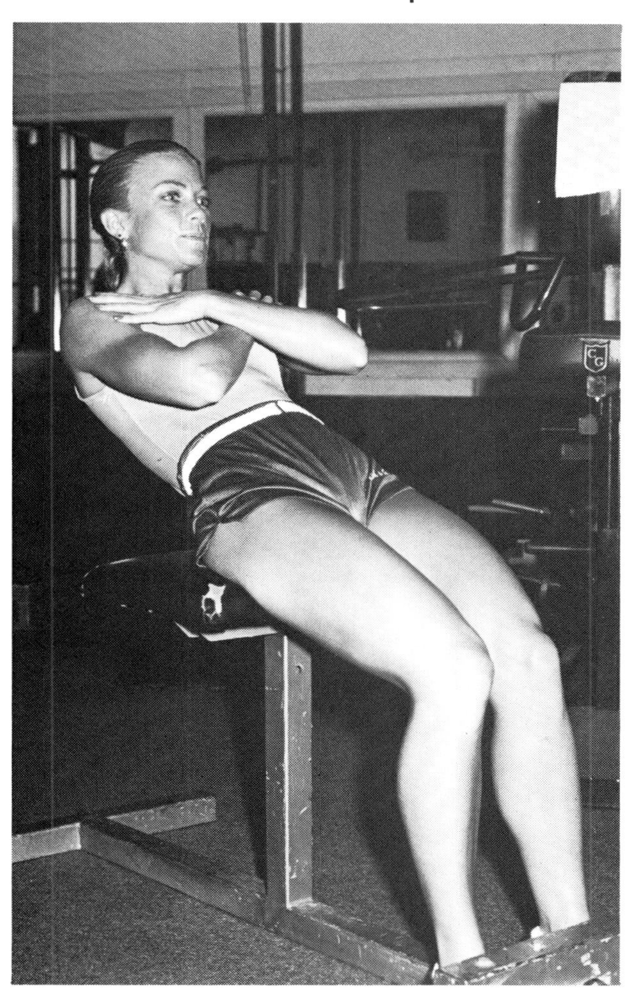

Roman Chair Sit-ups

General Comments: This has become one of the favorite exercises among Gold's Gym members for bringing out upper abdominal muscularity.

Starting Position: Sit on the padded surface of a Roman chair apparatus and slip your insteps under the toe bar near the floor. Cross your arms on your chest and keep them in this position throughout the movement.

Exercise Performance: Lean backward until your torso is a little below a line drawn at a 45-degree angle from the floor. This will be the limit of your range of backward motion. Then sit back up until you begin to feel stress being lifted from your front abdominals. This will be the limit of your forward range of motion. Simply rock back and forth between these two points to stress your upper abdominals.

Training Tips: For added stress on your abs you can place a thick block of wood under the foot end of the apparatus. You can also hold a light barbell plate across your chest, though this is not often done at Gold's Gym.

Intermediate-Level Workouts

In this section we present three additional progressively difficult training routines. If you have followed the programs presented at the end of Chapter 3, you will be ready for the first routine (Level 5, next page) in this section.

You should progress through these three routines, spending four to six weeks with each new workout. Once you have finished the Level 7 program you will have reached sufficient physical condition to be considered an advanced bodybuilder capable of handling the training schedules in Chapter 7.

Level 5

(Monday and Thursday)

Exercise	Sets	Reps
1. Hanging Leg Raise	2–3	10–15
2. Roman Chair Sit-Up	2–3	50–100
3. Incline Dumbbell Press	4	6–10
4. Parallel Bar Dip	3	10–15
5. Flat-Bench Flye	3	8–12
6. Seated Press behind the Neck	3	6–10
7. Side Lateral	3	8–12
8. Bent Lateral	3	8–12
9. Pulley Pushdown	3	8–12
10. Incline Triceps Extension	3	8–12
11. Barbell Preacher Curl	3	8–12
12. Concentration Curl	3	8–12
13. Barbell Wrist Curl	3–4	10–15
14. Barbell Reverse Wrist Curl	3–4	10–15
15. Seated Calf Machine (Toe Raise)	4–5	10–12
16. Donkey Calf Raise	3–4	12–15

(Tuesday and Friday)

Exercise	Sets	Reps
1. Bench Leg Raise	2–3	20–30
2. Crunch	2–3	20–30
3. Hyperextension	2–3	10–15
4. Dumbbell Shrug	3–4	10–15
5. Chin	4	8–12
6. Dumbbell Bent Rowing	3	8–12
7. Seated Pulley Rowing	3	8–12
8. Leg Press	4	10–15
9. Hack Squat	3	8–12
10. Leg Extension	3	8–12
11. Leg Curl	4	8–12
12. Reverse Curl	3–4	8–12
13. Dumbbell Wrist Curl	3–4	10–15
14. One-Leg Toe Raise	3–4	10–15
15. Calf Press	3–4	15–20

Level 6

Do Part 1 on Monday, Wednesday, and Friday during one week and on Tuesday and Thursday during the next. Do Part 2 on Tuesday and Thursday during the first week and on Monday, Wednesday, and Friday during the next. Continue alternating weeks like this *ad infinitum.*

PART 1

Exercise	Sets	Reps
1. Incline Leg Raise	2–3	20–30
2. Roman Chair Sit-Up	2–3	50–100
3. Side Bend	2–3	50–100
4. Decline Press	4	6–10
5. Incline Flye	4	8–12
6. Pec Deck Flye	4	8–12
7. Seated Pulley Rowing	4	8–12
8. Lat Pulldown behind the Neck	4	8–12
9. Dumbbell Bent Rowing	4	8–12
10. Stiff-Leg Deadlift	4	10–15
11. Upright Rowing	4	8–12
12. Seated Dumbbell Press	4	6–10
13. Front Lateral	3	8–12
14. Bent Lateral	4	8–12
15. Standing Calf Machine (Toe Raise)	4–5	10–12
16. Donkey Calf Raise	4–5	12–15

PART 2

Exercise	Sets	Reps
1. Incline Sit-Ups	2–3	20–30
2. Hanging Leg Raise	2–3	10–15
3. Seated Twisting	2–3	50–100
4. Front Squat	4	10–15
5. Lunge	4	10–15
6. Leg Extension	4	8–12
7. Leg Curl	5	8–12
8. Dumbbell Curl	4	8–12
9. Pulley Curl	4	8–12
10. Reverse Curl	4	8–12
11. Dumbbell Triceps Extension	4	8–12
12. Lying Triceps Extension	4	8–12
13. Dumbbell Wrist Curl	5	10–15
14. Barbell Reverse Wrist Curl	5	10–15
15. Seated Calf Machine (Toe Raise)	4–6	8–10
16. One-Leg Calf Raise	4–6	12–15

Level 7

(Monday-Thursday)

Exercise	Sets	Reps
1. Hanging Leg Raise	2-3	10-15
2. Incline Sit-Up	2-3	20-30
3. Side Bend	2-3	50-100
4. Incline Barbell Press	4	6-10
5. Parallel Bar Dip	4	8-12
6. Incline Flye	3	8-12
7. Dumbbell Bench Press	3	8-12
8. Chin behind the Neck	4	8-12
9. Front Lat Pulldown	4	8-12
10. Seated Pulley Rowing	3	8-12
11. Dumbbell Bent Rowing	3	8-12
12. Good Morning	4	10-15
13. Upright Rowing	4	8-12
14. Calf Press	4	10-15
15. Seated Calf Machine (Toe Raise)	4	8-12

(Tuesday-Friday)

Exercise	Sets	Reps
1. Incline Leg Raise	2-3	20-30
2. Crunch	2-3	20-30
3. Seated Twisting	2-3	50-100
4. Seated Press behind the Neck	4	6-10
5. Side Lateral	3	8-12
6. Front Lateral	3	8-12
7. Bent Lateral	4	8-12
8. Alternate Dumbbell Curl	4	8-12
9. Barbell Preacher Curl	4	8-12
10. Narrow-Grip Reverse Curl	4	8-12
11. Standing Barbell Triceps Extension	4	8-12
12. Decline Triceps Extension	3	8-12
13. Dip between Benches	3	10-15
14. Dumbbell Wrist Curl	4	10-15
15. Barbell Reverse Wrist Curl	4	10-15

(Wednesday-Saturday)

Exercise	Sets	Reps
1. Bench Leg Raise	2-3	20-30
2. Roman Chair Sit-Up	2-3	50-100
3. Hyperextension	2-3	50-100
4. Squat	5	10-15
5. Hack Squat	4	10-15
6. Leg Extension	4	8-12
7. Leg Curl	5	8-12
8. Lunge	3	10-15
9. Wrist Roller	4-6	—
10. Standing Calf Raise (Toe Raise)	3-4	10-15
11. Donkey Calf Raise	3-4	10-15
12. Calf Press	3-4	10-15

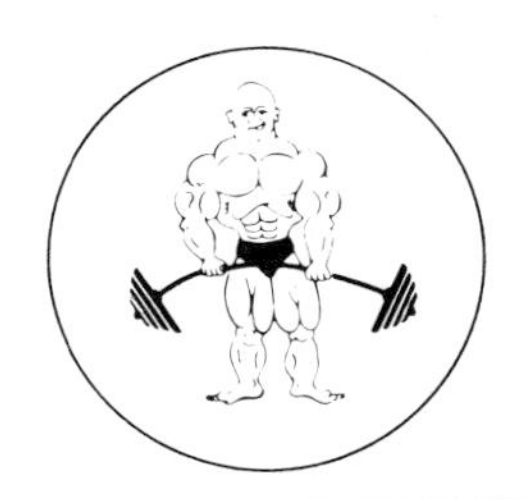

6 CONTEST-LEVEL TRAINING TIPS

Let's begin this chapter with a minilecture on bodybuilding public relations. While bodybuilding has achieved great public acceptance over the past few years—primarily through the film and television exposure given to it by Lou Ferrigno and Arnold Schwarzenegger—there are still many persons who look askance at bodybuilders. Give them one small opening, and they will go out of their way to ridicule you as being stupid, unathletic, plain weird, or any number of other negative descriptions.

As a bodybuilder, you have an obligation to maintain a good public relations posture, because any negative conduct on your part reflects negatively on all of us. Constantly talking about bodybuilding in public, wearing T-shirts that look like they've been spray-painted on (some fools dress like this even in subfreezing temperatures), or walking around with lats spread and every muscle in your body flexed to the max is definitely *not* the way to present bodybuilding to the general public in a positive light.

The great Bill Pearl (Mr. America and a four-time Mr. Universe winner) comments on proper bodybuilding public relations. "You'll do much more for both the sport and yourself by deemphasizing the fact that you're a bodybuilder," Bill said. "Your physique and latent physical power will be evident enough to everyone, even if you're dressed in a long-sleeved shirt and stand or sit totally relaxed at all times.

"Instead of projecting your body, work at projecting your intellect and your personality. Be friendly and relaxed around people and develop your skills as a conversationalist. This way the average person will see you as a likable human being rather than as a strutting peacock. And, believe me, this 'human' image does far more to promote our great sport than anything else you could do!"

Training Instinct

Every successful bodybuilder has developed over the years an instinctive ability to sense within a few days whether a new exercise or training technique is working well or a new dietary practice is having a desired effect on the body. Such training instincts are extremely valuable to bodybuilders, because they save them weeks and months of trial-and-error experimentation with a variety of bodybuilding and nutritional techniques.

The only way to develop an accurate training

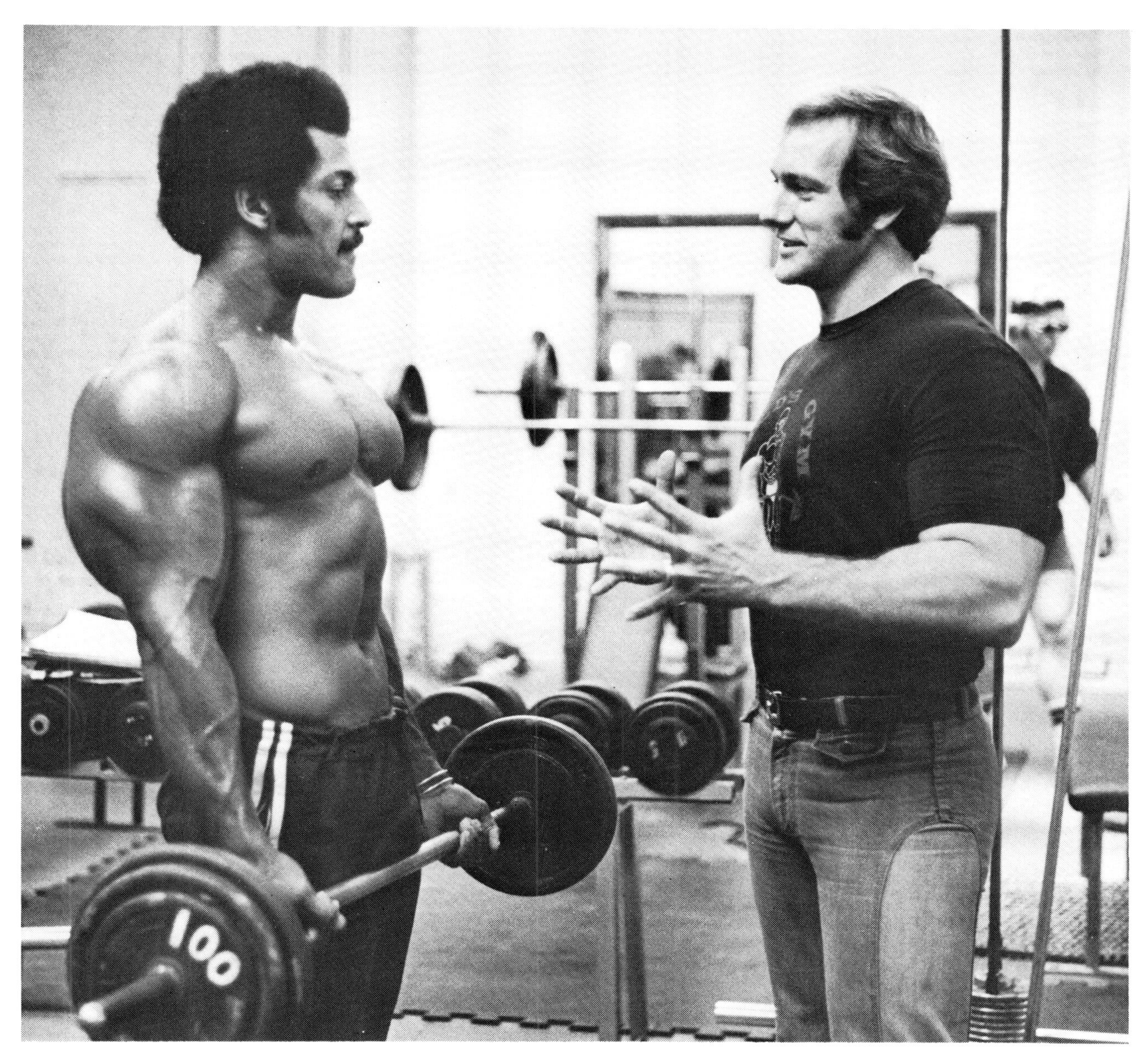

Ken Sprague (right) instructs Manny Perry (Mr. USA) on the intricacies of upper arm development, as if Perry needs advice on developing massive arms! *(Photo by Bill Reynolds)*

instinct is constantly to monitor the biofeedback signals that your body gives you. These signals can be as obvious as a great muscle pump from a particular set or as subtle as a good psychological response to a new training technique.

Muscle pump is probably the biofeedback signal that most bodybuilders monitor. Around Gold's Gym you constantly hear Lou Ferrigno or someone else saying, "Wow, I really got a good pump in my biceps with the new routine I'm on!" And a good pump (a tight, blood-congested feeling in a muscle) is a reliable signal that you've trained a particular muscle group optimally. Stiffness and soreness in a muscle group a day or two after training it also is a good sign that you really blitzed it into new growth.

Quite a few bodybuilders like to work for a "burn" in a muscle group. This burning sensation is caused by a build-up of fatigue toxins that is too great for the body to be able to eliminate the toxins quickly. Such a burn is

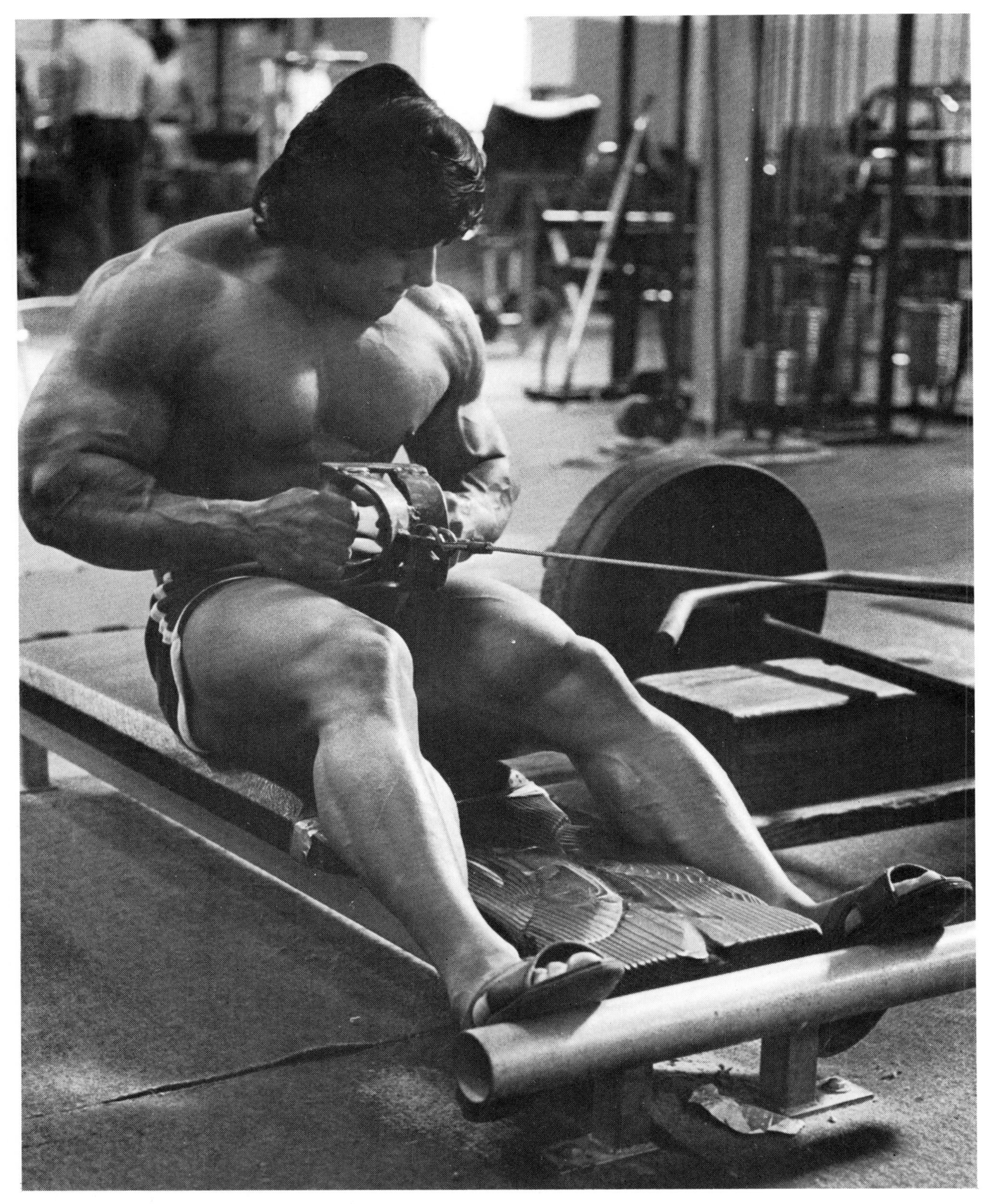

Massive Danny Padilla, "The Giant Killer," reps out on heavy Seated Pulley Rows at Gold's II. No one has equalled his huge muscle mass and perfect proportions. *(Photo by Bob Gardner)*

another sign that you've worked a muscle optimally. Usually this burning sensation also accompanies a good muscle pump.

To a great degree, increased strength in a variety of exercises also is a good indication that the muscles are growing. There is a linear relationship between muscle mass and the heaviness of the exercise weights you use for reps (usually a minimum of 4–5 repetitions) in your workouts. It is possible, however, to increase your strength dramatically for a single rep in any exercise without increasing muscle mass, because single-rep power is more a function of mind power and tendon-ligament strength than of muscle size.

There are tactile and visual factors that can also improve your training instinct. You can test your muscle density (hardness) simply by feeling each muscle group from time to time. Greater muscle density indicates that your training and dietary techniques are successful. It's also easy to see improvements in your physique in various poses in front of a mirror. Be wary of weighing or measuring yourself, however, because you can easily make weight and measurement gains while actually regressing in muscle quality.

Nutritional instinct is a little easier to develop than training instinct. What foods make you fatter? Are there certain foods that bloat your body with water? Which foods have you eaten that cut you up quickly? Is a low-calorie diet or a low-carbohydrate diet best for cutting up your body? Do certain supplements give you greater training energy? Simply answering these questions through a series of dietary experiments will quickly give you good nutritional instinct.

Within a year or two of monitoring your body's biofeedback signals you'll develop a feel for what does and doesn't work in your unique body lab. At that point you will have achieved true training instinct. It's difficult for a champion to explain to a novice bodybuilder how training instinct works, but the great professional champion Albert Beckles has attempted to tackle the task.

"When I inject some new technique into my routine I can feel how it works on my muscles immediately," Albert explained. "If it feels a certain way, I know that it's going to help improve my physique, and I retain it in my training philosophy. But if it feels another way, I know it's worthless and immediately reject it. It may take a year or two to develop this type of judgment, but it *will* come for you. And once you have it, you have every chance of eventually becoming a champion. Instinctive training ability is the most valuable weapon in a bodybuilder's arsenal."

Individualizing Routines

Obviously, we can't make up training programs for you *ad infinitum*. Sooner or later you'll need to take the plunge and make up your own workouts. And this will be greatly to your benefit, because by now you are beginning to learn more about your body and what makes it respond than we could ever know.

The first rule you should follow in formulating your routine is to include exercises for every body part. You should also use muscle priority training (explained in detail at the beginning of Chapter 4) on your lagging muscle groups by training them first in your routine when your mental and physical energies are at their highest. Following these two practices will assure you of maintaining a well-proportioned physique.

Next, you should be careful to avoid doing an excessive number of total sets per muscle group, which might ultimately cause you to overtrain. In precontest training you will always do more total sets in an effort to harden up your musculature, but in normal off-season muscle-building workouts you shouldn't exceed these tolerances for total numbers of sets for each muscle group:

Thighs and Back: 15–18
Chest and Calves: 12–15
Deltoids and Abdominals: 10–12
Biceps and Triceps: 8–10
Forearms: 6–8

Ordinarily, you needn't do any direct neck training, because the neck muscles tend to grow quite naturally from peripheral exercise for the shoulders and upper back.

Training frequency is also important. When following a general building cycle, you need not train a muscle group more than twice per week. Most commonly this is done on a six-day split routine, though some bodybuilders prefer to train on a four-day split during this cycle.

Next, it's generally best to train the larger muscle groups of your body early in your workouts. This is because the larger muscles require greater energy expenditures, and even when your energy reserves are low you can still train a small muscle group like your biceps. You would never, of course, be able to do justice to your legs late in your workout.

Here is a list of your muscle groups in descending order of size:

1. Thighs
2. Back
3. Chest
4. Calves
5. Deltoids
6. Triceps
7. Biceps
8. Forearms
9. Abdominals
10. Neck

Finally, when formulating your own routines, never do your arm workouts before you train your torso muscles. The reason for this will become abundantly clear in our discussion of preexhaustion later in this chapter. For now, however, simply understand that your arm muscles are smaller and weaker than those of your back, chest, and shoulders. As a result, arm strength limits the degree of exercise intensity that you can apply to your torso muscles. Training your arms first in a workout would further weaken them and aggravate the situation, so it's essential that you bomb your torso muscles prior to hitting your arms.

Slow Gainers

It won't take any bodybuilder long to discover that some men and women make exceptionally fast bodybuilding gains while others make exceptionally slow gains. A fast gainer—as exemplified by individuals like Casey Viator, Lance Dreher, Lisa Elliott, and the Mentzer brothers—can pack on muscle mass two or three times more quickly than a slow gainer.

Slow gains shouldn't discourage any bodybuilder, however. There are also a lot of slow gainers like Pete Grymkowski, Larry Scott, Laura Combes, and Frank Zane who have hit on formulas of training and diet that have ultimately made them into bodybuilding superstars. If you are a slow gainer, you can do the same thing by taking a persistent and scientific approach to your training.

Slow gainers are generally very prone to overtraining, so during the off-season they should never work out more than four times per week. And when they switch to a six-day split routine prior to a contest it should be one in which each major body part is trained only twice a week.

If you are a slow gainer, you will also find that you will make your best gains doing only one or two basic exercises per muscle group for as few as 6–10 total sets per body part. And you'll probably discover that your muscles respond most quickly to repetitions in the range of 5–6.

To clarify this, here is a typical off-season training routine for a slow gainer:

MONDAY-THURSDAY

Exercise	Sets	Reps
1. Incline Sit-Up	2–3	20–30
2. Hyperextension	1	10–12
3. Squat	5	5–8
4. Leg Curl	3	5–8
5. Seated Pulley Rowing	4	5–8
6. Lat Pulldown	3	5–8
7. Barbell Shrugs	3	8–10
8. Barbell Curl	3	4–6
9. Reverse Curl	2	5–8
10. Barbell Wrist Curl	4	10–12
11. Seated Calf Machine (Toe Raise)	5	8–10

TUESDAY-FRIDAY

Exercise	Sets	Reps
1. Hanging Leg Raise	2–3	10–15
2. Incline Barbell Press	4	4–6
3. Parallel Bar Dip	3	6–8
4. Flye	3	6–8
5. Military Press	3	4–6
6. Bent Lateral	3	6–8
7. Lying Triceps Extension	3	6–8
8. Barbell Reverse Wrist Curl	4	10–12
9. Standing Calf Machine (Toe Raise)	5	8–10

Be very sure to constantly try to increase the weights you use in every exercise, but not at the expense of strict exercise form. The stronger you become, the larger your muscles will be.

Full rest and recuperation are essential to a slow gainer. A full complement of sleep each night—as well as an afternoon nap, if possible—will be very valuable. And no slow gainer has ever been able to put on much muscle mass while running five or six miles per day, because such an energy expenditure is difficult to replenish each day. And without full recuperation, as explained earlier, your muscles simply won't grow, even as a result of a heavy workout.

Nutritionally, a slow gainer should follow the plan of eating five or six protein-rich meals per day as outlined in the section on weight gain diets in Chapter 4. This meal plan will allow your body to digest and assimilate the maximum amount of protein from your daily foods, which ultimately adds up to greatly augmented muscle mass.

Nonroutine Routines

Any way you cut the cake, your muscles are lazy little creatures. While they readily adapt to a new stress, they seldom like to do any more work than they are forced to do. They grow just enough in size and strength to accommodate the stress placed on them and then retain that level of mass and strength. Your muscles can become so used to a particular routine that, even though you are regularly increasing exercise resistance, they drag their feet in terms of adding mass and/or strength.

To circumvent this problem you might profit considerably from following a nonroutine routine in which you constantly vary the exercises, the numbers of sets and reps, the training poundages, and the exercise sequencing for each muscle group during every workout.

C. F. Smith, MD (Mr. Tennessee and a former fifth-place finisher in the Mr. America contest) was one of the first bodybuilders to advocate this method. Lou Ferrigno uses it extensively these days, calling it "muscle confusion training." And it literally does confuse the muscles, because they can never get used to any particular type of training and thus are constantly forced to grow in size and strength to accommodate each new challenge thrown at them.

Circuit Training

Circuit training has most frequently been applied to athletic conditioning, but it can also be applied in a bodybuilding setting when an athlete needs greater endurance. It is a method that builds a certain degree of strength and muscle mass along with super endurance. As such, you can see how this system can be so valuable to athletes. But bodybuilders can also use it to burn off body fat and reveal crisp contest muscularity.

In circuit training you must set up 10–20 stations around a gym at which you can do exercises for each muscle group. Then you proceed rapidly from station to station, doing 8–12 reps at each until you have completed a full circuit. You should rest only long enough between stations to move from one to the next. Then, after a full circuit, you can take a two- or three-minute break before continuing on to do two or three more circuits.

Here is a typical circuit of exercise stations that you can set up around your gym.

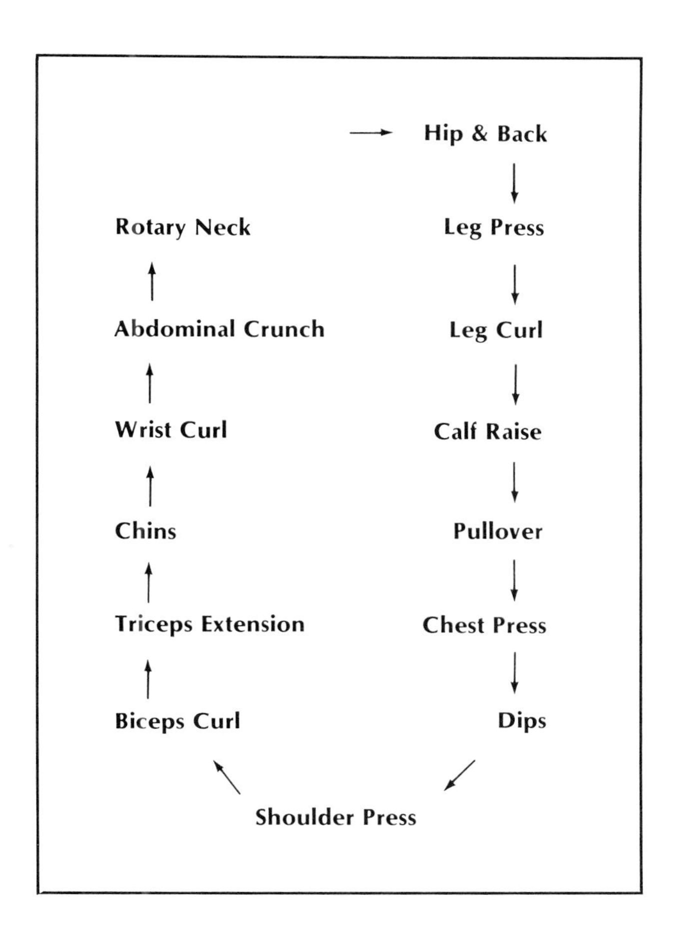

This circuit of 15 exercises should take no more than 15 minutes to complete. At first you will feel rather breathless and fatigued after only one circuit, but very quickly your cardiorespiratory endurance will improve, and you will soon be able to train virtually nonstop for an hour or more on this type of program.

PHA Training

Bob Gajda, winner of the 1966 Mr. America and 1967 Mr. Universe titles, was a student of exercise physiology at the time he was training to win his titles. He now has his PhD in physiology, operates a huge sports complex in Chicago, and is one of the world's leading experts on physical conditioning.

Gejda's mentor, Dr. Steinhaus, gave a lecture one day to Bob on Peripheral Heart Action, or PHA. Essentially, the human heart (which is merely a muscular pump) is not large or strong enough to pump all of the body's blood supply throughout the vascular system. As a result, it relies on hundreds of "peripheral hearts," which are the body's skeletal muscles. Every time a skeletal muscle contracts it squeezes blood past one-way valves in the vascular system, assisting the heart in circulating the blood.

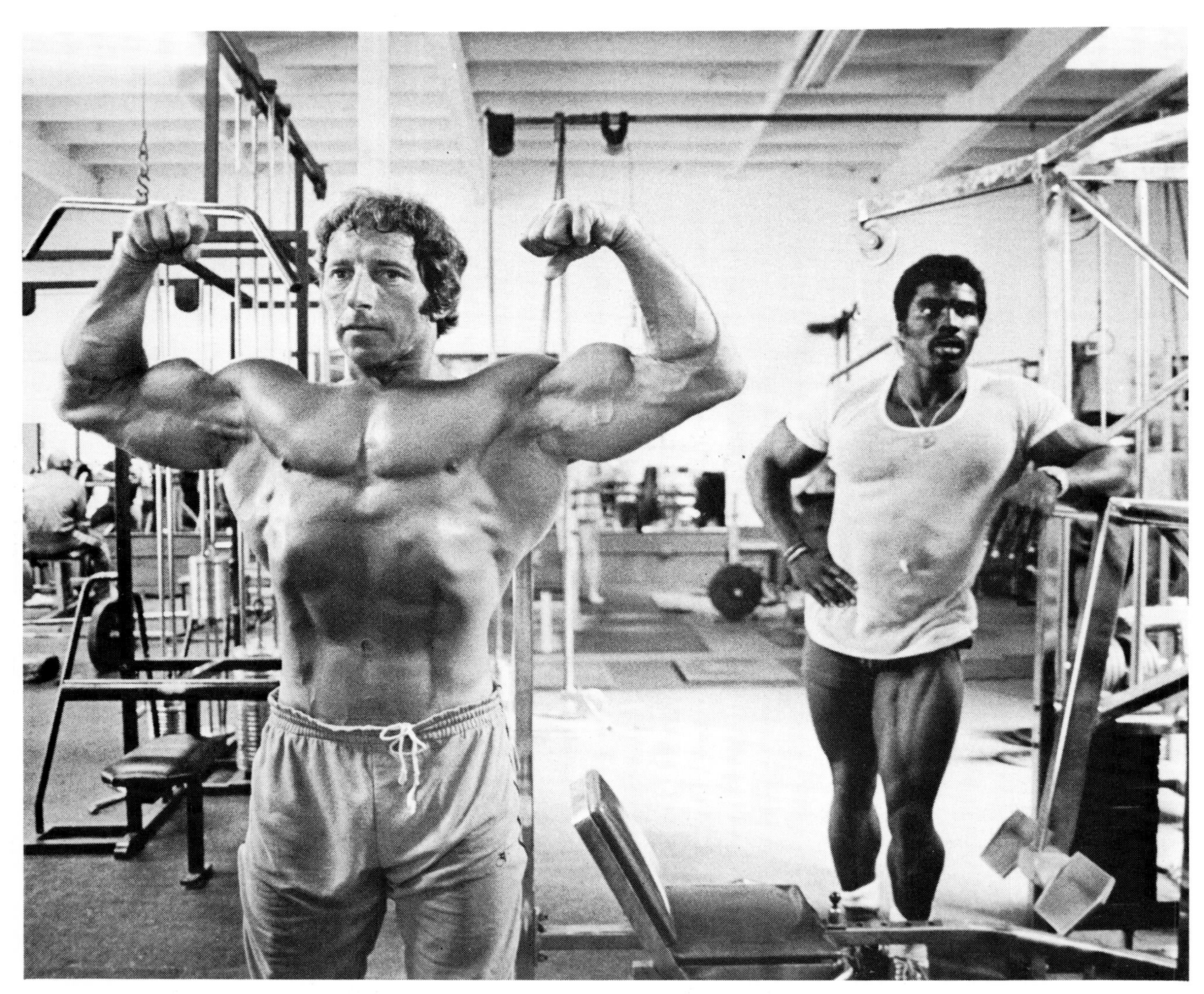

Robby Robinson checks out the upper body development of Ed Guiliani, Mr. Western America. *(Photo by Bill Reynolds)*

Without peripheral heart action, blood would pool in the lower extremities, since the heart-pump is unable to overcome gravity. An interesting example of this occurs when soldiers stand at attention in formation for an extended period of time. Eventually, so much blood pools in their legs that the brain is deprived of the oxygen that the blood normally supplies it. Then, the soldier—usually still perfectly at attention—faints and falls on his face.

From Dr. Steinhaus, Bob Gajda also learned that blood circulation, enhanced by peripheral heart action, also augmented the production of blood buffers, chemicals which cleansed the blood and simultaneously reduced fatigue and increased endurance. Gajda immediately saw an application for what Dr. Steinhaus told him to his bodybuilding training, and he soon developed his PHA systems.

Gajda's system was similar to the circuit training system just discussed except that he used shorter circuits of 4–6 exercises. In a public gym setting it's exceedingly difficult to set up circuits of 15–20 exercises, while 4–6-exercise circuits are not that difficult to hold together for 10–15 minutes. And Bob would use 6–10 such minicircuits in his PHA programs.

The object of PHA was to jump from one body part to another with each exercise. One was never to do two exercises in succession for one body part or for adjacent muscle groups, since this could induce a muscle pump, which was to be avoided. Maximum blood circulation was the object, and a pump was a sure sign of blood congestion, rather than circulation, in a muscle.

Since bodybuilders at the time were so pump-oriented, many openly ridiculed Gajda's PHA system. But using his own system, Gajda was able to use heavy poundages for 50–60 sets per muscle group with great results. He grew like a weed, and his supersharp muscularity was far ahead of its time. He was so good that he defeated the legendary Sergio Oliva in the 1966 Mr. America competition. And a year later in Warsaw, he easily won the Mr. Universe title.

Due to Bob Gajda's personal success, PHA training enjoyed a brief vogue during the late 1960s. Then, quite unfortunately, PHA fell into disuse. PHA has much to offer to today's champion bodybuilders, because no other system allows you to do so many total sets in one workout without becoming completely exhausted. And as a result, PHA will allow you to slice your physique to shreds—develop well-defined muscles—while maintaining a high degree of muscle mass.

As with circuit training, you will probably become very fatigued during your first two or three PHA workouts, because few bodybuilders are used to endurance-type training. Therefore, it's a good idea to do only a single trip through each circuit during the first couple of workouts. And then, as your endurance gradually improves, you can add a new series at each couple of workouts. Soon you can be breezing through 100- to 150-set workouts, getting huge and ripped in the process.

Here is a low-level PHA workout that you can use on three nonconsecutive days per week, just to get used to this type of training:

Series I	**Series II**
1. Bench Press	1. Seated Pulley Rowing
2. Leg Extension	2. Incline Sit-Up
3. Upright Rowing	3. Leg Press
4. Hyperextension	4. Barbell Curl
5. Pulley Pushdown	5. Seated Calf Machine (Toe Raise)
6. Barbell Wrist Curl	6. Side Lateral

Series III	**Series IV**
1. Incline Flye	1. Squat
2. Lat Machine Pulldown	2. Neck Strap Movement
3. Lying Barbell Triceps Extension	3. Front Barbell Raise
4. Leg Curl	4. Dumbbell Kickback
5. Bent Lateral	5. Standing Calf Machine (Toe Raise)
6. Stiff-Leg Deadlift	6. Dumbbell Press

Continued on next page

Series V	Series VI
1. Parallel Bar Dip	1. Seated Press behind the Neck
2. Reverse Barbell Curl	2. Incline Dumbbell Curl
3. Standing Leg Curl	3. Cross-Bench Dumbbell Pullover
4. Dumbbell Bent Rowing	4. Barbell Reverse Wrist Curl
5. Leg Press Machine Calf Press	5. Dumbbell Shrug
6. Seated Twisting	6. Pec Deck Flye

At first, you can go relatively slowly through one set of each series, building up within a week or two to doing a set of each series with only enough rest between exercises to move from one piece of equipment to another. Then gradually work up to doing three to five trips through each series, taking a two- or three-minute break between each fully completed series to set up your equipment for the next series.

When training for his Mr. America and Mr. Universe wins, Bob Gajda himself trained six days per week on his PHA system, using a modified split routine. To maintain the PHA effect, Bob actually trained each body part every day, but he alternated "upper body emphasis" days with "lower body emphasis" days.

Gajda's entire routine was so involved that it would be difficult to list the whole program on these pages. Here, however, are two typical series from each type of workout.

UPPER BODY EMPHASIS

Series I	Series II
1. Incline Dumbbell Press	1. Barbell Bent Rowing
2. Barbell Curl	2. Lying Triceps Extension
3. Leg Extension	3. Leg Curl
4. Seated Military Press	4. Decline Flye
5. Barbell Wrist Curl	5. Side Lateral
6. One-Leg Calf Raise	6. Hanging Leg Raise

LOWER BODY EMPHASIS

Series I	Series II
1. Squat	1. Front Squat
2. Lat Machine Pulldown	2. Flat-Bench Flye
3. Stiff-Leg Deadlift	3. Seated Calf Machine (Toe Raise)
4. Seated Twisting	4. Dumbbell Press

Bob Gajda would do up to 10 trips through each series, building optimum health, great physical endurance, superb strength, and an outstanding physique in the process. You could profit as much from PHA training yourself, if you give it a fair trial in your workouts.

Supersets

A superset is a grouping of two exercises done with little or no rest between movements, then followed by a normal rest interval. As such, supersets are a significant step up the ladder of training intensity from straight sets.

The most basic type of superset is done between antagonistic muscle groups, such as the biceps and triceps. Here is an example of a typical biceps-triceps superset (brackets enclose the exercises to be supersetted):

{ 1. Barbell Curl
{ 2. Pulley Pushdown

Similar supersets can be done for the lats and pecs (Lat Pulldown + Bench Press), the forearms (Wrist Curl + Reverse Wrist Curl), and thighs (Leg Extension + Leg Curl). The first supersets you do in your workouts should be for your biceps and triceps, since these are smaller muscle groups that require a relatively minor energy expenditure.

A more intense form of superset involves two consecutive exercises for the same muscle group. Here are several samples of this type of superset:

Biceps: Barbell Preacher Curl + Barbell Curl
Triceps: Lat Pushdown + Lying Triceps Extension

Deltoids: Side Lateral + Press Behind the Neck
Chest: Bench Press + Flye
Lats: Chin + Bent-Arm Pullover
Thighs: Squat + Leg Extension
Hamstrings: Stiff-Legged Deadlift + Leg Curl
Calves: Standing Calf Raise + Seated Calf Raise (Toe Raise)

Another step up the intensity ladder from supersets is trisets, which will be discussed in Chapter 8.

Cheating

In Chapter 4 we talked about training to failure and mentioned two methods for pushing a set past the point of normal muscular failure. One of these methods was cheating. Most beginning bodybuilders are advised to avoid cheating, (using extraneous body action to help lift up a weight), because they invariably cheat to make a set easier to finish. But if you can learn to cheat to make a set even harder than normal to finish, you will be able to take another large step up the bodybuilding ladder of intensity.

A Barbell Curl is one of the easiest bodybuilding movements on which you can effectively use cheating. Before you cheat, however, you must take a set of heavy Barbell Curls to failure. Then, when you can no longer do another repetition in strict form, use *just enough* body swing to curl the bar past the sticking point of the movement, after which you curl it under your own power to the finish point of the exercise.

It's essential as you cheat the bar up that you don't simply swing it from your thighs to your shoulders using little or no biceps strength. And you must avoid simply letting the barbell fall unimpeded from your shoulders back to the starting point of the exercise. Instead, you must mightily resist the downward path of the weight to take full advantage of the benefits of the negative aspect of the weight. Negative reps will be discussed fully in Chapter 8, but briefly for now, resisting the downward momentum of a weight actually has greater potential for building strength and muscle mass than lifting the weight in the first place.

After two or three cheating reps on the Barbell Curl, your biceps will feel like they're on fire. You will have pushed significantly past the point of normal muscular failure, consequently stimulating your biceps more than is normally possible. And, of course, they will grow more quickly from a set or two of cheating reps than from merely going to failure on each set.

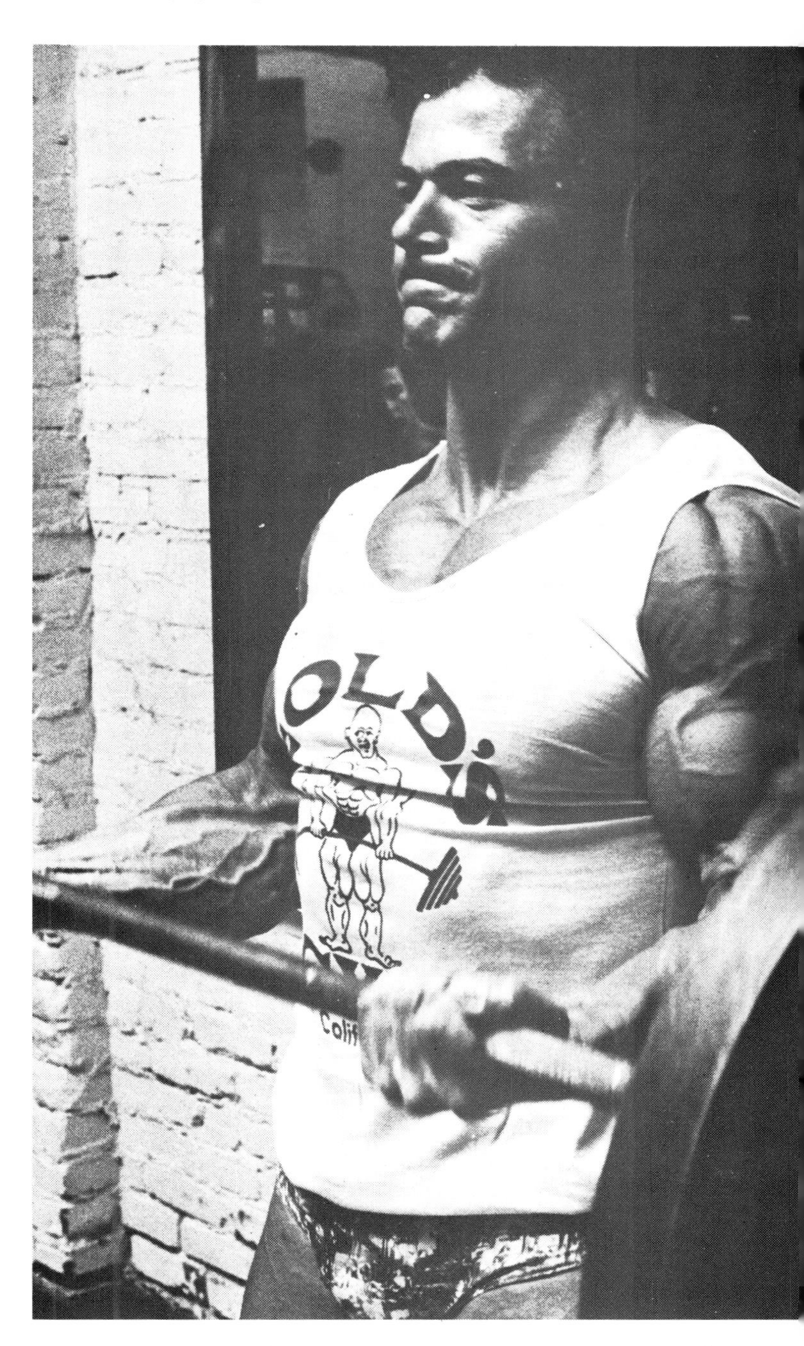

Alois Pek, a Czech bodybuilder, is typical of many of the foreign athletes who train periodically at Gold's Gym. Pek has won the Heavyweight Mr. Europe title. *(Photo by Bill Reynolds)*

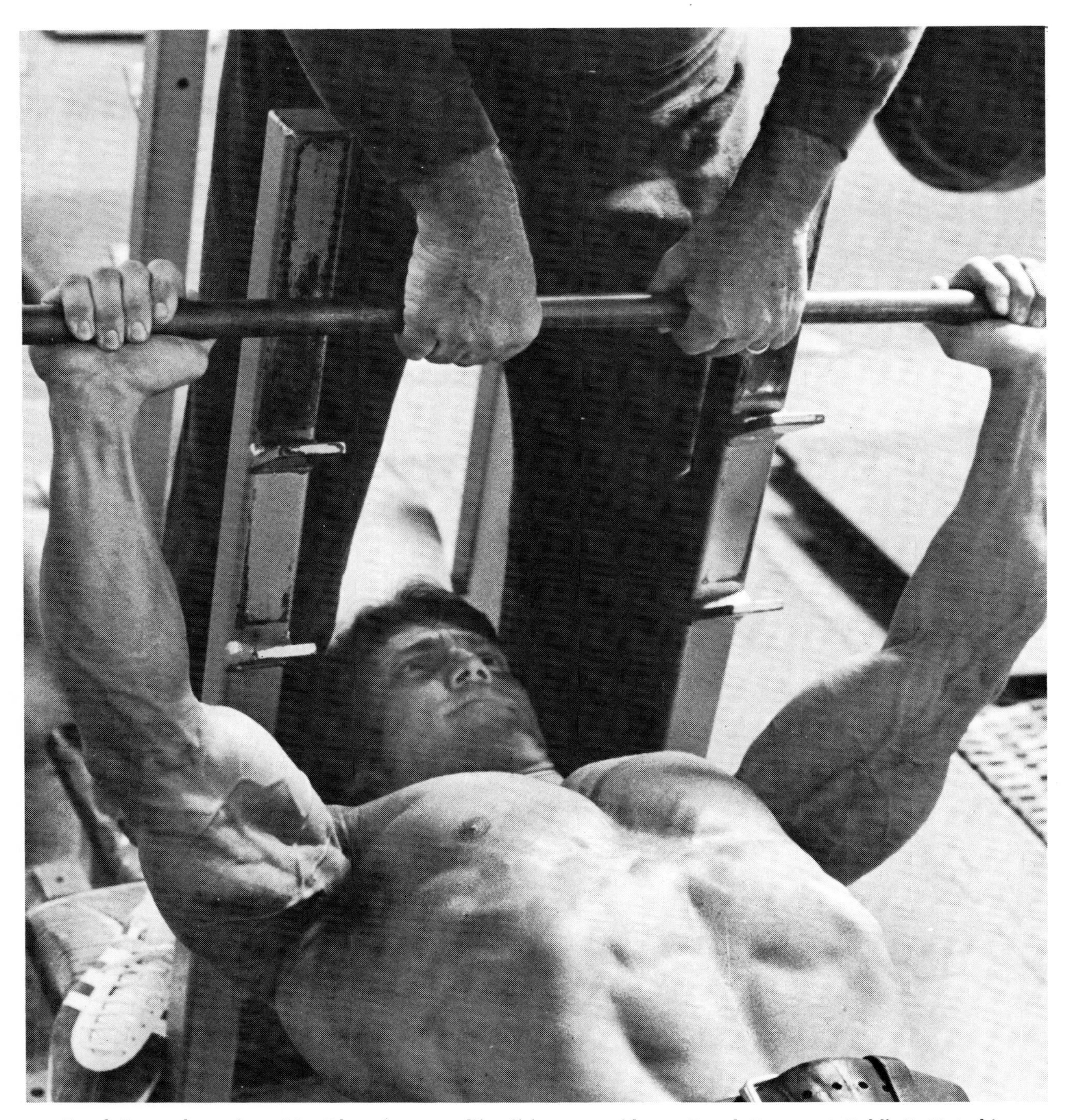

Frank Zane, three times Mr. Olympia, gets a lift-off for a set of heavy Bench Presses at Gold's II. Note his tremendous arm and torso development!

You can use cheating in a wide variety of movements, but never use more than the absolute minimum of extraneous body movement necessary to get the weight(s) past a normal sticking point. You will also probably find that you needn't cheat on more than the final one or two sets of each exercise you do in your routine.

Forced Reps

If you have a good training partner, you can use forced reps rather than cheating reps to push a set past the normal point of failure. With forced reps your training partner will pull up on your barbell, dumbbells, or exercise machine just enough to get you past the sticking point. And, in a way, forced reps are better than cheating, because your training partner can be more ruthless in applying the minimum necessary "assist" than you would probably be in applying your own cheating.

The Barbell Bench Press is a very good exercise on which to do forced reps, since your training partner will be spotting you during the movement anyway. As with cheating, you begin a set of forced reps by doing a full set to failure in strict form. Let's assume for now that on a set of Bench Presses you do seven full reps with 275 pounds before failing on an eighth repetition.

Failing on that eighth rep merely means that at that moment you are too fatigued to do a Bench Press repetition with 275 pounds. But it's highly likely that you still have enough strength left in your chest, shoulder, and triceps muscles to do a rep with 265 pounds. Even though you're tiring rapidly, you could do a second additional rep with 255 and a third with 245 pounds.

So, to force yourself past failure on the Bench Press set under discussion, you must find a way to instantaneously lighten the barbell by 10 pounds on the first extra rep, 20 pounds on the second, and 30 pounds on the third. And the way to do this is to have your training partner pull up on the center of the bar just enough on each extra rep to get it past the sticking point. And when your partner does this, he or she has given you a forced rep.

You will need to do only two or three forced reps at the end of a set to receive great benefits. You needn't do forced reps on more than one or two sets per body part during each workout for maximum results. And, generally speaking, you'll find it better to use forced reps on basic exercises than on isolation movements.

Preexhaustion

A bit earlier in this chapter, when discussing how to formulate your own individual routines, we recommended always doing your arm training *after* your torso work. The reason for this was that the smaller arm muscles are weaker than the large torso muscles, and therefore the arms often fatigue and limit the degree to which you can bomb your chest, back, and shoulder muscles. And we promised to reveal a method through which you can eliminate the problem of having your arms act as weak links in your torso exercises, thereby bombing your pecs, delts, and lats unmercifully. This technique is preexhaustion.

If you are doing a set of Presses Behind the Neck, your triceps will fail and terminate the movement before your front delts have been stimulated fully. But if you first do a set of a deltoid isolation movement such as Side Laterals to preexhaust your delts and immediately superset it with Presses Behind the Neck, your triceps will momentarily be stronger than your deltoids, and you can really blast your delts with the Presses.

It's very important that you do the basic exercise *immediately* after the isolation movement, because the preexhausted muscle will recover very quickly and thus cancel the desired effect. You can use preexhaustion for your pectorals, deltoids, lats, trapezius, and thighs. (The thighs are appropriate for this technique because, when doing Squats, your lower back muscles usually give out before your thighs.)

Here is a list of preexhaustion supersets that you can try in your workouts:

Upper Pectorals: Incline Flye + Incline Press
Lower Pectorals: Decline Flye + Decline Press
General Pectorals: Flat-Bench Flye + Bench Press
Deltoids: Side Lateral + Press Behind the Neck
Trapezius: Barbell Shrug + Upright Rowing
Latissimus Dorsi: Pullover + Lat Machine Pulldown
Thighs: Leg Extension + Squat

Some bodybuilders use preexhaustion in every workout, particularly on lagging body parts. When you first start using it, however, begin with only one preexhaustion workout per week on one or two muscle groups. From there, let your training instinct guide you in deciding how much more preexhaustion you should use in your overall training philosophy.

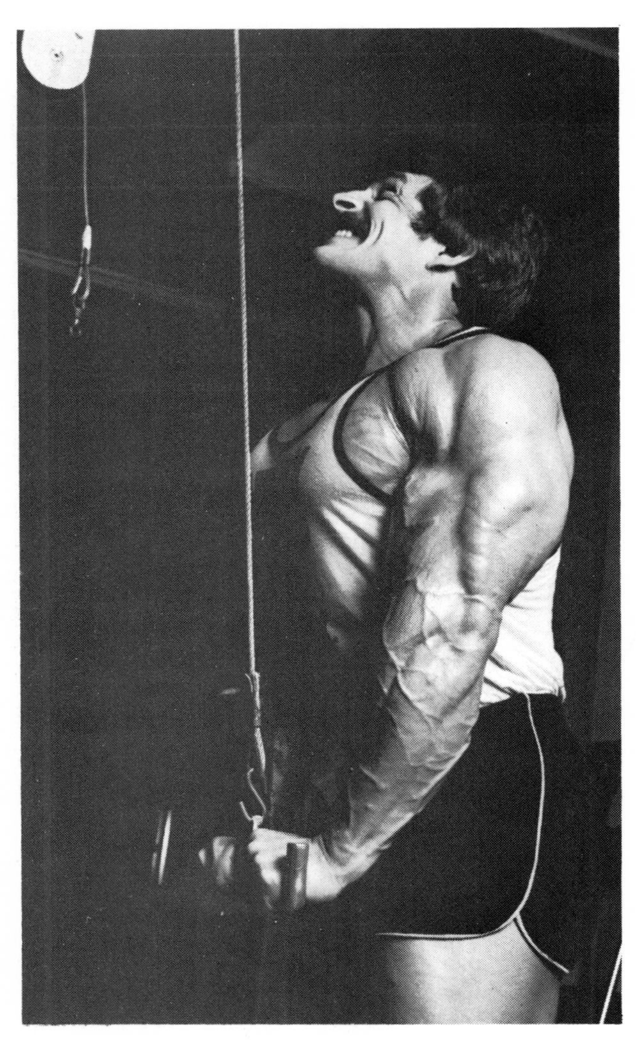

Mike Mentzer, advocate of the heavy-duty training system that incorporates the use of forced reps and negative reps. *(Photo by Peter Brenner)*

The Heavy-Duty System

Mike Mentzer, Gold's Gym member and Mr. America/Mr. Universe winner, has gotten a lot of mileage out of his heavy-duty system of training. He has, in fact, sold hundreds of thousands of dollars worth of courses and books on the system and currently has in the works videotapes advocating his bodybuilding practices.

In its barest essentials Mike's system advocates only three or four high-intensity workouts per week. A maximum of 4–6 sets are done for each muscle group, but the sets—many done on Nautilus machines—are carried to failure, pushed past failure with forced reps, and pushed even farther with negative reps. It's a very brutal style of training that Mike claims will build a great physique with only about three total hours of training per week.

Mike's system is based, to a very great extent, on the theories and recommendations of Nautilus inventor and promoter Arthur Jones. It has produced a quality bodybuilder here and there, but one must remember that while still a teenager and training "conventionally" Mike Mentzer had already developed a phenomenal physique, won the Mr. Pennsylvania title, and placed in the top 10 at the Mr. America show. Some bodybuilding experts have argued that Mike Mentzer would have become a superstar regardless of the training system he used.

Undeniably, the heavy-duty system is based on scientific fact, but it has produced only a handful of champions in comparison with conventional bodybuilding training. Still, your body might respond quite well to such workouts. You should give them a fair trial and then use your training instinct to decide whether or not this training system is appropriate for you.

Weightlifting and Powerlifting

Many bodybuilders have competed in Olympic weightlifting competitions and powerlifting meets. The heavy training required to excel in these competitive disciplines imparts a ruggedness to a bodybuilder's physique that can be attained in no other manner. One look at the physique of two-time Mr. Olympia winner Dr. Franco Columbu—an avid weightlifter and powerlifter—will convince you of this fact. And Ms. America Laura Combes can actually do *reps* in the Bench Press as a training exercise with a weight well in excess of the world record for a single-effort Bench Press in her weight class!

Teaching you how to become a weightlifter or powerlifter is well beyond the scope of this book. If these activities interest you—and we hope that they do—you can receive such instruction from Dr. Columbu's fine book, *Winning Weightlifting and Powerlifting* (Contemporary Books, 1980). It's an inexpensive training manual that will greatly assist you in mastering these two "iron sports."

Advanced Nutrition

Entire books have been written about nutrition in a bodybuilding context, so here we will touch on only those areas that will be most valuable to you. And we encourage you to augment your knowledge of diet by reading the nutrition books listed in the Bibliography at the end of this book, as well as the articles on nutrition presented regularly in *Muscle & Fitness, Muscle Mag International,* and the various other bodybuilding magazines. You will find the articles by Norman Zale and Bernard Centrella to be most valuable.

In this section we will cover three major topics: protein requirements, vegetarian bodybuilding, and the revolutionary new cytotoxic diet. Added to the dietary knowledge presented in chapters 2 and 4 (and later in Chapter 9), this new data will give you a fairly good idea of how to eat as a bodybuilder. Supplement this knowledge with further readings, and you will soon be a complete expert in bodybuilding nutrition.

Protein Requirements

There is considerable debate over how much protein an active bodybuilder should consume each day. The FDA has recommended a minimum daily requirement of one gram of protein per kilogram (2.2 pounds) of body weight. Bodybuilders eat from as little as 30–40 grams of protein per day to more than 300 grams daily.

Valerie Mayers, Ms. Empire State, has built muscle mass and gotten into superb shape on only 30–40 grams of protein per day. The great Bill Pearl has reached superb condition past the age of 50 while consuming 40–50 grams of protein entirely from lacto-vegetarian sources each day. On the opposite end of the scale Dave Johns (a Mr. America and Mr. Universe winner who has been coached by Bill Pearl) has consistently eaten 300 grams of protein per day and occasionally up to 400 grams. Dave routinely eats 50 eggs per day!

You will probably make your best muscle-building gains by eating one gram of protein per pound of your own body weight. And you can determine the protein content of foods by referring to a variety of nutrition books, such as the *Nutrition Almanac* (McGraw-Hill, rev. ed., 1979).

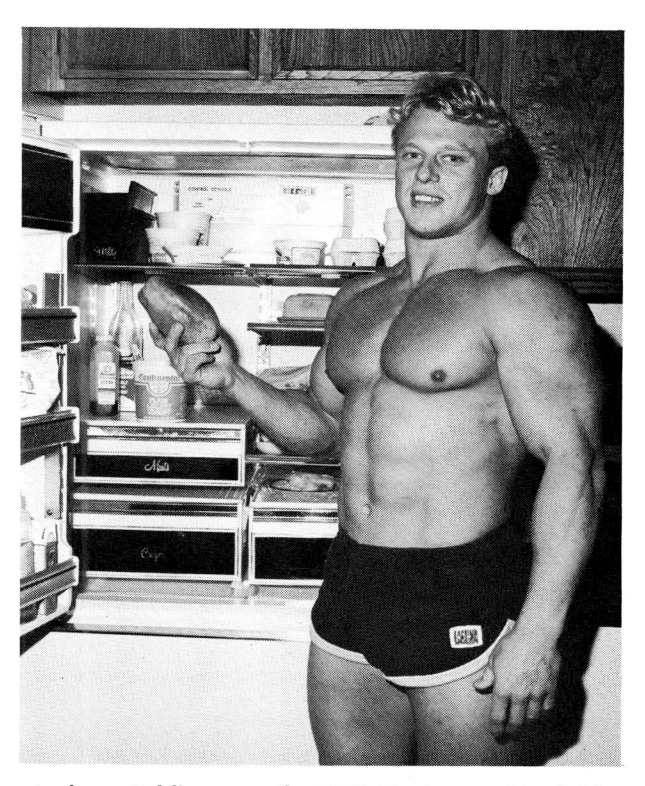

Andreas Cahling won the IFBB Mr. International title while following a vegetarian diet. Here's his well-stocked lacto-ovo-vegetarian refrigerator. *(Photo by Bill Reynolds)*

Generally speaking, protein from animal sources is of a higher biological quality and is therefore more assimilable than protein from vegetable sources. Animal-source proteins have a greater content of the eight essential amino acids that cannot be manufactured in the human body. Virtually all vegetable proteins are missing one or more essential amino acids. Only soybeans have all the essential amino acids, but even in soybeans some of them are available in only negligible amounts.

Vegetarian Bodybuilding

There are a number of successful lacto-ovo-vegetarian bodybuilders (men and women who follow a vegetarian diet supplemented with animal protein from milk products and eggs). Bill Pearl is chief among these bodybuilders. Two others who come immediately to mind are Andreas Cahling (Mr. International) and Roy

Hilligen, who won the Mr. America title during the early 1950s and then made a sensational comeback at the age of 55 to place third in the Mr. International competition.

Andreas Cahling argues eloquently in favor of a vegetarian lifestyle for bodybuilders and other athletes: "Overall, vegetarianism is healthier. The body system is cleaner, and there's less burden on the gastrointestinal tract. Vegetarian eating is more in harmony with the human body's chemistry than eating as a carnivore or omnivore. A vegetarian's digestive system is more efficient at processing the nutrients that he or she consumes.

"A vegetarian lifestyle is more ecologically balanced, and you're living in greater harmony with nature. Living animals are not forced to die simply so you can win a bodybuilding trophy. You are no longer at the mercy of the powerful meat-producing industry, which certainly has no concern for your health and well-being. It's less expensive to eat as a vegetarian bodybuilder, and raw vegetarian foods require far less preparation time than cooked animal flesh.

"As a successful vegetarian bodybuilder, I can testify that I have no problem gaining muscle mass, and it's much easier for me to maintain lean body mass. I have greater training energy—for both weight workouts and aerobic sessions—and I recuperate much more quickly from exercise sessions than when I used to consume flesh.

"*In toto,* I live a more harmonious and balanced life than ever before, and I've never made better bodybuilding gains than I have since I've become a vegetarian athlete. I can heartily recommend a vegetarian lifestyle to all bodybuilders!"

If vegetarianism is of interest to you, a book called *Are You Confused?* (Health Plus, 1971) by Dr. Paavo Ariola would be a good introduction to the subject.

The Cytotoxic Diet

In early 1981, the amazing cytotoxic diet was first publicized in *Muscle & Fitness* magazine by Bill Reynolds, editor-in-chief. This diet was brought to his attention by James Braly, MD, of the Optimum Health Labs in Encino, California. It is Dr. Braly's contention that a wide range of physical and psychological maladies are caused by mild to serious allergies to a wide variety of foods. He believes that eliminating allergenic foods from the diet will eliminate—or at least greatly relieve—these maladies.

Some of the allergy-provoked symptoms that he cites include joint pains; muscle weakness; depression; insomnia; irritability; asthma; chest, sinus, and nasal congestion; chronic fatigue; sore throat; restlessness and hyperactivity; excessive water retention throughout the body; acne; hunger and binge eating; anxiety; aggression; and arthritis. Bill Reynolds suffered from several of these problems for quite a period of time before being "cured" by Dr. Braly.

The allergy test is almost foolproof. A blood sample is taken and centrifuged to remove the plasma, red blood cells, and white blood cells. Then tiny drops of white blood cells are put on microscope slides with concentrated samples of more than 150 foods. After two hours the slides are examined under a microscope. If the body is not allergic to a food, the white blood cells will retain their normal configuration. But if there is an allergic reaction, the blood cells will become structurally distorted, or—in the case of a severe food allergy—the cell walls will rupture.

Bill Reynolds was allergic to 40 foods, primarily milk and grain products, eggs, chicken, and a random sampling of fruits, nuts, and vegetables. Significantly, as you will soon learn, the foods to which he was allergic were the ones that he ate most frequently.

"The reason you eat these foods so frequently," Dr. Braly counseled, "is that you actually have an addiction to them. To illustrate how a food addiction works, let's examine how smoking tobacco becomes an addiction, because the cases are identical. No one who ever began smoking cigarettes liked the taste of tobacco or the body's reaction to the first few cigarettes. But the nicotine in tobacco is a powerful poison, and the body's defense systems are forced to go into high gear to fight off the toxins. Thus, for a few minutes after smoking a cigarette, a smoker feels a physical and mental boost from the increased chemical activity of the body.

"The same thing happens when you eat an

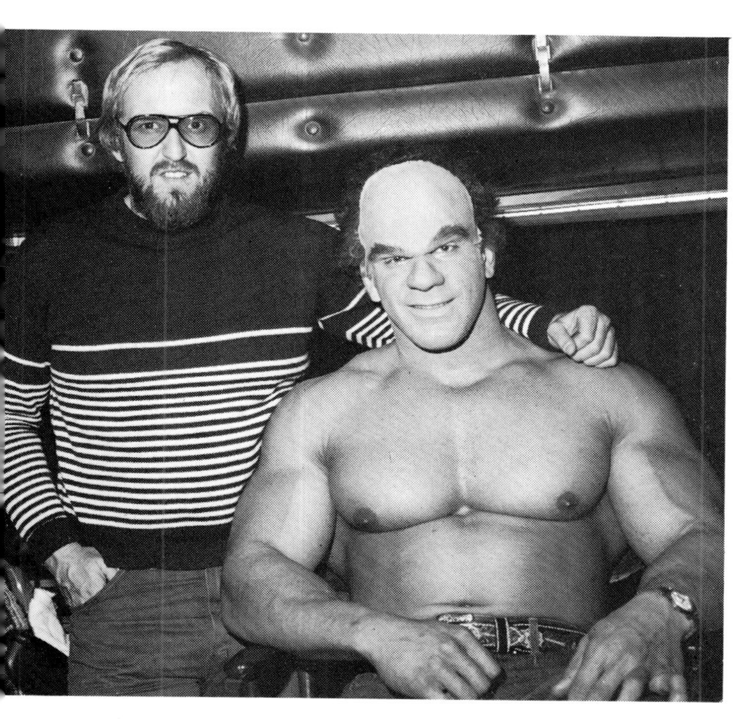

Co-author Bill Reynolds will go anywhere for a hard-hitting bodybuilding article. Here he interviews Lou Ferrigno, on location and partially made up for his "The Incredible Hulk" television role. *(Photo by Carla Ferrigno)*

allergenic food. The food is toxic to your body, and it causes the body's defense mechanisms to swing into action. And you feel a definite boost. Unfortunately, these toxins have long-range harmful effects on the body.

"Food allergies are most often manifested in the body as inflammations, which is why arthritis is a common by-product of food allergies. And since inflammations hold a great deal of water in the body, a bodybuilder could look bloated onstage, even if he had the bare minimum of body fat.

"Keep in mind here that we are not talking about acute allergic reactions to foods, such as a person breaking out in hives a few minutes after eating strawberries. We're talking about insidious, low-intensity food allergies, the symptoms of which are often confused with other types of diseases.

"The reason, therefore, that we eat some foods all of the time," Dr. Braly continued, "is that they give us a lift. You feel good when you eat them, or at least you feel good for a short time after eating a certain food. So, subconsciously, you begin to crave that food, because it's the one that makes you feel better. And often such foods will also alleviate the allergy symptoms temporarily.

"Within a few weeks of eliminating the allergenic foods from your diet, you'll notice some drastic changes in your physical and psychological well-being. One immediate result is a marked weight loss. Some patients lose up to 10–15 pounds in two or three weeks. This is primarily water that's flushed from the system once the allergy-induced inflammations have abated.

"The key to successfully following the cytotoxic diet is eating simply. Since you won't know for sure what is in most restaurant dishes, you'll have to eat mostly at home, and primarily you'll need to eat basic, simple meals. Something like beef stroganoff or macaroni and cheese will be virtually impossible to eat because of the wide range of ingredients in each of these dishes.

"If you can stay strictly on a cytotoxic diet for three to four months, most of your allergies will be eliminated. After three months you can reintroduce each of the allergenic foods into your diet, noting what allergy symptoms they induce. Usually they won't cause any problems. If that's the case, you can begin to include them rotationally in your overall diet."

Incidentally, Dr. Braly believes that eating a food too frequently, even when you are not initially allergic to it, can cause you to develop an allergy to that food. Therefore, on the cytotoxic diet, he suggests that no single food be eaten more often than once each four days.

Dr. Braly offered a concluding bit of advice to all bodybuilders: "Most individuals are allergic to milk products and/or grains. Even if you can't take a cytotoxic test, it would be a good idea to drop these two food groups from your diet. If you do, you probably will notice a considerable improvement in your physical and mental health in only two or three weeks."

If you would like to take this test, you should consult allergists in your area to see if they can give you the cytotoxic test.

Aerobics and Bodybuilding

Most bodybuilders include some form of aero-

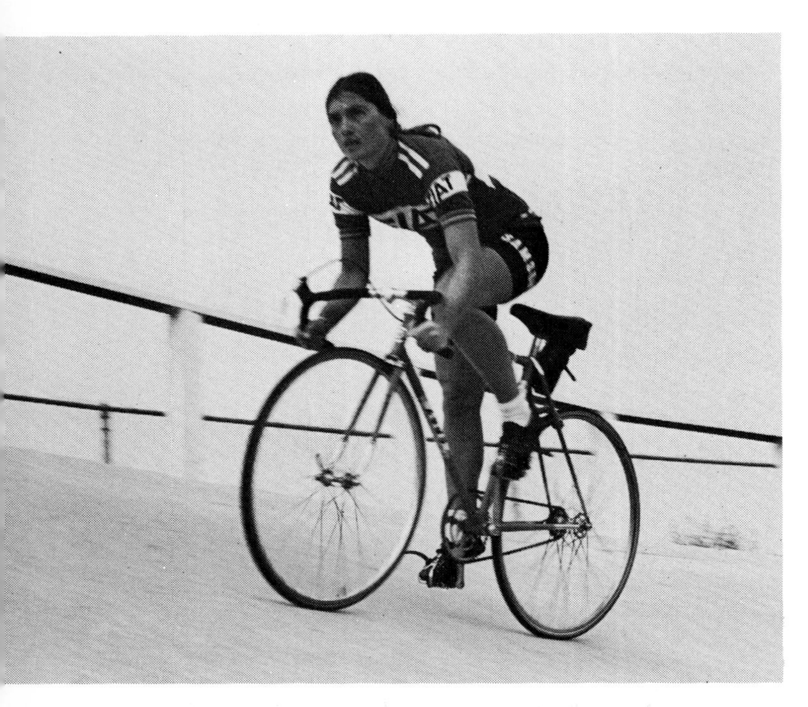

Bodybuilder Sue Barnett maintains a high level of off-season cardiorespiratory condition with daily bicycle rides. Sue became so adept at cycling that she now competes in that sport, too. *(Photo by Peter Brenner)*

bic training year-round in their overall bodybuilding training philosophies. Generally, this consists of one or two sessions of running or bicycling each week in the off-season and daily aerobic workouts when tuning up for a competition. The incomparable Laura Combes actually does two bodybuilding workouts and *two or three* aerobic sessions daily prior to a contest, since it's difficult for her to achieve a low level of body fat.

The word *aerobic* derives from the ancient Greek word meaning *with air.* Aerobic exercise, then, is low-intensity physical activity carried on for an extended period of time within the body's ability to supply oxygen at least as fast as the working muscles are burning it up. Anaerobic exercise, on the other hand, burns up oxygen so quickly that the body can't keep up with the expenditure and goes into an oxygen debt. Once this oxygen debt is sufficiently large, the body actually forces you to terminate the exercise.

The most common forms of aerobic exercise are running, cycling, swimming, dancing, fast walking, and playing racquet sports. Such activities develop superior cardiorespiratory endurance and burn off calories at a much faster rate than do the processes of your own basal metabolic rate. There are actually scientific studies that indicate that aerobic training burns off body fat at a faster rate than does an equivalent amount of anaerobic activity.

Here is a listing of the number of calories expended in a half-hour of continuous activity in six popular types of aerobic activity:

Aerobic Activity	Calories Expended
Running (10 mph)	450
Bicycling (15 mph)	300
Handball or Racquetball	300
Swimming (2½ mph)	275
Fast Dancing	240
Walking (2 mph)	140

Competitive bodybuilders do aerobic workouts to burn off extra calories and help define their bodies even more than is possible through bodybuilding training and adhering to a tight precontest diet. Arnold Schwarzenegger and Laura Combes run. Frank Zane takes long walks in the desert near his home in Palm Springs. Tom Platz and Andreas Cahling ride bicycles up and down a bike path along the beach at Santa Monica. Boyer Coe and Suzie Green pedal stationary bikes. Lisa Elliott loves to dance and take aerobic dance classes. In short, virtually all bodybuilders burn off extra calories close to a contest by doing daily aerobic workouts.

It's essential that you allow at least two or three hours of full rest between aerobic sessions and bodybuilding workouts. If you don't rest at least this much, you won't be able to do justice to one type of workout or another.

Many bodybuilders immediately groove on a particular type of aerobic activity, then stick with it for years. Many others are bored by aerobics. If you fall into the second group, adopt *variety* as your watchword. Constantly switch from one type of aerobic exercise to another, and you'll have fewer problems maintaining interest in your aerobic workouts.

Chest Expansion

The larger a male or female bodybuilder's rib cage, the larger will appear his or her torso, particularly in a side-chest pose. Since the rib cage consists of the sternum and ribs, all of which are bones, it would seem impossible to enlarge the rib box. But through a combination of special deep breathing movements and chest stretching exercises, you can lengthen the cartilages that attach the ribs to the sternum, thereby effectively lengthening the ribs and expanding the rib cage.

Enlarging the rib cage is a slow process under any circumstances, since the cartilages stretch very slowly. They stretch especially slowly once the body has ceased to grow, because the cartilages then begin to harden and are far less pliable than when you are still growing. The optimum age for rib cage enlargement, then, is from about 14 to approximately 17 or 18 years of age.

Rib cage expansion is accomplished by doing between one and three supersets of Breathing Squats and Breathing Pullovers. Do 25 reps per set of each movement and perform this exercise routine on three nonconsecutive days per week. Within three months, a teenage boy can add two or three inches to his rib cage expansion if he faithfully follows this program. A teenage girl should be able to add about half as much to her own expanded rib cage measurement. More mature individuals, while they can still expand their rib cages, will experience less rapid progress.

Breathing Squats have much in common with regular Full Squats, except that they are done with an exercise poundage no heavier than your own body weight. A light weight is used on the bar, because emphasis must be placed on inducing deep breathing via light high-rep Squats, rather than adding muscle mass to the thighs by doing heavy low-rep Squats.

Start your set of Breathing Squats with a light barbell held across your shoulders and your body set for a normal Squat. Take three slow, extremely deep breaths, pulling in all of the air possible and expelling all of it that you can from your lungs on each breath. Hold the third breath and squat down completely, expelling your breath only when you are once again fully erect. Repeat the breathing and squatting procedure until you have completed 25 repetitions, at which point you should be rather breathless.

Tom Platz demonstrates Breathing Squats, holding his breath at the start (top) through the squat (bottom).

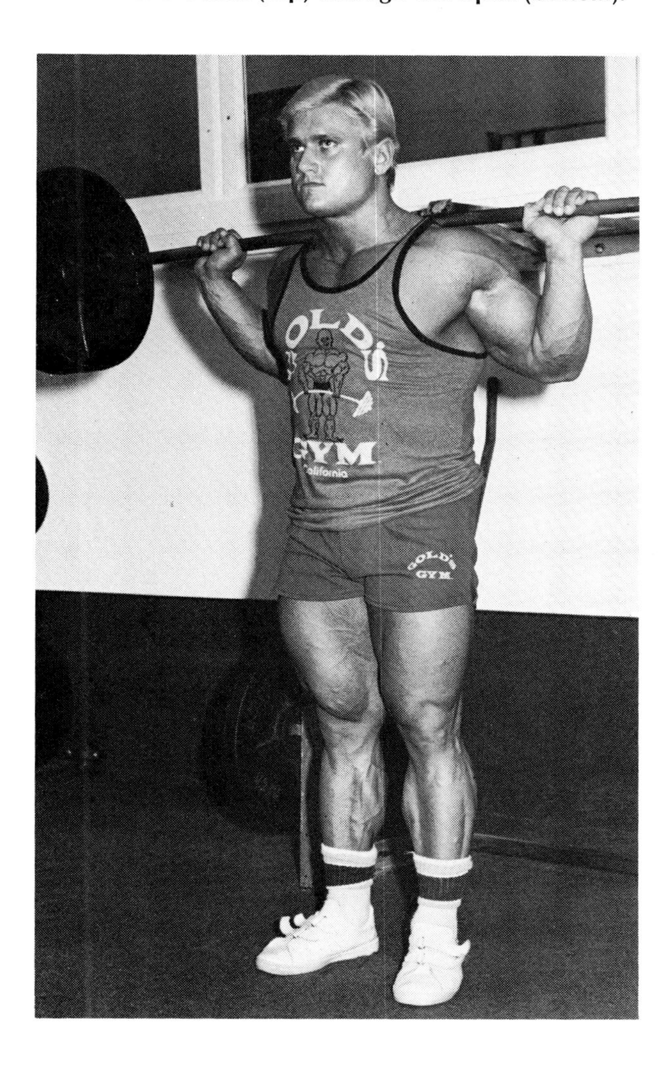

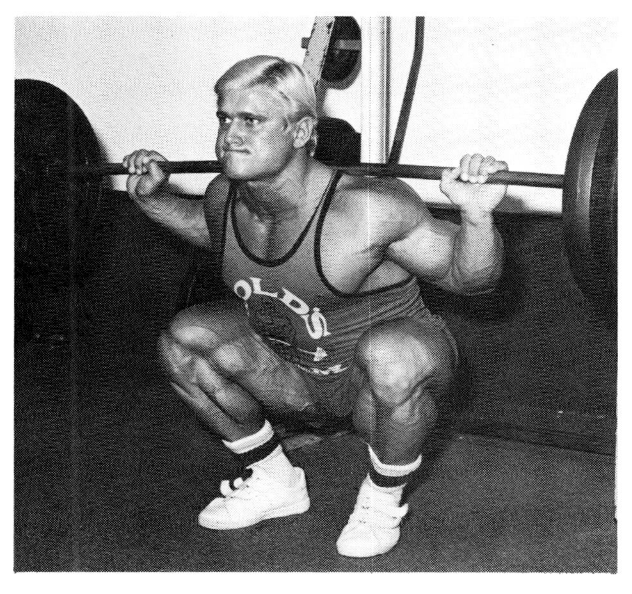

Before each of the first 10 reps of your set of Breathing Squats, take in three huge breaths. For the next 10 reps of your set, take in four maxed-out breaths. And for your final five reps, breathe in and out five times on each repetition. As soon as you have finished your 25th repetition, place the barbell back on your squat rack and immediately lie down on a flat bench to do 25 reps of Breathing Pullovers. Then rest for three or four minutes before repeating the superset, if you are to do another one.

For your Breathing Pullovers you will need a light barbell, one in the range of 10–15 percent of your body weight. Lie on your back on the flat bench, being sure that your head hangs off one end of the bench and your feet are planted firmly on the floor to balance your body on the bench during the movement. Take a shoulder-width grip on the barbell so that your palms are facing toward the foot end of the bench as you support the barbell at arms' length directly above your chest, precisely as for the start of a Barbell Bench Press. Stiffen your arms and keep them held perfectly straight throughout the movement.

From this basic starting position, lower the barbell in a semicircle backward to as low a position behind your head as is comfortable. As you lower the barbell, breathe in as deeply as possible. Once you have reached the low position, hold your breath and return the barbell along the same arc as it was lowered back to the starting point. Only then should you exhale. Repeat the movement for a total of 25 repetitions.

This combination of Breathing Squats (to stimulate deep breathing) and Breathing Pullovers (to stretch the cartilages of the rib cage) will gradually expand your rib box. Beginning-level bodybuilders need do only one superset of these two movements. Intermediates should do two supersets, and more advanced bodybuilders should do three such supersets for best results.

Coping with Training Injuries

The rate of serious injuries in bodybuilding is exceedingly low. Broken bones, torn cartilages and ligaments, ripped tendons, and torn muscles—injuries that are commonplace in many sports—are seldom seen in bodybuilding training. When they are they should be treated immediately by a physician.

If you assiduously follow the suggestions for warming up in Chapter 2 and consistently use the correct biomechanical positions recommended in the exercise descriptions in chapters 3, 5, and 7, you will probably be able to avoid every common type of bodybuilding injury. If you are injured, however, you will need to know how to heal the injury quickly so it doesn't retard your bodybuilding progress.

The most common training injuries are muscle strains (particularly in the lower back muscles) and sore joints. A strained muscle can be caused by poor biomechanical positioning during an exercise, poor concentration when using a heavy weight, or poundages that are too heavy when the muscles have not been thoroughly warmed up. Sore joints can be caused by each of the above factors, plus poor diet and general overuse.

Should you feel a muscle or joint strain while training, apply ice to the painful area for approximately 10 minutes each hour during your waking hours for the first day following the injury. Ice cubes wrapped in a towel will work admirably. The ice will keep down swelling in the injured area, and excessive swelling can retard the healing process.

After the first 24–36 hours of cold applications, you should apply heat to the injured area periodically for three or four days to help speed the healing process. A hot water bottle wrapped in a wet towel is one of the best ways to apply heat to an injury, because the damp fabric conducts heat very efficiently.

Once you have rested an injured joint or muscle you can begin to exercise the injury with very light weights and high repetitions. If you feel any significant or persistent pain at the injury cite, back off the weight a little. Otherwise you can gradually add weight to the movements affecting the injured area, until the injury is fully rehabbed.

Chronic joint pain can be caused by a high consumption of refined carbohydrates. It can also be caused by poor form in handling heavy weights, particularly by bouncing or jerking a heavy weight. Use a smooth steady motion with your heavier exercise poundages, and you'll have a minimum of joint problems.

Overtraining

One of the biggest roadblocks to any bodybuilder's success is overtraining, a condition in which the body becomes so supersaturated with training that the muscles refuse to grow. When an athlete is severely overtrained, his or her health can actually break down, and hard-earned muscle mass will dissipate. Horrors!

Overtraining seldom occurs when a bodybuilder takes short, high-intensity workouts and frequently changes training programs to avoid boredom in training. Usually it occurs when a bodybuilder either takes too lengthly workouts or remains on the same training schedule for a long period of time.

Overtrained bodybuilders will exhibit one or more of these symptoms:

- Apathy toward training
- Chronic fatigue
- Irritability, insomnia
- Elevated morning pulse rate
- Unexplained weight loss
- Chronic joint and/or muscle pain
- Lack of gains in muscle mass and/or strength

Having three or more of these symptoms indicates a relatively severe case of overtraining.

To cure overtraining you should begin by taking a complete, one-week layoff from bodybuilding training. Totally avoid the gym, but feel free to remain physically active. Go swimming, play racquetball, climb a mountain, or bicycle 20 miles a day, but stay away from the weights altogether. During your layoff, plan a new and shorter bodybuilding routine to follow once you get back into the gym. Reduce your total number of sets per body part by at least 20%, but make a corresponding 20% increase in training intensity by using heavier weights and more forced reps in your workouts.

Inexperienced bodybuilders probably overtrain more by prematurely adopting a six-day split routine than in any other way. If you have been training six days per week, drop back to only four workout days, and you'll immediately notice a quick growth spurt. Dennis Tinerino, winner of three Mr. Universe titles, trains only

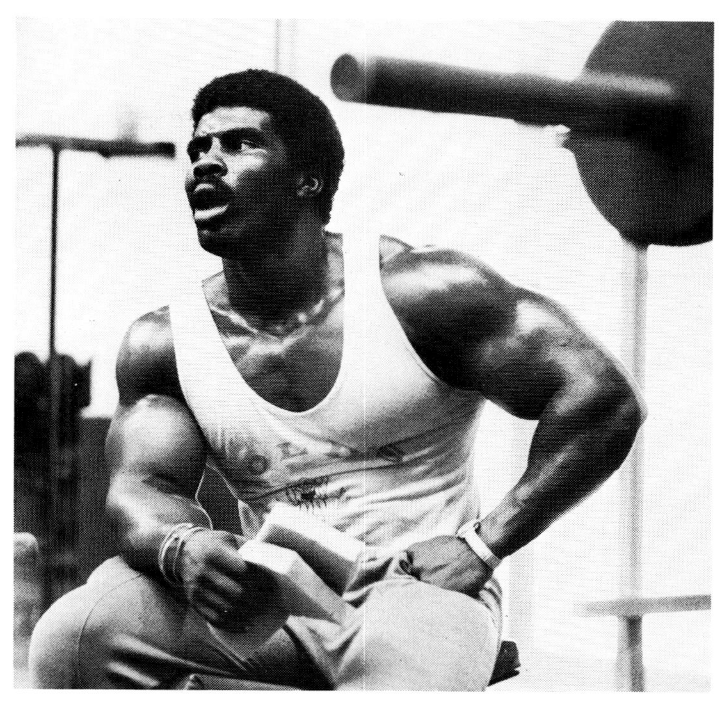

As he briefly rests between sets, the face of Robby Robinson mirrors the heart and soul of bodybuilding!
(Photo by John Balik)

four days per week when building muscle mass in the off-season from competition. The great Chris Dickerson trains five days per week in the off-season. How could you possibly expect to make good gains training six days per week when these two superb champions can't?

Once you are back in the gym you should also make a conscious effort to improve your diet, sharpen your mental attitude toward training, and closely monitor your recuperative processes. Bodybuilding is a holistic sport, and to make your best gains you must fit a number of jigsaw puzzle pieces together.

Layoffs

In addition to helping cure overtraining, there are a number of other reasons to take a layoff from hard training from time to time. One of the best times for a layoff is just following a competition.

"Right after a show, you're totally burned out," Danny Padilla (Mr. America, Mr. USA, Mr. Universe) said. "You've had to overtrain slightly to reach peak condition, so both your mind and body will be worn out. It's very likely that you will have developed a small, nagging injury or two. This is a great time to take a layoff to recuperate totally. It's always good, however, to remain physically active during a one- or two-week layoff from training."

Many bodybuilders find that taking a one-week layoff every 4–6 months allows them to make better progress in their general training. And any time you have a serious training injury you may need to take an extended amount of time off from your bodybuilding training to allow the injury to heal fully.

If you have taken a short layoff, the first workout or two after you return to training should be taken at less than peak intensity in order to avoid muscle soreness. And if you have been on an extended layoff, you may need a gradual break-in period lasting from a week to as much as a month.

Stress Management

One of the least understood obstacles to continued bodybuilding success is negative stress. The world's foremost stress researcher and expert is Hans Selye, MD, an Austrian-born, Canadian scientist. Dr. Selye has identified two types of stress—*distress* (negative stress) and *eustress* (positive stress)—that elicit similar physiological responses within the body but have drastically different effects on health and well-being.

Having a loaded gun pointed menacingly at you—a very pure example of distress—causes your pulse rate to quicken, your blood pressure to shoot upward, and your respiration rate to accelerate. But making love, which is usually (though not always) a good example of eustress, evokes the same physiological responses. Which situation is destructive and which constructive to your physical and mental health and sense of well-being? The answers are obvious.

Dr. Selye further points out that perceptions of distress and eustress vary widely from individual to individual, and he identifies two basic personality types. To the laid-back personality type, a life of total leisure would be eustressful. To a gung-ho type, however, such a lifestyle would be distinctly distressful. To such a personality type, a hard 10-hour day in the office is eustressful.

The trick to stress management, then, is to recognize which external stimuli are distressful and which are eustressful to you and then to minimize the first and maximize the second. When you do this successfully you will make excellent bodybuilding gains. You will also feel very happy.

The best way to identify situations of personal distress and eustress is to keep lists of each. Then, if you discover that consistently being around a certain person keeps you irritable and on edge, you can simply avoid that individual. If you find that playing a particular electronic video game relieves your feelings of distress, save up your quarters and go for it!

Flexibility

There are three major reasons why all bodybuilders should do regular stretching workouts:

1. *Stretching improves muscular development.* A muscle cannot be developed fully unless it is trained hard over its full range of motion. Stretching gradually but significantly lengthens the range of motion of most muscular groups. Exercise over a longer range of motion yields greater muscular development.

2. *Stretching prevents injuries.* Most everyday types of injuries and athletic injuries are caused either by trauma (a fall, a car accident, a 250-pound football player crashing into you, etc.) or by overextension of a joint, muscle, or connective tissue (e.g., muscle pulls, sprains, strains, etc.). Bodybuilders who follow regular and progressive stretching programs suffer at least 20% fewer overextension injuries than those who don't. So, to prevent injuries it seems essential that stretching be a regular part of advanced bodybuilding training.

3. *Stretching is a good warm-up before, and cool-down activity after, other types of training sessions.* A preworkout stretching program warms up the joints and muscles and improves neuromuscular coordination. And after a workout, stretching will prevent postworkout muscle soreness, as well as promote faster physiological recovery from a workout.

While everyone should stretch, you will quickly discover that some individuals are more adept at stretching than others. Don't let this discourage you if you seem especially tight, because even within individual age and sex groups there will be wide variation in native flexibility. Everyone should simply work with what nature gave him or her in terms of native flexibility. Generally speaking, however, women will be markedly more flexible than men, and children will be far more flexible than adults.

During the past couple of years several bodybuilders—most notably World Cup winner Boyer Coe—have discovered that stretching is an excellent supplement to bodybuilding training. "It builds bigger, better quality muscles," Boyer recently told us. "The first time I seriously used stretching workouts was prior to the last Olympia. Everyone there remarked that I'd improved 25%–30% since the previous Olympia, which was to them a remarkable improvement. They wanted to know my secret. If I'd told them 'stretching,' they'd probably have laughed at my statement. But I'm convinced that stretching is a superior adjunct to bodybuilding training."

How to Stretch

At times we're totally amazed at the abuse men and women subject themselves to in their stretching exercises. They stretch so hard that their muscles scream with pain and they almost scream out loud themselves. Or, they bounce forcefully into a stretch, unknowingly losing much of the value of stretching in the process. Correctly applied, stretching is a *gentle* form of exercise, and unless you pursue it gently you will lose out on most of the benefits stretching offers.

Because it's easy to injure yourself by overextending the range of motion of a joint or muscle, nature has provided your body with two protective mechanisms. Both of these are specialized types of neurons (nerve endings). One type senses when a muscle is being overstretched and signals this fact by feeding pain signals to the brain. In a moment, when we tell you exactly how to stretch, you'll clearly see the role that these neurons play in a perfect stretch.

The second type of stretch-sensation neurons are part of a protective mechanism called the *stretch reflex.* If a relaxed muscle is stretched too quickly, it can easily be torn. The stretch reflex prevents this. When the second type of stretch-sensation neurons sense that a stretch is progressing too quickly toward a full range of motion, the mind reflexively begins to contract the stretched muscle. And this acts as a shock absorber, quickly slowing, then halting, the stretch before the muscle can be injured. This is somewhat like the way your thigh muscles flex to absorb the shock of landing when you jump off a table onto the floor. It's important here to understand that the stretch reflex causes a muscle to contract and *shorten.*

When you stretch a muscle group ballistically (that is, in a bouncing manner) the stretch reflex is activated and the muscle shortens to stop the stretch. So, while it may seem logical to some that bouncing would intensify a stretch and bring faster results, such ballistic stretching actually has the opposite effect. Because of the stretch reflex, the stretched muscles actually shorten and you come up far short of reaching a fully stretched position.

To fully stretch a muscle (or joint) you must *slowly ease into the stretch* in order to circumvent the stretch reflex. Take 30–40 seconds to move slowly into a stretch to the point at which you just begin to feel slight pain in the stretched muscle. This is the maximum point to which you should stretch. Many stretching experts call this the *pain edge.* And if you stretch much past this pain edge, you can actually begin to pull tiny muscle fibers apart, literally injuring yourself by going well past the pain edge in a stretch. The next day you'll find that your muscles are brutally sore.

So, now you have enough physiological information to understand the perfect stretch. Regardless of the flexibility movement you use, take 30–40 seconds to ease slowly into the stretch. Then, once you encounter the pain edge, back off one or two degrees on the stretch until the pain has just disappeared. You'll need to move back almost imperceptibly to accomplish this, but once you've reached this *stretching zone,* hold the stretch in that position for 20–30 seconds (work up eventually to one or two minutes in this position).

Breathe shallowly, though with normal

rhythm, when holding a stretched position. Finally, relax the stretch and either repeat it a minute later or move on to another stretching movement.

If you are to receive maximum benefit from stretching, you must play with the pain edge enough to discover your unique stretching zone for each exercise. It's only while holding a flexibility movement in this stretching zone that you will accrue the greatest benefit from a program of stretching. Stretching does *not* have to hurt you to be beneficial. In fact, stretching to the point of pain can actually be counterproductive.

Stretching Progression

Anyone who has never undertaken a stretching program—even if that person has otherwise been very active physically—should begin very easily on the program outlined in this article. And he or she should progress very patiently and slowly. As we've mentioned, you can actually injure your muscles and become extremely sore if you push too hard. Proper stretching is virtually effortless, and yet you will slowly and steadily gain flexibility from even what seems like the easiest flexibility program.

Beginners to stretching should back far away from the pain edge in their first stretching efforts and hold each stretch for only 20 seconds. They should also do only one repetition of a single stretching exercise for each muscle group. From this beginning point, *slowly* add to the duration of each stretch (until you can hold it for a full minute) and to the severity of each stretch (until you have held it in the upper range of the stretching zone, just microns from the pain edge).

Once you reach this point you can either add repetitions to a stretch (but begin a second repetition of any stretch by holding it for only 20 seconds, then gradually work it up to 60 seconds duration), or add another stretching movement for the same body part to your program (again, begin it with a duration of only 20 seconds). At a maximum you will probably need no more than one or two one-minute stretches in each of two flexibility exercises for each body part. Such an all-out program could take you 30–45 minutes to complete. For our purposes, however, we recommend doing a one-minute stretch in one exercise for each body part, a workout that you'll be able to complete in 10–15 minutes.

Related Activities

Yoga, which is also a philosophy of life, is one of the best forms of stretching. And yoga can improve your overall flexibility far past the point that the programs in this book can take you. Many professional athletes—as well as a number of bodybuilders—have turned to yoga for their stretching regimen. Yoga can be learned through classes or via self-study. Some of the best books currently on the market include B. K. S. Iyengar's *Light on Yoga* (Shocken Books, 1979), Sandra Jordan's *Yoga with a Partner* (Arco Publishing Company, 1980), and Bikran Choudhury's *Bikram's Beginning Yoga Class* (J. P. Tarcher, 1978).

Bill Reynolds has personally taken classical ballet classes for the past three years and has found such classes an enjoyable way to achieve superior body flexibility. When he first started taking class at Gloria Yeager's Body Train in Woodland Hills, California, he could barely touch the middle of the length of his shins with his fingers when his legs were held straight. His hamstrings were that tight! Now he can stand on a chair with his legs straight and bend forward far enough to touch the middle of the length of his forearms to his toes.

Stretching Exercises

All of the stretches illustrated and described in this section are excellent for bodybuilders. By comparing the photos with the following exercise descriptions, you'll easily be able to learn every movement.

Standing Hamstring Stretch. This movement stretches the hamstring muscles at the backs of your thighs. Lock your legs and extend your arms overhead, clasping your hands. Keeping your legs straight, bend over and touch your hands to your feet. As you become more and more advanced, you will actually be able to lay your torso against your thighs in this position.

Hurdler's Stretch. This exercise stretches both

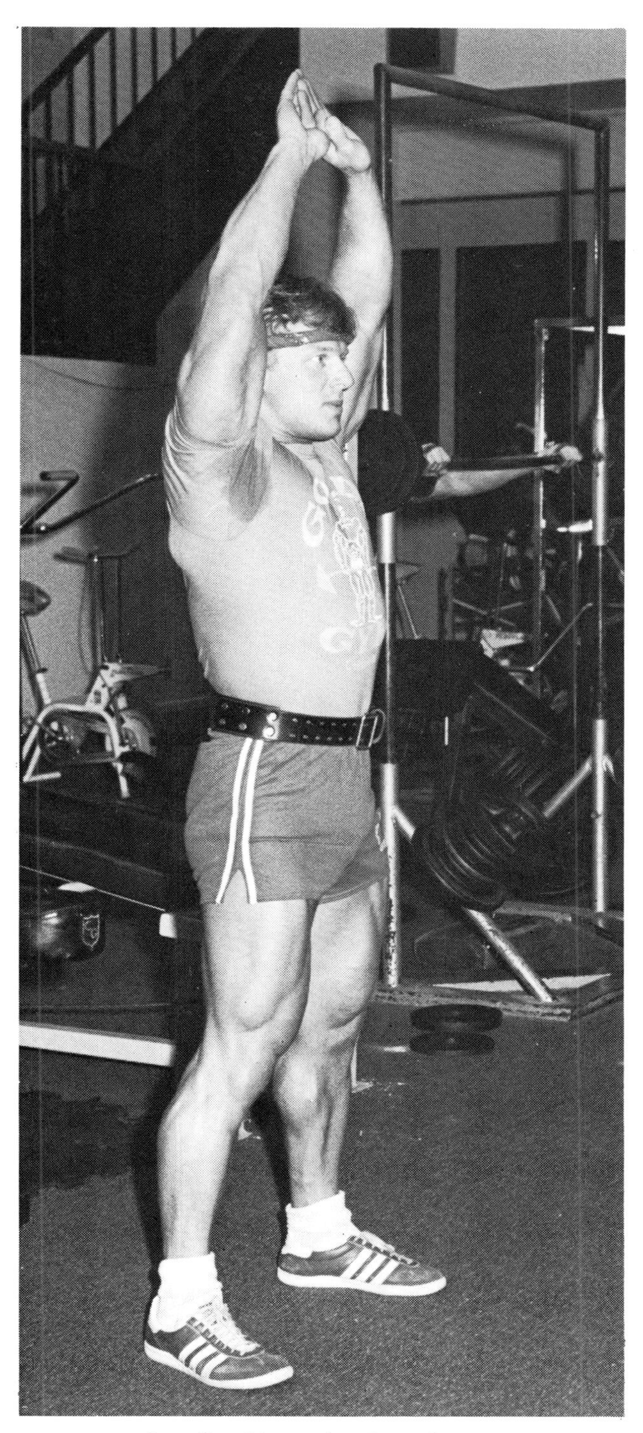

Standing Hamstring Stretch—start.

the hamstrings and the groin muscles. Sit on the floor (or on a mat, on the beach, or on your lawn). Extend your right leg forward and lock it straight throughout the movement. Your left leg should be bent at a 90-degree angle and lying flat on the floor behind your body. Your torso

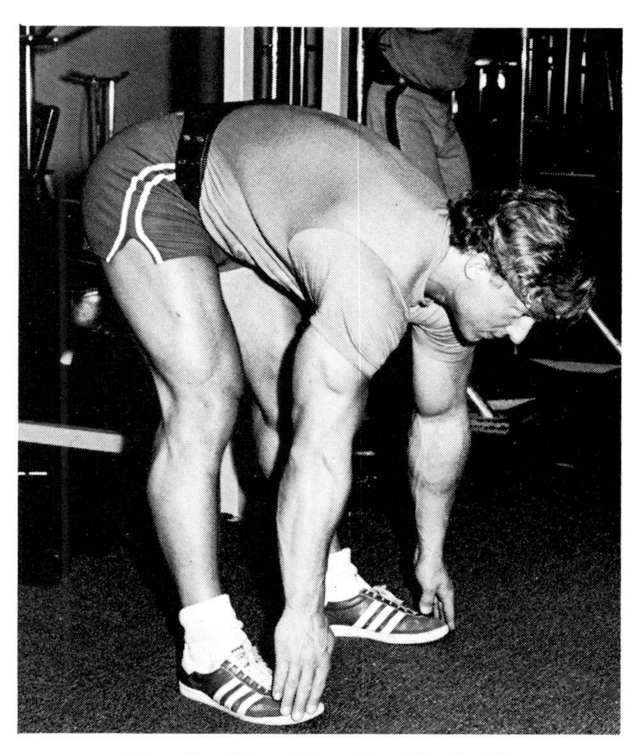

Standing Hamstring Stretch—finish.

should be upright and your arms extended directly forward, parallel to the floor. Bend slowly forward over your right leg and grasp your ankle to gently pull your torso down to rest along your extended thigh. After stretching with your right leg forward, do an equal amount of stretching with your left leg extended forward.

Seated Groin Stretch. This movement stretches all the muscles of the groin and inner thighs. Sit down and bend your legs as fully as possible, bringing your knees in toward your chest. (Ideally, your heels should be right up against your buttocks.) Position your knees close together. Grasp your knees with your hands. Be sure to keep your torso erect throughout the movement. Using your hands, slowly push your knees apart until they are as close to the floor as possible.

Lunging Stretch. This movement stretches the muscles of the hips, buttocks, and front thighs. Stand erect and place your hands on your hips. As illustrated, step forward with either leg and bend it fully while keeping the other leg fairly straight. Hold this position for the required length of time and then repeat the movement for the other leg.

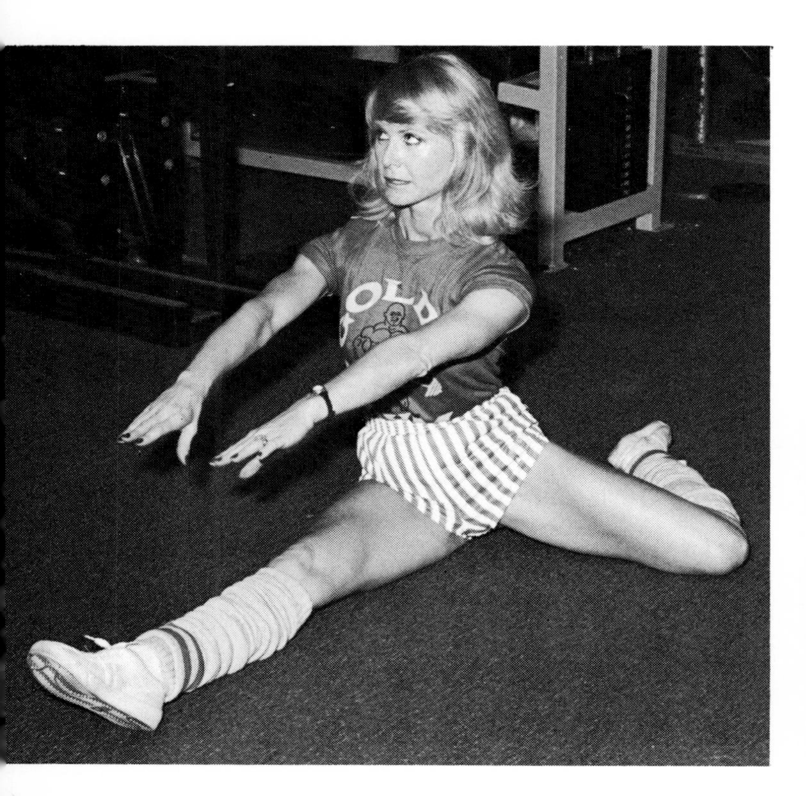

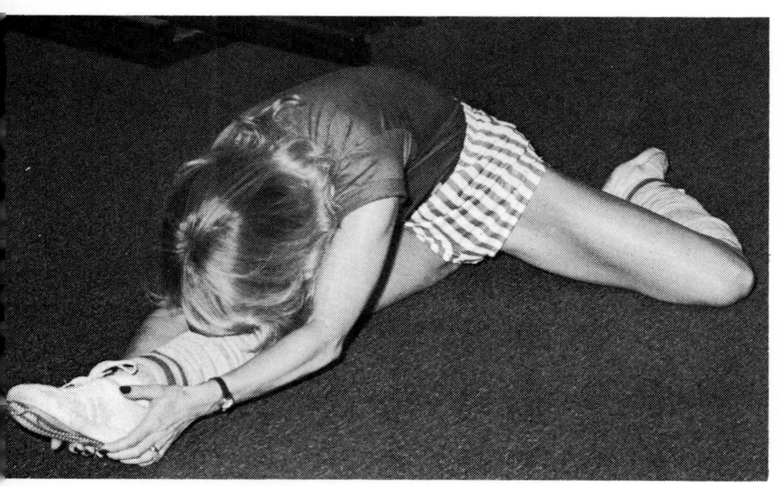

Hurdler's Stretch—start, top; finish, bottom.

Seated Groin Stretch—start, top; finish, bottom.

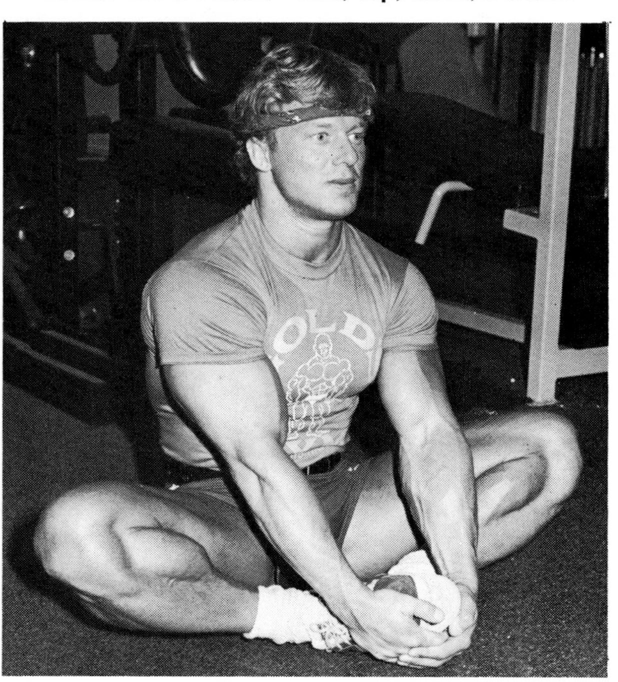

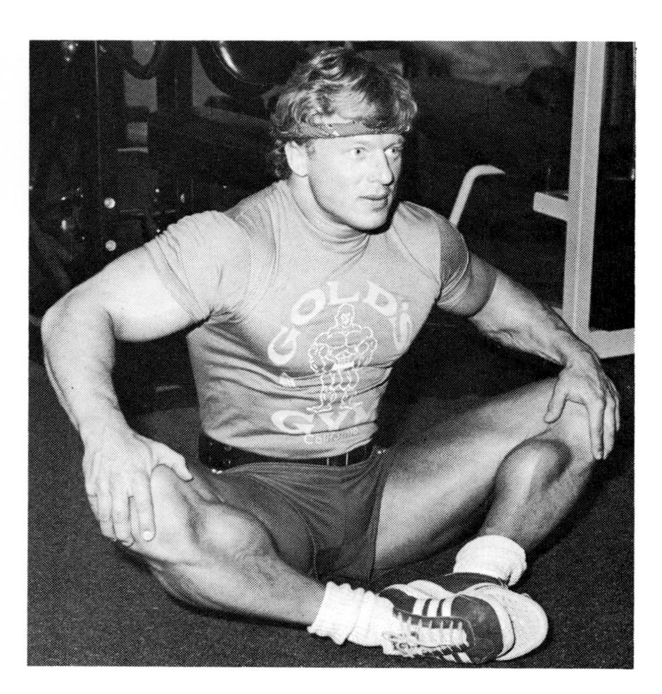

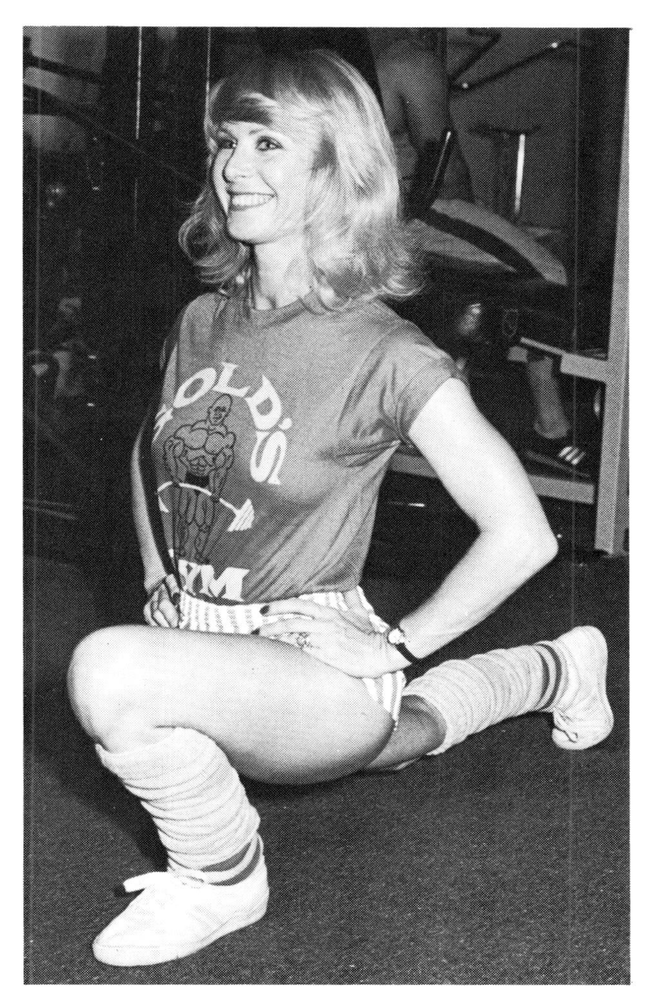

Lunging Stretch.

Thigh Stretch. This exercise strongly stretches the quadriceps muscles along the fronts of your thighs. Stand erect and balance on your left foot with your left leg held straight. Reach behind yourself and grasp your right ankle with your right hand, as illustrated. Pull gently upward on your ankle to stretch your thigh muscles.

Calf Stretch. This exercise stretches and tones all the muscles at the backs of your lower legs. Face a wall and place your hands against the wall at shoulder height. Walk backward with your feet until your right leg, torso, and arms make a straight line. Your left leg should be bent. Gently press your heel down to the floor. If you can comfortably place your heel flat on the floor, walk backward another 4–6 inches to intensify the stretch. Be sure to do an equal amount of stretching for each calf.

Twisting Stretch. This exercise stretches and tones the muscles at the sides of your waist. Stand erect and place your hands together in front of your chest as illustrated. Maintain this hand/arm position throughout the exercise. Trying to restrain the movement of your hips, twist your torso as far to the left or right as possible. Hold this position. Then twist as far to the other side as possible.

Front Abdominal Stretch. This movement stretches primarily the front abdominal muscles, but also the muscles of the hips and thighs. Support yourself on straight arms and straight legs with your hips pointed upward so that your legs make an approximate 90-degree angle with your torso. Keeping your arms and legs straight, lower your hips to a position as close as possible to the floor. Hold this stretched position for the required length of time.

Neck Stretches. These stretches influence all

Thigh Stretch.

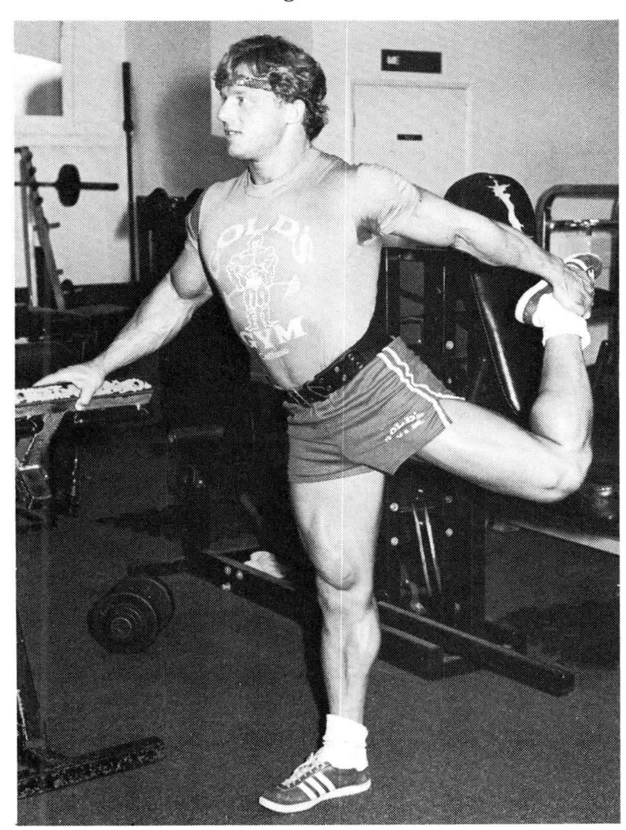

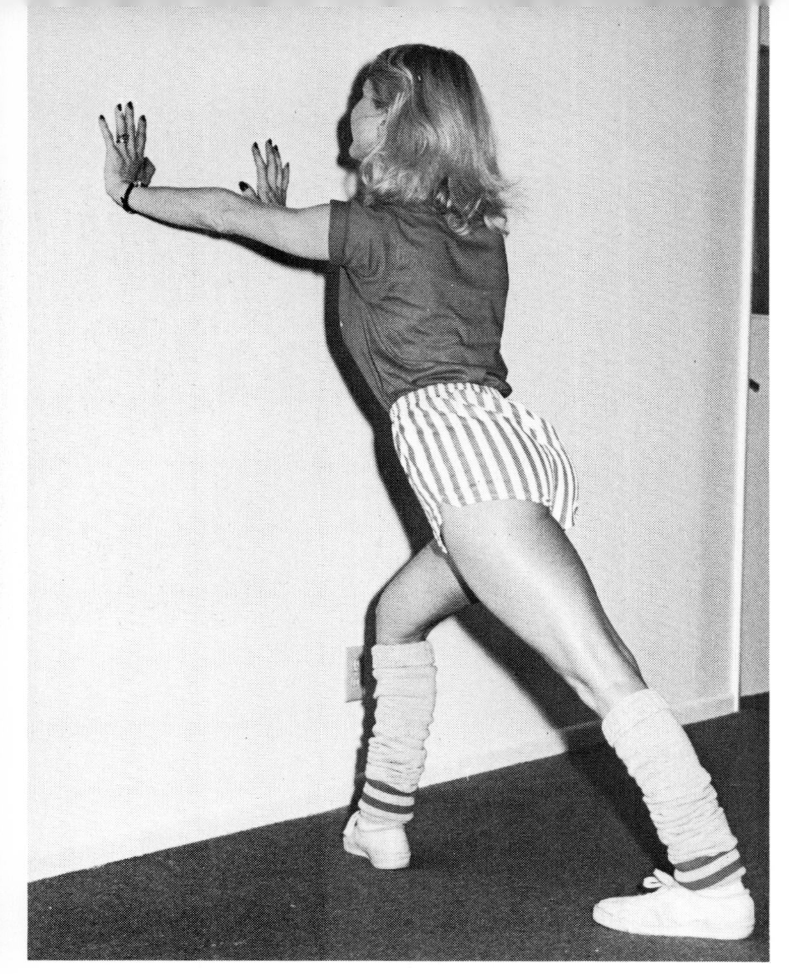

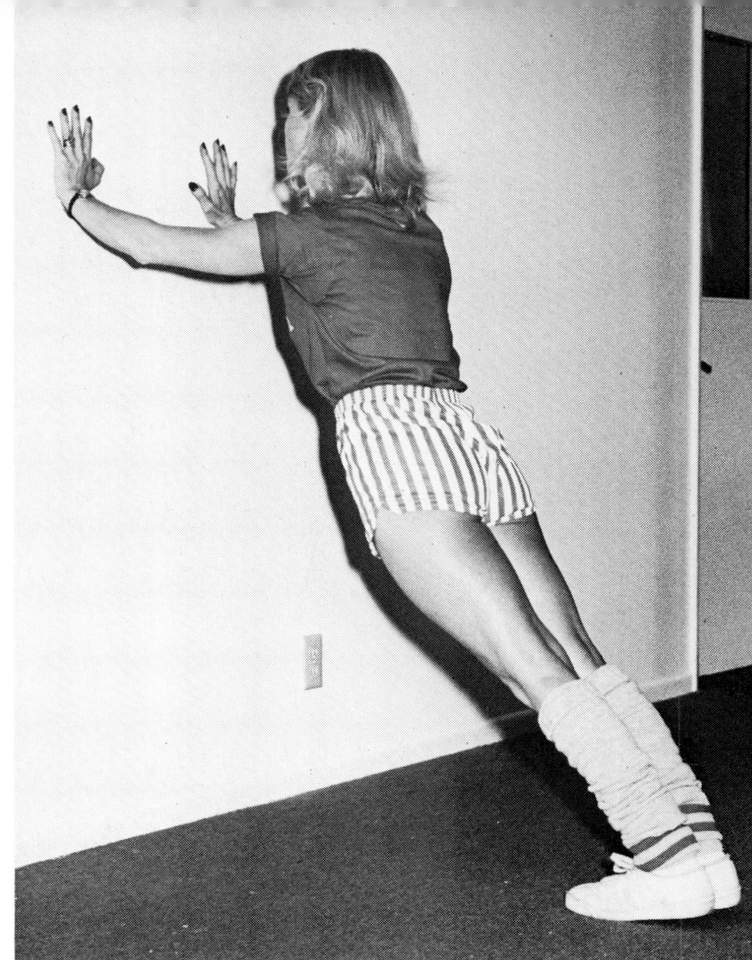

Calf Stretch—one leg, left; two legs, right.

Twisting Stretch—left turn, left; right turn, right.

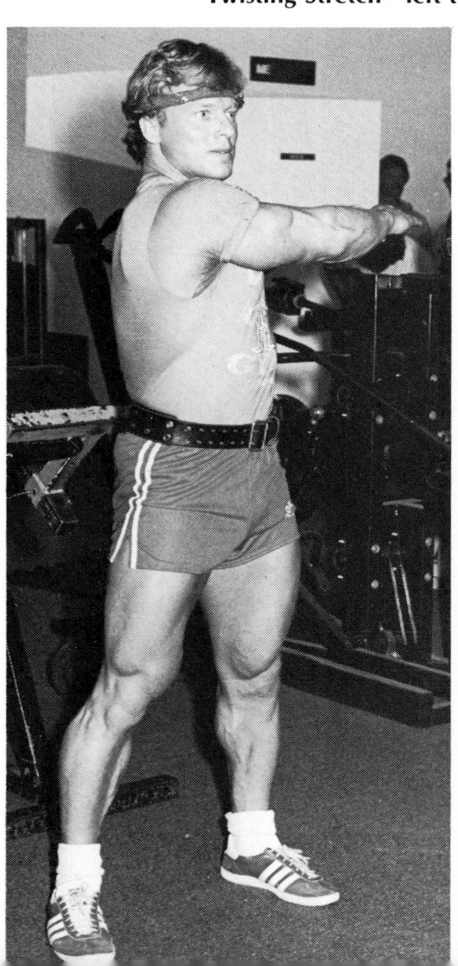

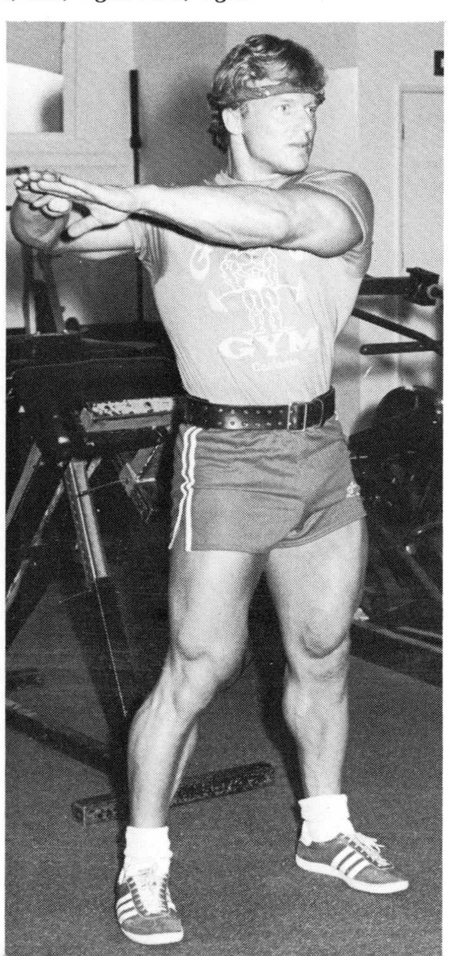

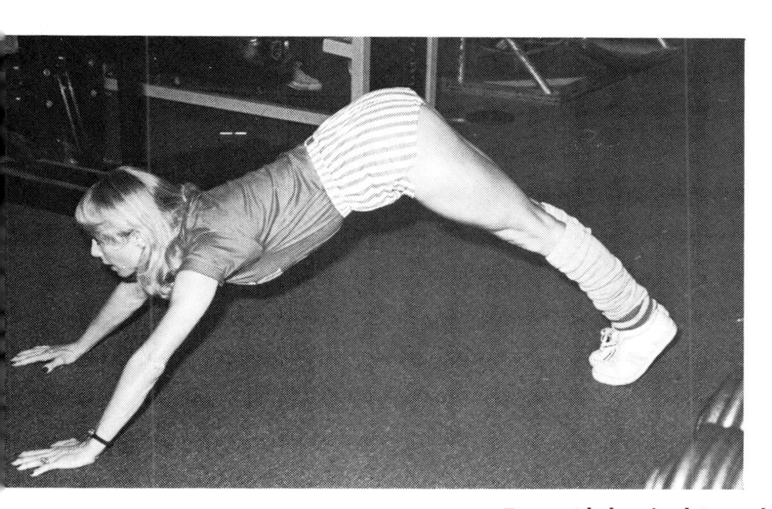

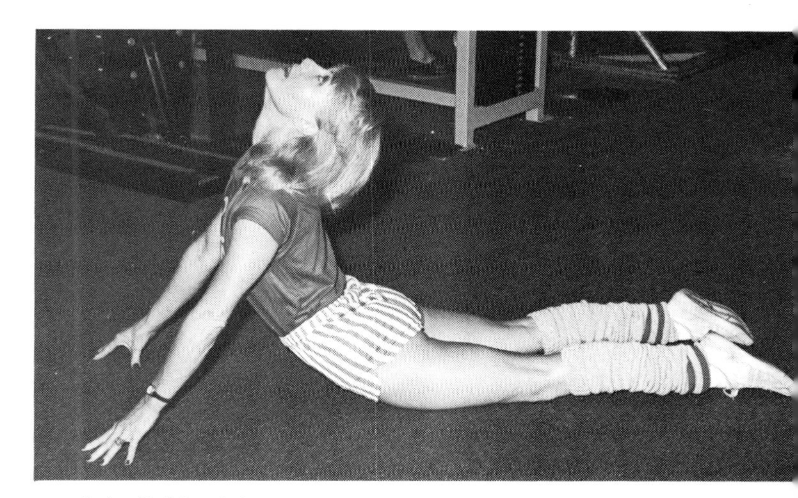

Front Abdominal Stretch—start, left; finish, right.

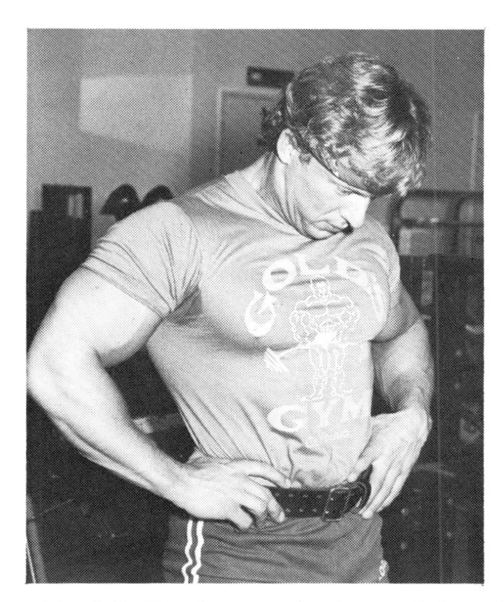

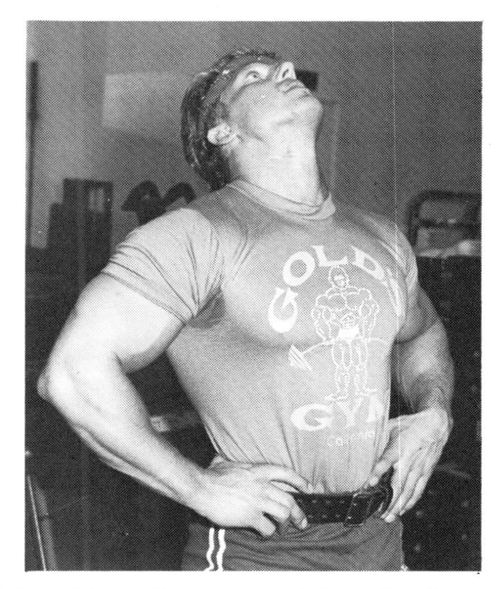

Neck Rolls—front to back, top left and right; side to side, bottom left and right.

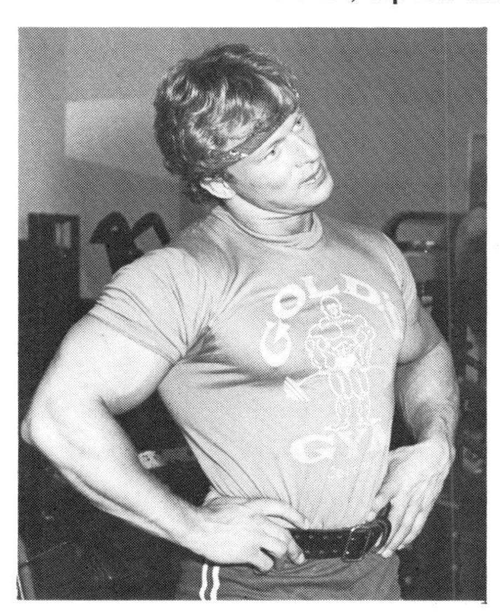

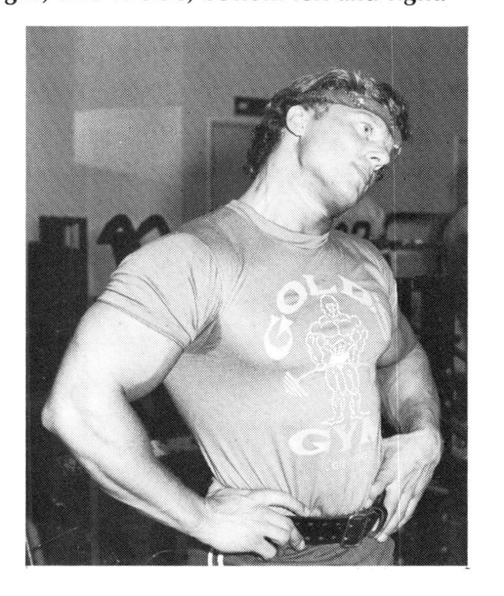

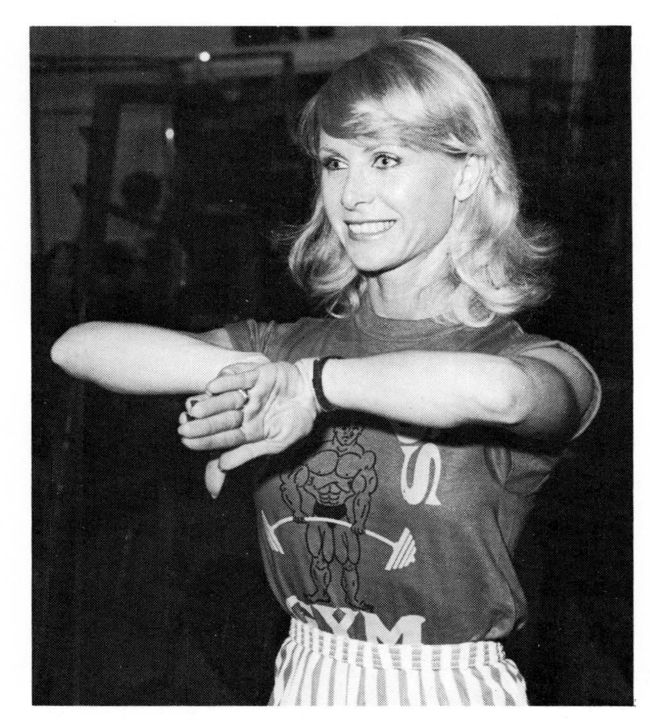

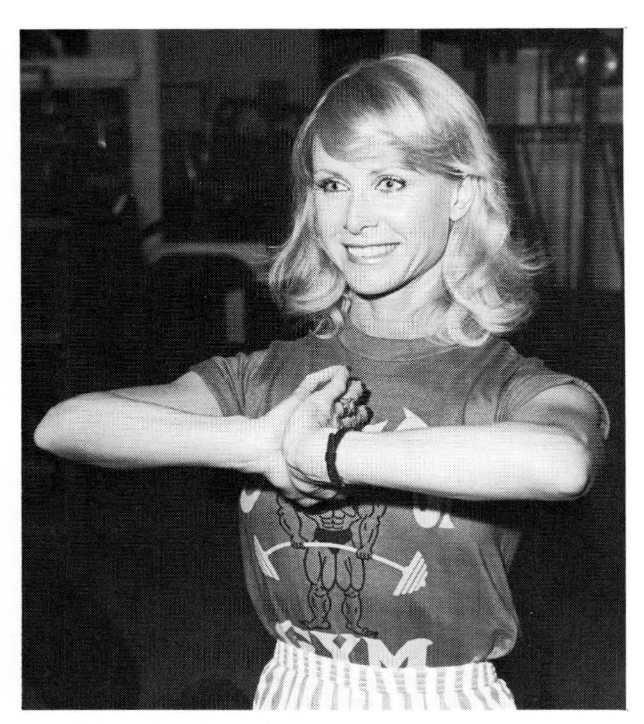

Finger/Wrist Stretches—palms out, left; palms in, right.

the neck muscles. Stand erect with your hands on your hips. Keep your legs, arms, and torso in this position throughout the movement. Tilt your head as far forward as possible and hold this position. Then tilt your head as far backward as possible and hold that position. Next tilt your head as far to the right side as possible and hold that position. Finally, tilt your head as far to the left side as possible and hold that position.

Finger/Wrist Stretches. These movements stretch all the muscles and joints of your fingers and wrists. Stand erect and place the tips of your fingers together with your palms facing inward. As an alternative you can place your fingers together with your palms facing outward. Press your wrists gently toward each other as illustrated to stretch the fingers and wrists.

Stretching Routine

The following is a good basic stretching program that you can try (do one or two repetitions of each movement).

Exercise	Starting Duration (in seconds)	Maximum Duration (in seconds)
1. Standing Hamstring Stretch	20	60
2. Hurdler's Stretch	20	60
3. Seated Groin Stretch	20	60
4. Lunging Stretch	20	60
5. Thigh Stretch	20	60
6. Calf Stretch	20	60
7. Twisting Stretch	20	60
8. Front Abdominal Stretch	20	60
9. Neck Stretch (to all four directions)	20	60
10. Finger/Wrist Stretch (to both sides)	20	60

In conclusion, here are five major points that you should remember when following this stretching program.

1. Stretch every day, if possible.
2. Progress slowly (stretching must be a *gentle* form of exercise).

3. Take 30–40 seconds to ease slowly into a stretch.
4. Find the pain edge and back off your stretch slightly. Hold it for 20–90 seconds in this stretching zone.
5. Do stretching exercises for every part of your body.

Lessons Learned from Bodybuilding Contests

You will soon be in good enough condition to enter your first bodybuilding competition, so it's essential to attend several of these events to familiarize yourself thoroughly with everything that takes place at them. This way you won't learn about essential procedures during or after your competition, when it's too late.

These bodybuilding competitions are advertised and/or listed in the "Coming Events" columns of *Muscle & Fitness, Muscle Mag International, Iron Man,* and most of the other bodybuilding journals. They are also frequently advertised via flyers and posters placed in gyms and spas in areas where contests are to be held. Additionally, once you are competing, you will be on the mailing lists of various promoters and will thus receive announcements of upcoming competitions from them.

You should order tickets for a bodybuilding

Lou Ferrigno on exhibition before a contest. *(Photo by Bill Dobbins)*

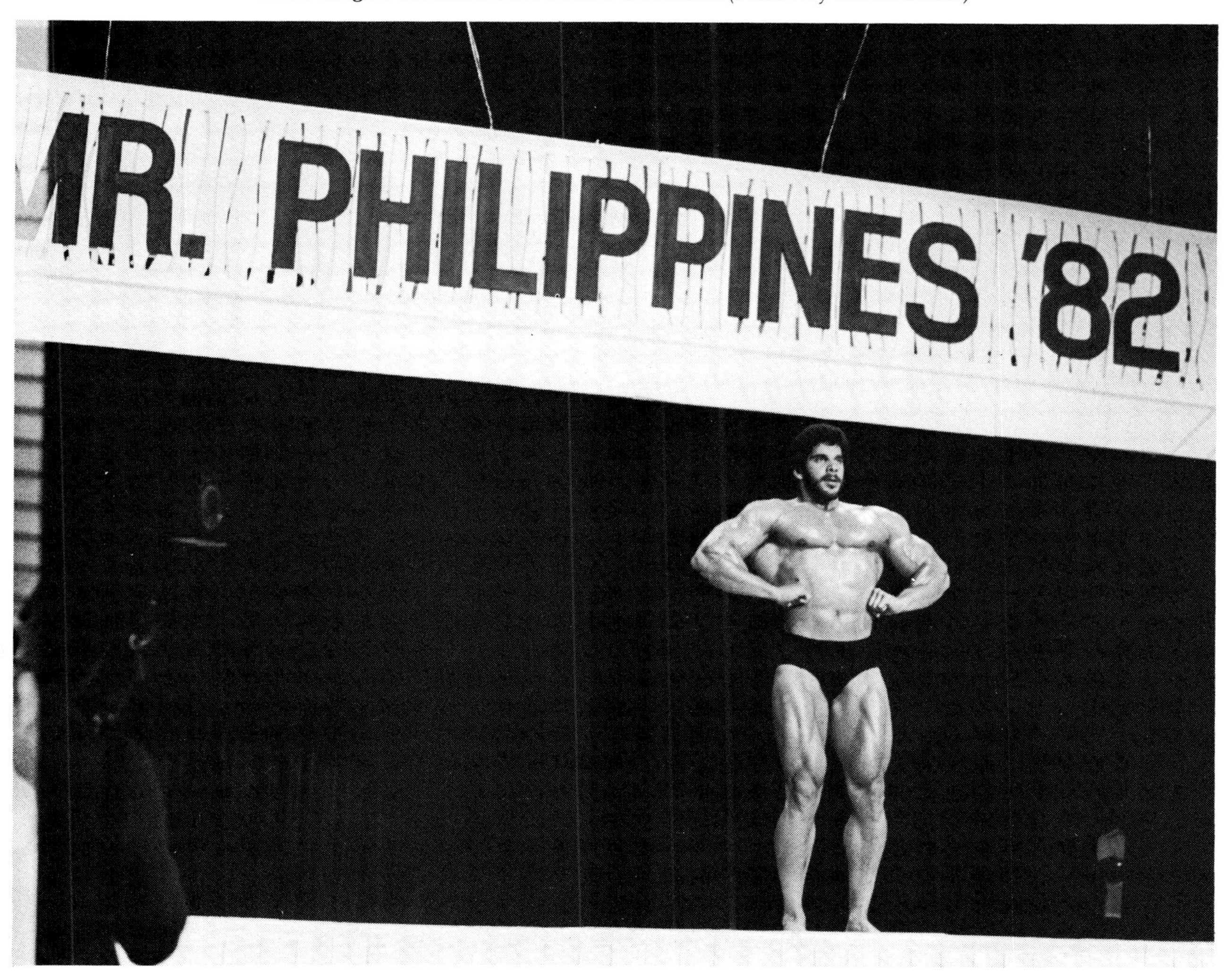

show as early as possible, so you can sit relatively close to the stage. If a contest is prejudged, as most are these days, be sure to attend the morning and/or afternoon prejudging sessions since this is where most of the real action of a bodybuilding competition takes place.

Competitions are conducted for men, women, and mixed pairs. Weight classes are usually used in men's and women's competitions to prevent smaller athletes from being compared unfairly with larger individuals. Frequently an overall winner will be chosen in a posedown among the various class winners, though this is more frequently done at or below the national level of competition than internationally.

Various age-group competitions are held for teenagers, athletes over 35 years of age, and bodybuilders over 40. These contrast with open contests in which athletes of any age can compete. Novice competitions also are held from time to time as an arena for athletes who have never placed in a bodybuilding competition. And junior contests are held in America for athletes who have never won a junior or senior title. (Internationally, however, the junior category corresponds to our own teenage division.)

The lowest level of competition is local, such as the Mr./Ms. Seattle, Mr./Ms. Manhattan Beach, or Teenage Mr./Ms. Omaha. Moving up to the state level, a bodybuilder would compete for such titles as Mr./Ms. California and Mr./Ms. Florida. Next in the hierarchy of bodybuilding competition are regional contests such as Mr./Ms. Pacific Coast, Mr./Ms. East Coast, and Mr./Ms. All-South.

A variety of contests are held on the national level. Among these are the Mr./Ms. America, Mr./Ms. USA, Mr./Ms. Teenage America, Mr./Ms. Over 40 America, Mr./Ms. Teenage USA, Mr./Ms. Over 40 USA, and Collegiate Mr. America. Increasingly, these contests are being referred to as championships, such as the American Women's Bodybuilding Championships and the National Teenage Championships.

There are numerous bodybuilding federations that sanction competitions, but Gold's Gym officially recognizes only three of these. Within the United States, the National Physique Committee, Inc. (NPC) sanctions approved men's competitions, and the American Federation of Women Bodybuilders (AFWB) sanctions approved women's competitions. International competitions are sanctioned by the International Federation of Bodybuilders (IFBB), which has more than 115 affiliated member national bodybuilding federations.

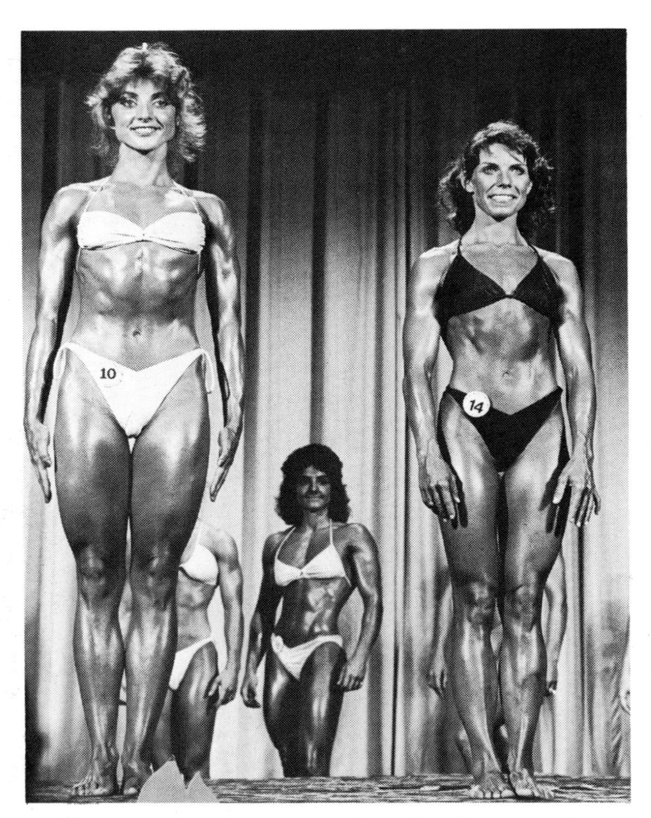

Round I relaxed facing poses by Kike Elomaa and Lynn Conkwright.

The IFBB System of Judging is used in virtually all competitions for men, women, and mixed pairs. Three major types of posing rounds are conducted, plus a posedown round among the top five competitors in which extra points can be earned in muscle-to-muscle combat. In each of the first three rounds a contestant can receive a maximum of 100 points or a possible total of 300 points after three rounds. In Round IV one additional point can be added by each of seven judges, bringing the maximum score to 307 points.

Each of the seven judges awards every athlete 1–20 points (though it's very uncommon for a bodybuilder to receive less than 10 points) in Rounds I–III, according to how they perceive the relative physical perfection of each competitor. Then the high and low scores are eliminated and the remaining five scores are totaled for a maximum round score of 100.

In Round IV, the posedown, each judge votes for only one contestant, and each first-place vote counts as one point, No scores are dropped in Round IV, so seven added points are awarded. Whenever total scores after three rounds are close, the posedown can be crucial, and leaders are occasionally upset in this final round of judging.

Round I consists of four "relaxed" facing poses (though competitive bodybuilders are seldom relaxed onstage) in which the athletes stand at attention facing forward, with their left sides to the judging panel, facing away from the judges, and with their right sides toward the judging panel. This round primarily reveals physical proportions (a balance of development among all body parts) and symmetry (overall

Round I relaxed side poses by Rachel McLish and Candy Csencsits at the '81 Miss Olympia.

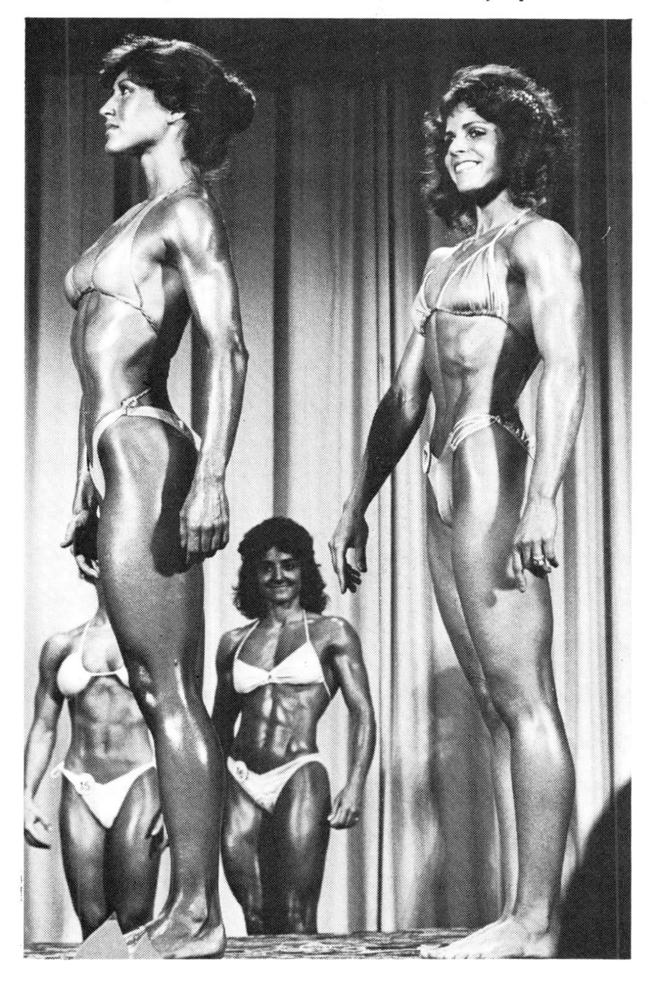

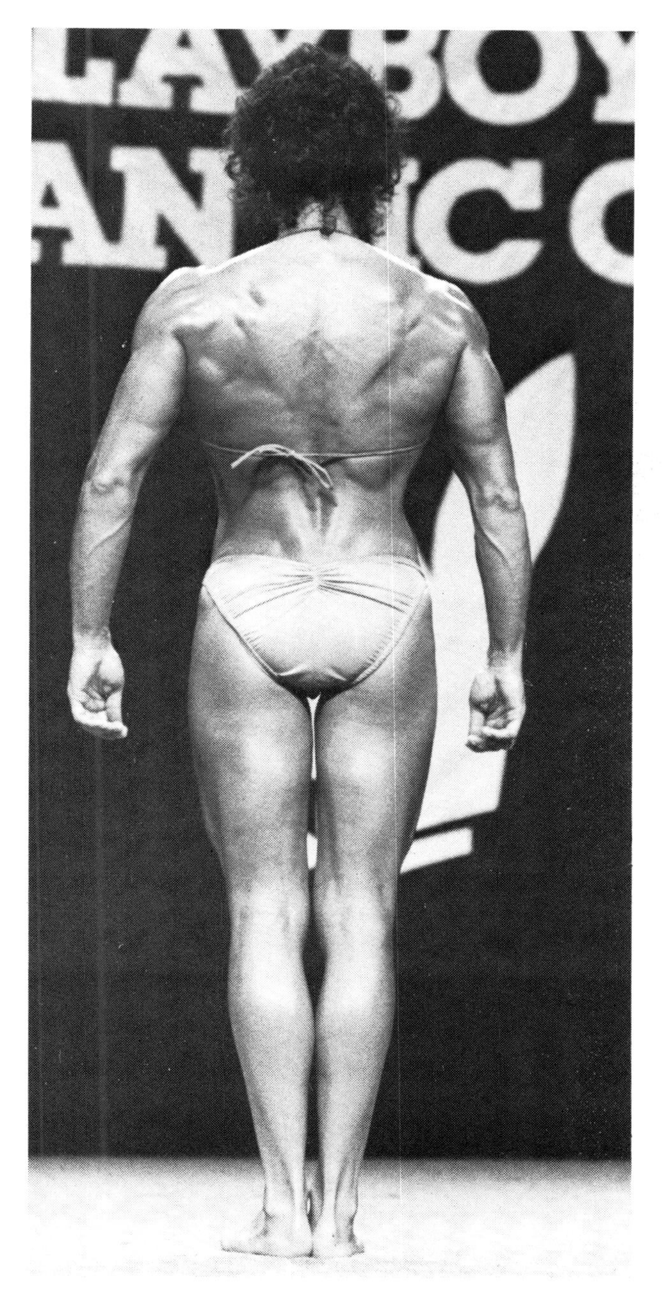

Relaxed back of Laura Combes, '82 Miss Olympia.
(Photo by Bill Reynolds)

body and muscle shape). Muscle mass and muscularity (an absence of body fat) are also revealed to a degree in Round I.

In Round II and Round III contestants are usually judged first as a group in each pose and then individually. Finally, comparisons are made in groups of two and three athletes prior to the final scoring by each judge. Round III, or the free-posing round, is conducted only with the athletes posing individually.

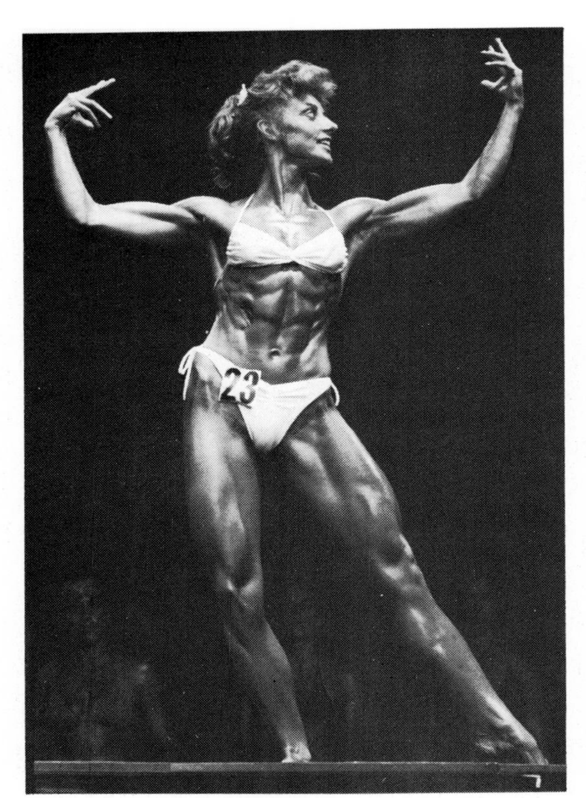

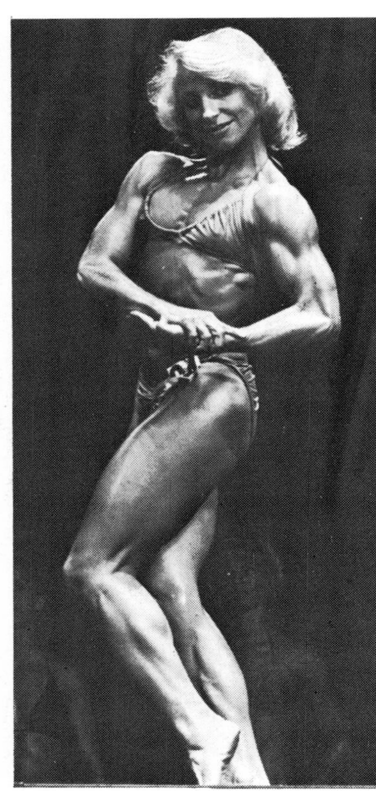

Round II, compulsory poses—Kike Elomaa, front biceps (left); Kay Baxter, side chest (right).

Round II, compulsory poses—Carla Dunlap, side triceps (left); Gail Shroeter, back biceps (right).

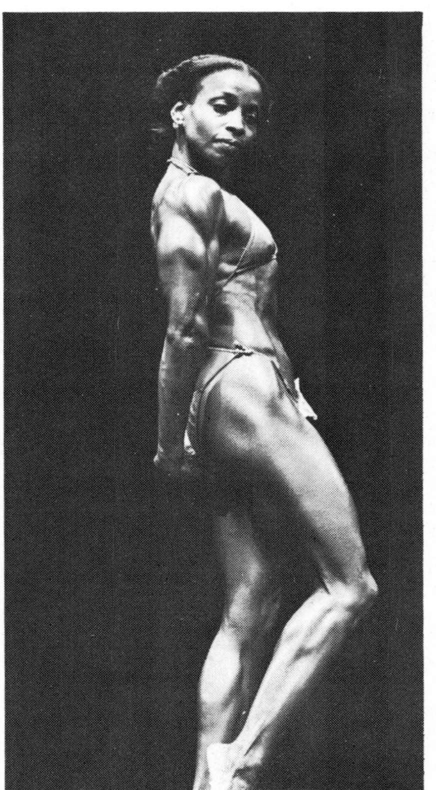

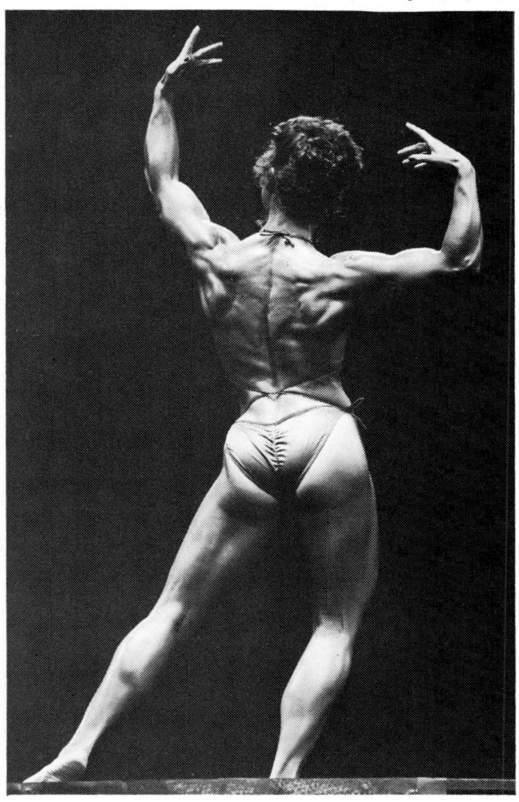

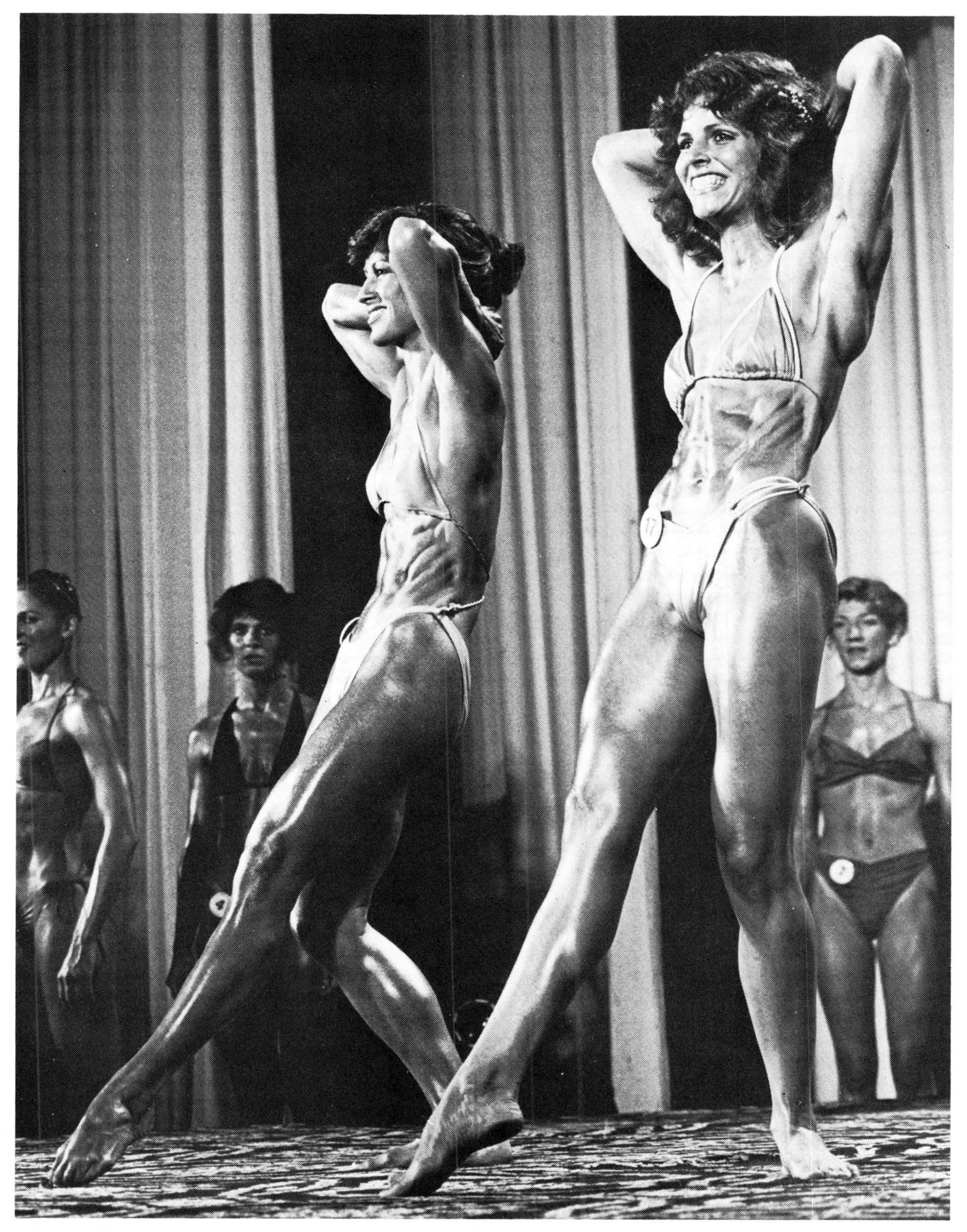

Round II, compulsory poses in comparison—Rachel McLish, left, and Candy Csencsits, right present ab and thigh poses.

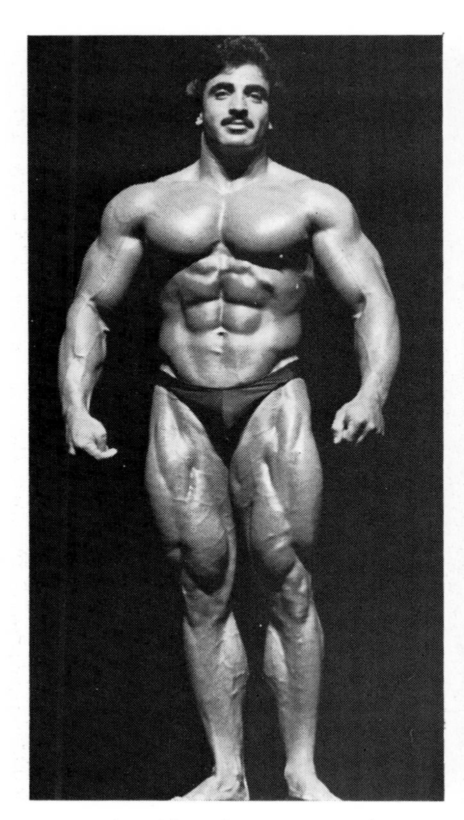

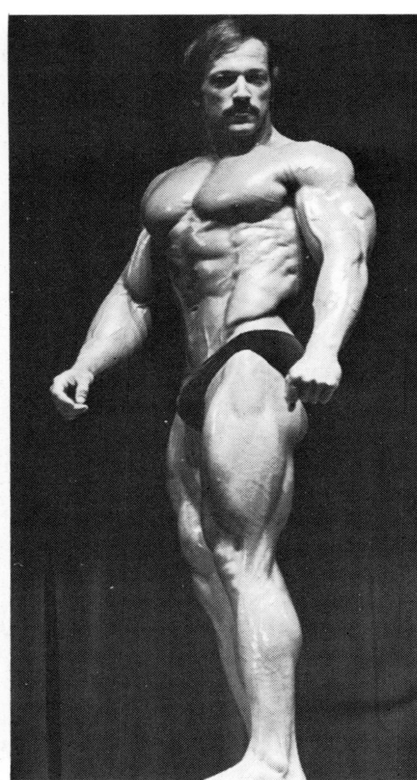

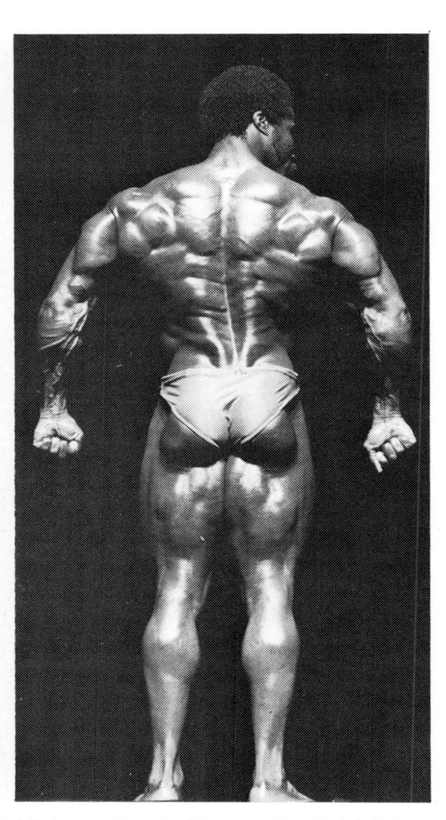

Round I, relaxed poses—Samir Bannout, front (left); Casey Viator, left side (middle); Robby Robinson, back (right); and Chris Dickerson, right side (below left). Round II, compulsory pose—Casey Viator, front double biceps (below right).

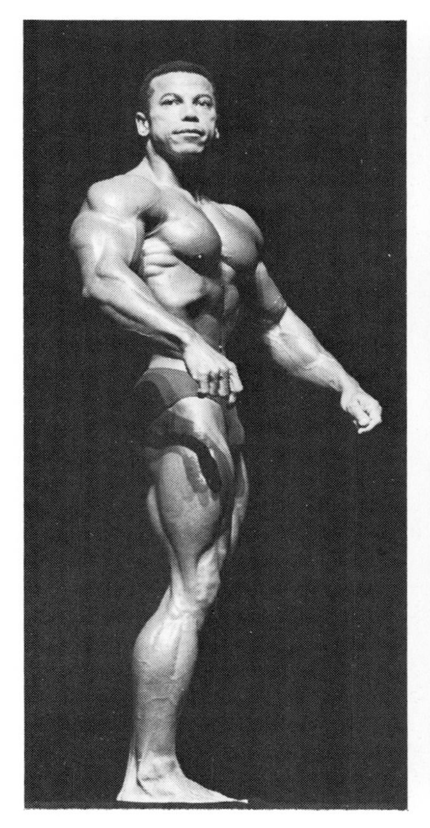

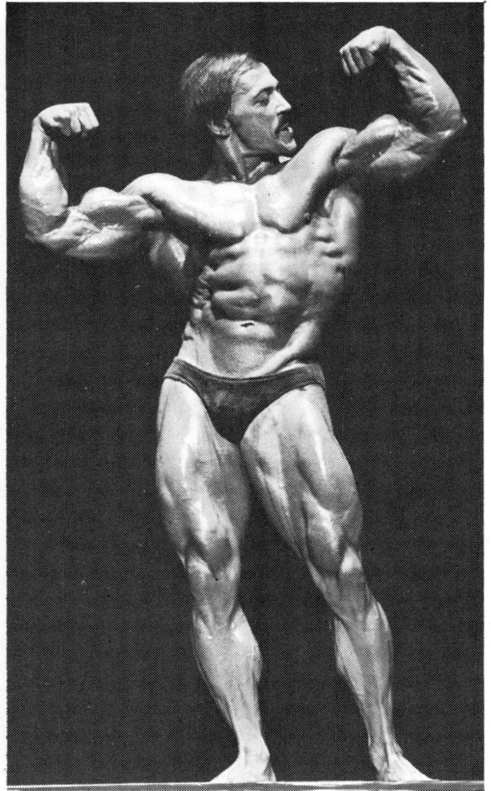

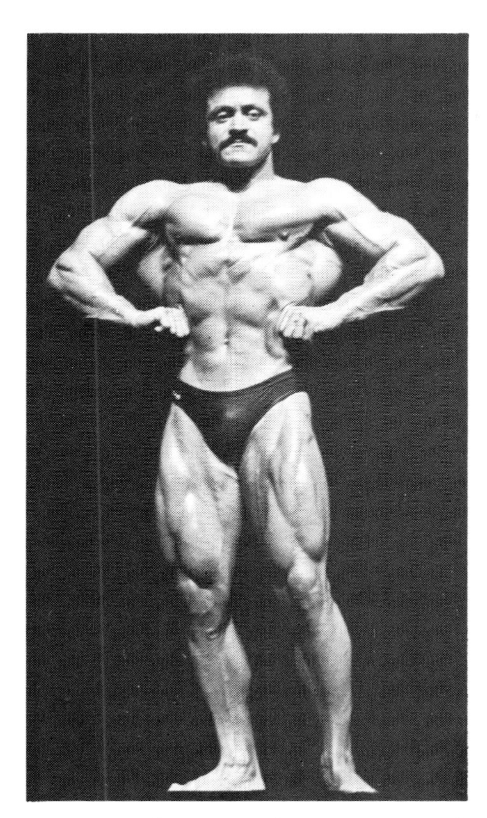

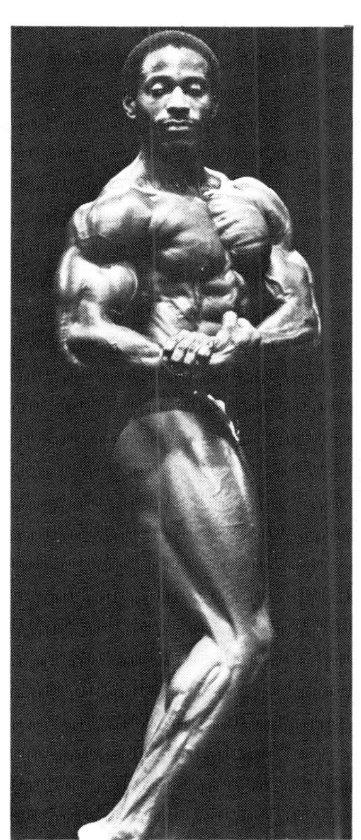

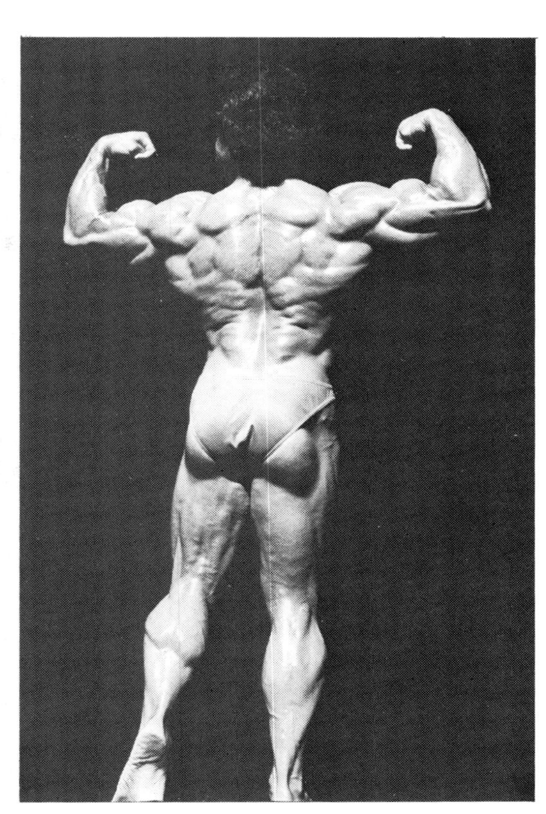

Round II, compulsory poses—Carlos Rodriguez, front lat spread (left); James Youngblood, side chest (middle); Samir Bannout, back double biceps (right); Roy Callender, back lat spread (below left); and Chris Dickerson, side triceps (below right).

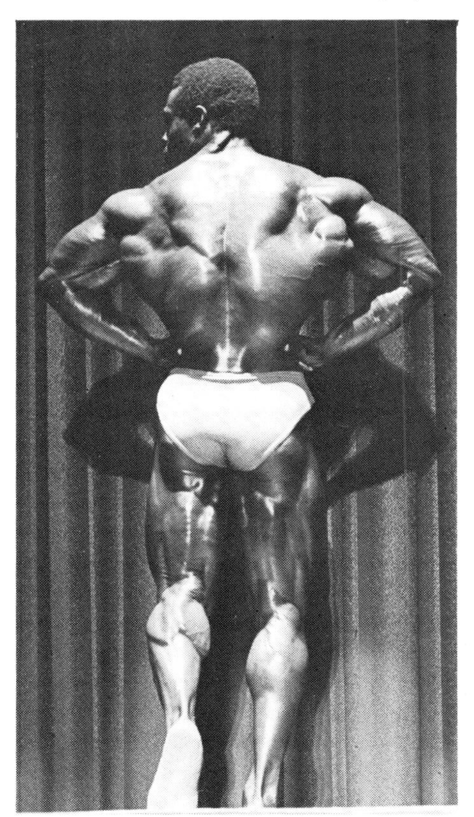

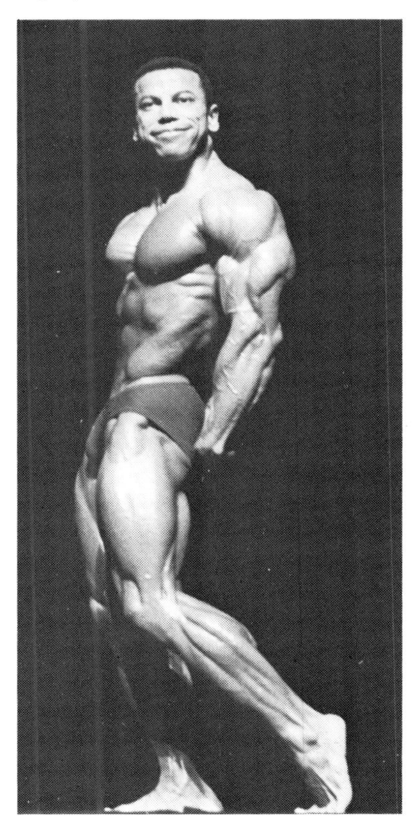

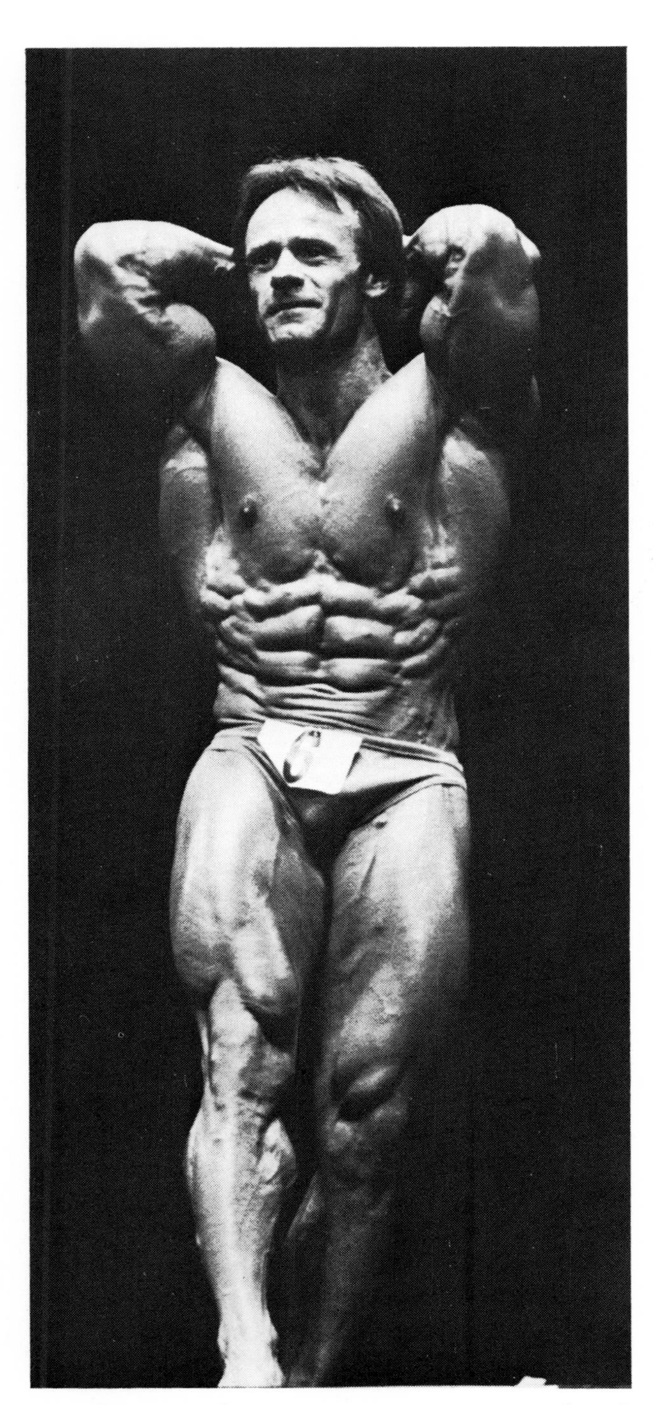

Round II, compulsory pose—Renato Bertagna, ab and thigh pose.

Round II consists of a series of compulsory poses that each contestant must execute. The compulsory poses for men, women, and mixed pairs at the time of this writing are illustrated on pages 166–172. These poses are changed periodically, however, so you should check with the meet promoter prior to competing to see which poses will be used. Or you can observe these poses in two or three competitions. These compulsory poses display every physical quality of a champion bodybuilder, but without allowing an athlete to hide weak points, as can be done in Round III.

The free-posing round brings out the creative abilities of each athlete, and this is the most important round to observe at each contest you attend. A huge variety of poses are done in this round, and the poses are designed by each athlete to display his or her body to maximum advantage. The poses are arranged with artistic transitions between each, and the whole is done to music. At its best, free posing is bodybuilding at its ultimate as an artistic endeavor.

Observe everything that occurs at each contest you attend and store up information to use when you begin to compete. You should especially observe the elation of each winner, because you too will soon experience this thrill of victory.

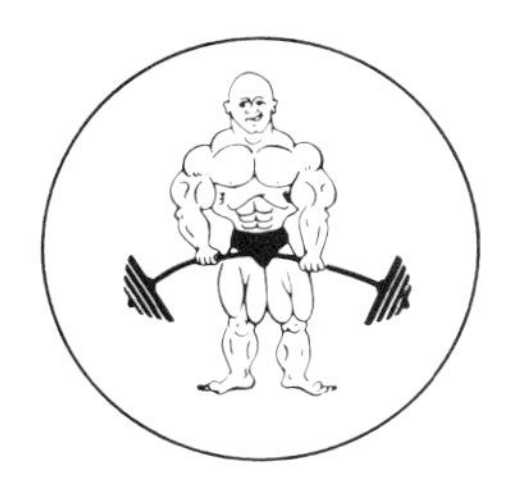

7 ADVANCED-LEVEL EXERCISES & WORKOUTS

This chapter contains illustrations and full descriptions of more than 30 additional bodybuilding exercises that you can add to the pool of movements from chapters 3 and 5. All told—and including the variations of exercises we have presented—this will bring your pool of bodybuilding movements to well over 100 exercises.

Without a doubt, you could easily continue bodybuilding profitably for life using only the exercises described in this book, but it would be much better for you to continue adding to the pool you have already developed. Through reading bodybuilding magazines and other books, observing accomplished bodybuilders in training, and discussing training with experienced bodybuilders, you can continually add to your exercise pool.

There are literally scores of bodybuilding movements for each muscle group, and the more you learn, the better. Each slight variation of a bodybuilding movement attacks a particular muscle from a slightly different angle. And the more angles of stress you place on a muscle group over a long period of time, the more complete your ultimate muscular development will be.

Finally, we will present two advanced-level training routines, one for the off-season and one for precontest training. If you have mastered the tips for formulating your own routines as presented in Chapter 6, you won't really need anyone else to do this for you. Still, you can profitably use these as examples in making up your own unique personal workouts.

Thigh Exercises

Sissy Squat

General Comments: This is a superb exercise for isolating the quadriceps muscles on the fronts of the thighs. Many champion bodybuilders do Sissy Squats to deepen the cuts separating each of the front thigh muscle masses. Very few bodybuilders use added resistance when they do Sissy Squats.

Starting Position: In the easiest version of a Sissy Squat you should stand between a set of parallel bar uprights. Grasp the uprights at about shoulder height with your arms slightly bent. Place your feet about six inches apart, toes directly forward. Your feet should be set slightly ahead of the bars you are grasping.

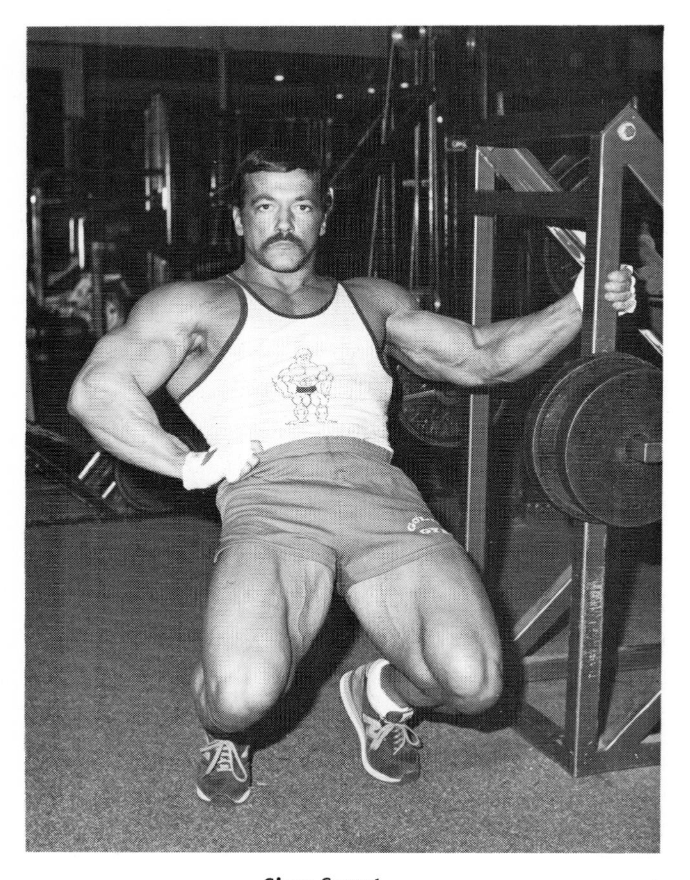

Sissy Squat.

Straighten your arms fully and stiffen your body so you are leaning back at an angle starting upward from your feet.

Exercise Performance: Consistently leaning your torso backward, simultaneously bend your knees and rise up on your toes. As you bend your knees fully, you should attempt to thrust them directly forward well over your toes. At the bottom position of the movement, your torso will be almost parallel to the floor. Using thigh strength alone, return to the starting position by straightening your legs. Repeat the movement for the desired number of repetitions.

Training Tips: Some bodybuilders prefer to do Sissy Squats while hanging on to an upright with only one hand. When you do the movement in this manner it is possible to hold a light dumbbell in the free hand to add a little resistance to the movement. Most bodybuilders do Sissy Squats at or near the end of their thigh training program, however, and at that point the thighs are so fatigued that the use of extra resistance is out of the question.

Partial Squats

General Comments: In Chapter 3 we described and illustrated the regular full Squat and described the muscles affected by it. Shorter-range Squats—such as Quarter Squats, Half Squats, Bench Squats, and Parallel Squats—work exactly the same muscle groups. The only difference is that the lower the range of motion you use in a Squat, the greater the amount of weight you will be able to handle.

Starting Position: Assume the same starting position as for a Squat.

Exercise Performance: Decide which depth you wish to squat to, then simply squat that far down and return to the erect position. For Bench Squats you place a low stool directly behind you and squat down until your buttocks touch it before standing erect again. In another variation of Bench Squats you simply straddle a flat exercise bench as you do the movement.

Training Tips: When you're doing Partial

Partial Squat.

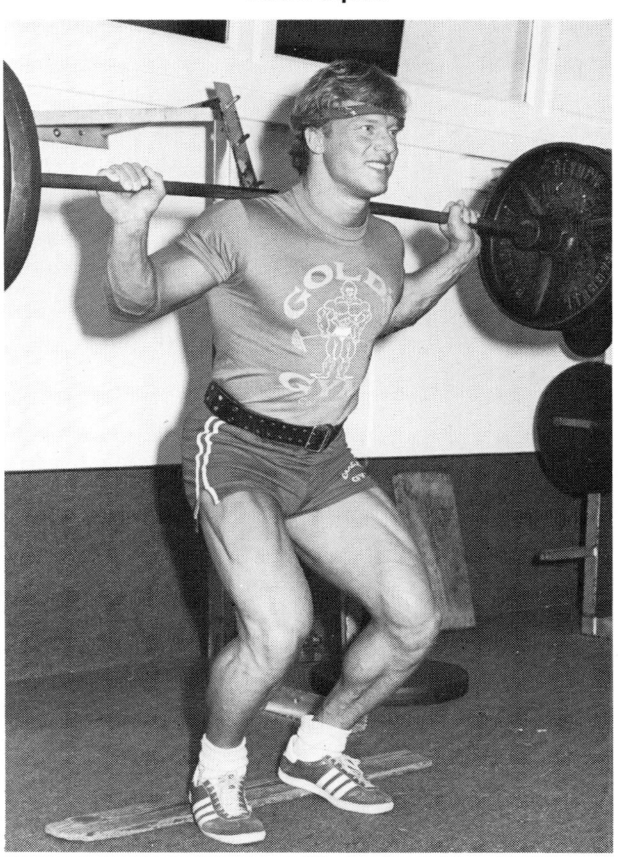

Squats, it is even more important to use a weightlifting belt than when doing Squats, since you will be using considerably heavier weights. Be sure that you don't violently bounce off the stool or bench, since that can lead to lower spine injuries. You should only lightly touch the bench before returning to an erect position.

Machine Squat

General Comments: This movement also affects the same muscle groups as a regular Full Squat. The advantage of using a machine lies primarily in eliminating the need to fight for balance while squatting. Additionally, you can place your feet up to a foot farther forward than when doing a regular Squat. Such a position isolates the buttocks from the movement.

Starting Position: Load up a Smith machine with an appropriate poundage, being sure that the bar is set at a position slightly below shoulder level. Step under the bar and position it comfortably across the trapezius muscles behind your neck. Set your feet about shoulder width apart and angle your toes slightly outward. Grasp the ends of the bar to keep your upper body in position during the movement. Release the bar.

Exercise Performance: Slowly bend your legs fully, then slowly return to the starting position by straightening your legs. Repeat the movement for the required number of repetitions.

Training Tips: In addition to the forward position of your feet mentioned above, you can experiment with wider and narrower foot stances. When you have no balance factor to worry about, you can experiment with a much wider variety of foot positions while squatting. You can also do Partial Squats on a Smith machine, provided you can put enough weight on it to justify doing short-range squatting movements.

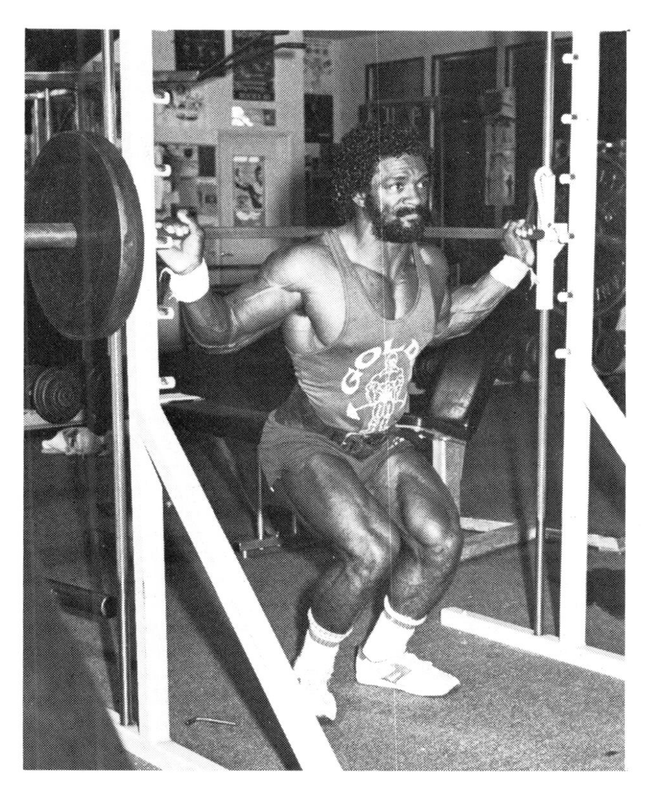

Machine Squat.

Back Exercises

Power Clean

General Comments: This is the movement in which you pull a barbell from the floor to your chest in preparation to do Military Presses. It is an excellent movement for adding mass to the trapezius muscles as well as for strengthening and muscling up the lower back.

Starting Position: Stand in front of a moderately weighted barbell with your shins just touching the handle of the barbell as it lies on the floor. Set your feet at about shoulder width with your toes pointed forward. Grasp the barbell handle a little wider than shoulder width on each side with your palms facing your shins. Bend your legs and flatten your back. Look directly ahead and keep your arms straight at the beginning of the movement. When you are in the correct starting position, your shoulders should be higher than your hips and your hips should be higher than your knees.

Exercise Performance: Begin pulling the barbell with relatively straight arms from the floor by beginning to straighten your legs. Then, as your legs near a straight position, begin to straighten your back. Finally, follow through by pulling with your arms to add final upward momentum to the bar. At the top of the bar's momentum, whip your elbows under the bar to catch it at your shoulders. With heavy weights

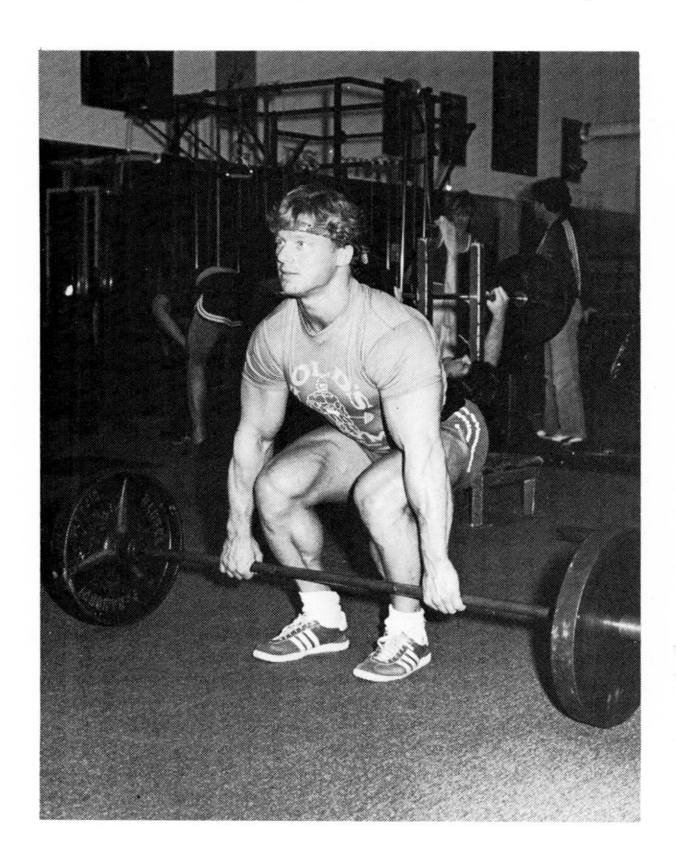

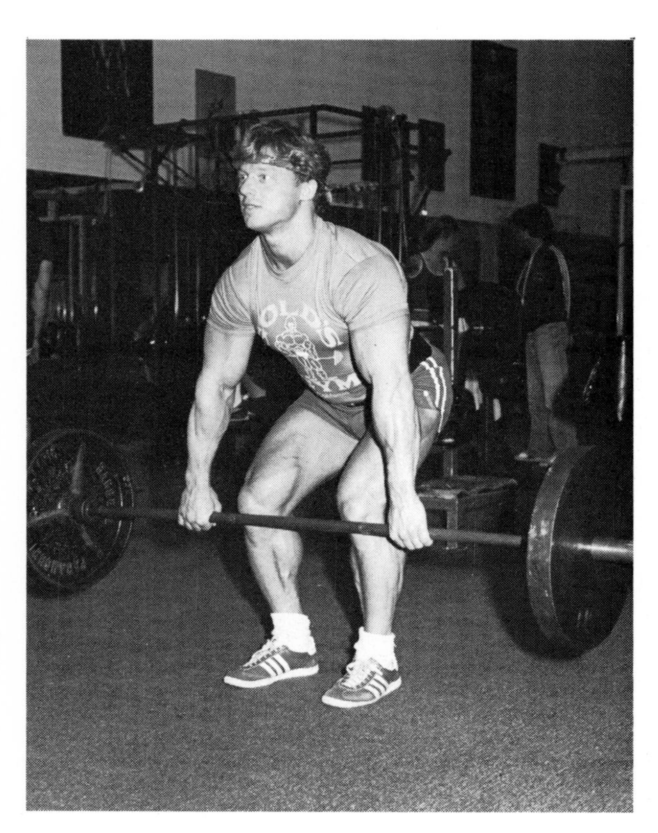

Andreas Cahling performing the Power Clean with strict form.

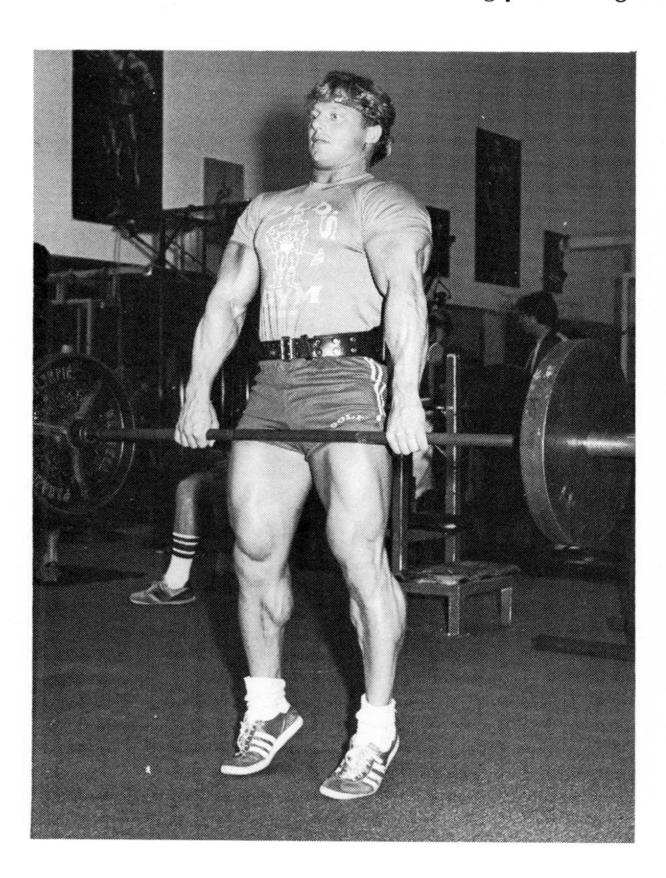

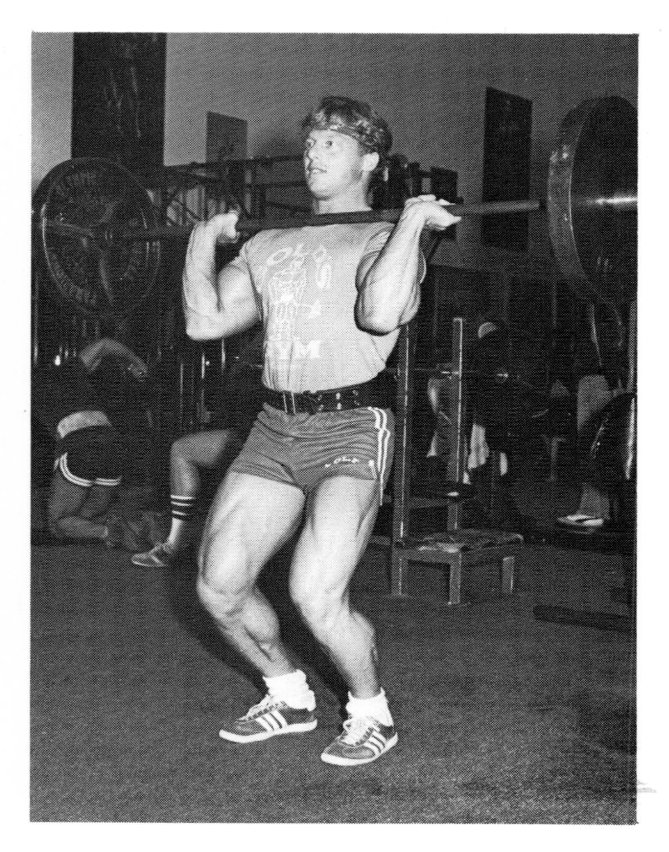

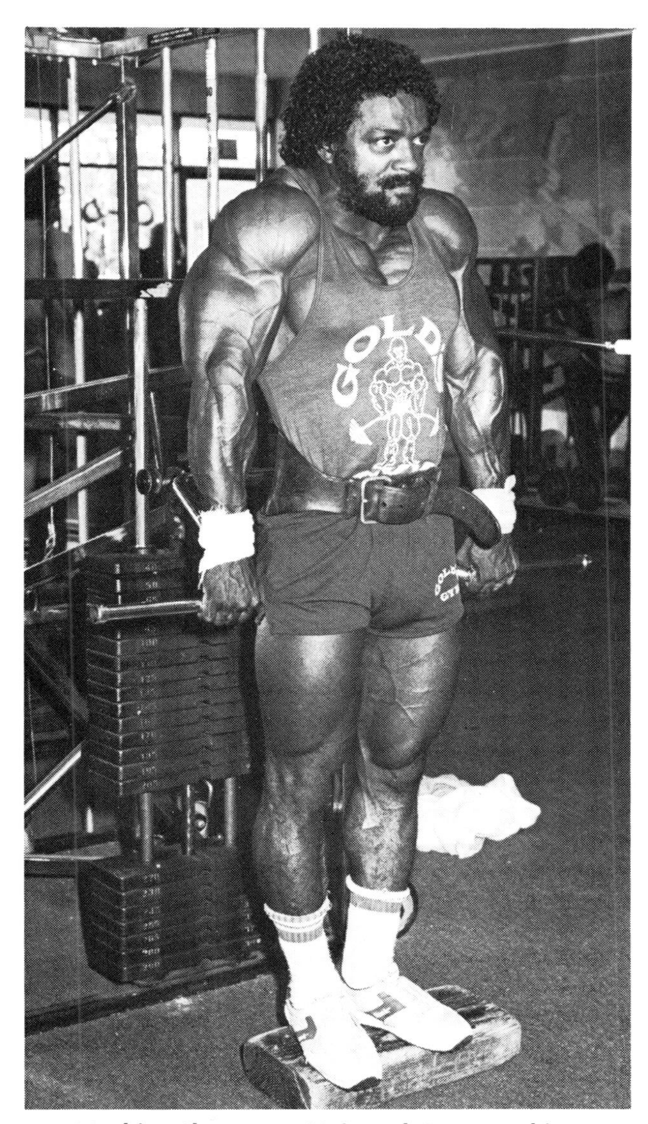

Machine Shrug on a Universal Gyms machine.

you can dip your knees a little to absorb the shock of the bar landing on your shoulders. Lower the barbell back downward along the same path you lifted it and repeat the movement for the required number of repetitions.

Training Tips: You can vary your grip on this movement for slightly different effects on your upper back and shoulder muscles. You can also lower the barbell just to your thighs on each repetition, forcing you to pull even harder to complete the next rep. This is called Cleaning from a "hang."

Machine Shrugs

General Comments: This is an excellent direct movement for stressing the trapezius muscles. It can be done either on a Nautilus machine especially made for doing Shrugs or on the Bench Pressing station of a Universal Gym machine.

Starting Position (Nautilus machine): Sit on the seat of the machine and extend your forearms between the pads, palms upward. Sit erect and sag your shoulders downward as far as possible.

Starting Position (Universal Gym machine): Stand between the handles of the machine, facing the weight stack. Grasp the handles of the apparatus with your palms to the rear. Stand erect and sag your shoulders as far downward as possible.

Exercise Performance: As on all shrugging movements, simply shrug your shoulders upward as high as possible, then return them to the starting position. Repeat the movement as many times as desired.

Training Tips: When using the Universal Gym machine, you can do the movement facing away from the weight stack as well. Shorter individuals may find that they need to stand on a thick block of wood when they do the exercise. With heavier weights, you may need to reinforce your grip with weightlifters' straps.

Bench Rows

Ganeral Comments: This is an excellent movement for strengthening the upper back muscles, particularly the lats, without placing any strain on the lower back. It is primarily a lat thickness movement.

Starting Position: Elevate a flat exercise bench to a height at which the barbell plates won't touch the floor in the low position of the exercise when you are doing the movement. Lie face down on the bench and have someone hand you a heavy barbell so that you can hold it in the same position as for a Barbell Bent Rowing motion. Stretch the barbell as close to the floor as possible.

Exercise Performance: Pull the barbell directly upward until its handle touches the underside of the bench. As you pull the weight upward, be sure that your elbows travel both outward and backward. Lower the weight slowly back to the starting position. Repeat the

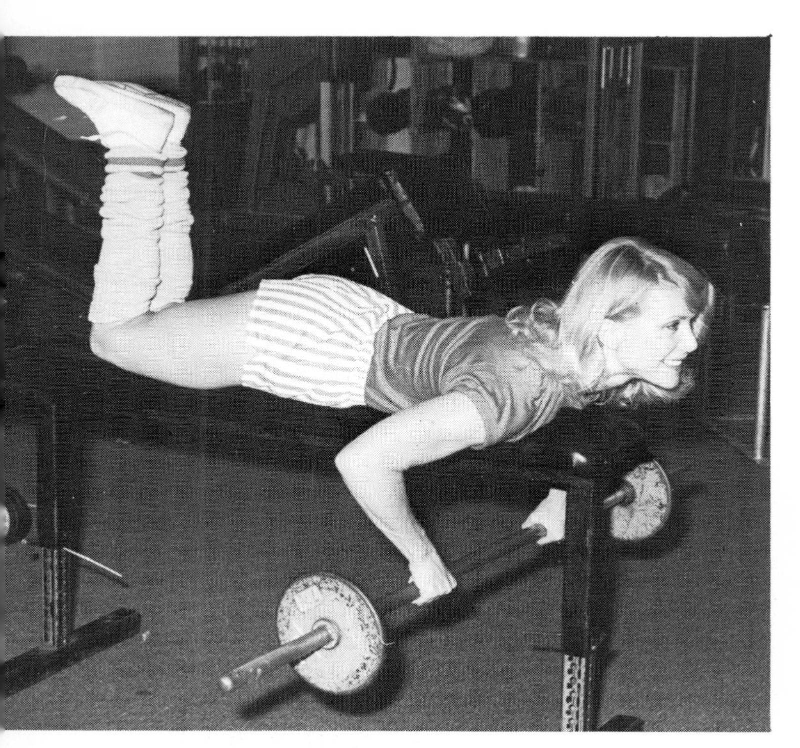

Bench Row.

movement for the required number of repetitions.

Training Tips: Vary the grip you use on the barbell. You can also use two dumbbells on this movement rather than a barbell. Some bodybuilders prefer to do this movement with the head end of the bench elevated slightly higher than the foot end to vary the stress on the lats.

Bent-Arm Pullover

General Comments: Pullovers work both the pectorals and the upper back muscles, but most bodybuilders nowadays use Bent-Arm Pullovers for latissimus dorsi development.

Starting Position: Lie on your back on a flat exercise bench so that your head hangs off the end of the bench. A barbell should be placed crosswise at the head end of the bench. Grasp this barbell with a narrow grip (about six inches between your index fingers) with your palms facing the ceiling.

Exercise Performance: Slowly pull the barbell in a semicircle from the floor up past your face until it rests on your chest. Throughout the movement, your elbows should be bent at a 90-degree angle and held as close together as possible while pulling the weight in a semicircle to your chest. Lower the weight back to the starting point and repeat the movement for the required number of reps.

Training Tips: With heavier weights you will find it easier to start the movement from your chest. You will also find the movement easier to do with heavy weights if someone restrains your knees to keep you flat on the bench when using heavy poundages.

Bent-Arm Pullover—start, top; finish, bottom.

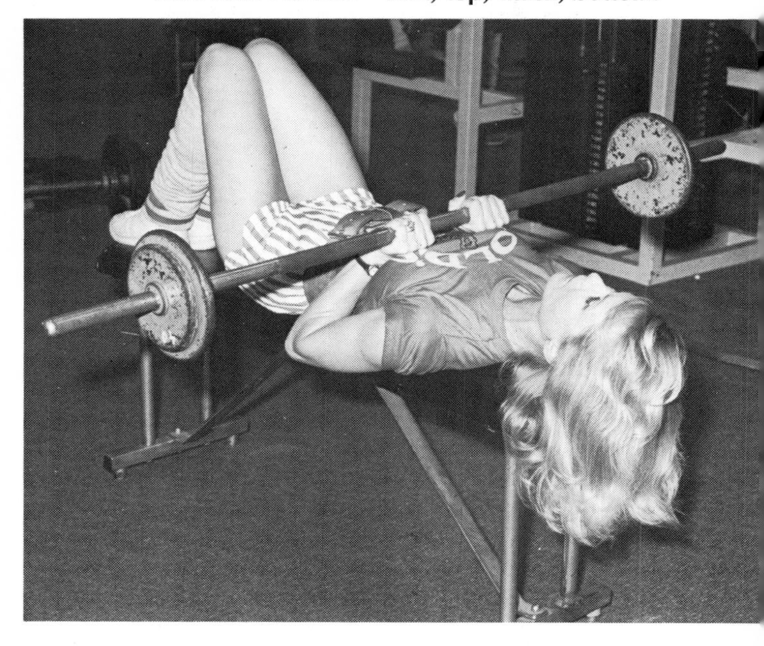

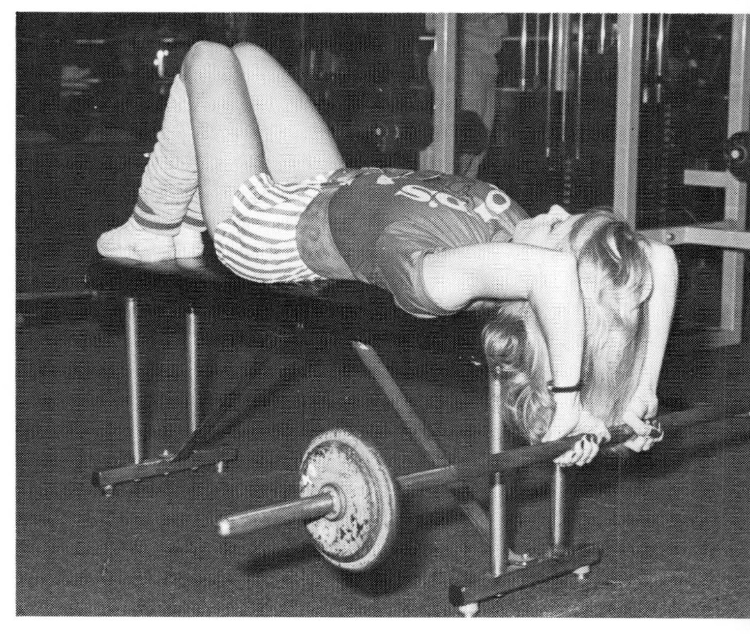

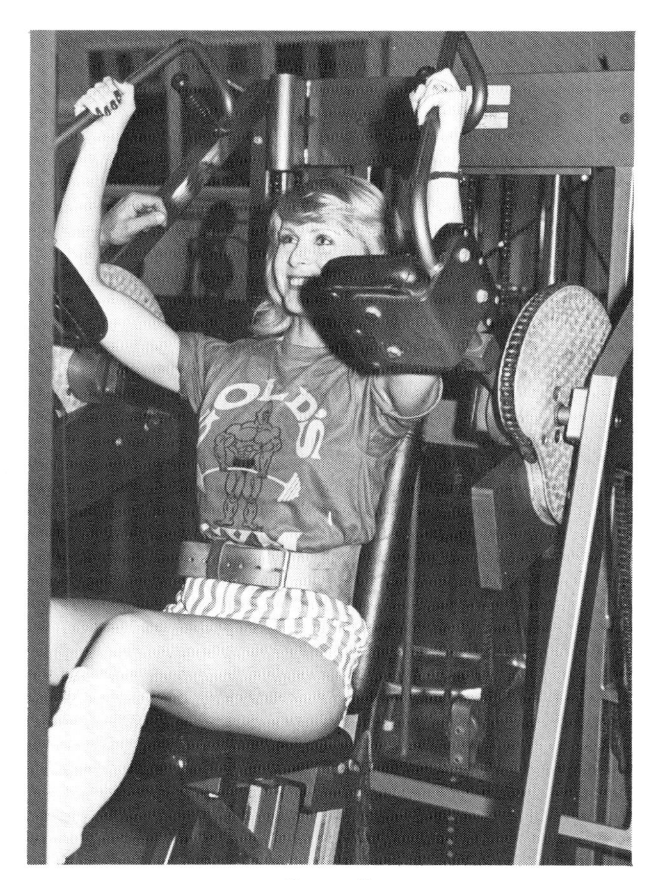

Nautilus Pullover.

Nautilus Pullover

General Comments: Without a doubt, more bodybuilders at Gold's use the Nautilus Pullover machine than do Bent-Arm Pullovers. The effect on the lats is the same with both machines.

Starting Position: Raise the seat of the machine high enough so that, when you sit in it, the middle of the cam on each side of the movement arm is on the same level as your shoulder joints. Fasten the lap belt around your hips and push down on the foot pedal to bring the movement arm of the machine into a position in which you can fit your elbows against the pads on each side. Rest your fingers on the bar that connects the two arms of the pads. Slowly release pressure on the foot bar to place full resistance against your elbows. Allow the weight to pull your elbows back behind your head as far as possible.

Exercise Performance: Push hard with your elbows to move the pads in semicircles forward and downward as far as possible. Return back along the same arc to the starting point and repeat the movement.

Training Tips: You can get a lot more out of this movement if you hold the contracted position of the exercise for two or three seconds.

Serratus Lever (Rope Crunches)

General Comments: You can use this movement to develop both your lats and your serratus muscles. Most bodybuilders use it to con-

Serratus Lever (Rope Crunch)—start, top; finish, bottom.

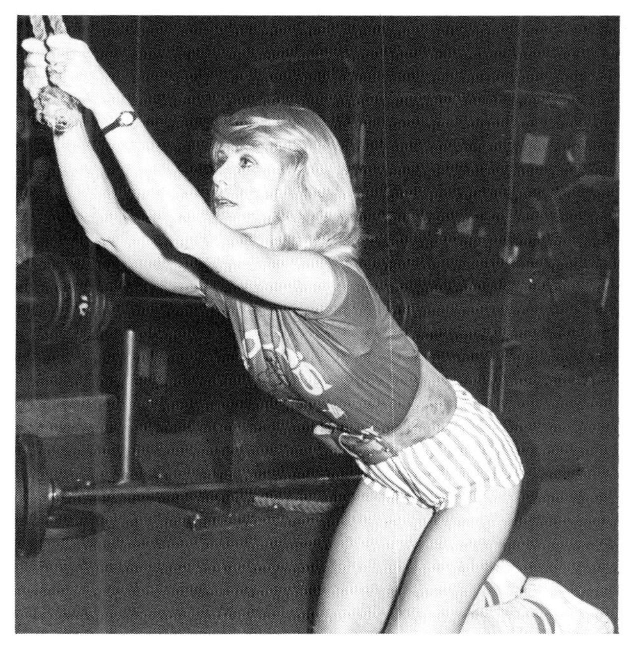

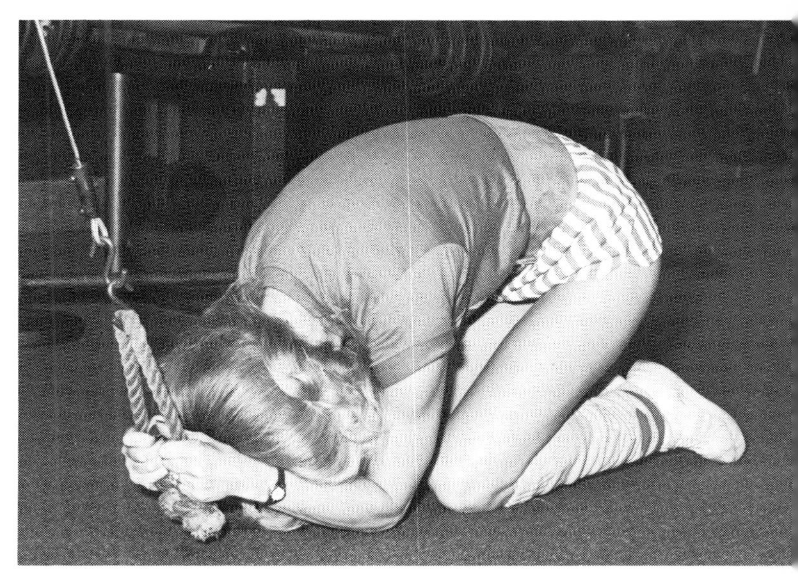

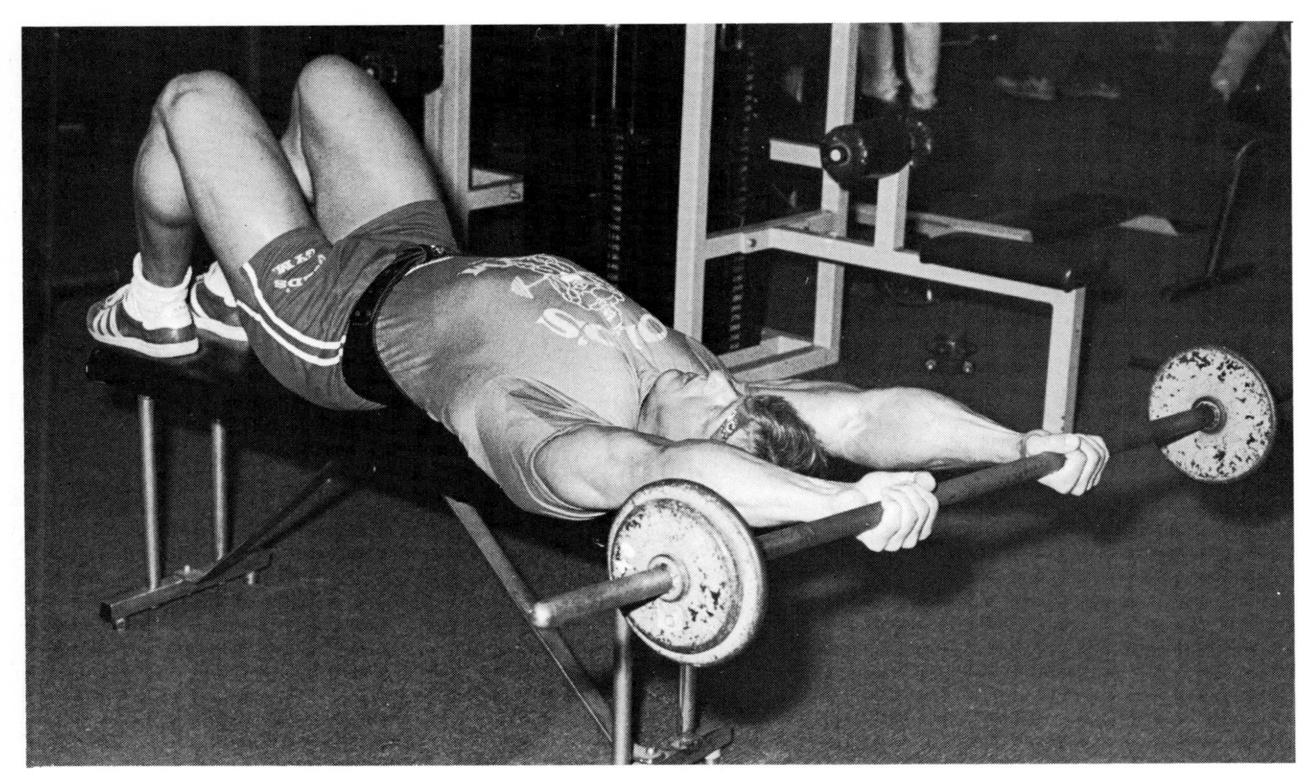

Stiff-Arm Pullover.

clude their abdominal routine, but you can also use it to finish off your lat workout.

Starting Position: Grasp a rope handle attached to a lat machine cable and kneel down about two feet back from the pulley. Straighten your torso and stretch your arms overhead as high as possible.

Exercise Performance: From the fully stretched position, bend over slowly while forcefully blowing out all of your air and executing a pullover motion with your arms. At the conclusion of the movement your hands will be on the floor and your face will be touching your hands. Return to the starting point and repeat the movement.

Training Tips: To stress the intercostals and one or the other side of the lats more forcefully, you can twist from side to side as you do this movement.

Chest Exercises

Stiff-Arm Pullover

General Comments: Bodybuilders usually use Stiff-Arm Pullovers in conjunction with Breathing Squats to enlarge the rib cage.

Starting Position: Lie on your back on a flat exercise bench, being sure that your head lies on the bench rather than off it as in a Bent-Arm Pullover. Take a shoulder-width grip on a light barbell, your palms facing your feet. Extend your arms directly upward to support the barbell in the same position as at the start of a Bench Press. Keep your arms straight throughout the movement.

Exercise Performance: Taking in a deep breath, slowly lower the barbell in a semicircle backward and downward to as low a position as possible behind your head. Return the barbell back to the starting point, exhaling as you do so. Repeat the movement.

Training Tips: You can experiment with a number of grip widths on this movement. You can also hold a single dumbbell in both hands.

Cross-Bench Pullover

General Comments: It's difficult to beat this

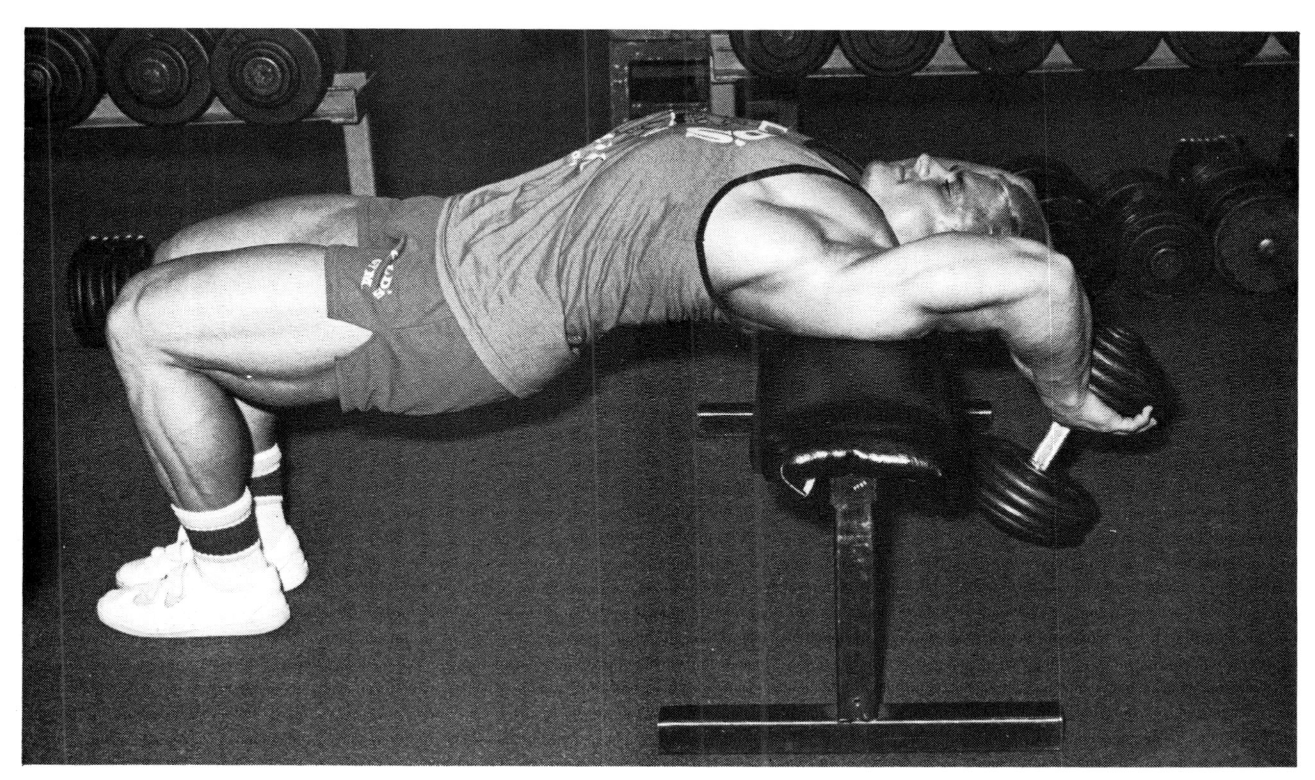

Cross-Bench Pullover.

movement for pectoral, latissimus dorsi, and serratus development. It is often done as a transitional movement between pecs and lats when bodybuilders are doing split routines in which they train their chest and back in one session.

Starting Position: Grasp a moderately weighted dumbbell with your palms against the inside plate so that the dumbbell handle hangs directly downward. Lie across a flat exercise bench with only your shoulders in contact with the bench and extend your arms directly upward so that the dumbbell is right above your chest. Place your feet a comfortable distance apart and bend your knees enough so that your hips are below the level of your chest.

Exercise Performance: While bending your arms slightly, slowly lower the dumbbell backward and downward in a semicircle to as low a position behind your head as possible. Return slowly to the starting point and repeat the movement.

Training Tips: Some bodybuilders do this exercise while lying lengthwise along a flat exercise bench, but it's not as effective as when done lying across the bench. When lying across the bench, you can get a more and more intense stretch the farther you lower your hips below the level of the bench when doing the movement.

Cable Crossover

General Comments: By doing Crossovers you can directly stress the entire pectoral muscle mass, but particularly the outer edges. Crossovers are used most frequently close to a competition in order to carve deep striations across the pecs.

Starting Position: Stand between the crossover pulleys and grasp one pulley handle in each hand. Place your feet about shoulder width apart. Your arms will angle upward at about 45-degree angles, and your hands should be facing downward throughout the movement. Bend your arms slightly and keep them bent throughout the movement. Bend slightly forward at the waist.

Exercise Performance: Slowly move your hands under tension downward in semicircles

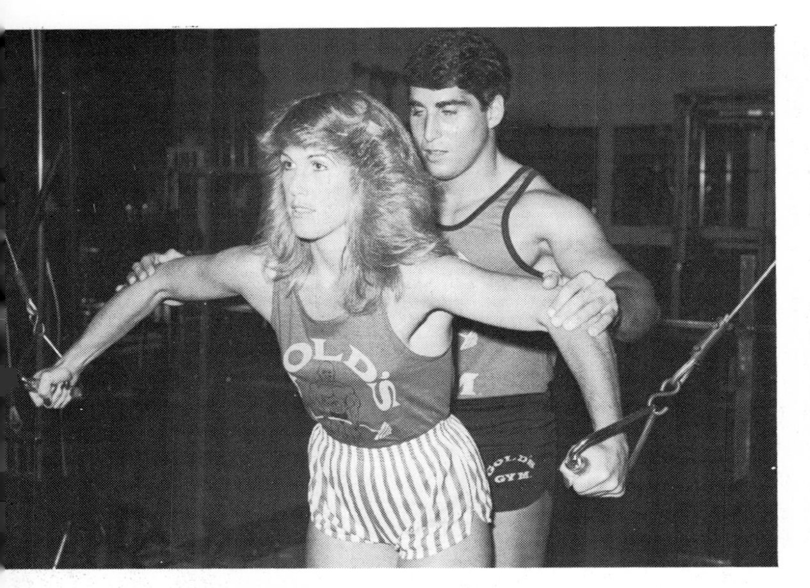

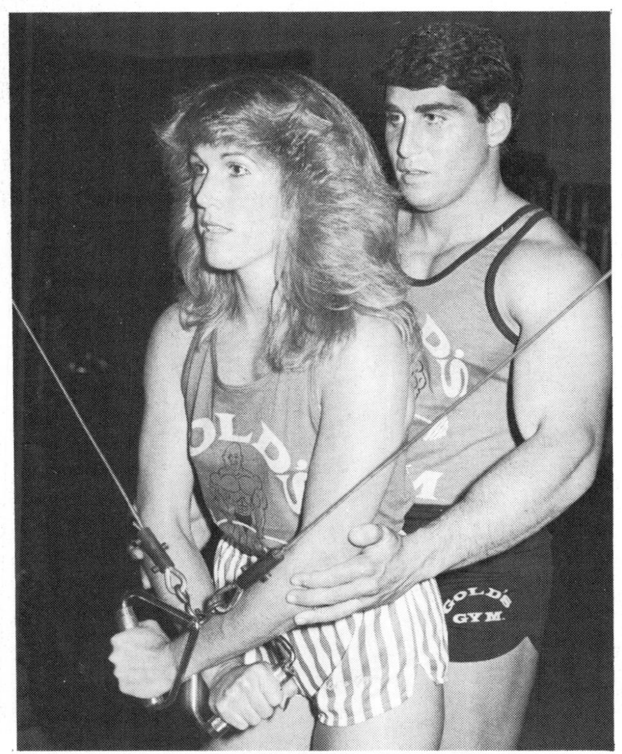

Cable Crossover—start, top; finish, bottom. Note partner's position for forced reps.

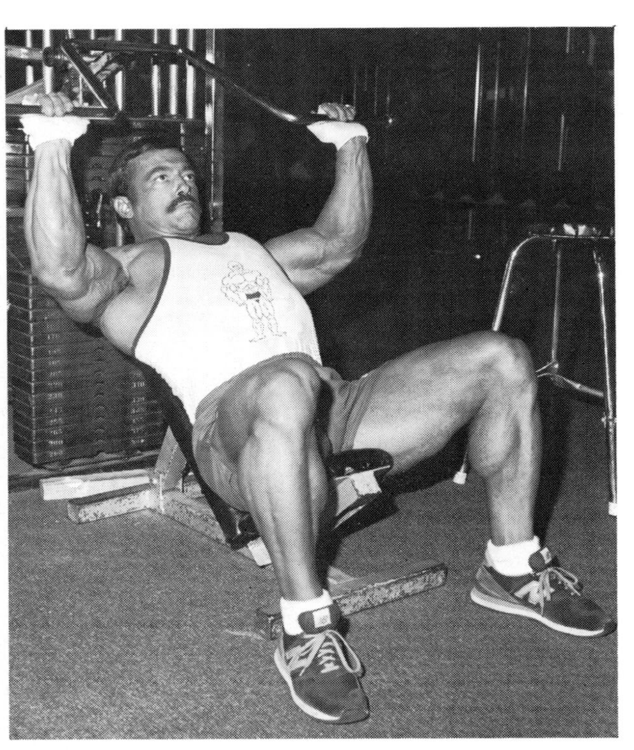

Incline Press on Universal Gyms machine.

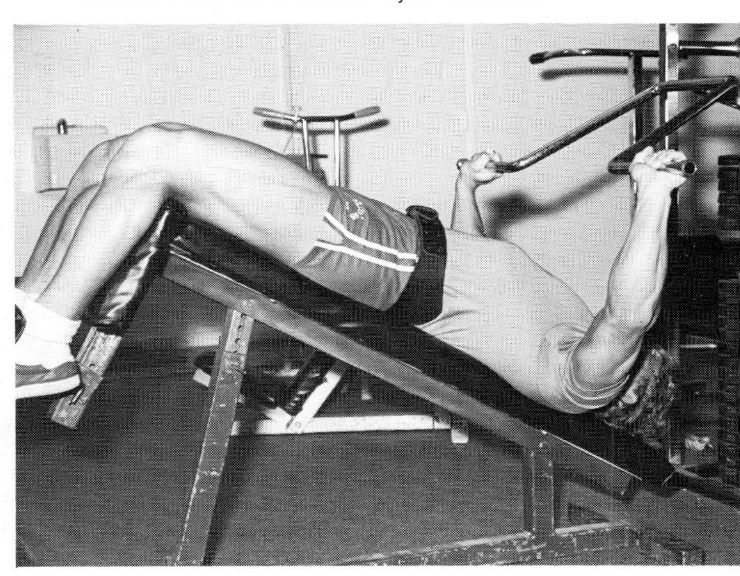

Decline Press on Universal Gyms machine.

until they touch each other four to six inches in front of your hips. Hold that position for three or four seconds, tensing your pectorals very hard as if doing a "Most Muscular" pose at a bodybuilding competition. Return your hands slowly to the starting point and repeat the movement for the desired number of repetitions.

Training Tips: The most common variation of this movement is done while kneeling between the pulleys, which makes the exercise somewhat more strict. You can also do Crossovers with one arm at a time.

Universal Incline/Decline Press

General Comments: At Gold's/Venice many

bodybuilders do machine Incline and Decline Presses at the bench press station of a Universal Gym machine. This involves placing a portable decline bench or incline bench beneath the movement arms of the machine and doing presses lying or sitting on such benches. The illustrations of these two movements will clarify the performance of such exercises. Depending on the relative height of the bench you use, you may need to place a block of wood or two under the head end of it to make the bench high enough to allow a complete range of motion.

Deltoid Exercises

Cable Side Lateral

General Comments: Virtually all Gold's Gym bodybuilders seem to prefer this movement for sharpening and adding mass to the medial and anterior heads of the deltoids.

Starting Position: Place your feet about shoulder width apart with the right one about two feet away from a floor pulley. Your right side should be directly toward the pulley. Reach over and grasp the pulley handle with your left hand and then stand erect. The pulley cable should then run across your body. Place your right hand on your hip and bend your left arm slightly. Maintain this right hand position and left arm flex throughout the movement.

Exercise Performance: Slowly raise your left hand in a semicircle outward and slightly forward until it reaches shoulder height. Slowly lower it back to the starting point and repeat the movement. Be sure to do an equal number of repetitions with each arm.

Training Tips: For a slightly different effect on your deltoid muscles, try running the cable behind your body instead of in front of it. Or raise your hand directly from the pulley without having the cable across your body. In this case the movement is somewhat like doing a Dumbbell One-Arm Side Lateral Raise but replacing the dumbbell with a pulley handle.

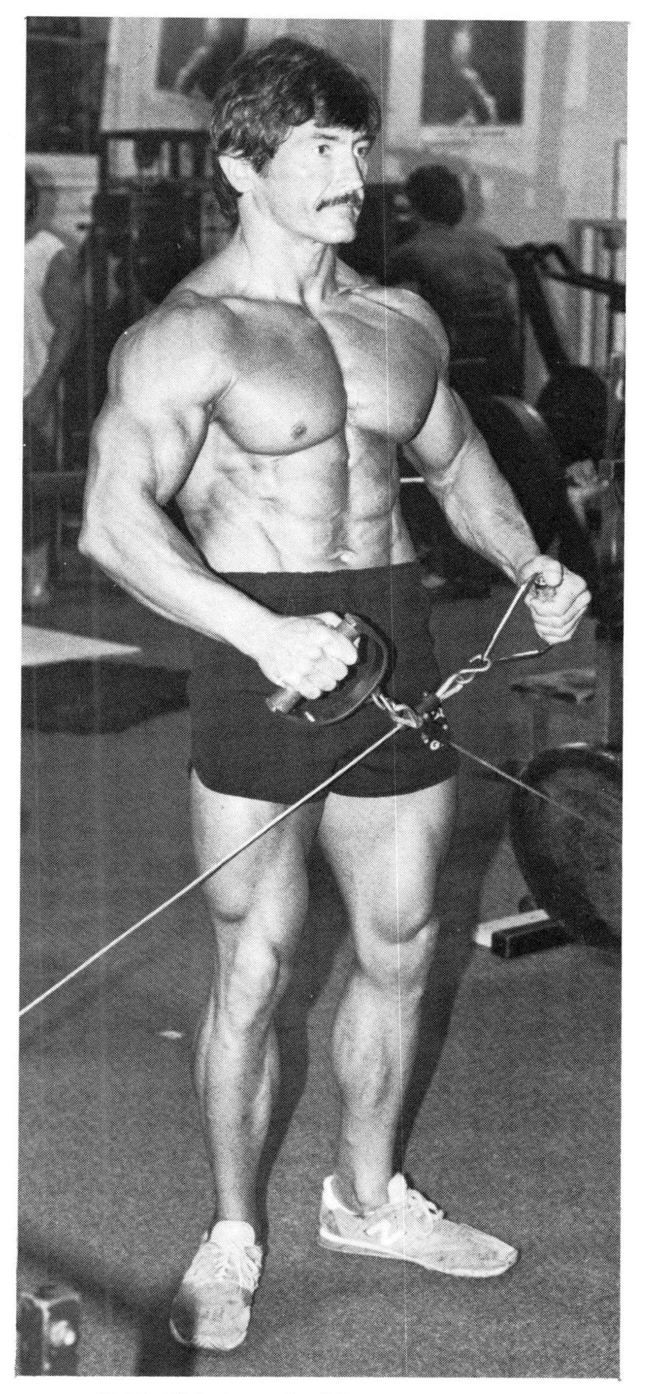

Cable Side Lateral with two arms—start.

Cable Bent Lateral

General Comments: This is quite an effective posterior deltoid movement, since it allows for continuous tension throughout the range of motion of the exercise. All bent lateral exercises are also secondarily effective in developing the upper back muscles.

Starting Position: Stand between a pair of low pulleys. Reach across your body with your right hand and grasp the pulley handle on the left side of your body. Next move over to the

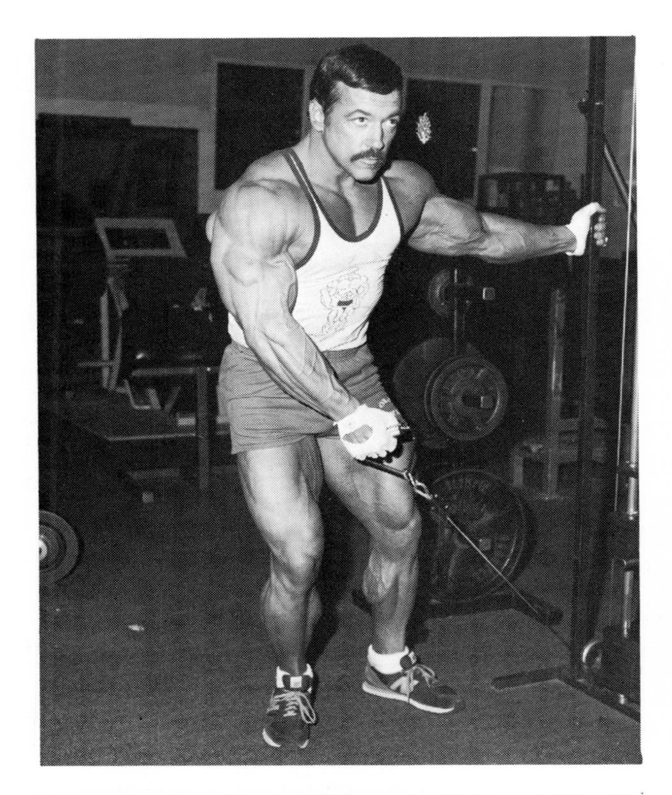

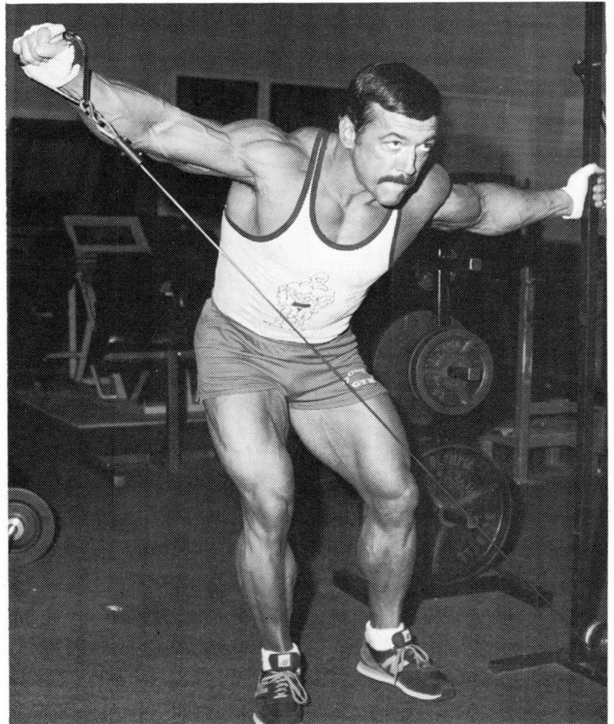

Cable Side Lateral with one arm—start, top; finish, bottom.

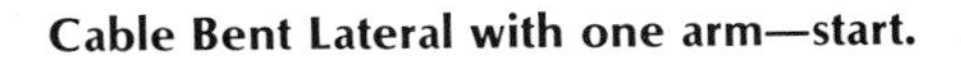

Cable Bent Lateral with one arm—start.

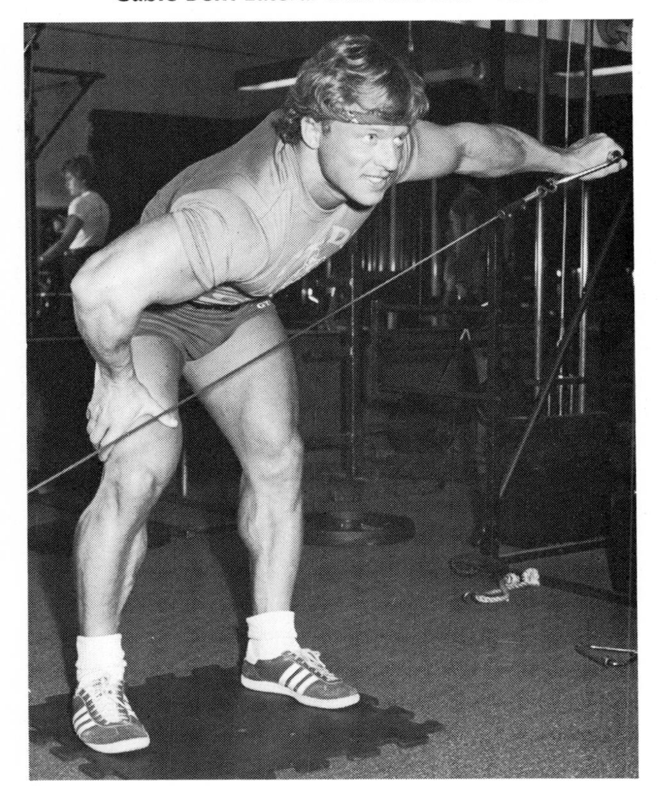

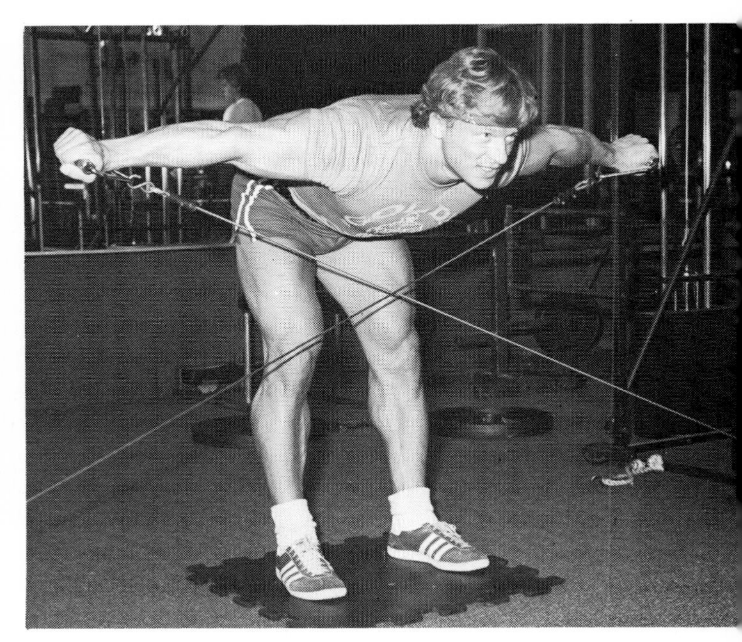

Cable Bent Lateral with two arms—finish.

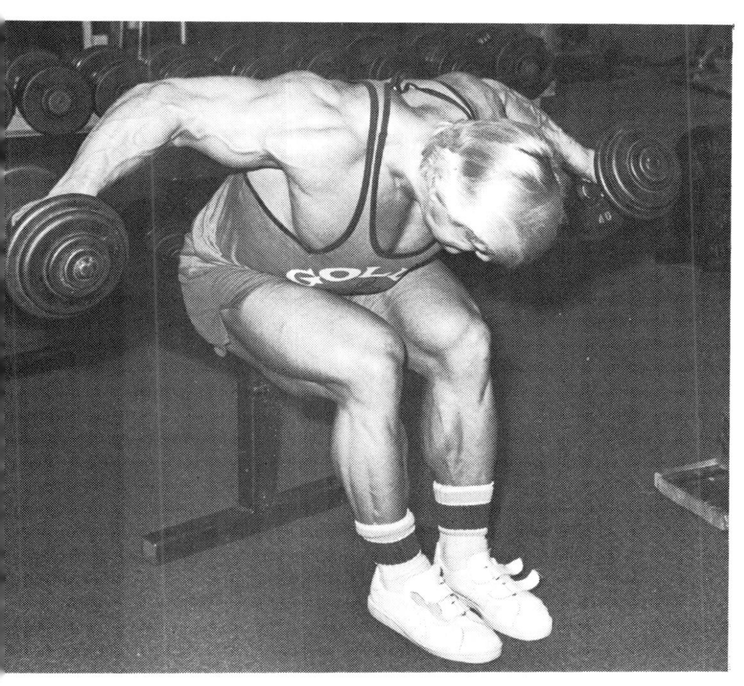

Seated Bent Lateral.

right far enough so you can grasp the handle on the right side with your left hand. Then center yourself between the pulleys and bend over until your upper body is parallel to the floor. Allow your arms to cross beneath your chest as far as possible.

Exercise Performance: From this basic starting position, raise your hands directly out to the sides in semicircles until they are a bit above the level of your torso. Hold this top position for a moment and then lower your hands back to the starting point. Repeat the movement for the desired number of repetitions.

Training Tips: Many bodybuilders do this movement with one arm at a time.

Seated Bent Lateral

General Comments: Because the legs are isolated from this movement, quite a few superstar bodybuilders like to use it to stress their posterior deltoids.

Starting Position: Grasp two light dumbbells and sit at the end of a flat exercise bench. Place your feet a comfortable distance apart and bend over at the waist until your torso is resting on your thighs. Hang your arms directly downward from your shoulder joints and bend your arms slightly throughout the movement.

Exercise Performance: Slowly raise the dumbbells directly out to the sides in semicircles until they are a bit above the level of your torso. Hold this top position for a moment and then lower your hands back to the starting point. Repeat the movement for the desired number of repetitions.

Training Tips: A somewhat similar movement can be done while standing, bending over, and placing the forehead on a padded surface of sufficient height to place the torso parallel to the floor.

Prone Incline Lateral

General Comments: This exercise is unique in that it stresses both the posterior and medial deltoid heads. Since it's done lying face down on an incline bench, it's virtually impossible to cheat while doing Prone Incline Laterals.

Starting Position: Grasp two light dumbbells and lie face down on a 30-degree incline bench. A 45-degree incline bench is acceptable, but it's not quite as good as using a lower incline. Dangle your arms directly downward from your shoulder joints, your hands facing inward. Bend your arms slightly and keep them bent throughout the movement.

Exercise Performance: Slowly raise the

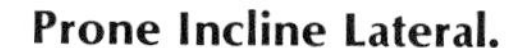

Prone Incline Lateral.

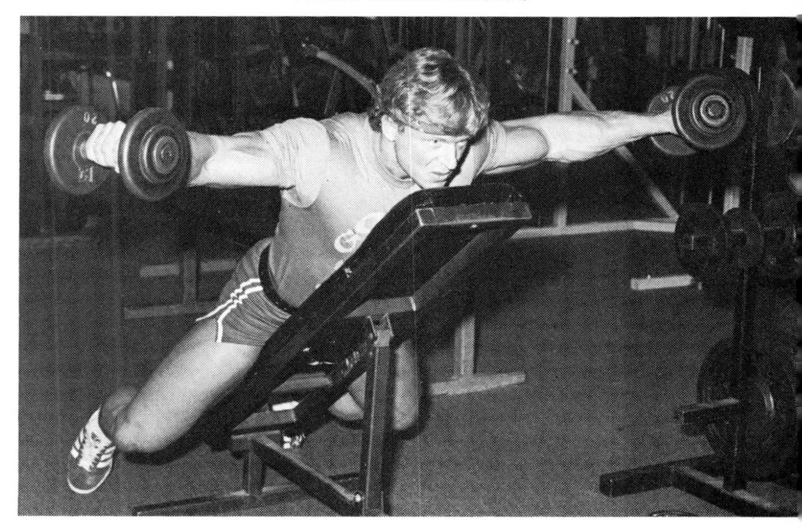

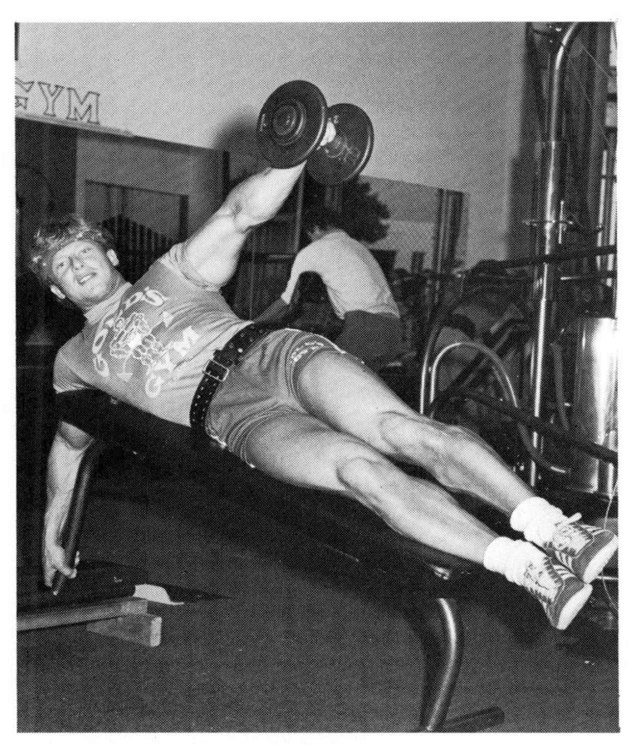

Side Incline Lateral.

dumbbells in semicircles directly upward to the sides until they are at shoulder level. Hold this top position for a moment and then lower them back to the starting point. Repeat the movement for the required number of repetitions.

Training Tips: In the same position you can also do Front Raises with the dumbbells, raising them either alternately or together.

Side Incline Lateral

General Comments: Virtually every superstar bodybuilder we have known has done this particular movement at one time or another to bulk and striate the medial heads of the delts.

Starting Position: It's easiest to do this movement on an abdominal board, but you can also do it while lying on a low incline bench. Grasp a light dumbbell in your left hand and lie on your right side on the board or bench. Bend your left arm slightly and keep it bent like this throughout the movement. With your palm down, rest the dumbbell on the board right next to your hip.

Exercise Performance: From this basic starting position, slowly raise the dumbbell in a semicircle directly out to the side until your arm is perpendicular to the floor. Lower the weight back to the starting point and repeat the movement. Be sure to do an equal amount of work for each arm.

Training Tips: You can also begin the movement with the dumbbell resting behind your back rather than in front of your hips.

Arm Exercises

Seated Dumbbell Curl

General Comments: By isolating your legs from this movement you can more strongly stress your biceps muscles doing Dumbbell Curls. And, as on all types of Dumbbell Curls, you can fully supinate your hands as you do the exercise.

Seated Dumbbell Curl.

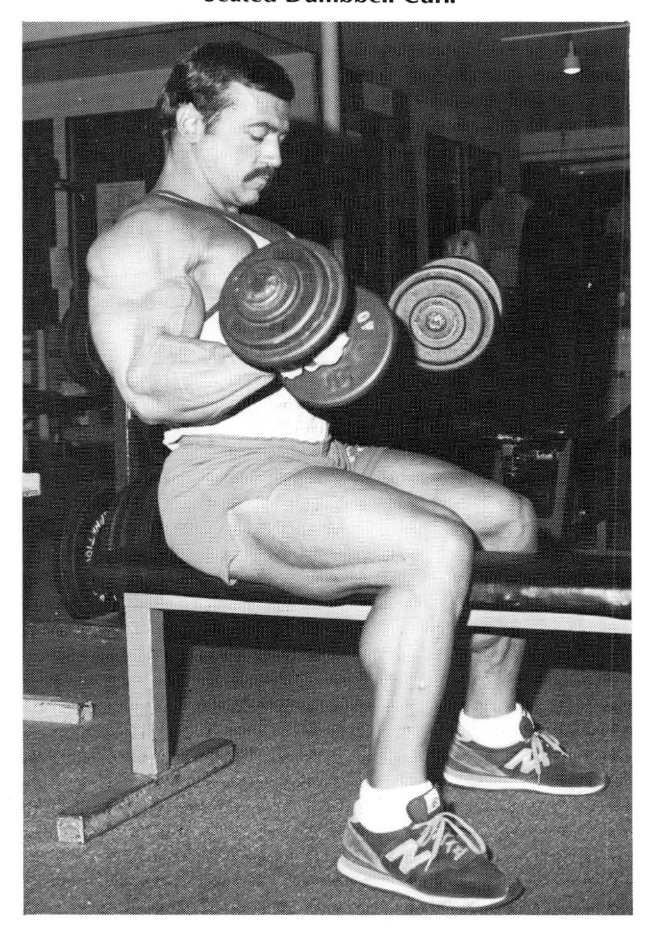

Starting Position: Grasp two moderately heavy dumbbells and sit at the end of a flat exercise bench with your feet planted firmly on the floor. Hang your arms directly down at your sides with your palms facing each other, and anchor your upper arms to the sides of your torso throughout the movement. Sit erect.

Exercise Performance: Slowly curl the dumbbells up to your shoulders, rotating your wrists so your palms are up at the conclusion of the movement. Return the dumbbells back to the starting point and repeat the movement for the required number of repetitions.

Training Tips: In addition to curling the dumbbells simultaneously, you can also curl them alternately while seated.

Barbell Concentration Curl

General Comments: All types of Concentration Curls accentuate biceps peak. Barbell Concentration Curls are especially good for achieving this.

Starting Position: Take a narrow grip on a barbell as if you planned to do a Barbell Curl with it. There should be no more than four or five inches between your hands as you grip the bar. Bend over at the waist until your torso is parallel to the floor. Hang your arms directly

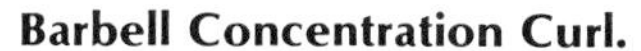

Barbell Concentration Curl.

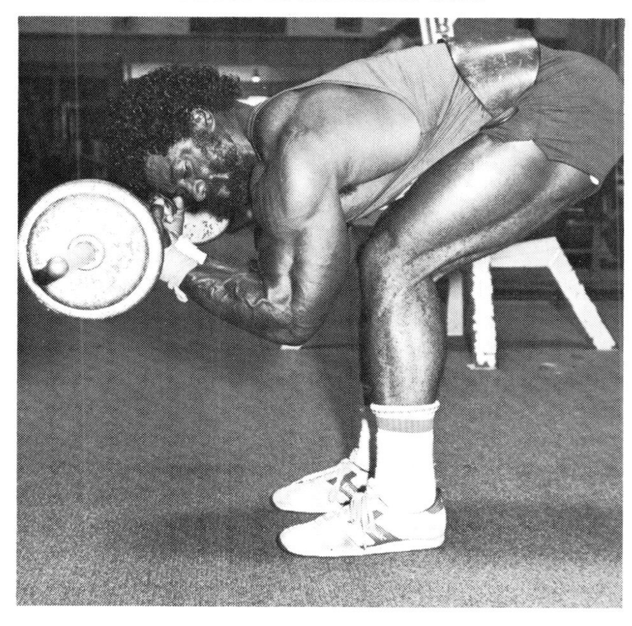

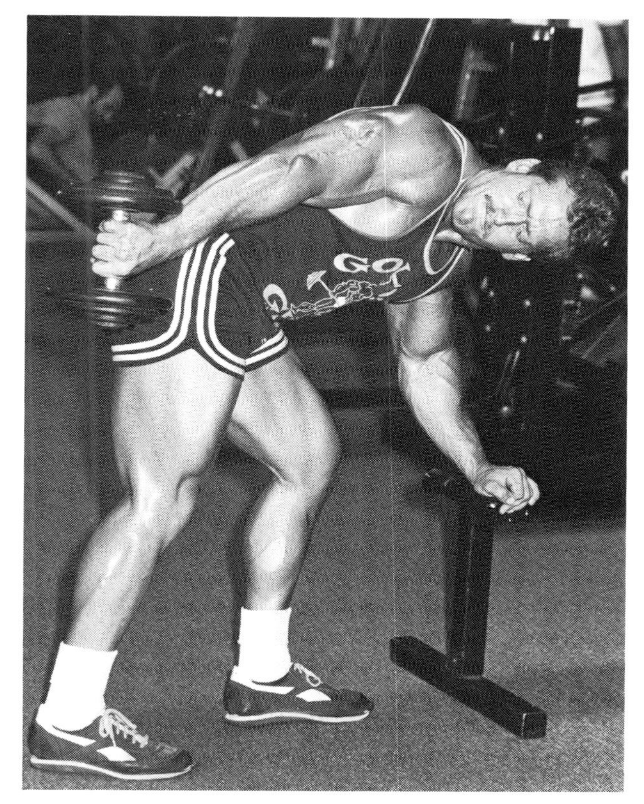

Dumbbell Kickback.

downward from your shoulder joints and keep your upper arms in this position throughout the movement.

Exercise Performance: From this basic starting position, slowly bend your arms and curl the barbell upward until it touches your upper chest. Return the weight to the starting point and repeat the movement.

Training Tips: If the barbell plates touch the floor before your arms reach full extension, you will have to stand on a high block of wood as you do this movement. You will also find this a very effective position in which to do Reverse Curls.

Dumbbell Kickback

General Comments: The best way to exert a very strong peak contraction effect on your triceps muscles is to do Dumbbell Kickbacks.

Starting Position: Grasp a light dumbbell in your left hand and bend over at the waist until your torso is parallel to the floor, using your

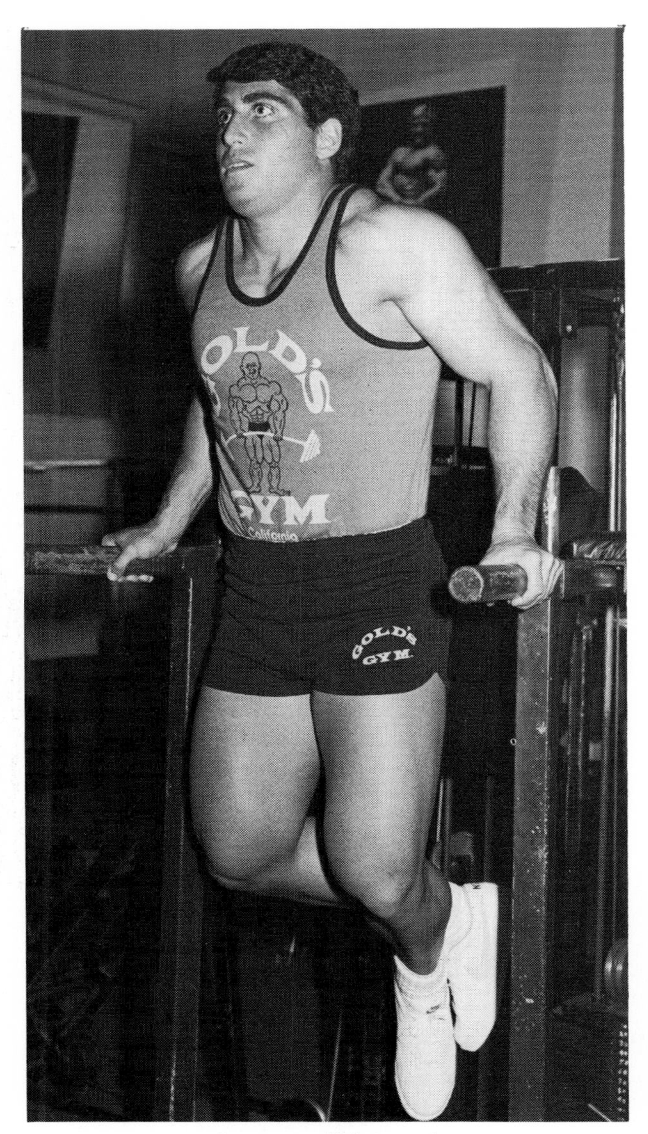

Triceps Parallel Bar Dip.

right hand, placed on a flat exercise bench, to support your torso in this position. Pin your left upper arm to your torso so it is also parallel to the floor. Allow your left forearm to hang down from your elbow so that it is perpendicular to the floor.

Exercise Performance: From this basic starting position, simply straighten your left arm. Hold this contracted position for a couple of seconds and lower the dumbbell back to the starting position. Repeat the movement for the required number of repetitions. Be sure to do an equal number of sets and reps for each arm.

Training Tips: This movement is occasionally done with two dumbbells simultaneously. It is also occasionally done with a single floor pulley.

Triceps Parallel Bar Dip

General Comments: This movement is very similar to doing Parallel Bar Dips for pectoral development, except that you must do the Dips with your torso held as upright as possible. When you do Parallel Bar Dips in this manner, you will very strongly stress your triceps. One well-known Gold's bodybuilder who does this movement is Mike Mentzer.

Standing Barbell Wrist Curl

General Comments: This movement was a favorite of Bob Birdsong (Mr. America and Mr. Universe) when he trained at Gold's Gym. It's a superb exercise for stimulating the powerful flexor muscles of the forearms under peak contraction.

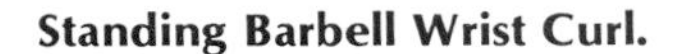

Standing Barbell Wrist Curl.

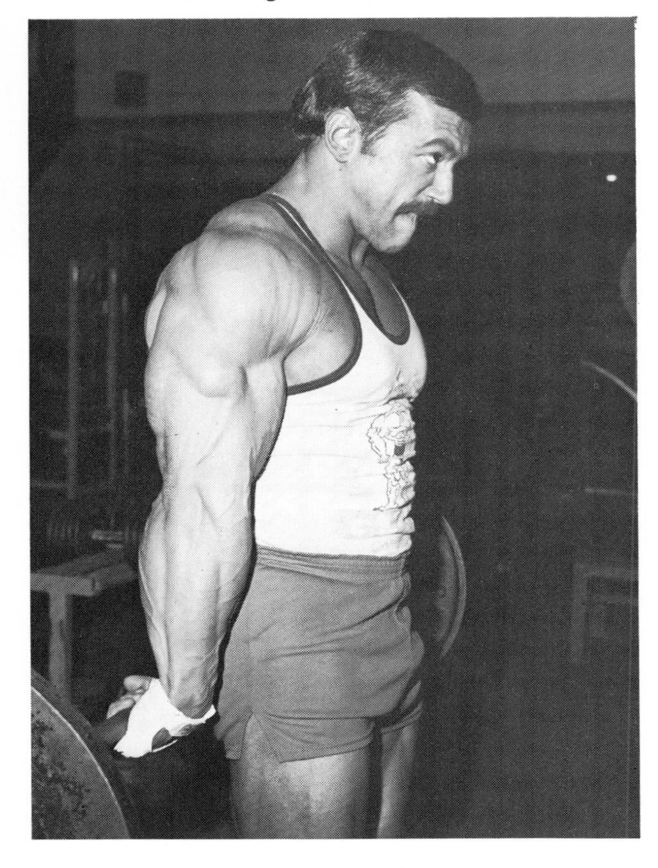

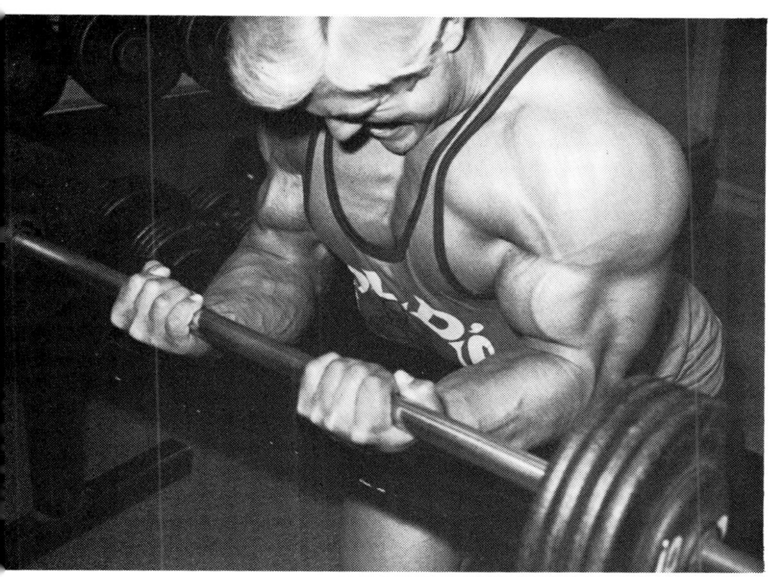

Cross-Bench Wrist Curl—palms up, left; palms down, right.

Starting Position: Place a moderately heavy barbell on the rack of a bench press bench. Back up to it and take a grip on it a little wider on each side than shoulder width. As you do this, it's important that your palms face toward the rear. Lift the barbell off the rack and step away from the rack a bit. Then hang your arms directly downward and keep them straight throughout the movement. The barbell will be resting across the backs of your thighs in this position.

Exercise Performance: From this position, simply flex your wrists to curl the barbell upward in a small semicircle to the highest possible position. Lower it back to the starting point and repeat the movement for the desired number of repetitions.

Training Tips: You can do a somewhat similar movement with two dumbbells. Simply hang them down at your sides with your palms facing inward. Then, from that position, slowly curl the dumbbells upward simultaneously in small semicircles.

Cross-Bench Wrist Curl

General Comments: This very strict movement can be done with the palms facing either upward or downward to stress the muscles of the forearms strongly.

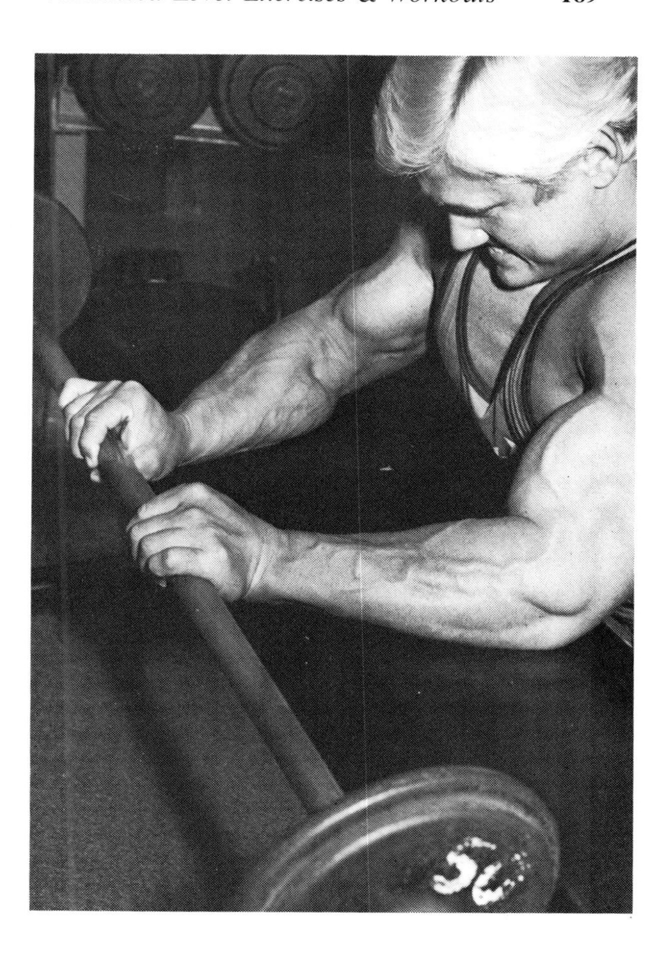

Starting Position: We'll describe the palms-up version here, and you can simply change your grip to do the other type of Wrist Curl. Take a shoulder-width grip on a barbell with your palms up. Kneel on one side of a flat exercise bench and run your forearms across the bench so that your wrists hang off one edge. Sag your fists downward as far as possible.

Exercise Performance: From this starting position, simply curl the barbell upward in a small semicircle to as high a position as possible. Lower the weight back to the starting point and repeat the movement for the required number of repetitions.

Training Tips: You can also do this movement with two dumbbells simultaneously or with one dumbbell at a time.

Calf Exercises

Jumping Squat

General Comments: The calf muscles are

stressed very strongly whenever you jump off the floor. So it stands to reason that jumping with weights held either in your hands or across your shoulders will build up your calf muscles.

Starting Position: Place a barbell across your shoulders as if preparing for a Squat. Alternatively, you can hold two moderately heavy dumbbells in your hands with your arms hanging down at your sides. Set your feet approximately shoulder width apart, your toes angled slightly outward.

Exercise Performance: Slowly squat to a point three or four inches above the position at which your thighs would be parallel to the floor. Then rise forcefully, actually jumping as high into the air as possible. Land on the floor and immediately begin to do another repetition. While you are doing Jumping Squats, be sure that you keep your torso as perfectly erect as possible.

Training Tips: This movement is a very good aerobic conditioning exercise when done in sets of 20–25 reps. You will also find it a good movement for slicing your thigh muscles to ribbons.

Nautilus Calf Raise

General Comments: You can use a Nautilus Omni machine and the waist belt that comes with it to exercise your calf muscles very effectively. This movement is very similar to a Donkey Calf Raise, but you won't need a heavy training partner to help you do the movement.

Starting Position: Set the weight stack pin so that you will be using a substantial poundage in this movement. Step into the waist belt and place it comfortably around your hips. Don't allow it to rest too high on your waist, since that belt position can be relatively painful with heavy weights. Fasten the ring on the belt to the end of the movement arm of the machine. There is a relatively simple type of clip with which you can do this. Stand erect with the weight and place first one foot and then the other on the step of the machine. Your feet should be set at about shoulder width, and your toes should be pointed directly forward.

Exercise Performance: Keeping your legs straight, sag your heels as far below the level of your toes as possible. Then rise up on your toes as high as you can. Repeat this movement for the required number of repetitions.

Training Tips: As with all calf exercises, be sure to do this with your toes pointed outward, inward, and straight ahead. Fairly strong bodybuilders will very soon be able to use more than the weight stack on the Omni machine. In such a case, you can add weight to the stack with special, long, locking pins.

Hack Machine Calf Raise

General Comments: This is another very effective calf movement that will add variety to your training routines.

Starting Position: Lie face down on a hack machine and grasp the handles at the lower part of the machine's sliding platform. Straighten your legs fully and place your toes and the balls of your feet on the edge of the platform at the bottom of the machine.

Exercise Performance: Sag your heels as far below the level of your toes as you can and then

Hack Machine Calf Raise done facedown.

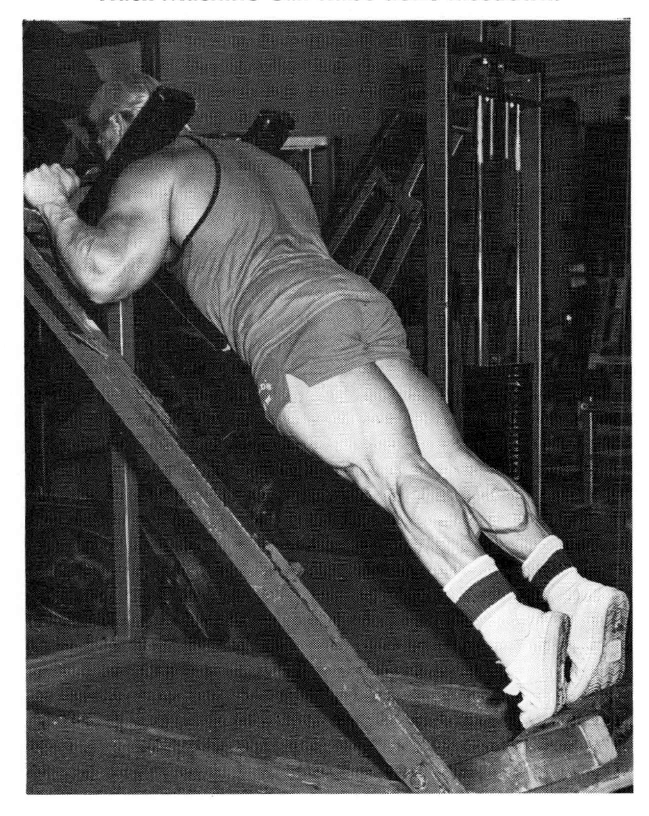

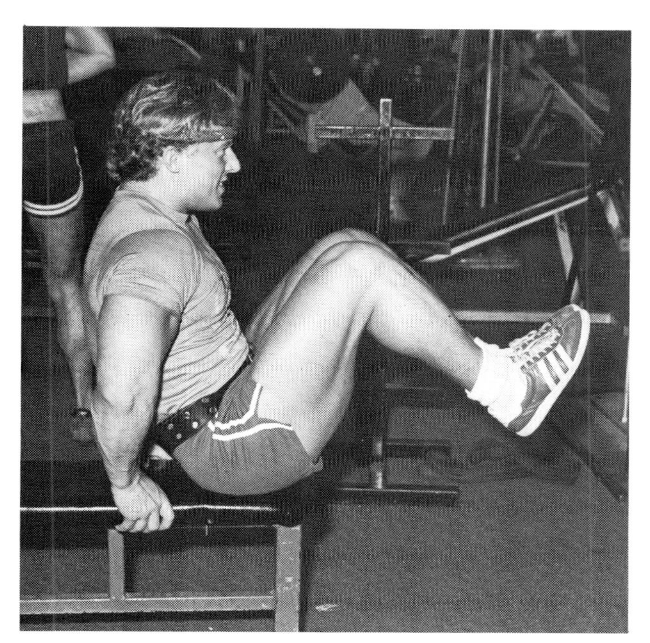

Knee-up.

rise up as high as possible on your toes. Repeat the movement for the appropriate number of repetitions.

Training Tips: In addition to varying the angle of your toes, try varying the space between your feet on the platform from time to time.

Abdominal Exercises

Knee-up

General Comments: This is a relatively low-intensity abdominal exercise that stresses primarily the lower abs. You'll need to do a lot of reps on it, but you'll find that Knee-Ups do a very good job of tightening your lower abs.

Starting Position: Sit at the end of a flat exercise bench and incline your torso backward to form a 45-degree angle with the floor. Brace your torso in this position throughout the movement by grasping the sides of the bench. Extend your legs forward so they make one long straight line with your upper body. Your feet should be just clear of the floor.

Exercise Performance: From this basic starting position, simultaneously bend your legs and pull your knees up to touch your chest. Lower back to the starting point and repeat the movement for the desired number of repetitions.

Training Tips: To hit your intercostals in addition to your front abdominals, you can twist your legs as you raise and lower them. Just be certain to twist alternately from side to side.

Bent-Over Twisting

General Comments: There's considerable debate among top bodybuilders about whether or

Bent-Over Twisting.

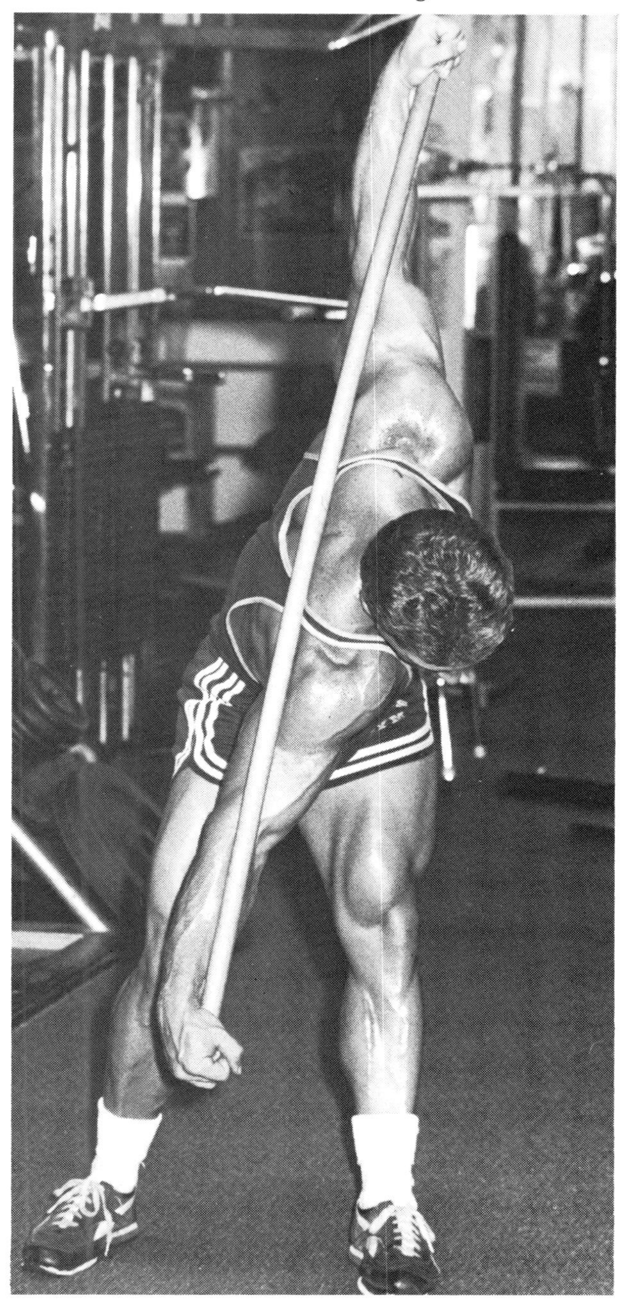

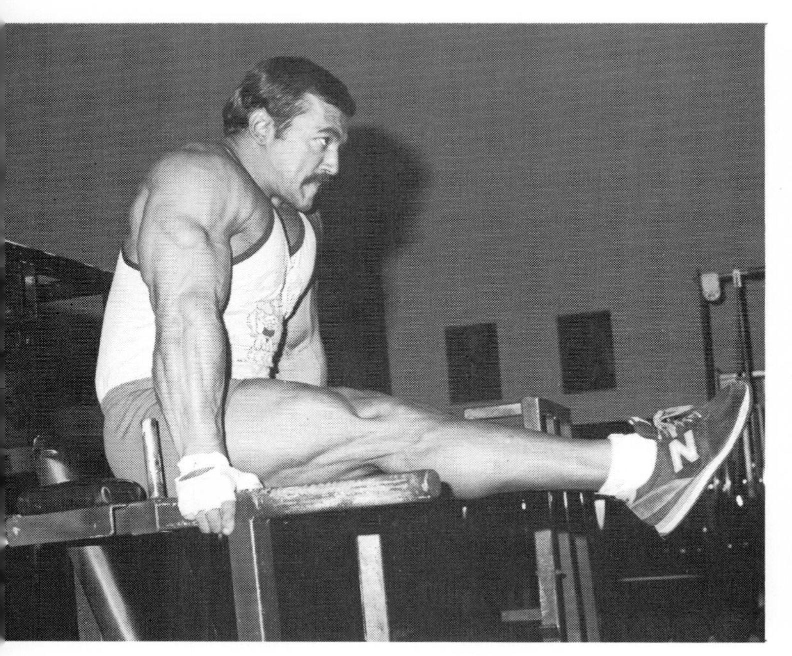

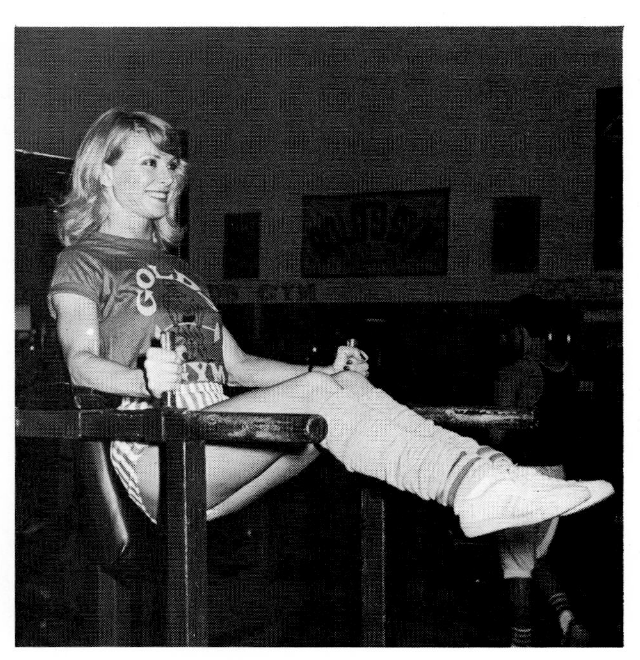

Parallel Bar Leg Raise—straight-leg finish, left; bent-leg finish, right.

not this exercise really does anything valuable, but we will present it nonetheless. Those who advocate this movement claim that it firms loose flesh on the lower back and the sides of the waist.

Starting Position: Place a broomstick or an unloaded bar across the back of your neck and wrap your arms around it. Place your feet on the floor a little wider than shoulder width. Bend over at the waist until your torso is parallel to the floor.

Exercise Performance: From this position, twist vigorously from side to side. From the front, it will look like your broomstick is a propeller on an airplane.

Training Tips: For slightly different effects on the muscles being exercised, you can bend over a little less when you do the movement.

Parallel Bar Leg Raise

General Comments: This exercise is a takeoff on a movement that gymnasts do on parallel bars. It's a very good exercise for the entire front abdominal wall, particularly for the lower abdominals.

Starting Position: Jump up on a pair of parallel bars and support yourself as if preparing to do Parallel Bar Dips. The only exception to this starting position is that you should be facing away from the wall and your legs should be pressed together and bent slightly. Keep your legs bent slightly throughout the movement.

Exercise Performance: Keeping your torso erect, slowly raise your feet in semicircles until your legs are parallel to the floor. Lower your legs back to the starting point and repeat the movement for an appropriate number of repetitions.

Training Tips: If you find this exercise difficult to do, you can bend your legs a little more. And once the movement becomes easy to do you can either hold a light dumbbell between your feet or wear a pair of iron boots.

Advanced-Level Workouts

You probably are already devising your own workouts by now, but we will present final off-season and precontest programs that you can use as examples in making up your own training routines.

OFF-SEASON WORKOUT

Monday–Thursday

Exercise	Sets	Reps
1. Parallel Bar Leg Raise	2–3	15–20
2. Incline Sit-Up	2–3	20–30
3. Bent-Over Twisting	2–3	50
4. Incline Barbell Press	5	10–4
5. Parallel Bar Dip	4	12–6
6. Flat-Bench Flye	4	6–8
7. Chin behind the Neck	5	10–12
8. Seated Pulley Rowing	4	12–6
9. Front Lat Pulldown	4	6–8
10. Barbell Reverse Curl	4	6–8
11. Cross-Bench Wrist Curl	4	10–12
12. Seated Calf Machine (Toe Raise)	4	8–10
13. Hack Machine Calf Raise	3	10–12
14. Calf Press	3	12–15

Tuesday–Friday

Exercise	Sets	Reps
1. Hanging Leg Raise	2–3	15–20
2. Roman Chair Sit-Up	2–3	50
3. Side Bend	2–3	50
4. Seated Press behind the Neck	5	10–6
5. Cable Side Lateral	3	6–8
6. Seated Bent Lateral	4	6–8
7. Seated Dumbbell Curl	4	6–8
8. Barbell Preacher Curl	4	6–8
9. Parallel Bar Dip	4	6–8
10. Incline Triceps Extension	4	6–8
11. Standing Barbell Wrist Curl	4–5	8–12
12. Reverse Wrist Curl	4–5	8–12
13. Nautilus Calf Raise	4–5	10–12
14. Standing Calf Machine (Toe Raise)	4–5	12–15

Wednesday–Saturday

Exercise	Sets	Reps
1. Bench Leg Raise	2–3	20–30
2. Crunch	2–3	25–50
3. Knee-Up	2–3	50
4. Leg Extension	4	10–12
5. Squat	5	15–6
6. Front Squat	4	10–6
7. Leg Curl	5	8–10
8. Stiff-Leg Deadlift	3	10–15
9. Jumping Squat	4	10–15
10. Cross-Bench Dumbbell Wrist Curl	5	10–12
11. Reverse Wrist Curl	5	10–12

PRECONTEST WORKOUT

Monday-Wednesday-Friday (A.M.)

	Exercise	Sets	Reps
1.	Hanging Leg Raise	3-5	15-20
2.	Incline Sit-Up	3-5	20-30
3.	Incline Dumbbell Press	4	10-12
4.	Pec Deck Flye	4	10-12
5.	Decline Flye	4	10-12
6.	Cable Crossover	4	10-12
7.	Cross-Bench Pullover	4	10-12
8.	Front Lat Pulldown	4	10-12
9.	Lat Pulldown behind the Neck	4	10-12
10.	Seated Pulley Rowing	4	10-12
11.	One-Arm Dumbbell Rowing	4	10-12
12.	Seated Dumbbell Press	4	10-12
13.	Cable Side Lateral	4	10-12
14.	Cable Bent Lateral	4	10-12
15.	Upright Rowing	4	10-12

Monday-Wednesday-Friday (P.M.)

	Exercise	Sets	Reps
1.	Seated Calf Machine (Toe Raise)	4-5	10-15
2.	Nautilus Calf Machine (Toe Raise)	4-5	10-15
3.	Calf Press	4-5	10-15
4.	Barbell Reverse Curl	4-5	8-10
5.	Standing Barbell Wrist Curl	4-5	10-15
6.	Cross-Bench Reverse Wrist Curl	4-5	10-15
7.	Seated Twisting	3-5	100
8.	Incline Leg Raise	3-5	20-30
9.	Roman Chair Sit-Up	3-5	50-100
10.	Knee-Up	3-5	50-100

Tuesday-Thursday-Saturday (A.M.)

	Exercise	Sets	Reps
1.	Hanging Leg Raise	3-5	15-20
2.	Incline Sit-Up	3-5	20-30
3.	Pulley Pushdown	4	10-12
4.	Incline Triceps Extension	4	10-12
5.	Dumbbell Kickback	4	10-12
6.	Dumbbell Preacher Curl	4	10-12
7.	Seated Alternate Dumbell Curl	4	10-12
8.	Barbell Concentration Curl	4	10-12
9.	Hack Machine Squat	4	10-15
10.	Leg Extension	4	10-15
11.	Lunge	4	10-15
12.	Sissy Squat	4	10-15
13.	Leg Curl	4	10-12
14.	Hyperextension	4	10-15

Tuesday-Thursday-Saturday (P.M.)

Repeat the Monday-Wednesday-Friday (P.M.). workout.

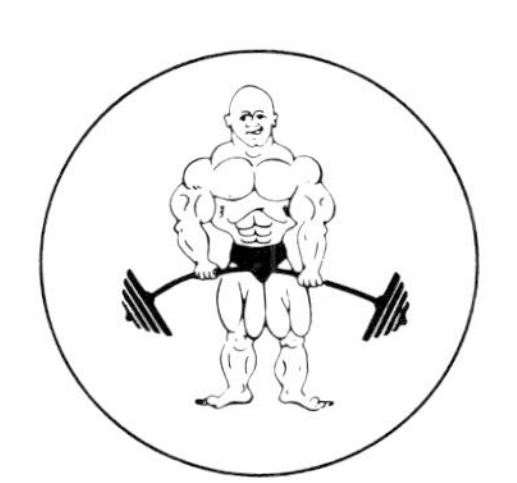

8 PRO TRAINING TIPS

If you have been following the advice in this book, in the order in which it is presented, you should have developed a fairly muscular physique and a good degree of strength by now. In fact, you may already have entered a bodybuilding competition or two and done fairly well. With a few more months of steady training—adding to your workouts some of the pro training techniques presented in this chapter—you should become a winner very soon!

The advice presented in this chapter is quite advanced, and no male or female bodybuilder with less than 1½–2 full years of steady training under his or her belt should expect to profit from these pro training methods. Inexperienced bodybuilders would quickly overtrain using any of the training tips presented in this chapter.

Many of the training methods we will discuss here won't work well for even an Olympian-level bodybuilder. As you are well aware, every body reacts differently to various training and nutritional stimuli. Review the discussion of training instinct at the beginning of Chapter 6 and use your own instincts to determine which of these pro-level training techniques will work well for you. Then systematically give each method a trial, rejecting those that are unproductive and including those that are most helpful in your overall training philosophy.

Augmenting Energy

Unless you subscribe to Mike Mentzer's heavy-duty system, as discussed in Chapter 6, your workouts will gradually grow longer as you progress from rank beginner to this advanced level of training. It's not unusual for champion bodybuilders to train 3–4 hours per day and six days per week. However, at Gold's Gym the average champion trains about two hours per day.

When doing such long workouts, physical endurance—or, more specifically, the ability to sustain a high energy level for two hours or more of training—becomes crucial. As you have progressed in your training, your body has gradually increased the energy reserves upon which you can draw during a workout. Still, there are three effective ways to increase your training energy even further.

The first of these is to follow the correct procedure for full body recuperation between workouts. You simply must get sufficient sleep every night, which will probably, at times, in-

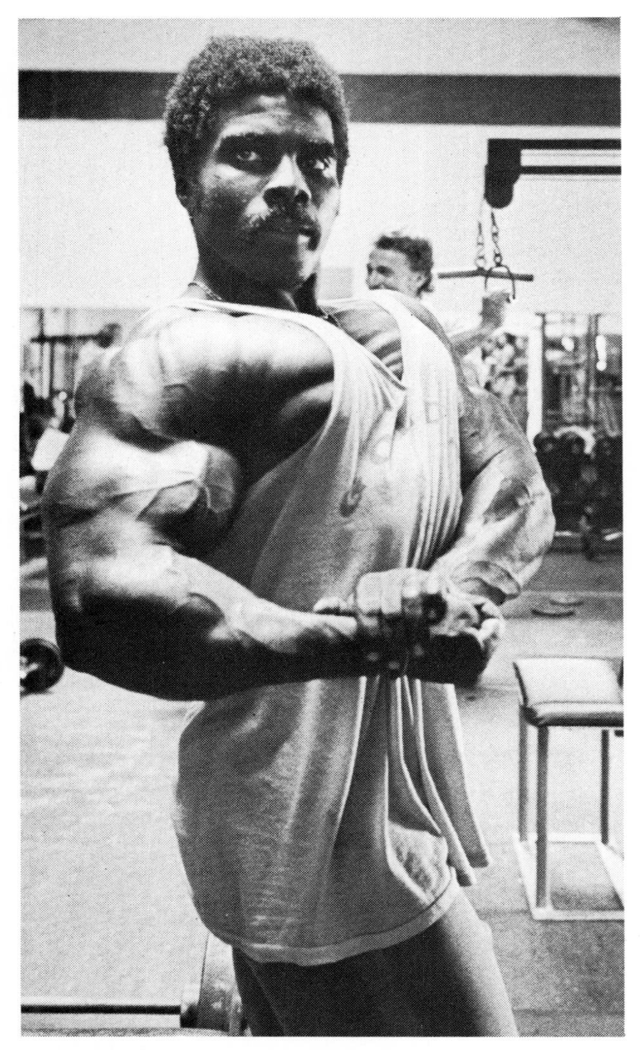

Robby Robinson displays the penultimate chest, arm, and shoulder development of a true superstar.
(Photo by Jack Neary)

volve sacrificing your social life. And it's essential that you avoid all possible stress in your bodybuilding lifestyle. Being constantly nervous and uptight can cause a tremendous mental energy drain, which in turn results in an incomplete physical recuperation between workouts.

Second, the maintenance of relatively low levels of body fat throughout the year will give you greater training energy than if you allow yourself to become overbulked between competitions. Body fat overloads every organ system of your body and greatly saps your energy reserves. As a general rule, male bodybuilders should never allow themselves to gain more than 8–10 pounds over their competition weight and female bodybuilders should remain within 4–6 pounds of their competitive weight.

The final energy augmentation technique involves food supplementation. Most top bodybuilders believe that consuming dessicated liver tablets increases training energy. They take at least 30 per day, and some champion bodybuilders have swallowed more than 250 dessicated liver tablets each day just prior to competition. Vitamin E (at least 400 IU per day) will also help improve endurance.

All women bodybuilders should take a chelated iron supplement, particularly while menstruating. Many women are iron-deficient, which results in poor oxygen transfer through the red blood cells in the vascular system. Hence, an iron supplement will improve the red blood cell count and augment energy by insuring efficient oxygen transfer from the lungs to the working muscles.

A few misguided bodybuilders have taken amphetamines to increase training energy, particularly before a competition. We condemn this practice. Amphetamines are highly addictive, they eat up hard-earned muscle tissue, and athletes have actually killed themselves while on amphetamines by pushing their bodies past the point of normal fatigue. The "speed freaks" always look stringy, emaciated, and ill onstage at a competition, and they're invariably beaten by healthy, well-muscled competitors.

Stretch Marks

If the muscle or fat tissue of the body expands in volume too quickly, it will stretch your skin to the point at which it tears. This results in reddish lines in the skin, which eventually turn to the color of scar tissue. Many champion bodybuilders have these stretch marks, particularly in the area where the pectorals tie in with the deltoids. A couple of the greatest male bodybuilding champions even have stretch marks on their forearms.

Women bodybuilders are not prone to incurring stretch marks from bodybuilding training. Most women, however, become familiar with stretch marks much earlier than do men. Women tend to get stretch marks around their hips and breasts during puberty. And many women who have had children have developed stretch marks on their stomachs from the rapid expansion experienced during pregnancy.

Stretch marks can be prevented or lessened in severity in two ways. First, never bulk up excessively by adding superfluous fat to your body. By slowly gaining weight—being sure that it is virtually all pure muscle tissue—you can avoid stretching your skin excessively. When you gain muscle mass at a normal rate your skin is naturally elastic enough to accommodate such growth without tearing.

If you begin to notice stretch marks on your skin you can minimize their severity by rubbing skin lotion containing vitamin E over and around the area where your skin is tearing. Vitamin E has great healing properties and can retard the spread of stretch marks.

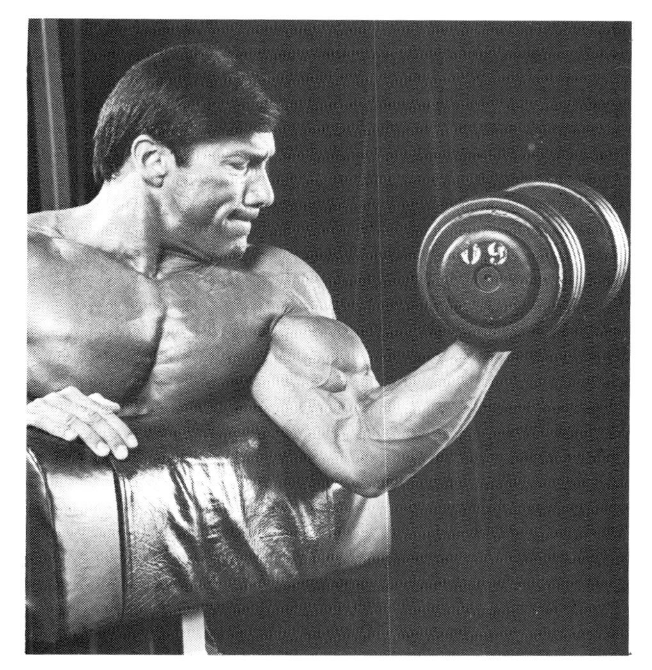

Boyer Coe: "What can be conceived and believed can be achieved. *(Photo by Mike Neveux)*

Visualization

Virtually all of the superstar bodybuilders at Gold's Gym use the mental technique called *visualization* to their advantage. This method allows bodybuilders to program the subconscious mind to assist them in reaching their training goals.

Visualization takes advantage of a psychological construct called *self-actualization.* Through self-actualization an individual's subconscious mind automatically makes decisions to allow something in which he firmly believes to come about, or to be actualized.

As an example, an obese man or woman visualizes his or her body being slim and muscular. Once the person has become convinced that this is what he or she will look like, the subconscious makes it easy to diet and exercise regularly. As a result, the overweight person quickly loses body fat and soon actualizes the visualized image.

Boyer Coe crystallized the visualization technique when he said, "What can be conceived and believed can be achieved." In essence, being able to conjure up a realistic image of what his body will soon look like, then constructively daydreaming about this image, Coe has been able to keep improving yearly for nearly 20 years. And the proof of the validity of this technique is in Boyer's competitive record. He has won 14 World Bodybuilding Championships.

Two other members or former members of Gold's Gym who have used visualization quite effectively are massive Tom Platz (Mr. Universe) and esthetically developed Frank Zane (Mr. Olympia 1977–78–79). Both of these great champions have spent many hours in developing realistically visualized images of themselves being in superb condition and winning big titles.

Most successful women bodybuilders also use this mental programming technique. Of those women who have trained at Gold's Gym, Rachel McLish (Ms. Olympia), Laura Combes (Ms. America), Deborah Diana (U.S. Champion), and Lisa Elliott (Ms. Eastern America) have used visualization very successfully.

The best time to practice visualization is while lying in bed before falling asleep each night. Then you can be assured of having 10–15 totally quiet minutes that are free from external distractions in which you can practice this technique. Or you can practice visualization at any other time during the day when you can be assured of peace and quiet (e.g., when sunbathing).

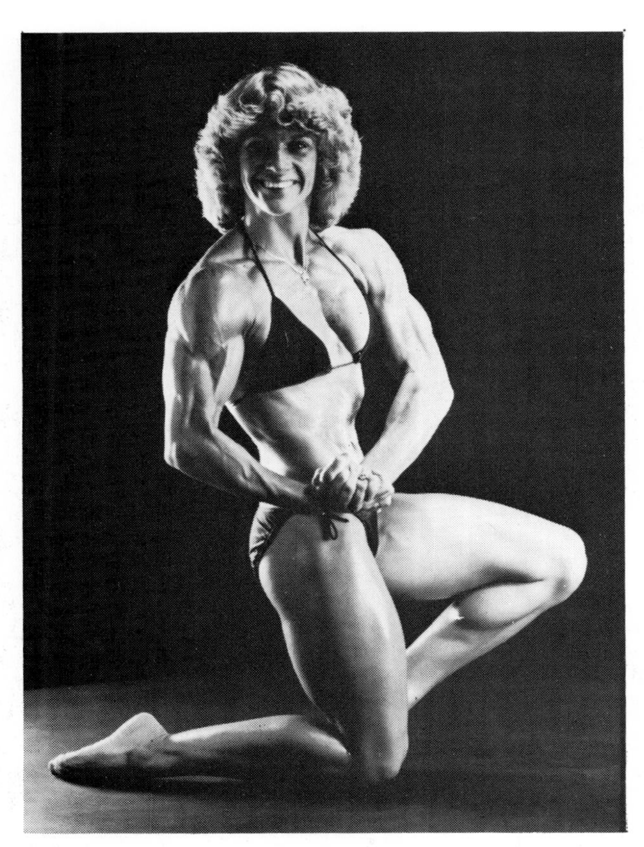

Lisa Elliot has successfully visualized winning contests.

For best results, you should practice visualization on a daily basis for at least 10 minutes at each session. Close to a competition, you can even practice this technique two or three times per day. For the last 4–6 weeks before competing, many elite bodybuilders spend an hour or more per day in performing such psychological contest preparations.

Your visualized image of yourself should be both realistically achievable and vividly imagined. Based on your progress in past months and years, develop an image of what you can realistically expect to achieve with six months or a year of dedicated training and dieting.

Then develop a vivid picture of this new self-image, complete in every detail. See each muscle contour and every semblance of vascularity. Actually *feel* yourself training with newly developed power and endurance. Relish the more massive and sharply delineated muscles you will have onstage at your next contest.

You should even develop an image of the contest itself, right down to the smell of body oil on yourself and other contestants. Enjoy going through your posing routine with your new body and revel in the audience's enthusiastic response to your efforts. And, above all else, visualize yourself triumphantly receiving the winner's trophy.

Faithful use of visualization will allow you to reach heretofore impossible heights of physical power and muscular development. It can also help you achieve excellence in other areas of your life (e.g., in school studies or personal relationships). Visualization will make your mind the most powerful weapon in your arsenal of bodybuilding techniques.

Trisets

Trisetting (or doing three exercises for a muscle group in quick succession with little or no rest between them) is an advanced technique that adds greatly to the intensity of your workout. Trisets are occasionally used on a stubborn body part during the off-season, but more frequently they are used during a precontest training cycle to intensify the workout you give any muscle group.

Trisets are best used with large muscle groups such as the thighs, back and chest or with three-faceted muscles like the deltoids (with anterior, medial, and posterior heads). Here is an example of a good triset for the thighs.

1. Leg Extension
2. Leg Press
3. Leg Curl

Done in quick succession, these three exercises will intensely stress every muscle group of the thighs, both anterior and posterior.

Considering trisets for three-faceted muscle complexes, here is one for the deltoids.

1. Side Lateral (medial head)
2. Press Behind the Neck (anterior head)
3. Bent Lateral (posterior head)

You will find that two or three of these trisets will give you an excellent shoulder workout. If you diligently used forced reps, as discussed in Chapter 6, you can actually stimulate your deltoids to the limit with only one of these trisets. Gold's members Mike Mentzer, Ray Mentzer, Casey Viator, and Rachel McLish train in this manner, and all four have won high-level bodybuilding championships.

On a continuum of bodybuilding training intensity, trisets are more intense than supersets but less intense than giant sets.

Giant Sets

Giant sets are series of 4–6 movements done with no rest between them to stimulate a single muscle group or two antagonistic muscle groups (e.g., the pecs and lats or biceps and triceps) at once. Giant sets are extremely intense, and few bodybuilders use them at any other time than during the last two or three weeks before competing.

A number of superstars (Lou Ferrigno is chief among them) never do giant sets, because the technique burns too much fat and muscle tissue, even for precontest training. Others rely on giant sets to add the final iota of muscle hardness and detail needed to win a big title. The legendary Robby Robinson (Mr. America, Mr. World, Mr. Universe, and one of the most successful pro bodybuilders of all time) uses giant sets for this purpose.

The least intense form of giant sets is a grouping of four exercises. Here is an example of such a giant set for the back muscles.

1. Hyperextension (erector spinae muscles)
2. Seated Pulley Rowing (latissimus dorsi thickness)
3. Barbell Shrug (trapezius)
4. Lat Pulldown (latissimus dorsi width)

And here is a giant set of four exercises for the biceps and triceps.

1. Barbell Preacher Curl
2. Pulley Pushdown
3. Seated Dumbbell Curl
4. Parallel Bar Dip (torso held erect)

For very large and complex muscle groups you can do a giant set consisting of five exercises. Here is an example of such a giant set for the back muscles.

1. Stiff-Leg Deadlift (erector spinae)
2. Chin (lat width)
3. Bent Lateral (upper back muscularity)
4. Dumbbell Bent Rowing (lat thickness)
5. Machine Shrug (trapezius)

Six-exercise giant sets are usually used for larger antagonistic muscle groups. This pecs/lats giant set is typical of that type.

1. Bench Press
2. Chins
3. Incline Flye
4. Seated Pulley Rowing
5. Parallel Bar Dip
6. Bent-Arm Pullover

Ultimately, you can use six-exercise giant sets to carve maximum muscular detail into a single large and complex body part. Here is an example of such a six-exercise giant set done for complete chest development.

1. Incline Dumbbell Press (upper pectoral mass)
2. Decline Flye (lower pectoral detail)
3. Cross-Bench Pullover (rib cage expansion)
4. Flat-Bench Flye (general pectoral shape)
5. Cable Crossover (inner pec mass, overall detail)
6. Parallel Bar Dip (lower pectoral mass and shape)

Again, giant sets are drastically harder than trisets. Among the various forms of giant sets, a four-exercise configuration is less intense than one with five exercises, and a five-exercise configuration is less intense than one with six exercises. Within each configuration, giant sets done for antagonistic muscle groups are less intense than those done for a single body part.

Staggered Sets

Generally speaking, bodybuilders must do a large number of sets (10–20 total) in calf and abdominal training each day, particularly just prior to a competition. And many bodybuilders find such calf and abdominal training boring. The answer to their problem is a training technique called *staggered sets.*

At Gold's Gym we dispense with the boredom of doing 20 sets of calf or abdominal exercises by interspersing a set of calf or ab work between each two or three sets done for another major body part. Since it doesn't take much time or energy to do an intense set of calf or waist movements, you can easily do this. And over the course of a 1½–2-hour workout, you can do 20 sets of calf exercises without even noticing that you've done it.

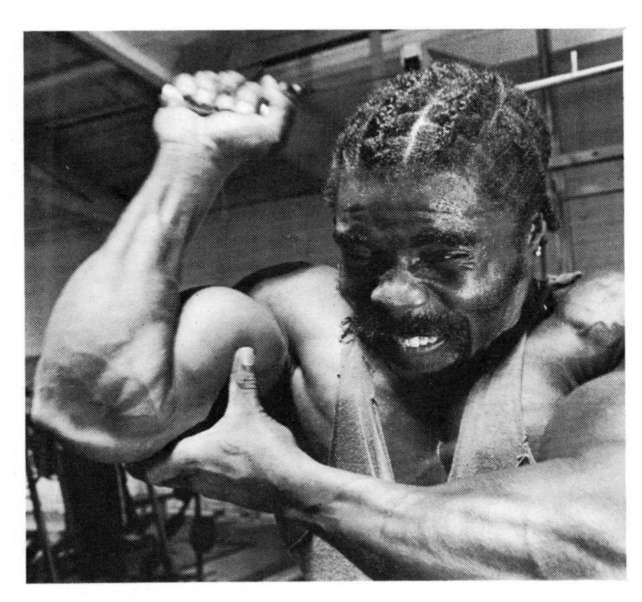

High-intensity training in action. Robby Robinson dramatically demonstrates how to build triceps mass, shape, and density!

As an example of how to do staggered sets, let's say that you want to do 15 sets of abdominal exercises during the following major chest and back workout:

Chest

1. Bench Press: 4 × 6–8
2. Incline Flye: 4 × 8–10
3. Parallel Bar Dip: 4 × 8–10
4. Pec Deck Flye: 4 × 8–10

Back

1. Chin: 4 × 10–12
2. Seated Pulley Rowing: 4 × 8–10
3. Lat Pulldowns: 4 × 8–10
4. Dumbbell Bent Rowing: 4 × 8–10

In this case you would do two sets of Bench Presses, then a set of Incline Sit-ups, or whatever other abdominal movement you intend to do. Next, you'd do two more sets of Bench Presses and another set of Incline Sit-ups. Continue like this, doing one intense set of abdominal exercises for every two sets of chest or back exercises, and you will be using staggered sets quite effectively.

Continuous Tension

One training technique that the champs rely on to produce the ultimate in muscular detail at contest time is continuous tension. When using this technique, you will move a weight slowly over the full range of motion of an exercise. Many bodybuilders also build added tension into such a movement by flexing the muscle group opposing the one they are training (e.g., the triceps when doing a Barbell Curl).

When you do an exercise with a quick movement, momentum robs a working muscle of much of its intended resistance. So, when you slow a movement down, you stress the muscle much more heavily. And as a result, you work the muscle harder and receive a better quality of muscular development when you use continuous tension.

The greatest exponent of continuous tension training who has worked out at Gold's Gym was Robby Robinson. Robby was able to make a set of Barbell Curls with 70 pounds feel as intense as a set done with a 150-pound barbell. And his 20-inch upper arm development featured incredibly peaked and ripped biceps!

Peak Contraction

The closer any muscle comes to being fully contracted, the larger the number of muscle cells that are contracted and the stronger a muscle is. It makes good sense, then, for you to keep the full amount of resistance on the muscle when it is fully contracted. Only when you do have weight on a contracted muscle will you be able to build a maximum degree of muscle mass and quality.

Unfortunately, however, at the completion point of many exercises no weight is on the working muscles. As an example, your biceps muscles are fully contracted in a Barbell Curl only when your arms are completely bent. And then the barbell is supported on your forearms, *not* pulling against the contracted biceps muscles.

By bending over and doing Barbell Curls in that position, you can get a peak contraction effect in your biceps, because in this position stress is still on your biceps when your arms are completely flexed. Other commonly used peak contraction exercises are Triceps Kickbacks, Side Laterals, Leg Extensions, Leg Curls, and Hyperextensions.

To achieve the ultimate in muscular detail for a competition, the superstars usually use both continuous tension and peak contraction in their workouts. Combined with a good precontest diet and high-quality training, these two techniques help produce the ultimate degree of muscularity displayed by bodybuilding greats like Frank Zane and Laura Combes.

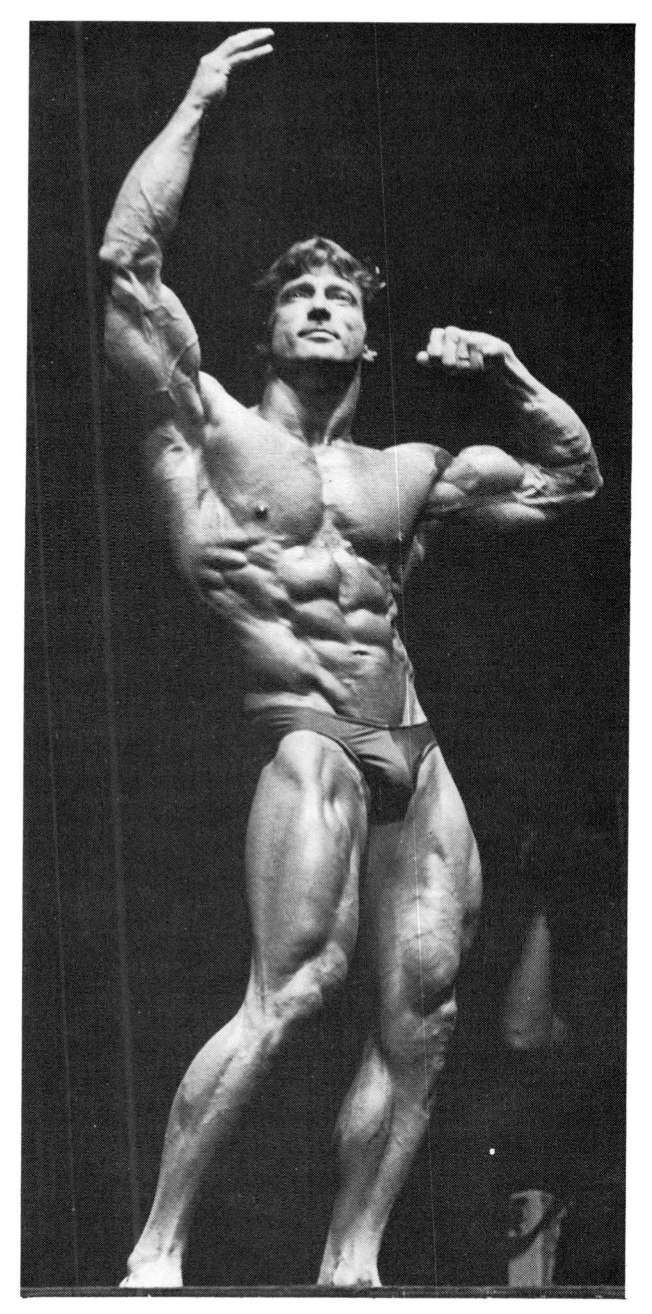

Frank Zane. *(Photo by Jimmy Caruso)*

Burns

One way to extend a set past the point of ordinary muscle failure, and therefore to stimulate a greater growth in muscle mass, is to use burns in your workouts. Usually when you fail to do a full rep you can still do several partial reps at either the beginning or the end of an exercise.

Burns are merely 5–10 of these partial reps done quickly and forcefully. These quick partial reps usually produce a fast buildup of fatigue toxins that makes the muscles "burn." Thus, these reps have been christened *burns*. And burns will greatly accelerate muscle growth.

One of the first champion bodybuilders to use burns was Larry Scott, who won the first two Mr. Olympia titles in 1965 and 1966. In recent years many of Gold's Gym champions have used burns, most notably Andreas Cahling and Rachel McLish, the first Ms. Olympia contest winner in 1980.

Negative Reps

About 20 years ago German physiologists discovered that the negative (downward) half of any resistance exercise has as much potential for strength improvement and muscular development as the positive (upward) half. So, in recent years, bodybuilders have made extensive use of negative reps in their workouts.

When you are doing pure negative reps a training partner or two will lift a weight 30%–50% heavier than you can normally use to the finish point of an exercise. Then you will lower the weight on your own while strongly resisting the downward momentum of the weight.

To use negative reps to help develop the ultimate in muscle mass and physical power, you should do one set of 3–5 negative reps on each basic exercise in your routine either once or twice per week. Used in this manner, negatives will increase your strength in all of your exercises, as well as your overall degree of muscle mass.

Unfortunately, pure negatives can wear your training partners out, so it's better to use a technique called *negative emphasis*. In its most basic form negative emphasis merely involves slowing down the negative half of a rep so that you'll be doing it half as fast as you do the positive half.

A more intense form of negative emphasis involves going up with two legs or arms on an exercise, shifting the weight to one arm or leg, and then resisting the downward force of the weight with that arm or leg. Obviously, you can do this type of rep only with machine movements in which the apparatus will not fall to the floor when you remove one arm or leg.

C. F. Smith, MD, a Mr. Tennessee winner and finalist in the Mr. America competition, frequently used this form of negative emphasis. As an example, when doing heavy Leg Extensions, C. F. would force the weight up with both legs and then resist the weight's descent with one leg. By alternating legs on every rep when using negative emphasis, C. F. was able to build enormous size and the ultimate in muscle density into his legs.

Stripping Method

Another way to push a fatigued muscle past the point of ordinary failure is to use the stripping method. As noted when discussing forced reps in Chapter 6, failing to complete a rep with a certain weight merely means you can't do a rep with that weight. Certainly you could do one or two reps with a lighter poundage, and a forced rep is a repetition done with a training partner pulling up on the weight to make it effectively lighter.

A different way to make a weight lighter is to have two partners strip a plate or two off each side. As an example, let's say you can do six reps in the Bench Press with 250 pounds before failing. When you fail, your partners can strip a 10- and 5-pound plate from each side. With 220 pounds you can do 2–3 additional reps. You can then have 20–30 more pounds stripped from the bar for a final 2–3 additional superhard reps.

Arnold Schwarzenegger (seven-time Mr. Olympia) used the stripping method quite extensively, particularly in his arm training. He also used stripping with dumbbells by going down the rack. This way you can use a pair of 50s for 5–6 reps, immediately a pair of 45s for 2–3 more reps, and finally a pair of 40s for 2–3 reps.

You can safely use the stripping method for two or three sets per muscle group once or twice per week. When you're going all-out in your precontest workouts, you can probably productively use stripping for four or five sets per muscle group at virtually every workout. Such a practice will give you a superb combination of muscle mass and sharp muscularity.

Quality Training

As you will recall from the discussion of progression in Chapter 2, one way to increase training intensity is to reduce the length of rest periods between sets. And this is exactly the principle behind quality training. By reducing their rest intervals between sets to as little as 10–15 seconds, and then combining this with a tight diet, champion bodybuilders are able to bring out superb muscular definition onstage at competitions.

When you gradually shorten the rest intervals between sets there is a temptation to lower the amount of resistance you use on each exercise. But to achieve the utmost in muscle density you must keep your poundages as high as possible. A tight diet makes this exceedingly difficult, but never allow your exercise poundages to drop by more than 20% when using quality training.

In the off-season you can rest 60–90 seconds between sets. Then, 4–6 weeks before competing, you should begin gradually to reduce your rest intervals. For the final two weeks prior to a competition you should be training at peak intensity.

Rest-Pause Training

It's an undeniable fact that using heavy training poundages produces the greatest possible degree of muscle mass. But your muscles are often limited in what they can do with heavy weights by the rapid buildup of fatigue toxins within the muscles.

By using rest-pause training in your workouts, you can prolong a set for 6–8 reps with a poundage that will ordinarily limit you to two or three reps. And as a result, you will be able to develop a much greater degree of muscle mass and physical power.

With 10–15 seconds of rest, your circulatory system can eliminate enough fatigue toxins to give a muscle group at least 50% of full recuperation. So, in rest-pause training, you will do 2–3 reps with a heavy weight, rest 10–15 seconds, immediately do 2–3 more reps, rest another 10–15 seconds, and finally force out an additional 1–2 reps. And such a set is the ultimate in training intensity.

At Gold's Gym Mike Mentzer has been the greatest exponent of rest-pause training, and he credits this method for developing much of his Herculean muscle mass. Mike recommends only one set of rest-pause work on one basic exercise per muscle group once per week.

Rest-pause training is such intense work that it will be productive only when used by advanced bodybuilders with at least two years of hard training behind them. Less experienced men and women will quickly overtrain with this method.

Over-the-shoulder view of Ray Mentzer blasting his bicep on a Nautilus Curl machine.

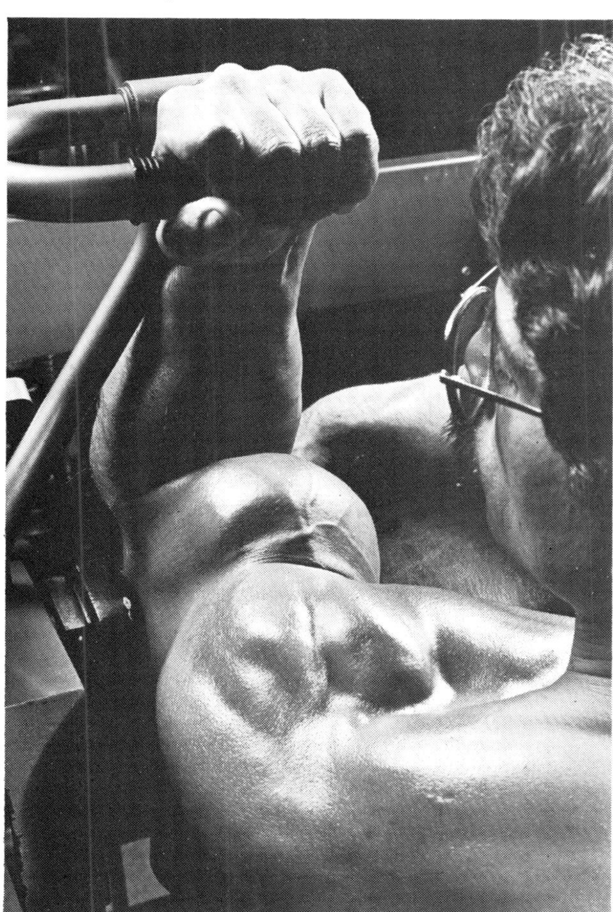

Double Split Routines

Very advanced bodybuilders tend to do a great number of total sets for each muscle group, particularly just prior to a competition. Because of this, they do exceedingly long workouts. Often these workouts become so long that a bodybuilder's energy reserves don't allow for sufficient training intensity toward the end of a gym session.

To allow for maximum energy availability throughout a training program, many advanced bodybuilders work out twice per day. Such a double split routine allows for shorter and more intense—albeit more frequent—workouts.

The most basic double split involves three extra workouts per week. In this program you do two workouts per day three times each week and one workout per day three times each week. Here is a double split performed by the legendary Robby Robinson.

M-W-F (AM)

Chest, Back, and Calves

M-W-F (PM)

Thighs, Abdominals, and Forearms

Tu-Th-Sa (AM or PM)

Deltoids, Biceps-Triceps, Calves, and Abdominals

A pure double split routine involves two workouts each day six days per week. Here is an example of such a double split routine.

M-W-F (AM)

Chest, Triceps, and Calves

M-W-F (PM)

Back and Abdominals

Tu-Th-Sa (AM)

Shoulders, Forearms, and Abdominals

Tu-Th-Sa (PM)

Thighs and Calves

Many superstar bodybuilders, such as Lou Ferrigno, never use a double split, because they lose muscle mass on one. Others, however, thrive on a double split, and Laura Combes actually trains as often as four or five times a day prior to a major competition!

Bodybuilding Publicity

The higher a bodybuilder goes in the competitive hierarchy, the more important good publicity becomes. There is no doubt that a relationship exists between the amount of public exposure a bodybuilder has had and his or her relative popularity. The greater the exposure a bodybuilder receives, the greater his or her popularity, and the better his or her economic value for giving exhibitions and seminars.

The main source of publicity for most bodybuilders is the various magazines associated with the sport. Articles in *Muscle & Fitness, Muscle Mag International, Muscle Digest, Muscular Development, Muscle Training Illustrated, Flex, Iron Man,* and other magazines give wide public exposure to various bodybuilders. These articles include personality profiles, training instruction stories, and reports of competitions in which a bodybuilder might have participated.

All bodybuilding magazines accept freelance contributions, so find a friend with some writing ability or write your own articles. Submit articles and relevant photos to the editor of one of the magazines, and if you are good enough and have something to say, you'll soon have plenty of publicity.

Good color and black-and-white photos also are essential for publicity as well as for studying your physique. In the next section of this chapter, we will tell you how to have good photos taken by a friend. Overall, however, you will get your best photos if the better bodybuilding photographers—John Balik, Mike Neveux, Denie Walter, Russ Warner, Gary Bartlett, and Chris Lund, for example—shoot you. And the better you get, the better your chances of attracting the attention of one of these photographers.

This principle also holds true with having articles written about yourself. The various magazines actively pursue elite bodybuilders. If you haven't won a national or international title, however, you may have to pursue the magazines yourself.

Bodybuilding Photography

As just stated, you will get the best photos of yourself if you have them taken by an experienced photographer who specializes in the field of bodybuilding. You can, however, get reasonably good photos without one of these photographers if you follow these 14 rules:

1. Be sure that you are in peak physical condition. If you don't have a good physique, you can't hope to get good photos of yourself.
2. Shave and spend enough time getting a deep, even tan if you are fair-skinned. A dark-looking bodybuilder looks harder than one who looks very pale.
3. Wear posing attire of a solid color that is harmonious with your general coloring. Patterned suits are quite distracting to the eye and detract from your physique. You also should avoid black or white attire, which will look too black or too white in black-and-white photos.
4. Be well groomed. Women should wear their hair pinned up so it doesn't hide any of their back or shoulder musculature.
5. Oil your body lightly with some type of vegetable oil (almond and avocado oil are both popular) that sinks into your skin. You should have on just enough oil to impart a glow to your skin. Nothing looks as bad on a bodybuilder as an excessively heavy coat of oil.
6. Choose a nondistracting background such as a beach, the sky, or a lakeside promontory. Avoid having trees, bushes, houses, and other distracting objects in the background. Be sure that you don't have a tree, rock, sailboat, or telephone pole "growing" out of the subject's head.
7. Choose a time of day when direct sunlight strikes the model at a 45-degree angle.
8. Have the model face slightly away from the sun. Be sure the camera is held on the same level as the subject's belly button.
9. Use a 35mm camera with a lens that can be adjusted for a precise focus. For cover photos it's better to use a camera that takes a

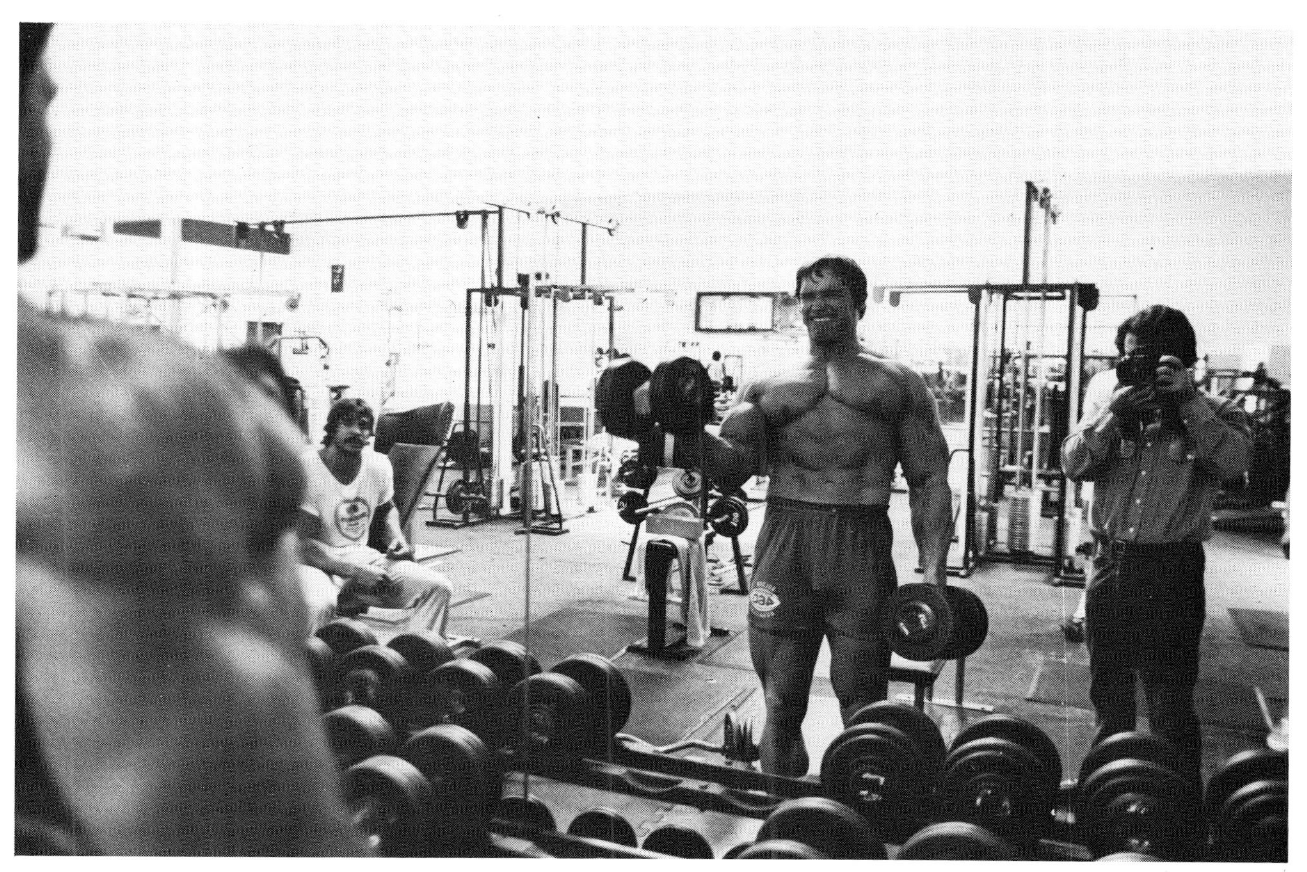

And this is how the greatest physique of all time was built. Photographer John Balik records for posterity the superb intensity of Arnold Schwarzenegger bombing his biceps!

larger-format negative or transparency (the 2¼ × 2¼-inch format, such as produced by a Hasselblad camera, is the most popular).

10. Use a shutter speed of at least 1/250th of a second, and preferably of 1/500th of a second. Slower shutter speed will result in a blurry photograph due to lens movement.

11. For black-and-white photos use Kodak Plus X film, for color slides use Kodak Kodachrome 64 film, and for color prints use Kodak Kodacolor film.

12. Be sure that the camera exposure is correct for the type of film being used. For color film, shoot one photo a half-stop higher than the correct exposure, one photo at the correct exposure, and one photo a half-stop lower than the correct exposure. If possible, have your lens aperature set at f5.6 or f8, the sharpest of the f-stop settings on most lenses.

13. Shoot several photos of each pose so that you are sure the model's eyes are open and he or she has a pleasant facial expression. Compared with the effort it takes to get into peak condition for a photo session, film and processing expenses are cheap.

14. Be sure that the model is relaxed. A nervous bodybuilder will look nervous in a photograph.

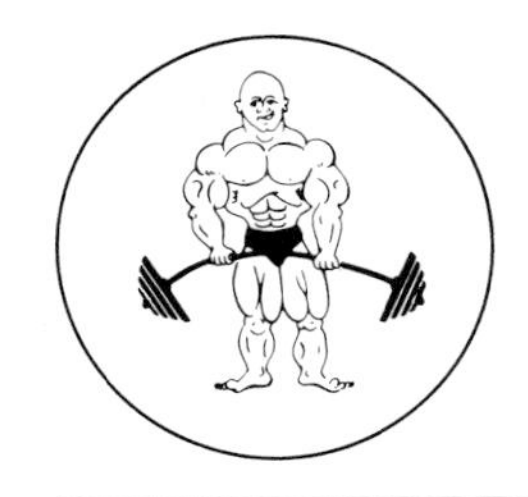

9 THE FULL CYCLE

In this chapter we will synthesize everything you've learned so far about bodybuilding training and diet in a discussion of cycle bodybuilding. Both off-season and precontest cycles will be discussed. We will also discuss contest grooming, tanning, posing, and bodybuilding pharmacology.

The Cycle Training Philosophy

Virtually all athletes follow a cycle training philosophy in order to reach a higher competitive peak than would ordinarily be possible. Cycle training involves building a conditioning base during the off-season, then honing that base through quality training to reach a sharp peak.

Track and field athletes who run the mile would burn out if they merely ran fast mile time trials. So during the off-season, milers build a base by running over their distance each day. They might run five or six miles per day at a relatively slow pace to improve their aerobic capacity to the point where actually running a mile becomes easier and easier.

Then, once they have developed a good physical conditioning base, they quality train by doing speed work to sharpen their ability to run a mile at a fast, anaerobic pace. A miler's speed work involves doing many repetitions at 220, 330, 440, 660, and 880 yards at a pace significantly faster than that segment would be run in an actual race. Runners take a rest interval between these repetition runs, and this interval is reduced the same as in bodybuilding quality training as an athlete approaches a peak. Runners call this type of speed work *interval training*.

While a runner is honing his or her base through interval training, he or she will usually maintain that base through periodical overdistance runs. This involves one or two longer and slower runs per week if a miler trains once per day. Better milers, however, usually run twice per day, overdistance in the mornings, and intervals in the afternoons.

Once a peak has been reached, a miler will cycle back into an off-season phase to begin building an even better base of conditioning. And through alternating off-season and precompetitive cycles, he or she can more quickly improve a mile time. The first below-four-minute mile was run by Roger Bannister, now a physician in his native England, at a time when

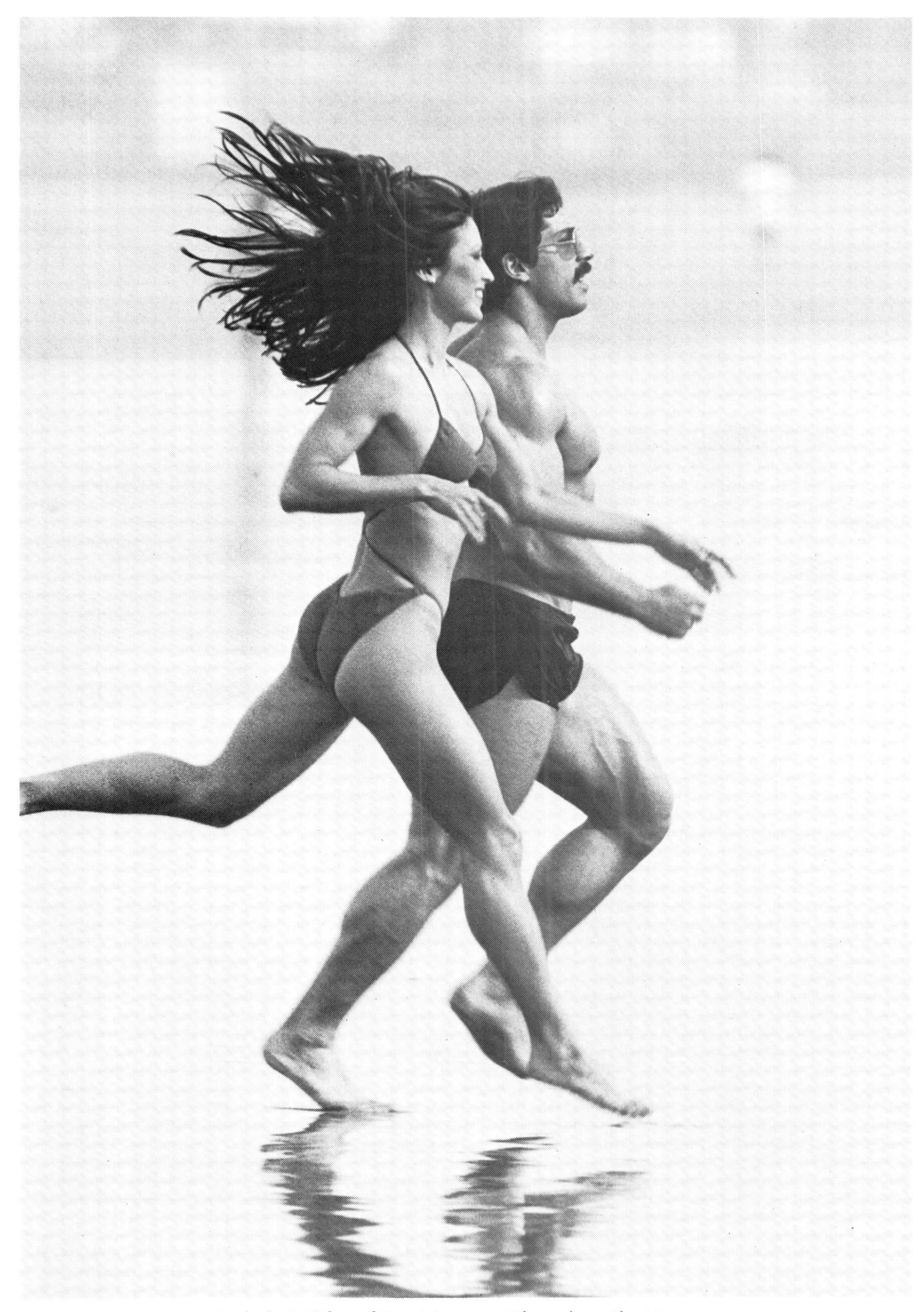

Rachel McLish and Ray Mentzer. *(Photo by Mike Neveux)*

interval workouts and cycle training were in their development stages. Today cycle training has reached maturity in track training, and the men's mile record is 12 seconds faster than Bannister's mark.

Over the past 15–20 years, bodybuilders have gradually evolved a mature cycle training philosophy as well, and this is one major reason why bodybuilders today are so much better than they were in the 1960s. Instead of building endurance in the off-season, however, they seek to develop greater strength and the increased degree of muscle mass that comes with it. Then, during the precontest phase, they attempt to hone this muscle mass through lighter quality training until it is fully defined.

Bodybuilders also cycle their diets in conjunction with their training, making the task of peaking—reaching their best physical form at the time of a contest—much more intricate than in other sports. During the off-season the diet is calculated to add the greatest possible degree of muscle mass, while close to a competition the diet is reduced in calories to minimize body fat for an optimum combination of muscle mass and muscular detail.

They do, incidentally, follow champion runners' example by training in a special way to maintain the best possible degree of off-season muscle mass during a precontest cycle. All of this will become much more clear as you read the following four sections of this chapter: off-season training, off-season diet, precontest training, and precontest diet.

The salient point we wish to leave you with in this section is that almost all champion bodybuilders follow a cycle training and dietary philosophy, because it allows them to combine an optimum degree of muscle mass with sparkling muscularity when totally peaked out. And, by alternating off-season and precontest phases, a bodybuilder can continue to add to his or her muscle mass, muscularity, and proportional balance over a period of 10 or more years.

Off-Season Training

You should have two main objectives during your off-season training cycle. The first of these, as just stated, is to add to overall body strength and mass. Second, you must attempt to gradually improve your weak point(s) during off-season training. Precontest training should be devoted solely to achieving peak contition, not to improving a weak body part or two.

Overload training should reach a zenith during the off-season. "Pick one or two basic exercises per muscle group and work each movement with maximum poundages in good exercise form," advises Tom Platz, the most massively muscular bodybuilder of all time. "Keep your reps in the range of 4–6 and consistently push to the point of failure on each set. Once each week, use forced reps to push your muscles well past the point of normal failure.

"Less experienced bodybuilders will probably make their best gains in the off-season on a four-day split routine, training each major muscle group twice a week. Bodybuilders with considerable training under their belts could gain fairly well on a six-day split, but still training each major muscle group twice per week. Only an Olympian-level bodybuilder could make good off-season gains on a six-day split routine in which each major muscle group is bombed three times a week. Even many Olympians can't handle that level of intensity during an off-season cycle."

All champion bodybuilders place considerable emphasis on the use of basic exercises during an off-season power- and mass-building cycle. These are the movements in which you can handle very heavy training poundages. Be certain, however, that you warm up thoroughly on each basic movement and that you use correct biomechanical position during the execution of an exercise. This will prevent you from being injured when using maximum training weights.

In addition to emphasizing basic exercises during the off-season cycle, most of the champs do many more barbell movements and fewer dumbbell and cable exercises in the off-season. Generally speaking, it's easier to use a very heavy training poundage on a barbell than on two dumbbells, so this use of barbells stands to reason.

Based on the foregoing suggestions, here are typical advanced-level off-season training programs for each major muscle group (calves, abs, and forearms are excepted):

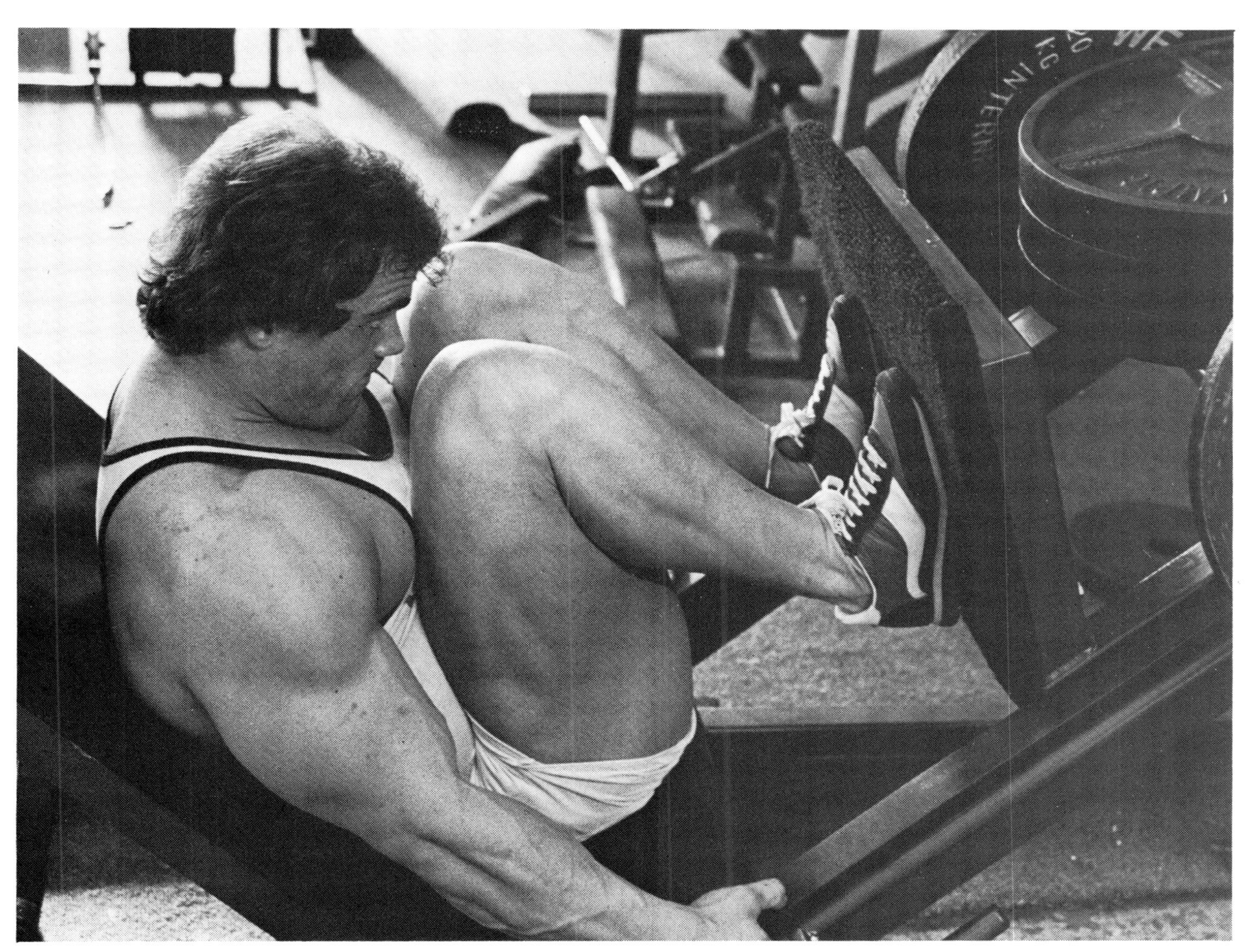

Gary Leonard starts Leg Presses on a 45-degree-angled machine.

Thighs

1. Squat: 5 × 12–14
2. Leg Press: 5 × 12–6
3. Leg Extension: 5 × 8–10
4. Leg Curl: 5 × 8–10

Back

1. Seated Pulley Rowing: 5 × 12–4
2. Barbell Bent Rowing: 5 × 12–4
3. Stiff-Leg Deadlift: 5 × 15–6
4. Barbell Shrug: 5 × 15–6

Chest

1. Incline Barbell Press: 5 × 12–4
2. Barbell Bench Press: 5 × 12–4
3. Parallel Bar Dip: 5 × 15–6

Shoulders

1. Press behind the Neck: 5 × 12–4
2. Upright Rowing: 5 × 12–6
3. Bent Lateral: 5 × 15–6

Biceps

1. Standing Barbell Curl: 5 × 12–4
2. Barbell Preacher Curl: 5 × 12–4

Triceps

1. Lying Triceps Extension: 5 × 12–4
2. Parallel Bar Dip: 5 × 15–6

Unfortunately, most of the body part routines presented in the various bodybuilding magazines are for precontest training, even though this usually is not stated. If you compare the foregoing genuine off-season routines with some that you see in the muscle mags, you'll understand why so many young bodybuilders are chronically overtrained.

In terms of improving a weak muscle group during the off-season, you can let your strongest body part(s) slide a bit to conserve mental and physical energy in each workout for an all-out blitz of your weak points. Rod Koontz (Natural Mr. America, Mr. USA), for example, once went nearly a year without doing back or biceps training so he could blast his then-weak thighs and calves. These areas were improved dramatically, and once he started training them again his back and biceps were up to par in less than three months. This approach won Rod his Mr. USA title on his first entry into national competition.

An intelligent bodybuilder analyzes photos of his or her physique after each peak, expressly to discover weak points. And from peak to peak these lagging muscle groups will change. It's always a good idea to have a full photo session each time you reach a peak.

If you have average or better genetic potential, any lagging muscle group will respond adequately.

Off-Season Diet

The off-season diet is somewhat relaxed, but still nutritionally well-balanced to promote perfect health. If you are not in good health, you simply can't make optimum gains in strength and muscle mass. You should, therefore, strictly follow the dietary advice presented in chapters 2, 4, and 6.

To give you an illustration of how a champion bodybuilder eats during an off-season cycle, we interviewed Dr. Lynne Pirie (an orthopedic surgeon who has won the light-heavyweight Ms. USA title and placed in the top three—competing as an amateur against professionals—in the World Women's Bodybuilding Championships) on the subject. Dr. Pirie's observations are valid for both women and men.

"As is the case with most high-level bodybuilders, both my training and diet are cyclical," Lynne revealed. "During the off-season I used to feel that I could indulge myself with ice cream and other treats whenever I felt like it, just as long as I kept up my protein intake and vitamin and mineral supplementation. Unfortunately, this practice led me to accumulate excessive levels of body fat, which was difficult to diet off prior to competition. Since it's so much easier to go up in body weight than it is to come back down, I finally decided to monitor my diet year-round and keep myself within 6–8 pounds of my competition weight at all times.

"By definition, an off-season diet is somewhat relaxed, in that sufficient calories must be taken in to allow all-out, heavy, mass-building workouts. But there is no valid reason for a bodybuilder to pig out during this dietary and training phase. Simply follow a well-balanced diet that is relatively high in protein, contains a low-to-moderate amount of fats, includes enough unrefined carbohydrates to meet all training energy requirements, and includes sufficient amounts of vitamins, minerals, and trace elements to maintain optimum health.

"You should make an effort to determine your daily caloric maintenance level, then avoid going more than 100–200 calories per day above this level in your food intake. Remember that you will add one pound of body fat for each 3,500 calories you consume in excess of your energy maintenance needs.

"My own maintenance level during the off-season is approximately 2,500 calories, so I normally consume 2,400–2,600 in my food each day during my off-season cycle. This maintenance level can vary widely, however, according to sex, body weight, relative Basal Metabolic Rate (BMR), and physical/mental energy expenditure levels. I know several women bodybuilders who routinely consume 4,000 calories per day and men who eat over 7,000 calories per day in the off-season without getting fat.

"Many bodybuilders feel that it's too much hassle to keep close track of how many calories they are consuming in the off-season, so they prefer to eat instinctively. In other words, they alter the amount and type of food they eat according to how they look and feel. If they are getting excessively pudgy, they will cut back on

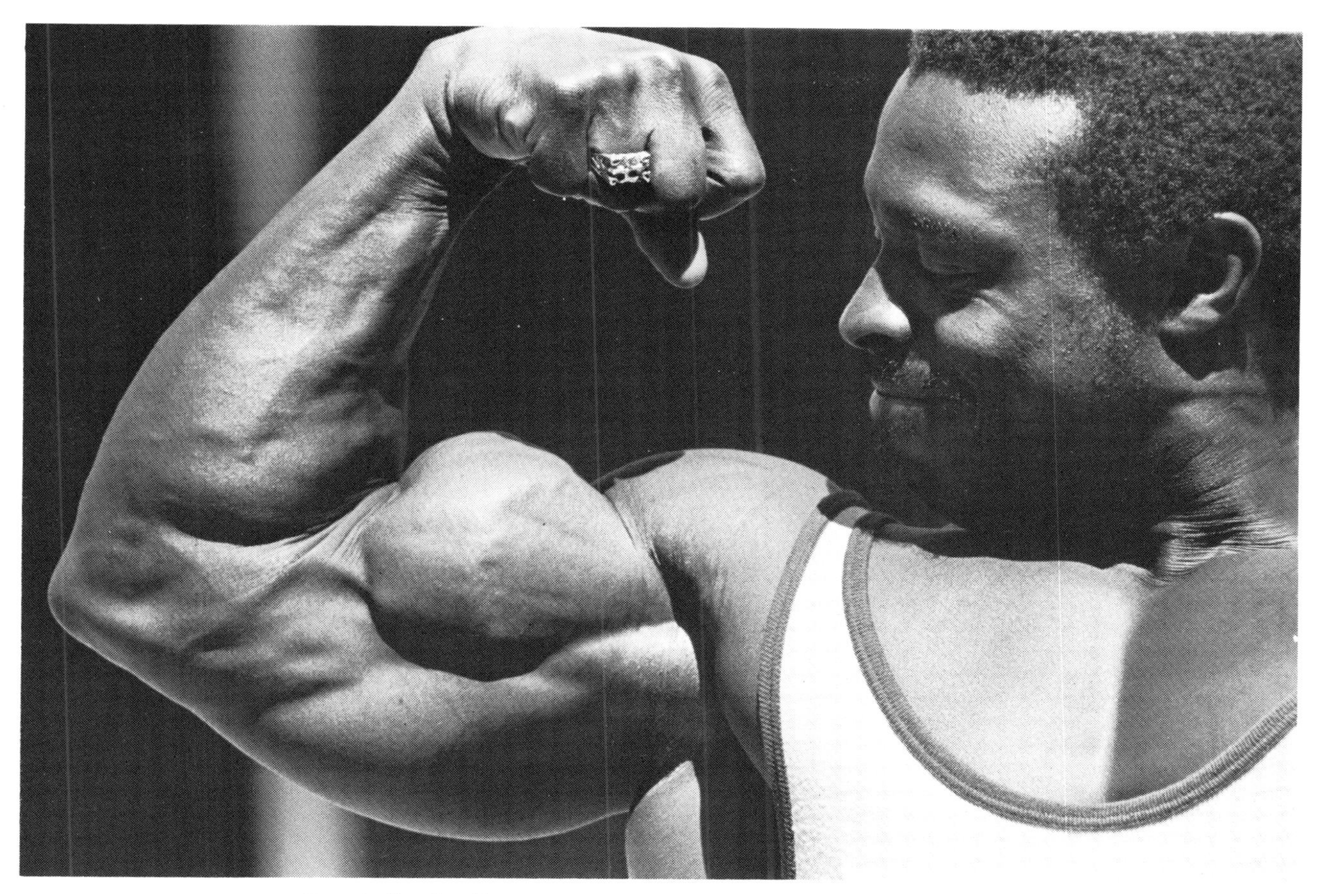

Roy Callender flexes a mighty biceps. *(Photo by Mike Neveux)*

calories. Or if their energy levels are too low, they will eat more calories and/or additional carbohydrate foods.

"Since a precontest diet is deliberately low in calories in order for your body to burn off fatty tissue and to expose the muscular development beneath it, my off-season diet is quite a bit higher in calories than the one I use prior to competition. As a result, I can include more fats in my diet. Due to the high calorie concentrations in fats, I must virtually eliminate fat from my diet prior to competing. In the off-season I might also treat myself once per week with a small serving of some type of junk food that I like, but otherwise I keep my junkouts totally under control.

"You will need adequate supplies of protein in your diet to build an optimum degree of muscle mass in the off-season. The FDA recommends consuming approximately one half gram of protein per pound of body weight, but I feel that most bodybuilders should consume an average of one gram of protein per pound of body weight. The highest quality proteins come from animal sources such as poultry, fish, eggs, meat, and milk products.

"Several well-known bodybuilders follow vegetarian diets, but I can't build muscle mass very quickly unless I consume animal proteins, which have a much better amino acid balance than vegetable-source proteins. Some vegetable proteins are acceptable in the off-season diet, however, particularly if they are consumed in conjunction with animal proteins that can complete the amino acid balance of vegetable proteins. The better vegetable protein foods are nuts, seeds, grains, corn, seed sprouts, legumes, beans, and potatoes.

"The best sources of carbohydrates in the off-season are fresh fruits, vegetables, grains, potatoes, nuts, and seeds. Fruit gives you a quick boost of energy, such as you might need just before or during a hard workout. For a sustained flow of energy, however, it is better to eat

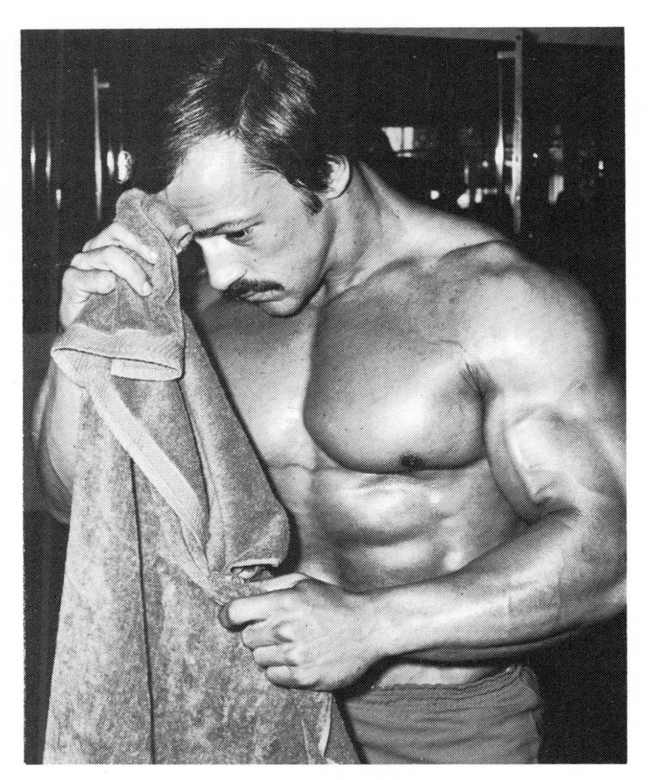

No one ever said that bodybuilding is easy! Massive Casey Viator (history's youngest Mr. America and now one of the top IFBB pro bodybuilders) takes a short break between exercises. *(Photo by Peter Brenner)*

complex carbohydrates—as found in rice, potatoes, and vegetables—which take a longer period of time to digest completely.

"Although I take vitamin and mineral supplements year-round, I take quite a bit less in the off-season than prior to a contest. When I'm on a strict diet it's much more likely that I'll develop nutritional deficiencies than it is during the off-season. So, during my precontest cycle, I supplement my diet fairly heavily with vitamin and mineral tablets and capsules.

"The easiest way to supplement your diet during the off-season is to use the convenient multipacks of vitamins and minerals distributed by various supplement companies. One or two multipacks per day will be more than adequate off-season supplementation. Incidentally, you'll assimilate your supplemental vitamins and minerals more efficiently if you take them with your meals.

"If you have a great deal of difficulty in gaining muscular body weight, you should investigate the use of a protein supplement *between* meals. Since your body can only efficiently digest 20–30 grams of protein per feeding, protein supplements are wasted when taken *with* meals. The best protein powders are made from milk and eggs, since these two foods are of much higher biological quality than the soya-based proteins commonly sold.

"Use a blender to mix up two or three protein drinks per day. To a base of 10–12 ounces of milk, add two tablespoons of protein powder and some type of soft fruit like peaches or bananas for flavoring. Blend it well, and drink the concoction two or three time a day.

"By eating intelligently during the off-season, you can maximize your overall bodybuilding gains. Rather than junking out like a pig—as many bodybuilders, even champions, do—you should maintain a balanced and nutritional diet. Then you will be well on your way to becoming a better bodybuilder!"

Precontest Training

To present an example of how a high-level bodybuilder trains prior to a contest, we interviewed Casey Viator, history's youngest Mr. America winner and one of the best professional bodybuilders today. His comments are valid for both male and female bodybuilders.

"My precontest cycle starts 12 weeks prior to a competition," Casey revealed. "Over the 12-week precontest cycle, I gradually and progressively tighten my diet and intensify my training. Rather than training each major muscle group twice a week as in the off-season, I work major body parts three days per week, and I do more total sets per muscle group during my precontest phase. The more total sets I do each week for a muscle group, the harder and more defined it seems to become.

"During my precontest cycle I also do more and more aerobic training to help burn off body fat to reveal the muscles under my skin in bold relief. A lot of bodybuilders like to run every day, but long, slow distance running tends to bore me. I would rather ride my bicycle up and down the bike path stretching along the Pacific Ocean beach from Santa Monica southward for 20 miles to Palos Verdes. Sometimes I'll also pedal a stationary bike for an hour as I watch television at night.

"To bring out optimum muscle mass and hardness, I *must* quality train by gradually shortening my rest intervals between sets. At peak precontest intensity, I'll average only 15–20 seconds rest between sets. To assist my quality training, I will use plenty of supersets close to a contest. Combining quality training with aerobic workouts and a tight precontest diet, I can achieve a super-muscular appearance while maintaining maximum muscle mass.

"When I am dieting strictly and quality training to the max, my workout poundages inevitably will drop. The secret to maintaining mass while achieving the best possible degree of muscle density is to fight to keep these poundages up as high as possible while still using strict exercise form on every repetition of every set. I train like a dog at this point—and it really hurts!—but if I give everything I have during the last few weeks before a competition, I'm inevitably in great shape onstage. But when I slack off a little, I never am able to reach peak condition.

"To bring out the ultimate in muscularity, I use as many peak contraction and continuous tension reps in my training as possible. To keep the momentum generated on a barbell or dumbbell by quick reps from robbing a muscle group of some of the intense stress it should be receiving, I move the weight in every set both slowly and with heavy added tension in my muscles over the full range of motion of every exercise.

"During the final six weeks before I compete, I spend an hour or more per day on my posing practice. Not only does this improve the flow of my routine, but it also helps a little to harden up my muscles. I even extend this hard muscle flexing into my actual bodybuilding workouts by tensing the muscles I'm working in several 6–8-second reps between sets for that muscle group.

"In my actual posing practice, I will hold each of the compulsory poses for up to 60 seconds at a time. Onstage when comparisons are being made, I often must hold a pose at maximum tension for 30–40 seconds without shaking like a leaf. The only way to acquire this ability is to frequently hold the poses for an even longer period of time when practicing."

To illustrate more precisely how he changes his training during a precontest cycle, Casey Viator gave us these off-season and precontest chest training schedules.

OFF-SEASON (twice a week)

Exercise	Sets	Reps
1. Incline Barbell Press	6–8	12–4
2. Bench Press	6–8	12–4
3. Parallel Bar Dips	5	10–5
4. Incline Flyes	5	12–6
5. Pec Deck Flyes	5	12–6

PRECONTEST (three times a week)

Exercise	Sets	Reps
1. Incline Dumbbell Press	5	8–10
2. Incline Flyes	5	10–12
3. Bench Press	5	8–10
4. Parallel Bar Dips	5	10–15
5. Cross-Bench Dumbbell Pullover	5	10–12
6. Cable Crossovers	5	10–12

"You should note several things from reviewing these two routines," Casey said. "See especially how I use mostly basic exercises in the off-season and a greater number of dumbbell and cable isolation movements prior to a contest, since the isolation exercises aid in bringing out a muscle's optimum number of striations. And note how I do more total sets for the body part each week, how I do a little higher reps, and how I use supersets prior to a contest and straight sets in the off-season.

"There is one more precontest technique that I use. Since I'm doing so many more sets each workout day, I switch to using a double-split routine for the final six weeks before a contest. Not only does this switch allow me to spend less time in the gym each workout, but the more frequent training also tends to speed up my metabolism and get my body more cut-up.

"Try to think of the training aspect of a peaking cycle as a snowball rolling down a hill. At first it is small and it rolls relatively slowly. But the further down the hill a snowball rolls, the larger it becomes and the faster it is moving. In the same manner, you will gradually increase the volume and speed of your workouts to peak out perfectly and win your next competition!"

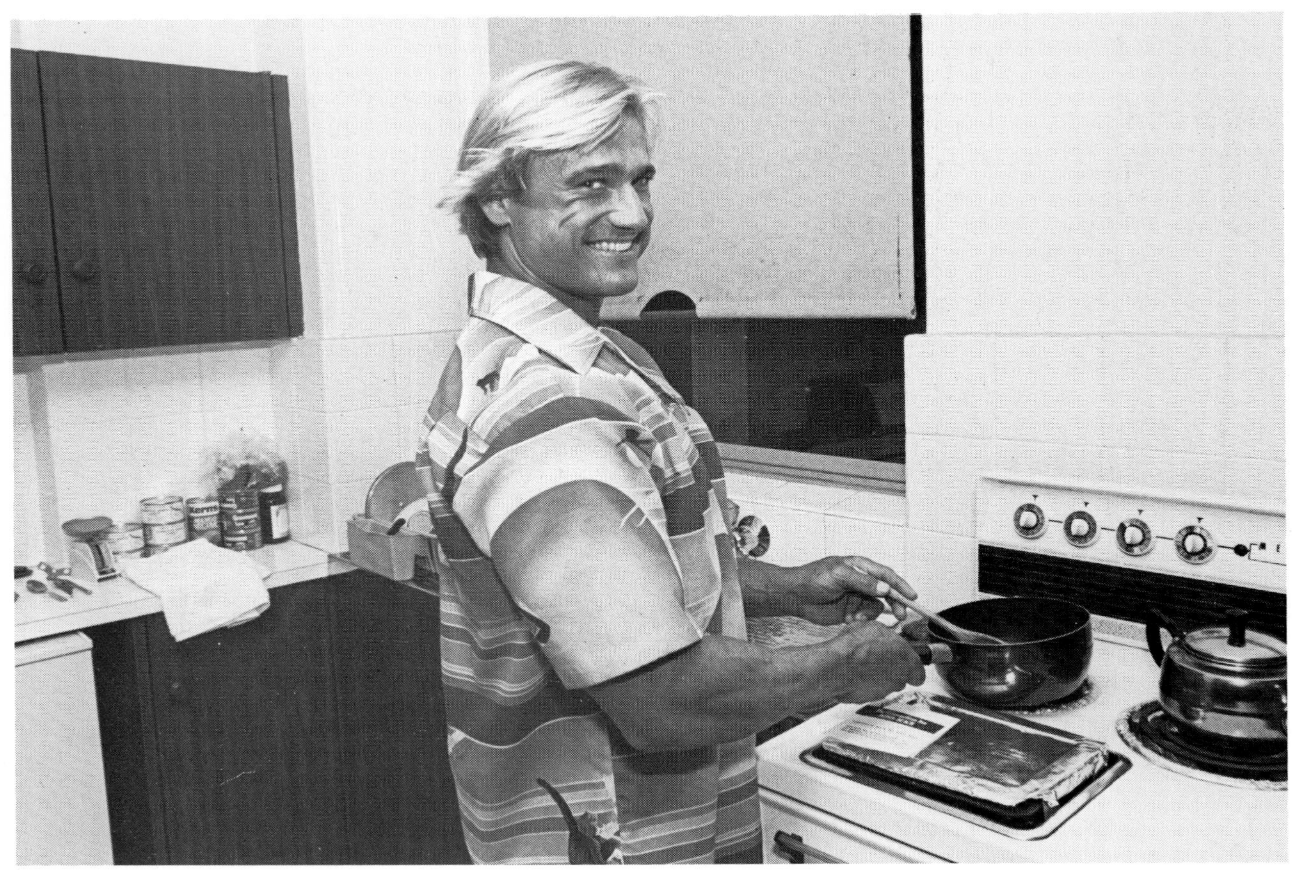

Tom Platz whips up a meal in his motel room in Sydney, Australia, a day before the 1980 Mr. Olympia competition. *(Photo by Mike Neveux)*

Precontest Diet

Two main types of precontest diets are followed by male and female competitive bodybuilders—low-carbohydrate and low-calorie. And, in recent years, the low-fat/low-calorie diet has become most popular.

For many years a low- to zero-carbohydrate diet was the mainstay of most bodybuilders trying to cut up. Depending on how fat a bodybuilder had become in the off-season, he or she would begin dieting 6–12 weeks prior to a competition. Using a carbohydrate gram counter (available in drugstores and health food stores), the dietary carbohydrate intake was reduced gradually, beginning with about 150 grams per day and gradually limiting the diet by 20–30 additional grams per week.

At a minimum, bodybuilders consumed 10–20 grams of carbohydrate each day on a low-carb diet. It's impossible actually to reduce dietary carbohydrate intake to zero, because even high-protein foods such as beef and chicken have traces of carbohydrate in them.

Even though a low-carb diet is high in fats, you will lose weight on it. Much of this weight, however, is lost in the form of body water retention diminishment. Each gram of carbohydrate holds approximately four times its weight in water inside the body. Therefore, a limitation of dietary carbohydrate consumption will result in a dramatic loss of body fluids during the first week of a low-carb diet. Thereafter the weight comes off much more slowly.

To give a clear picture of what a low-carbohydrate diet looks like, here is a sample one-day menu:

Breakfast—eggs fried in butter, steak, coffee or tea (with artificial sweetener), supplements.

Lunch—broiled chicken, salad with oil and vinegar dressing, iced tea, supplements.

Dinner—steak or baked ham, diet soda, supplements.
Snacks—hard cheese, cold cuts.

Note that sugar, grain products, milk, potatoes, rice, fruit, and vegetables other than salad greens have been deleted from this diet. Note also, however, that no limitation has been placed on dietary fat intake—no specific quantities have been recommended.

Numerous champion bodybuilders have gotten ripped to shreds on this diet in past years, and a few today still follow it. Unfortunately, though, the low-carb diet is not free of negative effects.

The most disastrous complication for most competitive bodybuilders is a noticeable loss of muscle mass, which can be sure death onstage at a bodybuilding competition. Training energy is extremely limited on such a diet, and everyone we've seen following a low-carb diet has been exceedingly miserable. Depression and irritability are quite common.

A low-carb diet also is hard on a person's health. It results in low blood sugar, adversely affecting the brain. Low-carb dieting can also be quite hard on the kidneys, particularly if accompanied by a restriction of liquid intake.

We recommend that you try a low-carb diet at least once to see how well it works for you, since all bodybuilders react differently to a variety of nutritional philosophies. It might be best, though, to try this diet at some time other than just before a contest. This way a competitive Armageddon can be avoided if the low-carb diet greatly diminishes your degree of muscle mass.

A far more sensible and workable precontest diet is the low-fat/low-calorie regimen discussed in the advanced nutrition section of Chapter 6. It guarantees a high degree of physical and mental health as well as a high degree of training energy. On a balanced low-calorie diet you can gradually reduce body fat levels without losing appreciable muscle mass.

Reread the part about low-calorie dieting in Chapter 6 to be certain you understand it, then try the diet a couple of times, comparing its effects on your body with the low-carb diet. Most contemporary champion bodybuilders prefer low-calorie dieting. You may agree.

Peaking Experience

Peaking perfectly for a competition is an art form. It takes experience and several attempts at peaking for competition to learn to peak precisely on schedule for a particular contest. Virtually no one reaches an optimum peak on his or her initial attempt. Moreover, it usually takes several tries to peak fully, since the first few peaking attempts tend to fall a bit short of a full peak.

The cardinal rule that you should follow in learning to peak correctly is *learn from every peaking attempt.* As you already know, myriad factors—such as diet, weight training intensity, and aerobic workouts—must be orchestrated precisely in order for you to peak perfectly. Therefore, your task over the next few contests is to learn exactly what effect such variables have on the way your body responds in approaching a peak.

You should make mental and/or written notes—even photographs—of how your body responds. You should also note how you need to look at checkpoints set a few days apart leading up to a show. This allows you either to accelerate or to retard your progress toward a peak, according to how much or how little body fat you see when you pose in front of the mirror.

With experience, you will learn how much more aerobic training you need and how much more strict your diet must become to accelerate the peaking process. And, if you are ahead of schedule, you will learn to moderate your diet, train heavier, and shorten your workouts to retard the arrival of a peak. Once you master these skills, you will be able to reach a 100% peak virtually every time you compete. And that increases your chances of being a consistent winner!

Contest Grooming and Training

Winning bodybuilders invariably look healthy and physically attractive onstage. And this winning look is largely a result of careful attention to personal grooming and tanning prior to a competition.

Grooming

You have no doubt developed a personal

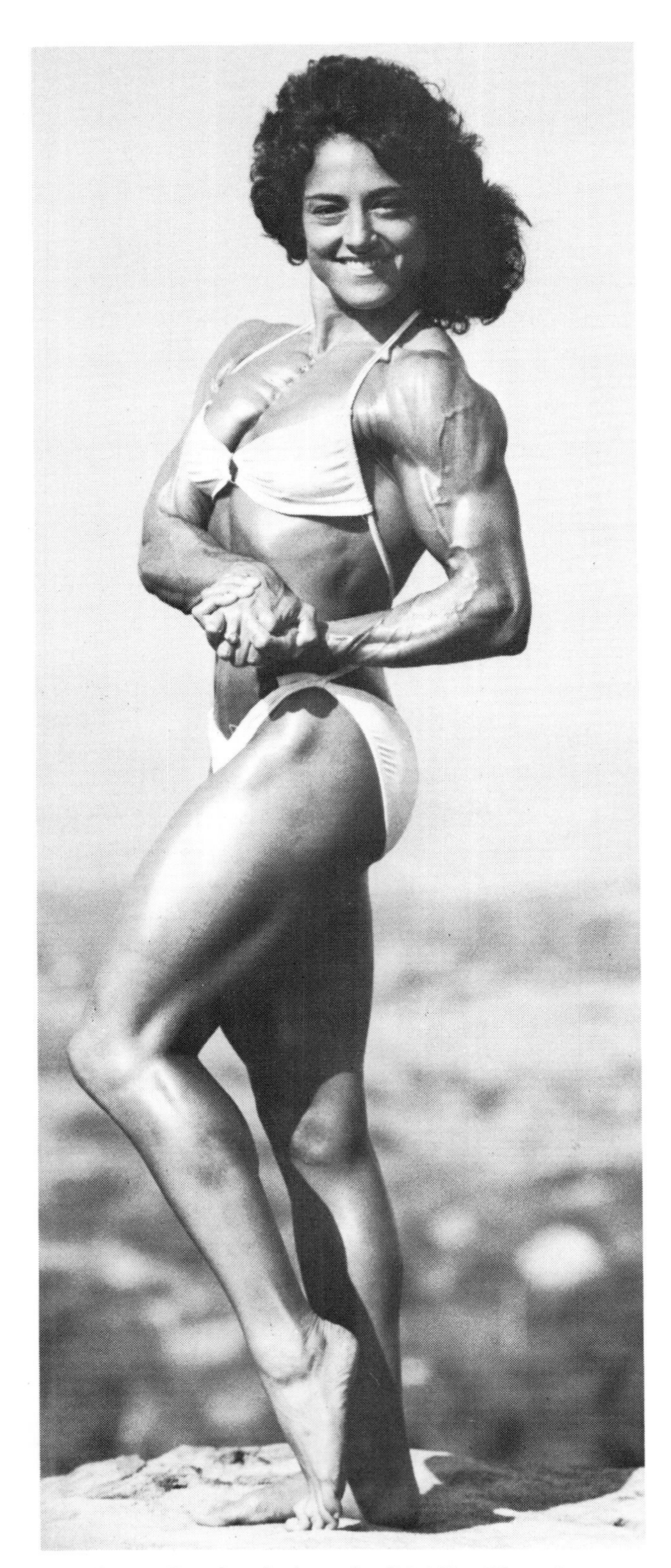

Laura Combes before the '82 Miss Olympia.
(Photo by Bill Reynolds)

hairstyle (or several hairstyles) to compliment your appearance. There is no reason why you shouldn't continue using this hairstyle. Women are required to wear their hair up off their shoulders, however, in order to avoid obscuring upper back and shoulder muscularity. As a result, you may need to work on developing an alternative hairstyle for use in competition.

Above all, avoid a harshly braided or otherwise severely styled hairstyle. The "soft" look is in for women bodybuilders. This can involve either a ponytail or an otherwise pinned-up style, such as Dr. Lynne Pirie and Laura Combes use, or a softly permed coiffure such as Lisa Elliott has adopted. As long as the hairstyle compliments your appearance, it will not detract from your placing in a bodybuilding competition.

A wide variety of flowers, headbands, and other hair ornaments have become popular with women bodybuilders. In some cases such adornments have been overdone. A subtle use of these ornaments can have a positive effect on your appearance, however.

Danny Padilla. *(Photo by Russ Warner)*

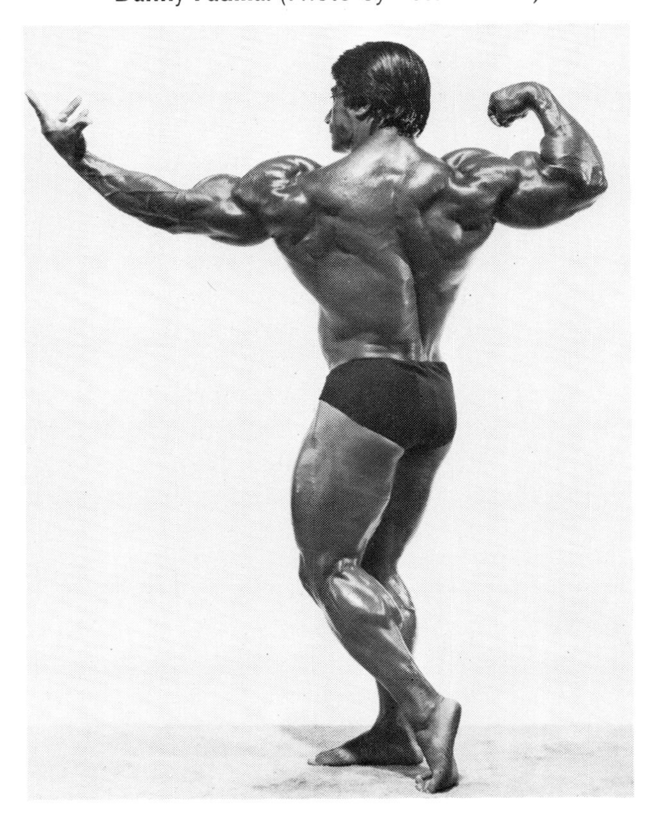

With male bodybuilders, facial hair is in. A neatly trimmed mustache, such as worn by Mike Mentzer, can add to a man's appearance and personal style. A neatly trimmed beard can also enhance a bodybuilder's appearance, though very few bearded bodybuilders have won major competitions.

Other than nonostentatious earrings and finger rings, you should avoid wearing jewelry onstage. Watches, necklaces, bracelets, waist and ankle chains, and any other such body adornment can be quite distracting to a judge. Even eyeglasses can be distracting, and we have seldom seen anyone wearing them onstage for that reason.

Posing attire should also be chosen to minimize distraction. This means avoiding patterned or multicolored posing suits. Instead, wear a solid-colored suit and be sure that the suit's color harmonizes with your own coloring.

Experiment with a variety of suit cuts to see which one does the best job of displaying your physique. These suits can be obtained through the ads of champion bodybuilders in *Muscle & Fitness* and a variety of other bodybuilding journals. Or you can find them in fashion stores and beach-wear-oriented boutiques.

If you experience difficulty in choosing an appropriate posing suit, don't be afraid to consult an experienced competitive bodybuilder or other expert. Make every effort to find appropriate posing attire. Your posing suit is the only piece of clothing you wear onstage, so select it carefully. You should also be sure to purchase two or three spare posing suits, since they quickly become oil-spotted and unusable.

Women often remove body hair as a normal course of action in their daily lives, but many men balk at doing so. A mat of body hair can obscure hard-won muscular development, however, so it's vital that you shave for contests.

To prevent razor burns and outright gashes that will show onstage, it's best to shave with a safety razor at least two weeks before a contest, then maintain the shave with an electric razor. Many champion male bodybuilders will maintain a body shave year-round in this manner.

Your first shave should be taken in a bathtub filled with hot water. If you can't figure out how to do it, ask your wife, girlfriend, or sister to show you how to shave down. You'll need someone to help you shave your back anyway.

Finally, the use of facial makeup is of concern to most women bodybuilders. We've even seen a few male bodybuilders use such makeup (in a more muted sense, however) onstage.

Bodybuilding stage makeup should be used relatively heavily—the same as theatrical stage makeup—since the lights onstage will dull the drama of ordinary makeup. The amount of makeup you use is something with which you must experiment. Try varying amounts at each contest, relying on a perceptive friend to tell you how it looks. Then, once you have developed a winning makeup formula, stick with it.

Tanning

The darker a bodybuilder's skin, the harder he or she looks, so a deep and natural tan is essential for fair-skinned competing bodybuilders. Even many black bodybuilders—such as Serge Nubert—also lie in the sun, even though their skins are very darkly hued. Nubert believes that the hot sun dries out his skin, making it much tighter and thinner looking.

It's best to begin sunbathing 4–6 weeks before a competition, so you have plenty of time to acquire a deep, even tan. This way, one or two overcast days during the last precontest week won't spell disaster to your onstage appearance.

If you haven't been in the sun much, stay out no longer than 10–15 minutes on each side of your body. Then add about 3–5 minutes per side with each additional exposure to the sun, up to approximately 60 minutes per side. This will allow you to tan gradually without receiving a painful sunburn.

In most latitudes the sun is most directly overhead between 11:00 a.m. and 1:00 p.m., so it's best to lie out during these hours. Use a suntan lotion to keep your skin soft and supple and don't be afraid to apply a sunscreen to your nose, lips, and other areas that burn easily. When you're lying on your back you can protect your eyes by placing moist cotton balls over your eyelids.

Some bodybuilders use a prescription drug called Trisoralen to enhance skin pigmentation. Trisoralen should be used only under the strict supervision of your physician, however, since it does have side effects. Trisoralen is not, incidentally, available in Canada.

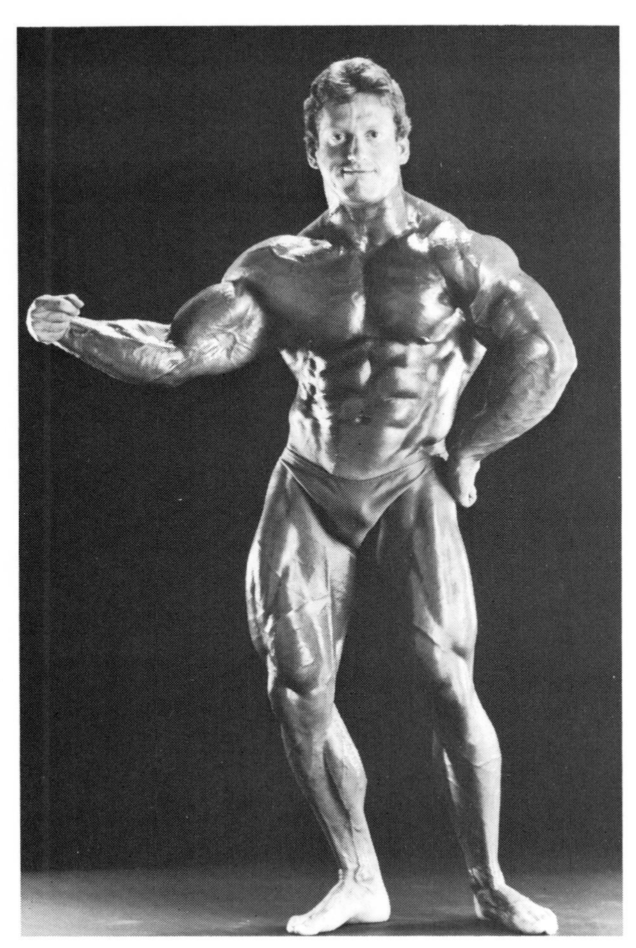

Bob Jodkiewicz.

During the winter and at other times when the sun isn't cooperative, you can profitably use a tanning salon to acquire a sunlamp tan. Many bodybuilders have used such salons and gotten good tans with them, but overall nothing can equal a natural tan acquired through exposure to the sun's rays.

Various chemical "quick-tan" preparations are occasionally used by bodybuilders, but most of these result in an odd orange- or yellow-looking tan. If you have no other alternative, however, you can use one. Be sure to wear rubber gloves and use cotton balls to apply these chemicals. You must also apply less cream to thick-skinned areas such as over the knees or elbows, since these patches of skin "tan" more quickly. And don't forget to do your face!

The use of body makeup is another alternative. One brand of makeup, Indian Earth, is very good, and you can buy it at many cosmetic counters. It gives the skin a very acceptable temporary coloring, and it takes oil well. It actually does look a bit streaky when the oil is first applied, but when it soaks into the skin the makeup regains its smoothly colored appearance.

A number of bodybuilders use a combination of natural sun, artificial light, chemical agents, and/or makeup to achieve an optimum tan. One look at the superb natural tan of a Tom Platz, however, and you'll easily be convinced that a 100% natural tan is best.

Oiling

A lot of contests are lost through thoughtless application of body oil. Properly applied, the oil will highlight your muscular development. Improperly utilized, however, body oil can obliterate your hard-earned muscularity.

Avoid using mineral oils, which lie on the surface of the skin in a thick layer. Instead, use vegetable oils, which soak into the skin and then gradually flow out with the perspiration to give a glow—rather than a sheen—to the skin. Almond and avocado oil are both good.

Apply oil lightly and evenly all over your exposed skin and rub it into the skin. It's difficult to do this for yourself, so don't be shy about bringing an "oiler" with you to a contest. Such an assistant can easily see how smoothly your oil is applied, adding oil to flat spots and blotting up excessive concentrations of it with a towel.

Like every other facet of competitive bodybuilding preparation, oiling should be practiced. Get together with your oiler a few days before competing, and be sure that he or she can oil you correctly. With the right application of body oil, your physique can look much more impressive under the lights than it would without the oil.

Pumping Up

Prior to going onstage to compete in the prejudging session—as well as before posing in the evening show—all bodybuilders pump up. A light workout backstage will force blood into your muscles, making them look larger and more impressive. Excessive pumping, however, can smooth out the cuts in a muscle group.

You should pump up for no more than 15–20 minutes before going onstage, and you should place most of your emphasis on pumping up a weak body part or two. Go ahead and do one or two light, high-rep sets for each muscle group, but on your weak points you can do as many as 6–8 total sets when pumping up the area.

Posing

Many bodybuilders—some of them champions—don't take the four semirelaxed facing poses used in Round I of the IFBB judging system very seriously. They *are* poses, however, and as such they should be practiced regularly and assiduously.

The best bodybuilders have discovered small variations of foot stance, body twist, shoulder and arm placement, and so forth that allow them to look good from all angles. Work on these in front of a two-mirror setup that allows you to see your back. Observe every angle the way individual judges will, and you'll be ahead of competitors who don't.

The best first-round posers have a confident and aggressive appearance onstage. This is partly developed by good theatrical presentation and is partly an inner confidence born of regularly practicing visualization, imagining onstage charisma, during the weeks leading up to a contest. Only regular posing practice, experience, and visualization ability will give you this winning appearance.

Since one third of your contest score is given in Round I, it's essential to practice these four facing poses hour after hour, day after day. They seem simple enough, but don't neglect them.

Another third of your score will be presented in Round II, so the compulsory poses must also be mastered. Additionally, some or all of these poses will appear in your Round III free-posing routine, so they become doubly important.

Again, subtly different body positions can greatly improve a compulsory pose. You can easily prove this to yourself by cutting out magazine photos of 15–20 champion bodybuilders doing a double-biceps pose. By placing these photos side by side, you can easily see subtle differences in how each athlete assumes the pose. Moreover, you will no doubt discover that no two bodybuilders do a pose identically.

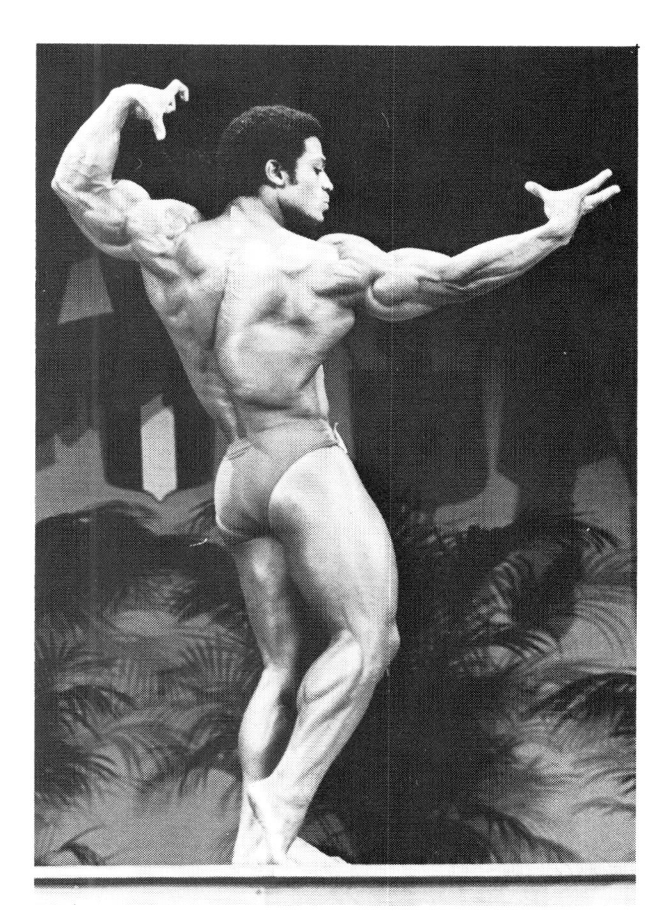

Mohamed Makkawy.

Take a clue from this revelation and practice faithfully each of the compulsory poses until you have evolved a stance for each that displays your body at its best. Only then will you be ready to enter a competition and do your best.

Some champions, such as Chris Dickerson, have actually developed transitions between compulsory poses, so they essentially have developed a routine, and this is to their advantage. The order in which you do your compulsory poses is strictly prescribed, but the transitions between them are subject only to your imagination and creative abilities.

The free-posing round displays a bodybuilder's physique in its best light. It also allows for the utmost degree of creativity and originality. As such, it is the zenith of bodybuilding posing as an art form. It will take many months of concerted effort and diligent research to develop the perfect free-posing routine for your unique physique, personality, and personal flair.

Begin developing a free-posing routine by

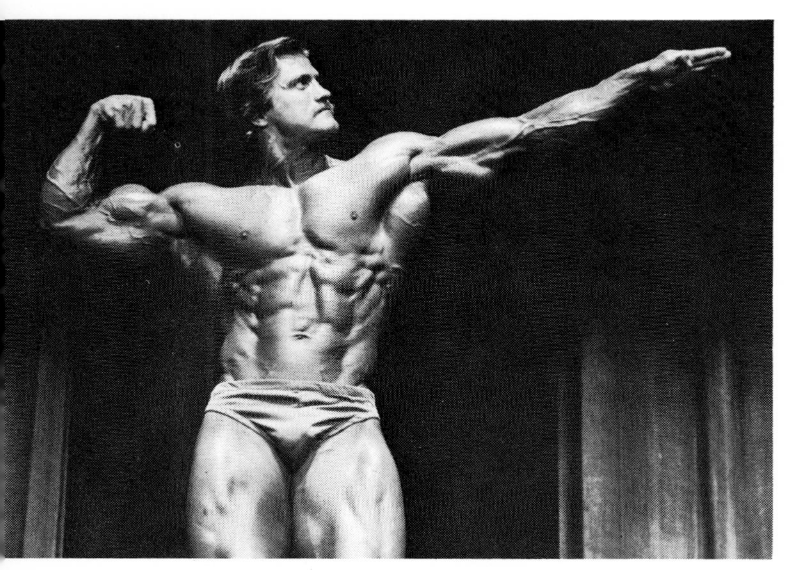

Roger Callard. *(Photo by Craig Dietz)*

James Youngblood holds up his 1981 Mr. America trophy.

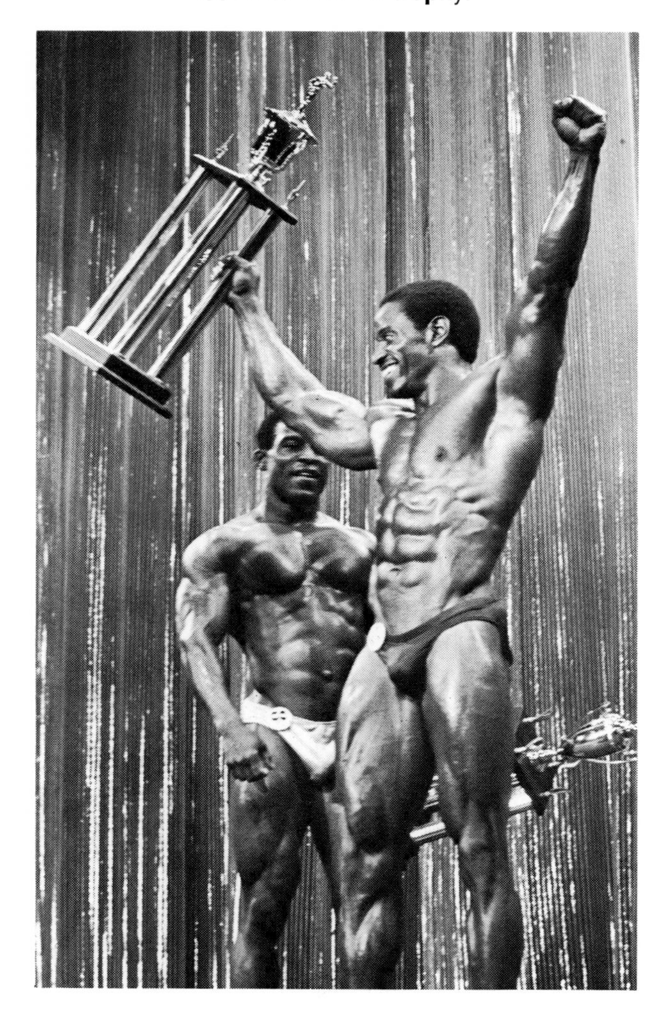

observing various poses done by bodybuilders at competitions you attend or as depicted in bodybuilding magazines. As with your compulsory poses, adapt these stances to your own use, selecting only those that make your physique appear at its best. Unlike the compulsory round, no one will force you to do a pose you don't favor in Round III. Therefore, don't include any poses that aren't really outstanding.

The more time you spend in front of a mirror, the greater number of totally unique poses you will come up with. And these highly individualized poses are what identify particular champion bodybuilders. You should constantly seek to develop them.

A novice competitive bodybuilder will need 12–15 good poses in his or her repertoire before beginning to develop a free-posing routine. The mistake many novices make is in attempting to do 25–30 poses, 15–20 of which do little or nothing for their physiques. Only an Olympian-level bodybuilder can profitably do so many poses. It takes years of practice and experience to reach the level of posing ability at which you can do that variety of poses.

Among your poses should be at least two or three that display your back, left side, and right side, in addition to the front of your body. Frequently novice competitors will display their physiques primarily from the front. You'll never see a Rachel McLish, Eddie Corney, or Chris Dickerson make such an elementary mistake. A well-developed bodybuilder who can display his or her physique from a wide variety of angles has the best chance of winning a high-level title.

As you develop your individual free-posing stances, you should also be observing the artistic transitions that accomplished bodybuilders use to move from pose to pose. You can see these at higher-level contests, or you can purchase films of better bodybuilders posing through ads in various bodybuilding magazines. With time and patience you can gradually piece together your various poses using these transitions, as well as a few transitions that you devise on your own.

Many very good bodybuilders hire the services of a choreographer to help assemble routines precisely suited to particular music. Call a dance studio or two and ask for help. Or you can do it on your own. Either way, your routine should reflect your unique personality and sense of style. And this takes time and patience. The more you practice and compete, the better you will become at free-posing.

Your musical selection should be recorded on a cassette tape. It's always a good idea to bring an extra tape with you to a competition, because sound systems sometimes eat tapes for dinner. Having a spare can save you the embarrassment of posing either to someone else's music or with no music at all.

The final type of posing that you must gradually master is used in the posedown. It is quick and aggressive posing designed to attract a judge's eye and favor. It's extremely difficult to describe such posing, so we recommend that you attend several contests and observe the posedowns. In this way you can clearly see how it's done and pattern your own posedown routine on what you have seen.

Overall, posing is a skill that *must* be mastered. Frequently, we have seen superbly developed bodybuilders lose to less impressive competitors who displayed themselves to greater advantage. If you've got the goods, learn how to flaunt 'em!

Bodybuilding Pharmacology

In recent years bodybuilders have used more and more drugs in an effort to appear even more impressive at a competition. This issue has moral overtones, but it is a fact of life, so we can't avoid discussing it. We certainly don't recommend drug usage, but we would be remiss if we didn't present the information.

The decision to use various bodybuilding drugs should be entirely yours. We certainly don't wish to influence you to use drugs, but if you are deciding to use them, you should be careful to follow these four guidelines:

1. No drug should be used without the supervision of a physician, and this supervision should include all relevant physical exams and testing procedures. Many bodybuilders make the mistake of self-administering prescription drugs purchased on the black market.

2. Be aware that every drug listed in the *PDR (Physician's Desk Reference,* a medical reference book that describes all American prescription drugs in detail) has at least one side effect, and every drug involves a certain degree of risk to its user. Before deciding to use any drug, thoroughly investigate these side effects and health hazards.

3. Avoid using all bodybuilding drugs until you have built a national-caliber physique. Using drugs, especially steroids, to build up muscle mass is dangerous. If used at all, they should be used only for short periods of time to peak for major competition.

4. Women should avoid the use of steroids, and no woman should ever use androgenic drugs. Androgenics will definitely masculinize a woman, and steroids have the potential to do the same.

There are seven general classes of bodybuilding drugs—anabolic steroids, androgenics, stimulants, depressants, appetite depressants, thyroid supplements, and analgesics. Each of these drugs will be discussed in detail on the following pages.

Anabolic Steroids

Anabolic steroids are artificial male hormones with the muscle-building anabolic component enhanced and the masculinizing androgenic component minimized. Such steroids were developed to assist malnourished World War II POWs to regain lost strength and body weight. Today they are frequently used in geriatric medicine to strengthen enfeebled elderly patients.

The muscle- and strength-building characteristics of anabolic steroids were discovered during the 1950s by strength athletes, weightlifters, and bodybuilders. During the 1960s and 1970s they became more and more commonly used, until today most top male bodybuilders use them from time to time. Even a few women have experimented with steroids.

While there is little doubt that anabolics increase strength and muscle mass, they have a number of side effects, some of them potentially catastrophic. Here are 12 side effects listed for steroids in the *PDR*:

1. Liver and kidney dysfunction and damage.
2. Possible liver, kidney, and prostate cancer.
3. Testicular atrophy and increased or decreased libido (in men).
4. Masculinization and clitoral enlargement

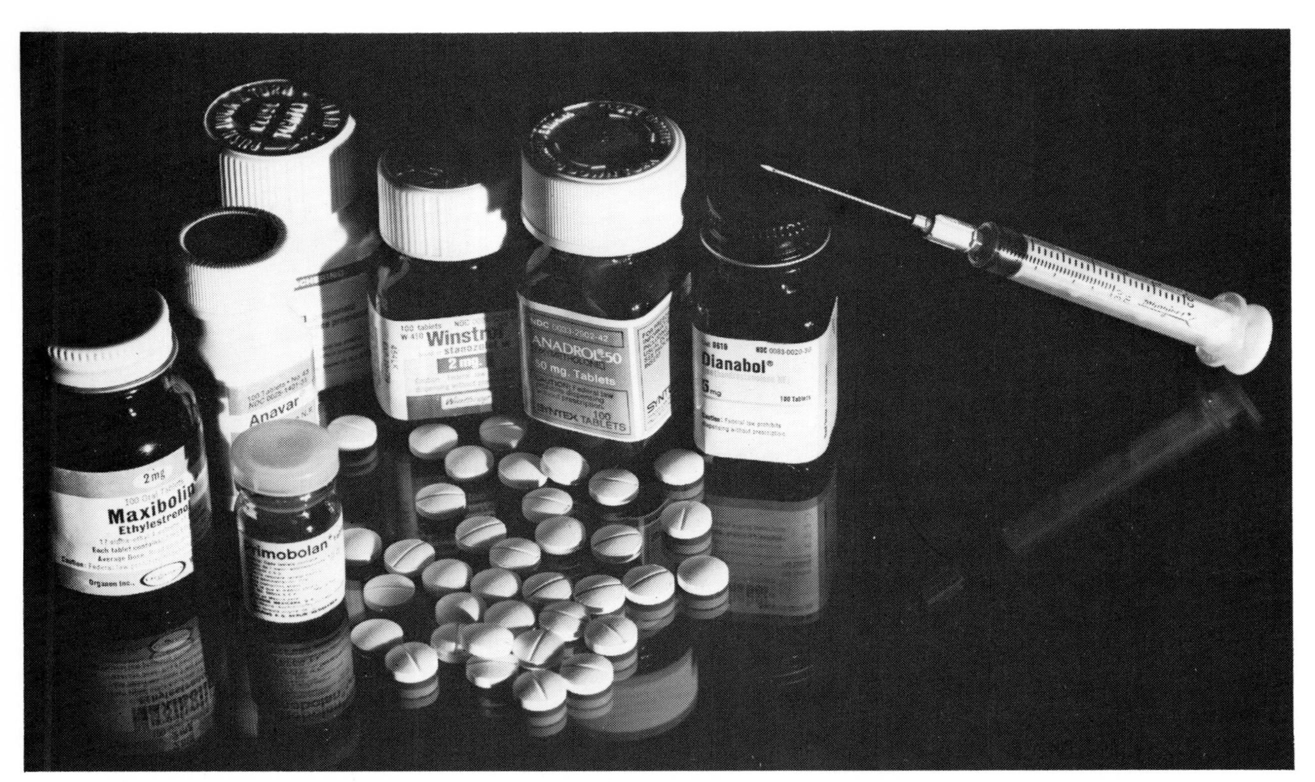

A variety of anabolic steroids and the hypodermic needle needed to administer them.

(in women). Such enlargement, incidentally, is largely irreversible.

5. Masculinization of a fetus.
6. Premature closure of bone growth plates in pubertal individuals (which results in a stunting of height).
7. Water retention and consequent high blood pressure.
8. Acne.
9. Hair loss.
10. Osteoporosis (a weakening of the bones caused by a depletion of bone calcium).
11. Increased aggression.
12. Death.

The biggest mistake you can make in using steroids is to stay on them for more than 6–8 weeks at a time. The longer you take steroids, the more you must take to achieve an anabolic effect. This is because your body gradually decreases its natural production of testosterone when you are on steroids.

The more steroids you take and the longer you're on them, the greater chance of incurring side effects. And death should certainly be avoided! Moreover, if you have taken steroids long enough, your own testosterone production will be so low that you'll lose most of your muscle mass gains once you go off the drug. It can take up to 10 weeks to regain normal testosterone output.

The most commonly used steroids are orally administered tablets like (Dianabol, Winstrol, and Anavar). Such drugs as Deca-Durobolin and Therabolin are taken via intramuscular injections. Most top bodybuilders seem to favor using injectable steroids, believing that they cause less water retention in the body and are less destructive to the liver and kidneys.

Overall, steroids are nothing to play with indiscriminantly. They are potentially dangerous prescription drugs that must be taken with care and discretion.

Androgenic Drugs

Some bodybuilders take pure testosterone injections. Testosterone has a mild anabolic effect and greatly magnified androgenic effects compared to anabolic steroids. These drugs don't provide nearly the anabolic effect of steroids. And water retention and aggression are dramatically increased. Under the circumstances, then, androgenic drugs should be avoided by all bodybuilders.

Stimulants

There's usually quite a temptation for bodybuilders to use some type of stimulant when energy is low due to rigid dieting and hard, frequent training during the last few weeks prior to a show. The mildest stimulant is caffeine, which doesn't seem to cause any deleterious effects to a competing bodybuilder. As a result, we often see bodybuilders at Gold's with a plastic cup of coffee in their hands as they arrive to work out.

Up the scale, and far more injurious (to say nothing of being illegal), are amphetamines and cocaine. Some bodybuilders do use such hardcore stimulants, but they pay a price in doing so. Such stimulants eat away at muscle tissue, causing a bodybuilder's physique to look lean and stringy rather than fully developed and crisply defined. These drugs are also highly addictive, so avoid them at all costs.

Depressants

Depressants, or "downers," are used by a few bodybuilders to sleep better than normal when nervous prior to a contest. One or two bodybuilders also use them to fortify a diet, saying, "If I eat, I can't get off on downers. So I have to avoid food when I use them!"

Depressants, particularly when consumed with alcohol, can be life-threatening. Additionally, they can cause you to sleep so much that you may skip workouts and it becomes difficult to get fully cut up for a competition. And, finally, when taking depressants frequently, it's difficult for a bodybuilder to maintain good training drive. We certainly don't recommend their use.

Appetite Depressants

These drugs are the amphetamines, cocaine, and other stimulants discussed in the foregoing section on stimulants. Again, they are addictive and will eat up your hard-earned muscle mass.

Thyroid Supplements

Many bodybuilders take synthroid, dessicated porcine thyroid, and other types of thyroid supplements to speed up their basal metabolic rates and burn off additional body fat to gain deeper cuts. These thyroid supplements do burn fat, but they're indiscriminate in what they burn; they also consume muscle mass, as do stimulants. Therefore, to achieve maximum muscle mass with good cuts, it's best to avoid thyroid drugs and merely maintain a good precontest diet for a longer period of time.

Thyroid supplements also have a number of undesirable side effects. Tachycardia (irregular heartbeat) is one side effect, and it can lead to a heart seizure. Insomnia and spontaneous perspiring are two additional side effects.

One problem with thyroid supplements is that your body's thyroxine output is lessened when you're on the supplements. As a result, some bodybuilders balloon drastically in weight once they go off the supplements. Then it's even more difficult—and it often requires even more artificially added thyroxine—to get acceptably cut up for a subsequent competitive appearance.

Analgesics

Analgesics are pain killers. They include such drugs as aspirin, Darvon, and morphine. In milder forms you can probably safely use analgesics, but you should definitely avoid the use of heavy pain killers. They can mask pain so efficiently that it's possible to injure a joint or muscle even further. Pain is nature's way of telling you that something is wrong, and the signals should be heeded.

Many bodybuilders have recently begun to use DMSO (dimethyl sulfoxide), an inexpensive industrial solvent, to deaden pain. It works for some people and doesn't for others. Investigate and give it a try for minor overtraining pains.

Go For It!

This is as far as we go together. We urge you to continue reading about the sport and learning everything you can about the various aspects of bodybuilding. Then be persistent, and you'll soon be an outstanding bodybuilder. Go for the gold with Gold's Gym!

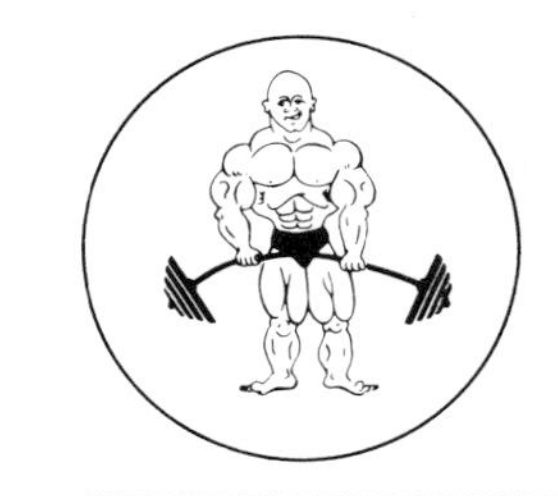

10 THE GOLD'S GYM CHAMPIONS

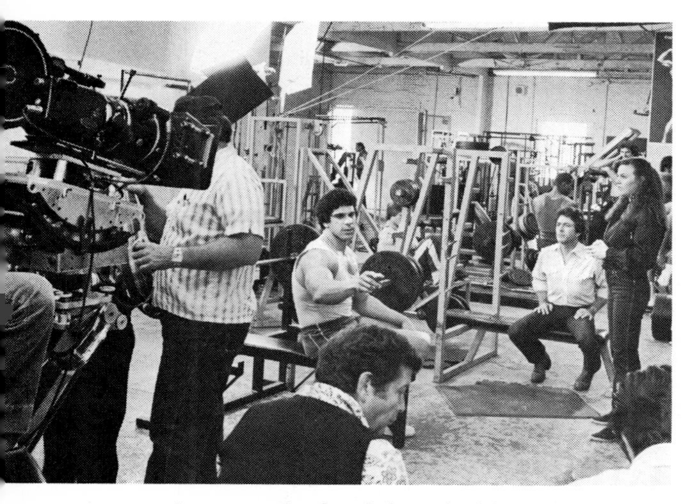

In one episode of the television series "The Incredible Hulk," Lou Ferrigno played dual roles as the Hulk and an aspiring bodybuilder who's managed by Bill Bixby (seated to Ferrigno's left.) Naturally the bodybuilding scenes were filmed at Gold's Gym. *(Photo by John Balik)*

In this innovative concluding chapter to *The Gold's Gym Bodybuilding Book* we will profile more than 150 top male and female bodybuilders who have worked out at Gold's Gym through the years at one or more of its three locations—at 2006 Pacific Avenue in Venice, California; at 1452 2nd Street in Santa Monica; or at its current location, 364 Hampton Drive in Venice. If the chapter reads like a *Who's Who In Bodybuilding,* that is simply because virtually every top American bodybuilder—as well as a large number of international champions from other countries—have trained in Gold's at some point in their careers.

With each short personality profile, we will present a body part routine from the champion profiled. There are at least 10 different routines for every body part, except for the neck which very few bodybuilders train directly. For the arms, chest, back, shoulders, and thighs you will have more than 20 routines per body part from which to choose as you experiment to discover what types of training programs work best for your unique body.

Photos of virtually all of these great champions are included either within this chapter or elsewhere throughout the book. Unfortunately, we couldn't obtain photos of a handful of these champs. You will also notice that there are far more male bodybuilders presented than female bodybuilders. Rest assured that this is not a sexist gambit on our part, but rather the consequence of women's competitive bodybuilding being such a new sport.

It's possible that we might have overlooked a handful of champions while researching and compiling this chapter. Such omissions were entirely unintentional.

Brian Abadie

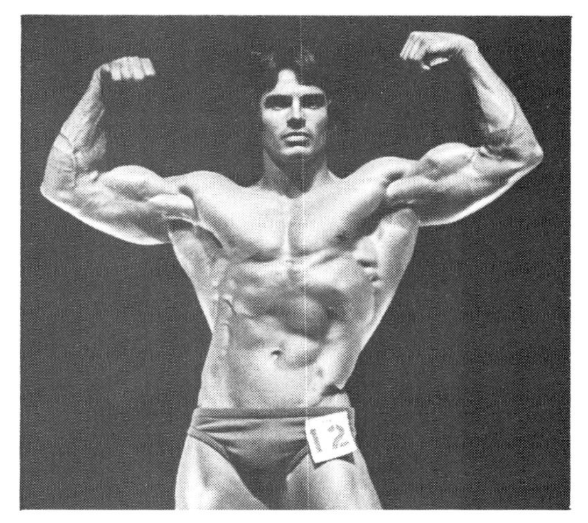

Brian Abadie. *(Art Zeller)*

Originally from Louisiana, Brian won the Junior Mr. California competition in 1977. With his symmetrical, muscular, and esthetic physique, he could have gone much further in bodybuilding had he desired to continue training for competition. For a time, Brian served as manager of Gold's Gym, and he was well known for his great leg strength. At a body weight of slightly under 200 pounds, he has squatted two reps with 600 pounds.

Because he was such a phenomenally powerful squatter, Brian didn't need to emphasize that movement much in his thigh routine. So, he placed most of his energies on shaping exercises. Here's one thigh routine he used while training at Gold's:

1. Squat (warm-up only): 1 × 20–30
2. Hack Squat: 4–5 × 10–15
3. Leg Extension: 4–5 × 10–15
4. Leg Curl: 6–8 × 10–15
5. Lunge (precontest only): 4–5 × 15

Dale Adrian

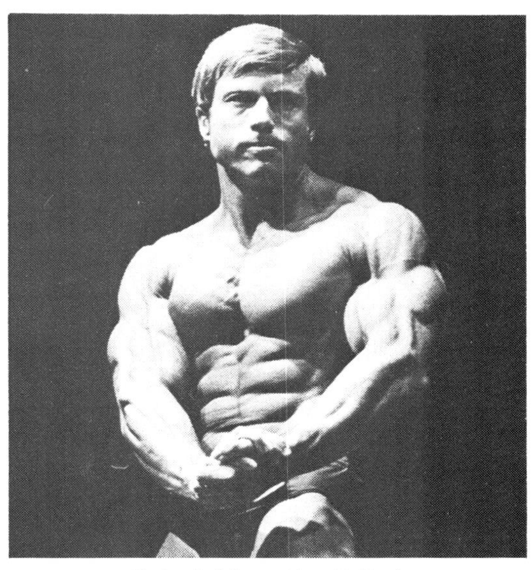

Dale Adrian. *(Art Zeller)*

Dale won the 1975 Mr. California and Mr. America competitions, creating quite a sensation in the process. He's been in semiretirement but plans a big comeback as soon as job pressures abate.

Adrian's legs were phenomenally impressive, and he's the only athlete to win the "Best Legs" subdivision four consecutive years in the Mr. California competition. Here is a Dale Adrian thigh workout:

1. Hack Squat: 6–10 × 10–20
2. Squat: 6–10 × 10–20
3. Leg Extension: 8–10 × 15–20, supersetted with . . .
4. Sissy Squat: 8–10 × 20
5. Leg Curl: 6–8 × 10–15

Obviously, Dale believes in doing a high number of sets for each muscle group, and he also uses quite substantial poundages in each exercise once he is fully warmed up. As an example, he uses 250 pounds for Leg Extensions and 150 pounds for Leg Curls in the above program. Try that sometime!

Madeline Almeida

Pert Madeline Almeida has won the Ms. Eastern America title and placed high in the Ms. America competition. At 5′0″ in height she packs 95 pounds of well-defined and shapely muscle mass on her body at contest time. Blessed with naturally balanced proportions and symmetry, Madeline could go much higher in competitive bodybuilding if she continues to train in her usual high-intensity manner.

Here is a typical Madeline Almeida thigh routine (all sets are done to failure, most with forced reps and some with negatives):

1. Leg Extensions: 4 × 10–12
2. Leg Press: 4 × 10–12
3. Leg Curls: 3 × 10–12
4. Lunges: 2 × 10–15

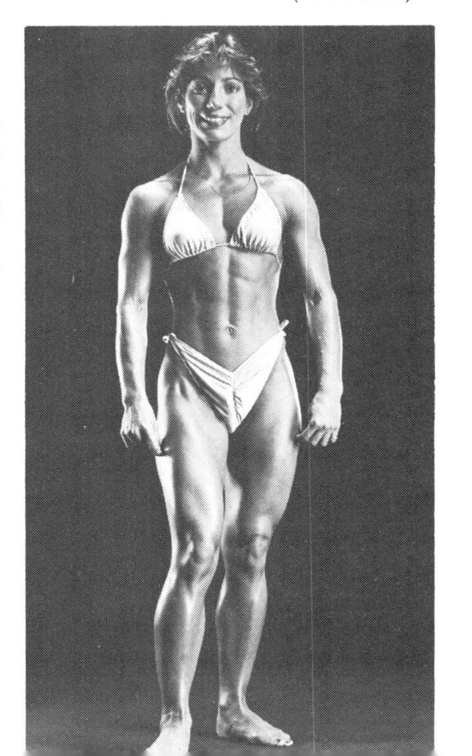

Madeline Almeida.

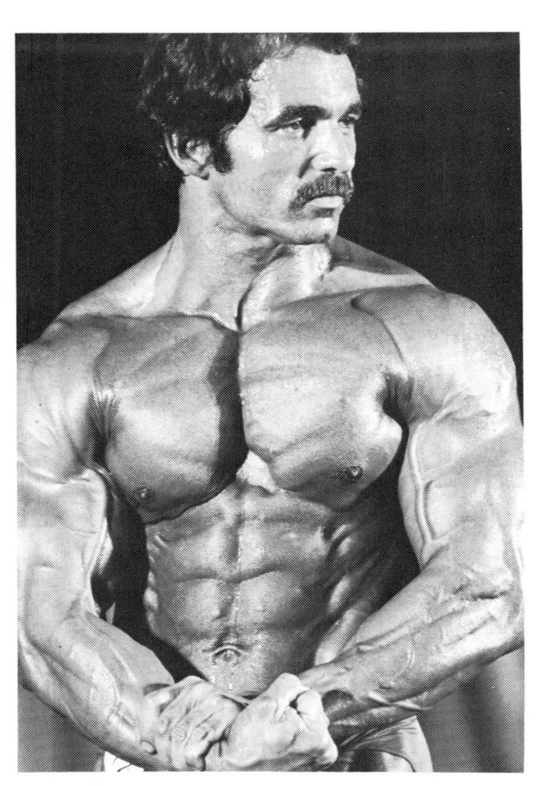

Billy Arlen.

Billy Arlen

A three-time All-American halfback on the Sam Houston University football team that won the 1966 NAIA National Championships, Arlen was first inspired to train with weights by viewing a Steve Reeves muscle movie at the age of 15. As a bodybuilder he has won the Mr. Texas title and has been in the final three in the Mr. USA, Mr. America and IFBB Mr. International competitions. He is definitely one of the best amateur bodybuilders in America.

Arlen prefers to do about 15–20 total sets per body part on a six-day split routine (each major muscle group is hit three times per week) prior to competition. He also prefers a lot of variety in his workouts, as indicated in this deltoid routine.

1. Seated Press Behind Neck: 3 × 8–10
2. Seated Bent Laterals: 3 × 8–10
3. Dumbbell Presses: 2 × 8–10
4. Side Laterals: 2 × 8–10
5. Cable Side Laterals: 2 × 8–10
6. Cable Bent Laterals: 3 × 8–10

A resident of Houston, Texas, Billy Arlen is married and works as a high school teacher and football coach.

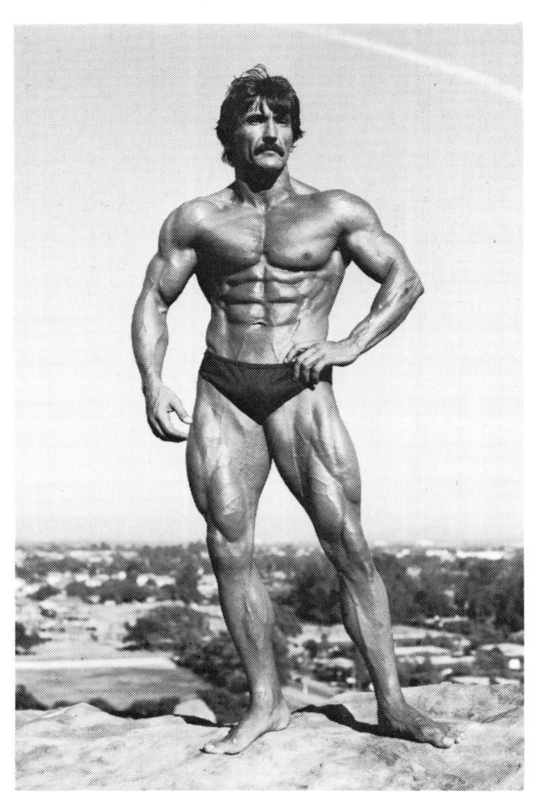

Mike Armstrong.

Mike Armstrong

Originally from Alabama, Mike moved to southern California during the early 1970s specifically to train at Gold's Gym. And he has worked out extensively at all three Gold's Gyms in the Venice-Santa Monica area. A teacher in the Los Angeles school system, Armstrong has won the Mr. Alabama, Mr. San Pedro, Mr. Southeastern, Mr. Olympic (he stresses that the title name ends with a "c" rather than an "a") and Mr. Region III titles. At 5′9″ and 192 pounds at contest time, Mike Armstrong displays a very muscular, symmetrical, and classically proportioned physique.

Mike has deeply etched abdominals, and he gave the authors this three-days-per-week abdominal routine:

1. Hanging Leg Raises: 3 × 30–20 (to failure each set)
2. Twisting Cable Crunches: 4 × 20–30 (he does 20–30 reps, each to the left side, right side, and directly forward, all three directions to failure)
3. Weighted Sit-Ups: 40 lbs., 5 × 10 (to failure), plus 20–30 additional reps each set with no added weight.

"Virtually all bodybuilders make the mistake of training their abdominals aerobically, that is with very high reps and low intensity," Armstrong stated. "It's better to treat them just like any other muscle group. Use weights to train them, and do so with high intensity."

Bronston Austin, Jr.

A native of Illinois, Bronston has spent considerable time training at Gold's Gym. He was originally a powerlifter who registered official lifts of 625 pounds in the Squat, 510 in the Bench Press, and 670 in the Deadlift at a body weight of 198 pounds. As a bodybuilder, he has won the Mr. Midwest, Mr. Central States, and Mr. Western America titles. Bronston has also won his class at the Mr. America competition and placed second behind Johnny Fuller in the 1980 Light-Heavyweight Mr. Universe contest.

One of Bronston Austin's favorite back routines is as follows:

1. Seated Pulley Rowing: 5–8 × 5–8
2. T-Bar Rowing: 5–8 × 5–8
3. Barbell Bent Rowing: 5–8 × 5–8
4. One-Arm Dumbbell Bent Rowing: 5–8 × 5–8
5. Nautilus Pullover: 5–8 × 5–8
6. Lat Pulldown: 5–8 × 8–10

A teacher by profession, Austin has a master's degree. He is married and has two children.

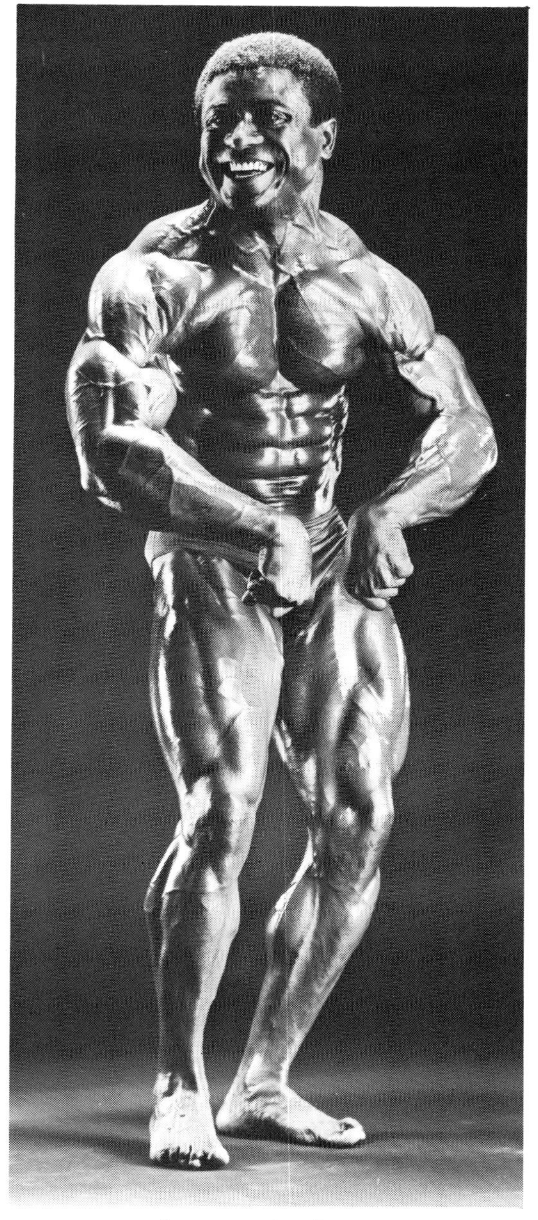

Bronston Austin.

Richard Baldwin

Owner of his own gym in Tallahassee, Florida, Richard has spent considerable time training at Gold's Gym for high-level competitions. He's won Mr. Florida, Collegiate Mr. America, his class in the Mr. America contest (twice), and has twice placed second in the IFBB Mr. Universe contest. At 5′8″ in height he packs an esthetic 180 pounds of superhard muscle on his physique.

Here is a deltoid program that Richard Baldwin contributed.

1. Press Behind the Neck: 6 × 6–10
2. Bent Lateral: 5 × 8–10
3. Cable Upright Rowing: 5 × 8–10
4. Dumbbell Press: 3 × 6–10, supersetted with. . .
5. Front Raise: 3 × 8–10

"On most exercises I do a light set, three hard sets at a steady weight, and a final pump set," Richard concluded.

John Balik

John Balik, the outstanding bodybuilding photographer who took all of the exercise photos and many other photos in this book, was a very successful competitive bodybuilder during the late 1960s. John won the Junior Mr. Los Angeles, Junior Mr. California, and Mr. Western USA titles. He also placed third in the 1967 Mr. California competition, won by Chris Dickerson.

Balik's super color and black-and-white photography has long been one of the strongest features of *Muscle & Fitness* magazine, and he has photographically illustrated numerous other bodybuilding books. John even finds time to write magazine articles on his special area of interest, bodybuilding nutrition.

Here is a typical John Balik chest training program (chest is worked twice during an eight-day training cycle):

1. Incline Flyes: 3 × 5–10
2. Bench Press: 3 × 5–10
3. Cable Crossovers: 3 × 5–10

"Actually, I train every body part differently from workout to workout, since that builds maximum variety and interest into my training sessions," John commented. "For my chest I normally do three sets each of three or four exercises, choosing from a pool of 10–12 movements."

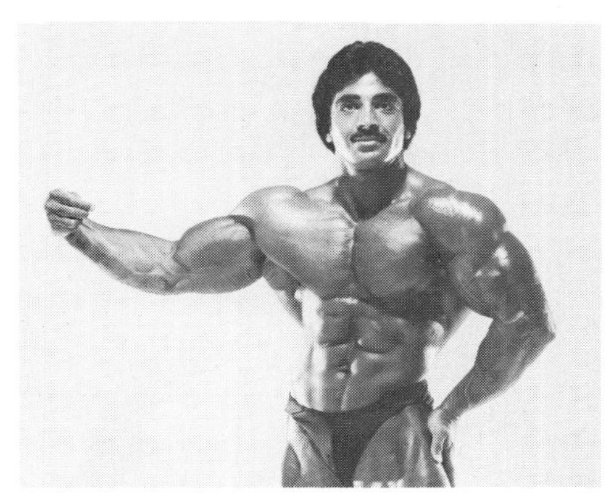

Samir Bannout.

Samir Bannout

Born in Beirut, Lebanon, Samir was by his own admission "an incredible pencil neck" before taking up bodybuilding training. His knees were actually larger than his pipestem thighs. But through many years of hard bodybuilding training, "The Lion of Lebanon" succeeded in adding more than 100 pounds of quality muscle tissue to his puny frame. His physical excellence—particularly his superb symmetry and muscle shape—eventually won for him the titles of Mr. World and Mr. Universe. Still in his mid-20s, Samir has his best years ahead of him.

Bannout believes in a combination of heavy basic exercises and lighter shaping movements in training each muscle group. Following this philosophy, here is one of Samir's most effective thigh workouts, which he performs at Gold's twice a week in the off-season and three times per week prior to a competition:

1. Squat: 1–2 warm-up sets, then 5–6 progressively heavier sets of 6–8 reps up to a max of about 500 pounds.
2. Hack Squat: 4 × 10–12
3. Leg Extension: 4 × 10–12
4. Leg Curl: 5–6 × 10–12

Prior to a contest Samir will also include four or five sets and 15 reps of Lunges. And he does some sprinting to bring out maximum thigh cuts.

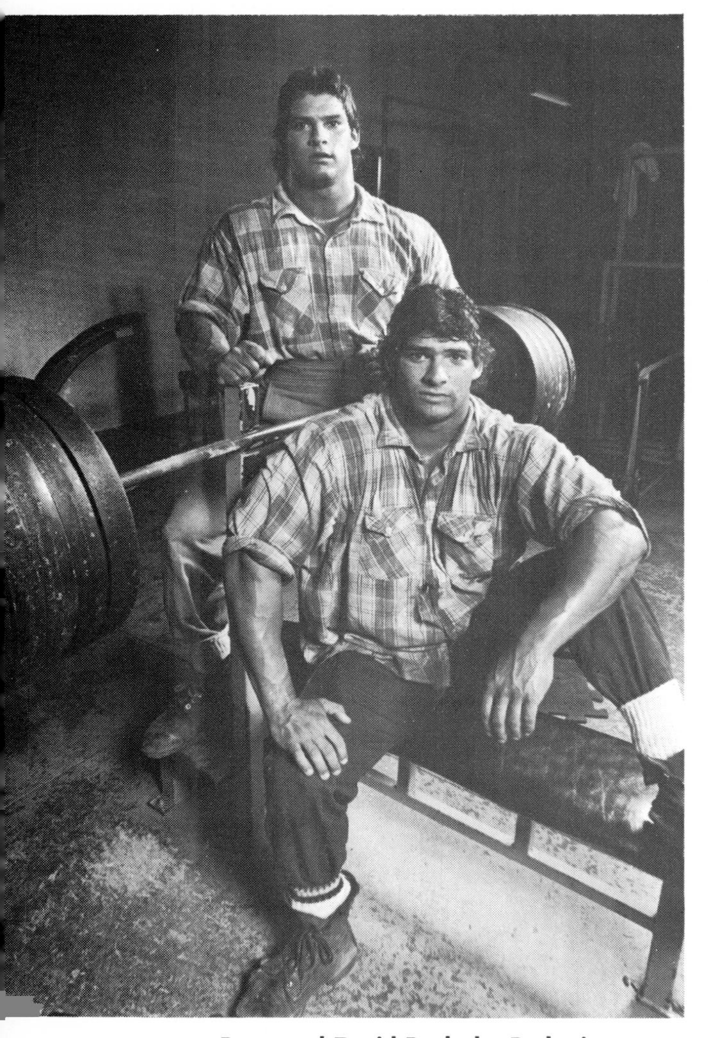

Peter and David Paul, the Barbarians.
(Mike Neveux)

The Barbarians

Two of the most colorful characters ever to stomp through Gold's Gym are The Barbarians, Peter and David Paul, "the world's most powerful twin human beings." While neither has yet competed as a bodybuilder, both Peter and David are thickly developed and phenomenally strong. How's a Reverse-Grip Bench Press with 500+ pounds sound for power?

Since The Barbarians don't follow a set routine, we present below several of their typical philosophical quotes:

- The man who sees the invisible will do the impossible. We cannot be defeated because we refuse to admit defeat. No force on earth can oppose us. Like the starving wolf, we will die before we will back down. We do not believe—we *know!*
- There's no such thing as overtraining. It's a word used by the weak-minded. There is only undereating, undersleeping, and the failure of will.
- The mind and body are one. As one grows, so does the other. The bigger and stronger the body becomes, the more intelligent the mind.

Clarence Bass

An attorney from Albuquerque, New Mexico, Clarence is well known for his ability to get his body fat level down to 2%. He's won his class at both the Past-40 Mr. America and Past-40 Mr. USA competitions, and he's long been a top-level judge and National Physique Committee official.

While Clarence does most of his training in his own well-equipped home gym, he bombs away at Gold's Gym whenever in Los Angeles. Here's his favorite thigh routine:

1. Nautilus Leg Extension: 1 × 8–10
2. Vertical Leg Press: 1–2 × 10–12
3. Hack Machine Squat: 1 × 10–15
4. Horizontal Leg Press: 1 × 10–15
5. Nautilus Leg Curl: 2 × 10–15

This thigh workout is essentially done as a giant set, with very little rest between sets.

Kay Baxter

Kay is one of the true pioneers of women's bodybuilding, having won titles as long ago as 1978. Among her titles are Ms. Southwest, Ms. Southern Pacific, and Ms. Gold's Classic. Kay has also placed second in the 1981 World Women's Professional Bodybuilding Championships. Consistently featured in bodybuilding magazines and a threat to win any bodybuilding competition she enters, Kay has been an AFWB State Representative and judged the Ms. America contest.

Kay gave the authors of this book the following biceps routine, which she consistently uses at Gold's Gym.

1. Cable Preacher Curl: 4 × 12–15
2. Standing Barbell Curl: 4 × 10–12
3. Incline Dumbbell Curl: 4 × 10–12
4. Dumbbell Concentration Curl: 4 × 15–20

Kay Baxter has a degree in physical education and is an accomplished professional singer.

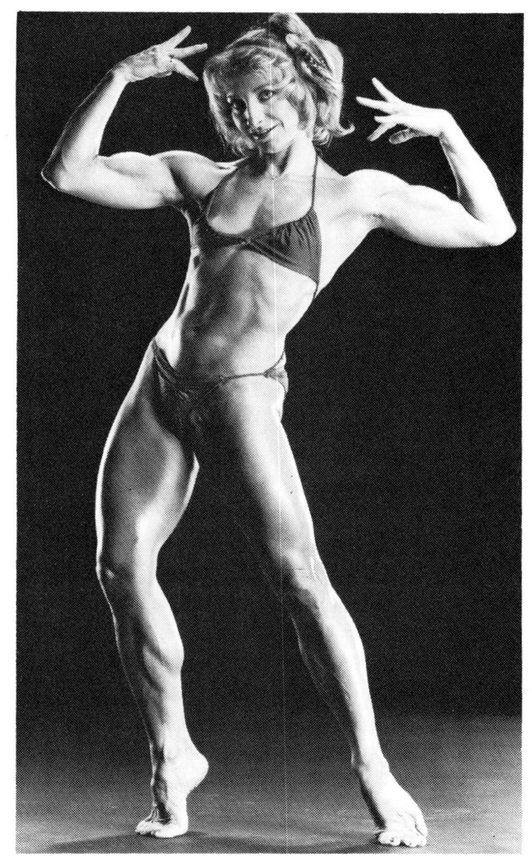

Kay Baxter.

Ray Beaulieu

Ray has won Mr. Canada twice, placed in the top five in the Lightweight IFBB Mr. Universe competition, and won numerous smaller titles. As an airline employee, he can fly down to Gold's frequently at minimal cost. At 5′3½″ in height, Ray packs on 165–170 pounds of fairly hard muscle mass in the off-season, so it's ordinarily a bit of a struggle for him to reach the Lightweight Class limit of 70 kg. (154½ lbs.). He does so with a low-calorie diet of natural foods and ends up extremely cut-up in the process.

We solicited Beaulieu's forearm program, which is as follows:

Monday-Wednesday-Friday

1. Barbell Reverse Curl: 4–5 × 8–10
2. Dumbbell Wrist Curl: 4–5 × 10–15

Tuesday-Thursday-Saturday

1. Barbell Wrist Curl: 4–5 × 10–15
2. Barbell Reverse Wrist Curl: 4–5 × 10–15

"The forearms are very tough muscle tissue—like the calves—so they need near-daily training like in my routine," Ray commented. "With persistence, however, this training program will give you forearms that look like bowling pins."

Ray Beaulieu

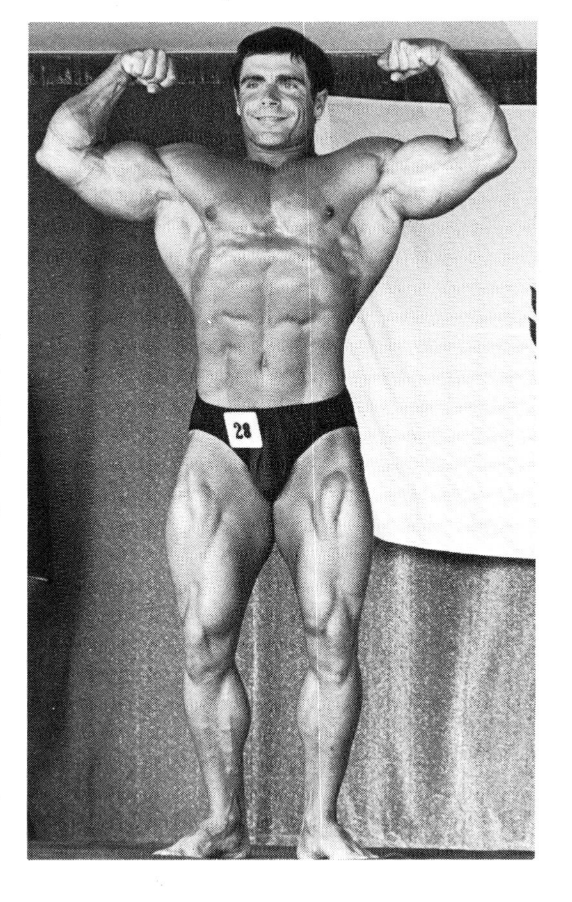

Darcy Beccles

One of the most outstanding bodybuilders ever to spend a summer training at Gold's was Barbados native Darcy Beccles. Darcy has won the Mr. Caribbean and Mr. World titles, and he has one of the greatest differences in girth between chest and waist ever seen in the sport. For a time, Beccles was Robby Robinson's training partner, and the dynamic duo pumped iron like a well-oiled machine.

Darcy has had to work exceptionally hard on his calves. Here are the routines he used when training at Gold's.

Monday-Wednesday-Friday

1. Seated Calf Machine: 4–6 × 10–15
2. Donkey Calf Raise: 4–6 × 15–20
3. Seated Calf Press: 4–6 × 15–20

Tuesday-Thursday-Saturday

1. Standing Calf Machine: 4–6 × 10–15
2. Dumbbell One-Leg Calf Raise: 4–6 × 15–20
3. Lying Calf Press: 4–6 × 15–20

Darcy also recommends stretching and flexing the calves several times per day.

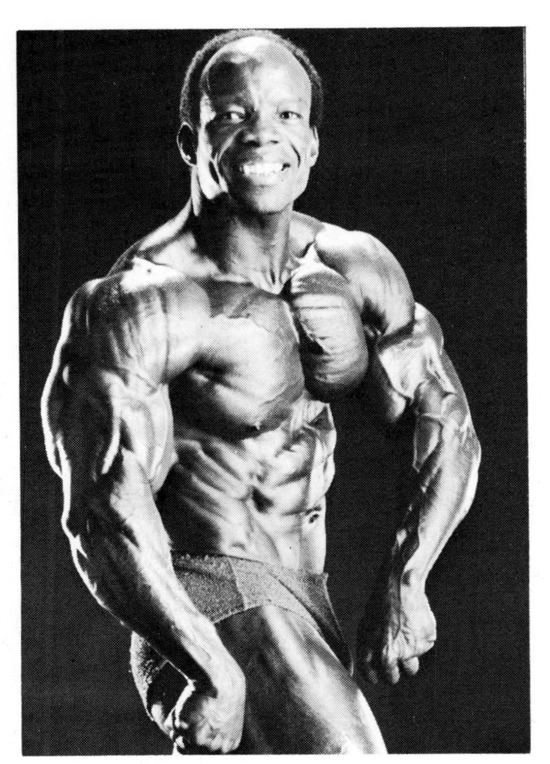
Albert Beckles.

Albert Beckles

Originally from the island of Barbados in the Caribbean, Albert has lived most of his life in England. One of the elite pro bodybuilders of the current day (at age 45!), Albert has won Mr. Britain (twice), Mr. Europe, Mr. Universe, the New England Grand Prix, the World Professional Championships, and the Night of the Champions pro event. An accountant, Beckles is retired from government service, but he still trains in a fully equipped gym at the British Ministry of War in London where he worked.

Albert's most notable feature is his biceps development, but he seldom trains that body part. Therefore, we present his chest workout, as we observed it done when he trained at Gold's Gym.

1. Dumbbell Bench Press: 5 × 10–12
2. Flat-Bench Flye: 5 × 10–12
3. Weighted Dip: 5 × 10–12
4. Cross-Bench Dumbbell Pullover: 5 × 10–15

"My normal off-season poundage for Dumbbell Bench Presses is 180 pounds in each hand," Albert noted. "But prior to a contest I use only 120-pound dumbbells, due to my tight diet and faster training."

To achieve his startling muscularity, Beckles diets for up to three months on a low-fat and nearly zero-carb diet. It's a tough nutritional regimen to follow, but it obviously works!

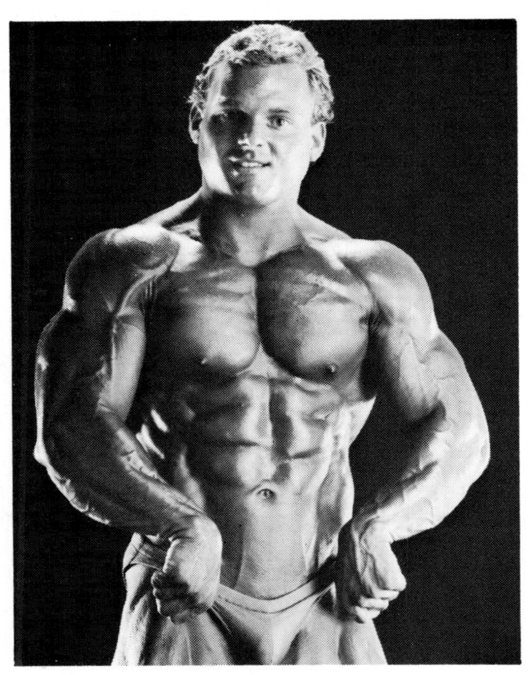
Tim Belknap.

Tim Belknap

One of the most massive and powerful bodybuilders of all time, Belknap roared out of Illinois to win the 1981 Mr. America title. And it was quite an accomplishment for a diabetic kid who once weighed only 95 pounds and was so weak that girls could beat him up! Now he can do 10 reps with 675 pounds in the Squat and six reps with 505 pounds in the Bench Press. Truly, Tim is a future superstar.

Belknap contributed the following abdominal routine that he used regularly while training at Gold's Gym.

1. Crunch: 5 × 20–30, supersetted with. . .
2. Cable Leg Raise: 5 × 20–30
3. Side Bend: 5 × 30–50

To watch Tim Belknap train twice a day for the America on less than 900 calories of food intake a day was an awesome sight!

Ulf Bengtsson

Ulf is a high-level Swedish bodybuilder who frequently spends his summers at Gold's in order to peak maximally for the fall international competitions. A former Mr. Sweden and Junior Mr. Scandinavia, Bengtsson has been a finalist in several Mr. Universe and Mr. International competitions. Ulf's esthetically developed physique is widely envied.

Bengtsson contributed the following precontest thigh routine, which he does three days per week.

1. Squat (warm-up only): 1–2 × 15–20
2. Hack Machine Squat: 4–5 × 10–15
3. Sissy Squat: 4–5 × 10–15
4. Leg Extension: 4–5 × 10–15
5. Lunge: 4–5 × 10–15
6. Nautilus Leg Curl: 6–8 × 10–15

Reggie Bennett

Reggie moved from Texas to California specifically to train at Gold's Gym. She has won her class in the Texas Cup Championships, Ms. Texas (twice), and Ms. South Texas (twice). She is 21 years of age, 5'7" tall, weighs 125 pounds in contest condition, and sports 14-inch upper arms. A former powerlifter, Ms. Bennett has best lifts of 240 pounds in the Squat, 170 in the Bench Press, and 350 in the Deadlift. Also a champion arm wrestler, Reggie has never been defeated by a woman and has beaten most of the men she's arm wrestled.

Reggie Bennett contributed the following precontest abdominal routine, which she performs five or six days per week.

1. Knees-to-Chest Crunch: 3 × 30
2. Gravity-Boot Hanging Crunch: 3 × 15
3. Roman Chair Sit-up: 5 × 30 (no added weight)
4. Roman Chair Sit-up: 5 × 15 (with added weight)
5. Seated Twisting: 5 × 50
6. Hanging Leg Raise: 3 × 15

"I also use an electronic muscle stimulator on my abdominals every other night for 30 minutes just before going to bed," Reggie revealed.

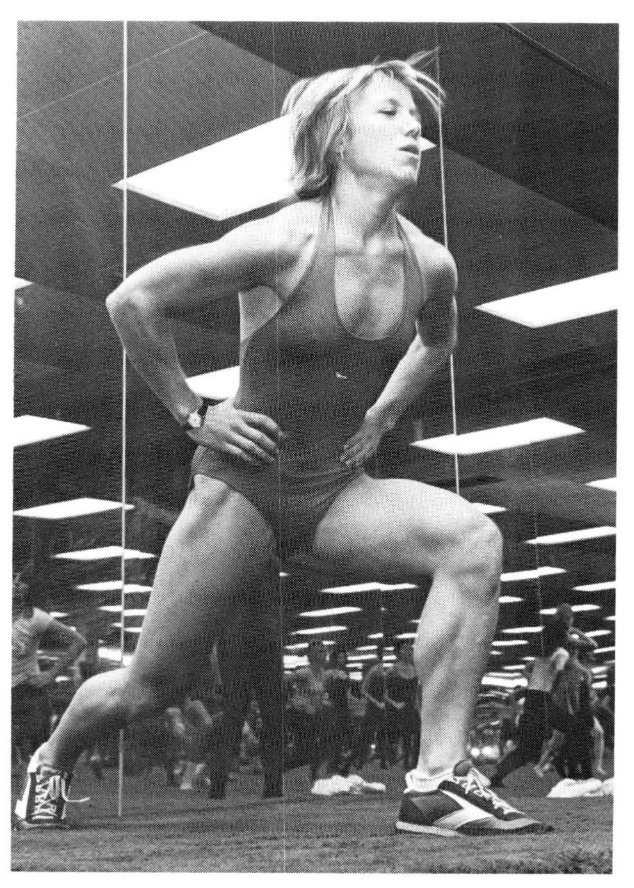

Stacey Bentley.

Stacey Bentley

Stacey is one of the early pioneers of women's bodybuilding. After moving from Pennsylvania to train at Gold's she placed in the top five in the first World Women's Bodybuilding Championships promoted by Gold's Gym in Los Angeles in June 1979. Then she won the 1980 Zane Pro Invitational Championships and placed in the top five at the 1980 Ms. Olympia show. A born-again Christian, she is currently retired from competition.

Here is a typical Stacey Bentley precontest back workout, which was done three days per week:

1. Deadlift: 5 × 12–15
2. Dumbbell Bent Rowing: 5 × 12–15
3. Hyperextension: 5 × 12–15
4. Lat Pulldown: 3 × 6–8
5. Seated Pulley Rowing: 3–5 × 8–12

Stacey dieted on as few as 800 calories per day prior to competition and did plenty of aerobic training to reach peak muscular definition.

Renato Bertagna.

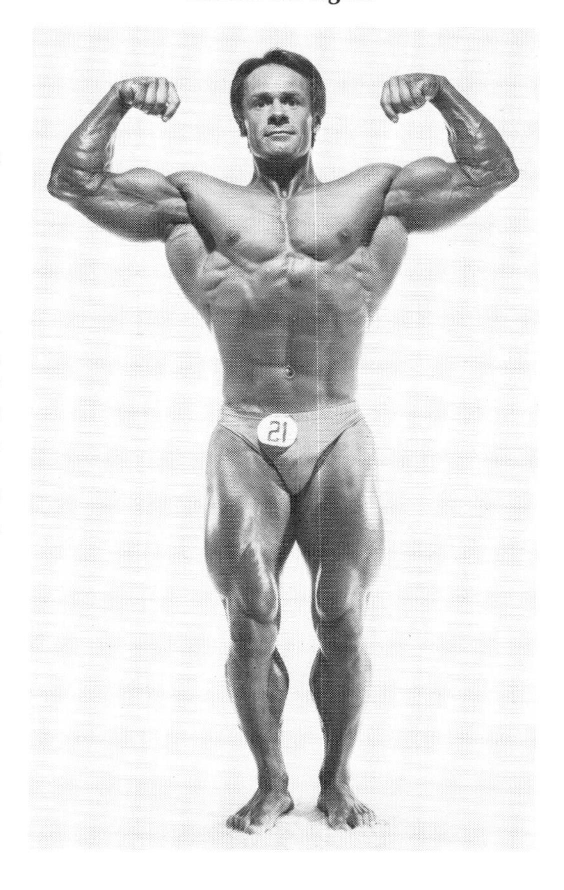

Renato Bertagna

Bertagna has won the IFBB Mr. Universe and Mr. International titles, as well as Mr. Italy and Mr. Europe. A mechanic living in Milano, Italy, Renato has never turned professional, and he continues to terrorize lightweight competitors in international contests with his thickly developed and well-proportioned physique. When in California, he frequently trains at Gold's Gym.

Renato believes in training all of his body parts hard, and his forearms are no exception to the rule. Here are his routines for forearm development:

Monday-Thursday

1. Reverse Barbell Curl: 4–6 × 8–10
2. Barbell Wrist Curl: 4–6 × 12–15

Tuesday-Friday

1. One-Arm Dumbbell Wrist Curl: 4–6 × 12–15
2. Barbell Reverse Wrist Curl: 4–6 × 12–15

With attention to detail such as this, it's easy to see why Renato Bertagna has been so successful in international competition.

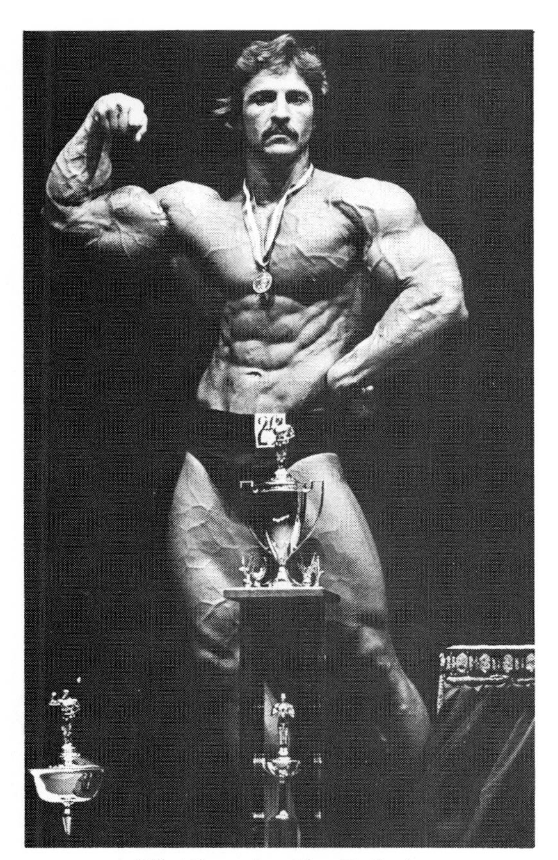

Clint Beyerle. *(Art Zeller)*

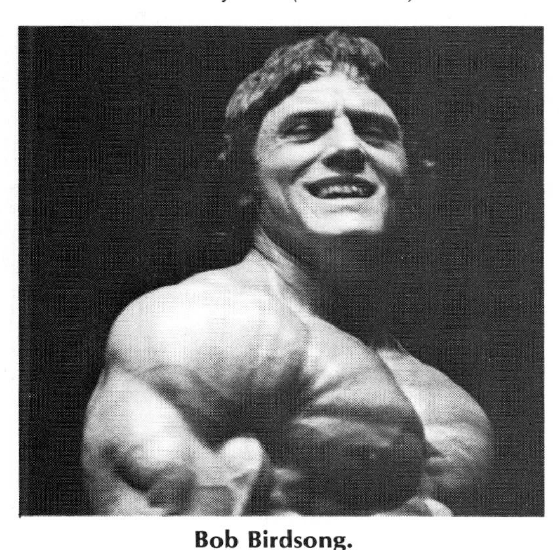

Bob Birdsong.

Karl Blömer. *(Benno Dahmen)*

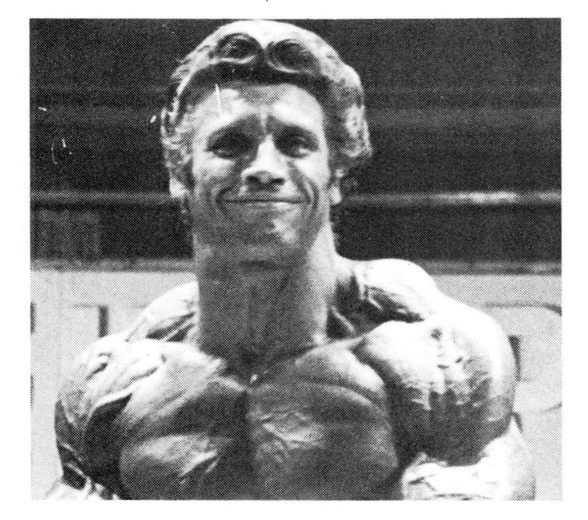

Clint Beyerle

Winner of the prestigious Mr. USA title and a former second-place finisher in the Mr. America competition, Clinton is a practicing chiropractor, an amateur pilot, and a general *bon vivant.* He's particularly noted in bodybuilding circles for his extreme vascularity. The veins in his arms, shoulders, and chest look like a relief map of the Los Angeles freeway system.

Dr. Clint follows a relatively low-carbohydrate diet year-round but reduces his carb intake virtually to zero for four to six weeks before a competition in order to bring out his best cuts. During the off-season he reserves Sunday as a junk food day but follows a good bodybuilding diet the other six days per week.

Beyerle's deltoids are undoubtedly his best body part, and here is one of his off-season shoulder routines:

1. Press Behind the Neck: 6–8 × 8–2 (up to 270 lbs.)
2. Side Lateral: 4–5 × 8–10
3. Dumbbell Press: 4–5 × 8–10
4. Cable Bent Lateral: 5–6 × 8–10

Bob Birdsong

One of the most popular Gold's Gym members during the mid-1970s was Bob Birdsong, Mr. Pacific Coast, Mr. America, and Pro Mr. Universe. After a four-year retirement to study for a Christian ministry, Birdsong recently made a successful comeback as a pro bodybuilder, placing well in the Mr. Olympia contest and other high-level events. He works as a traveling youth counselor all over the Pacific Southwest, traveling from a home base in Palm Springs, California, where he lives with his wife and child.

Bob Birdsong's balanced and super-muscular physique was complemented by terrific forearms. Here are the forearm workouts he often performed at Gold's:

Monday-Wednesday-Friday

1. Barbell Wrist Curl (Bench Supported): 5 × 15
2. Reverse Wrist Curl: 5 × 15
3. One-Arm Dumbbell Wrist Curl (Supported): 5 × 15

Tuesday-Thursday

1. Barbell Wrist Curl: 5 × 15
2. Standing Barbell Wrist Curl (Behind Back): 5 × 15

Karl Blömer

A gym owner and successful nightclub entertainer in Köln, Germany, Blömer enjoyed his greatest success as a bodybuilder during the early 1970s. With a well-proportioned and super-ripped physique, he won the Mr. Germany, Mr. Europe, and Middleweight IFBB Mr. Universe titles. Then in 1978, when well past the age of 40, he trained for most of the year at Gold's to make a comeback. Although he succeeded in achieving his lifetime best condition that year, Karl was unable to place in the top three at the IFBB Middleweight Mr. Universe competition, won by another Gold's athlete, Tom Platz.

Karl had wide and thick lat development, which was achieved through using routines like this:

1. Front Chin: 5 × 10–15
2. Seated Pulley Rowing: 5 × 8–10
3. Pulldown Behind Neck: 5 × 8–10
4. One-Arm Dumbbell Bent Rowing: 5 × 8–10

Keith Bogoff

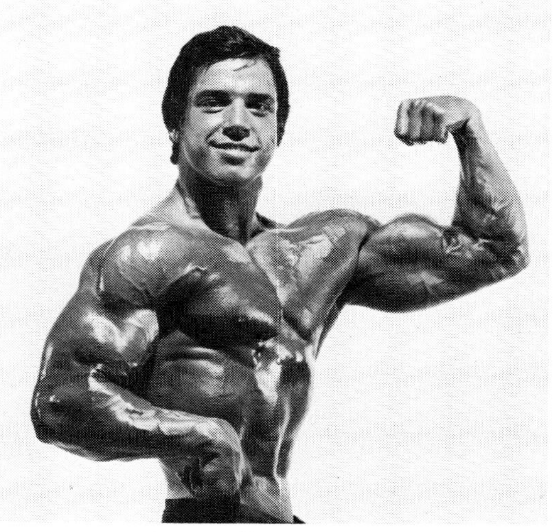

Keith Bogoff. *(Russ Warner)*

Keith has trained for months at a time on several occasions at Gold's Gym. An exceptional young ice hockey player, Bogoff chose bodybuilding over the National Hockey League, eventually winning the Mr. Michigan and Mr. Mid-West titles. A friend and training partner of Samir Bannout, Keith has a very well-proportioned and symmetrical physique, and he can diet down to very muscular condition prior to competition.

Here are the forearm routines that Keith Bogoff has used at Gold's:

Monday-Wednesday-Friday

1. Zottman Curl: 4 × 8–10
2. Barbell Wrist Curl (supported): 4 × 10–15
3. Barbell Reverse Wrist Curl (supported): 4 × 10–15

Tuesday-Thursday-Saturday

1. Dumbbell Wrist Curl (One-Arm, supported): 5 × 10–15
2. Wrist Roller: 3-4 windings in each direction

With his powerful forearm development, Keith would no doubt have a much improved slap-shot if he returned to playing hockey.

John Brown

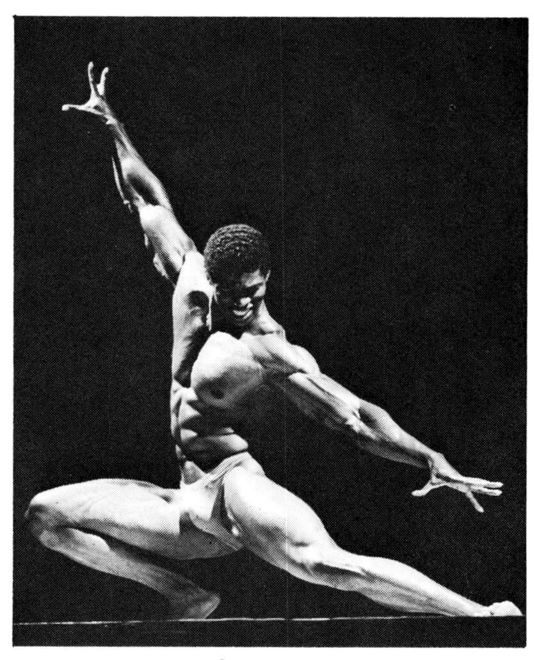

John Brown.

A college art student from Fullerton, California, Brown occasionally trains at Gold's Gym. John has won the NABBA Mr. Universe and WABBA Mr. World titles, and he is noted as one of the world's most outstanding posers. Overall, John trains quite heavy and primarily on basic exercises. As an example, he can Bench Press more than 500 pounds, more than twice his massive 225-pound body weight.

Here is one off-season chest routine we have observed John Brown using at Gold's.

1. Bench Press: 8–10 × 12–4
2. Barbell Incline Press: 6–8 × 12–4
3. Weighted Dip: 4–6 × 8–10
4. Flat-Bench Flye: 4–6 × 8–10

If you ever have the chance to see John Brown pose, take it! His routine is a work of art.

Gerard Buinoud

Gerard Buinoud.

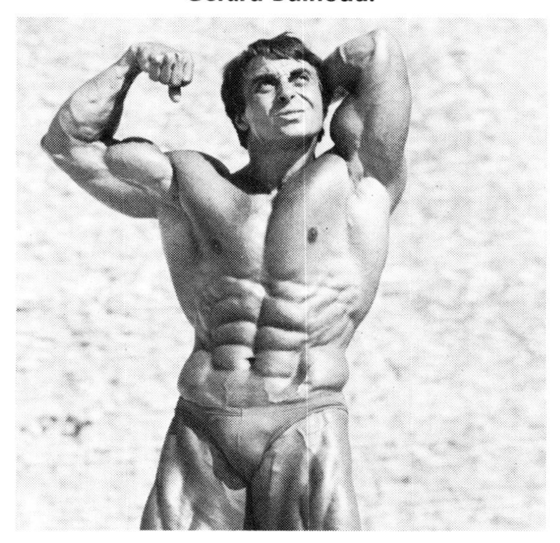

Buinoud, a fireman from Lyon, France, trains every summer at Gold's in preparation for the Fall international shows. And his training paid off with an IFBB Mr. Universe title in 1981. Gerard has now turned pro and will no doubt continue to shine with his special brand of onstage charisma contest after contest.

At 5′6″ in height, Buinoud competes at about 175 pounds of ripped-to-shreds muscle, but as a confirmed chocoholic, he can balloon up to over 200 pounds quite easily in the off-season. Scarfing down a kilogram (2.2 pounds) of chocolate at a sitting is sort of routine for Gerard. But he pays a price for this indulgence. For two months prior to competing, he eats only meat, fish, water, vitamins, and minerals.

Gerard Buinoud's chest is particularly impressive, with an unbelievable number of deep striations across his pecs. Here's one of his favorite precontest, pectoral training schedules:

1. Barbell Bench Press: 12–15 × 10–15
2. Barbell Decline Press: 12–15 × 10–15
3. Incline Flye: 8–10 × 10–15
4. Parallel Bar Dip: 8–10 × max reps on each set

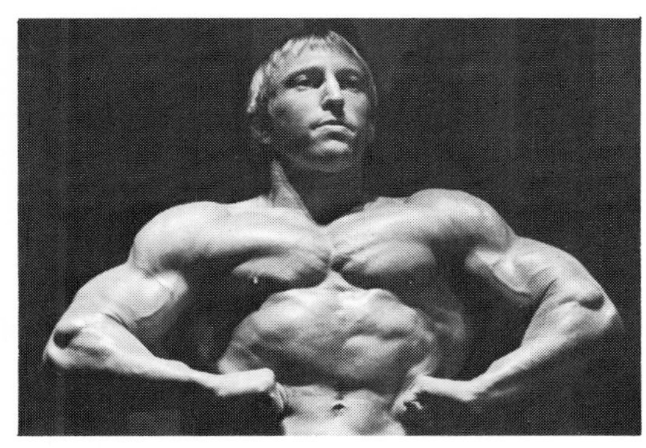

John Burkholder.

John Burkholder

A gym owner in Seattle, Washington, John trains at Gold's when passing through Los Angeles. He has won the Mr. Washington, Mr. Pacific Northwest, Mr. USA, and Mr. North America titles and has been a finalist several times in his class at the Mr. America contest. Burkholder also is an accomplished contest promoter who uses top guest posers and routinely packs the house for his Seattle shows.

John contributed the following intermediate-level deltoid routine that male and female bodybuilders can use twice per week:

1. Military Press (warm-up): 1–2 × 10–15
2. Seated Press Behind the Neck: 4–5 × 6–8
3. Bent Lateral: 3–4 × 8–10
4. Cable Side Lateral: 3–4 × 8–10

"The Seated Press Behind the Neck is your basic exercise," Burkholder commented. "It should be pushed quite hard. Go to failure on at least the final two sets."

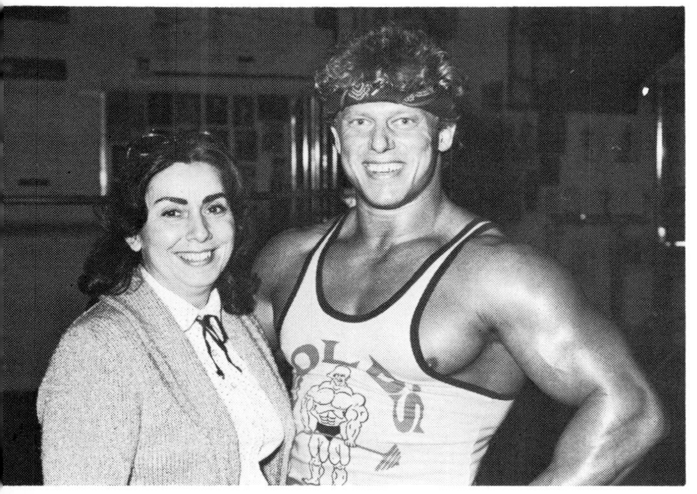

Andreas Cahling with Gold's Gym manager, Joyce Sprague.

Andreas Cahling

Andreas is a Swedish bodybuilder who emigrated to America specifically so that he could train at Gold's. He has, in fact, applied for American citizenship so that he can stay. In Chapter 1 we discussed his remarkable success story, and here we wish to show you Andreas's dramatic "before" and "after" photos, vividly illustrating that a once-pencil-neck kid can add a phenomenal amount of muscle mass and win the Mr. International title. Andreas also contributed this deltoid routine, which he performs twice per week in the off-season and three times per week during his precontest cycle:

1. Machine Press (light for a warm-up): 2–3 × 10–15
2. Seated Press Behind the Neck: 3 × 6–8
3. Seated Bent Lateral: 2 × 8–10
4. Standing Dumbbell Side Lateral: 2 × 8–10
5. Cable Side Lateral: 2 × 8–10
6. Cable Bent Lateral: 2 × 8–10
7. Front Barbell Raise: 2 × 8–10

Andreas obviously believes in doing a limited number of sets on a wide variety of exercises for each body part, but he does make every set count by doing forced reps and plenty of burns.

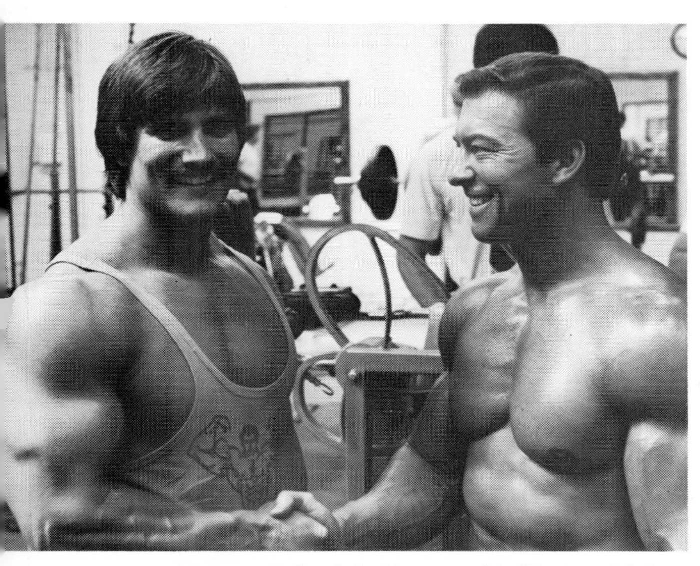

Roger Callard (left) meets his lifetime idol, Larry Scott (the first Mr. Olympia).
(Bill Reynolds)

Roger Callard

A former college football player and world-class sprinter from Michigan, Callard won numerous titles, including Mr. Western America, Mr. USA, and his weight class in the Mr. America show twice. A carpenter by trade, he has also had a successful acting career, appearing in numerous television films and series.

Roger had an esthetically balanced and very muscular physique when he was in top shape. This is the type of chest workout he favored while training at Gold's Gym:

1. Incline Barbell Press: 6 × 12–8
2. Cross-Bench Dumbbell Pullover: 5 × 12
3. Decline Dumbbell Press: 5 × 10
4. Decline Flye: 4 × 10
5. Cable Crossover: 4 × 15

Powerful enough to do six strict reps with 420 pounds in the Bench Press, Roger generally eschewed such heavy powerlifting-style training for concentrated isolation movements with moderately heavy weights to max out his pec development.

Roy Callender

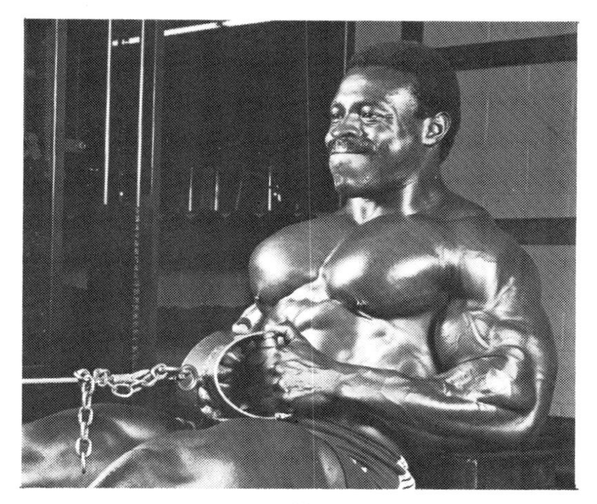

Roy Callender.

A native of Barbados who now lives in Canada near Montreal, Roy has occasionally trained at Gold's Gym. He is one of the most massively muscular bodybuilders of all time. Among his titles are Mr. Canada, Mr. International, Amateur Mr. Universe, Pro Mr. Universe, and the pro Diamond Cup Championship. Callender has also placed in the top five at the Mr. Olympia contest, and he remains one of the most formidable IFBB pro bodybuilders.

One of Roy Callender's most impressive body parts is his chest. Here is one of his superset pectoral routines used in precontest training.

{ 1. Dumbbell Incline Press: 4–6 × 8–12
{ 2. Incline Flye: 4–6 × 10–12
{ 3. Parallel Bar Dip: 3–5 × 10–12
{ 4. Straight-Arm Pullover: 3–5 × 15–20
{ 5. Flat-Bench Flye: 3–5 × 10–12
{ 6. Cable Crossover: 3–5 × 10–15

Roy and his wife, Maggie, have one daughter.

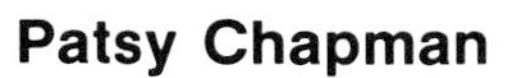

Patsy Chapman

Patsy was a Michigan State University coed when she bested a field of 47 contestants in the 1979 Best-in-the-World Championships. Patsy won as a result of superior natural symmetry, weight-trained muscles, and an eye-catching posing routine. She competed several other times through 1979 but is now out of competition. Currently living in Texas, Patsy Chapman is a police officer.

Patsy's chest program at the time she won the Best-in-the-World Championships was as follows.

1. Bench Press: 5 × 10 (105–125 lbs.)
2. Flat-Bench Flye: 5 × 10 (20s)
3. Incline Barbell Press: 5 × 10 (65–75 lbs.)

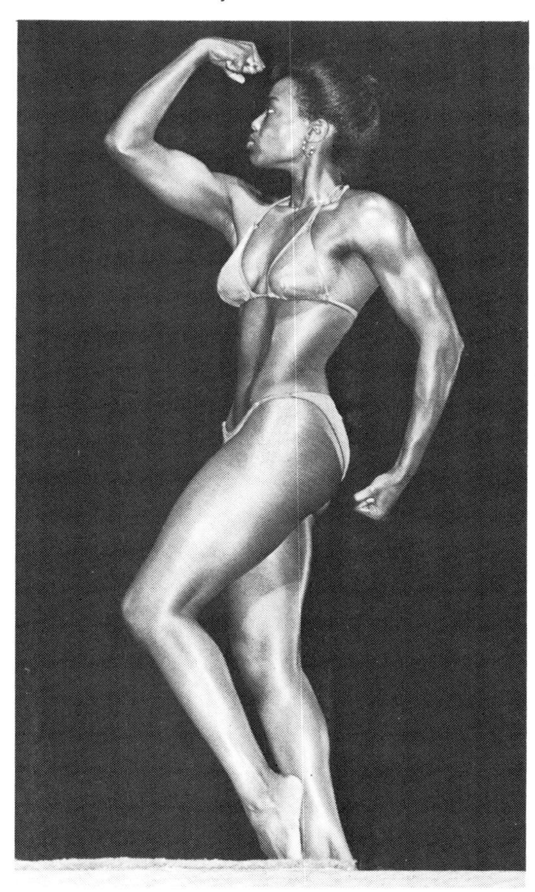

Patsy Chapman. *(Bill Dobbins)*

Roy Chaves

Roy was born in British Guiana, but has spent most of his life residing in England, where he has won the Mr. Britain title. In 1978 Chaves trained for six months at Gold's Gym in preparation for the IFBB Mr. Universe competition in Acapulco, Mexico. Training on a double-split routine, doing up to 40 total sets per body part and eating little but skinned and broiled chicken breasts, Roy came into the Universe ripped to the bone. He placed in the top three and won the Ben Weider Trophy as the IFBB's most improved amateur bodybuilder for 1978.

Chaves trained his calves during the second half of his double-split routine each day using these schedules.

Monday-Wednesday-Friday

1. Standing Calf Machine: 5 × 15–20
2. Calf Raise On Hack Machine: 5 × 15–20
3. One-Leg Calf Raise: 5 × 15–20

Tuesday-Thursday-Saturday

1. Seated Calf Machine: 5 × 15–20
2. Donkey Calf Raise: 5 × 15–20
3. Calf Press: 5 × 15–20

"I believe in stretching and flexing my calves throughout the day," Chaves commented. "It helps to sharpen them up for competition."

Roy lives in London and works as a bodyguard.

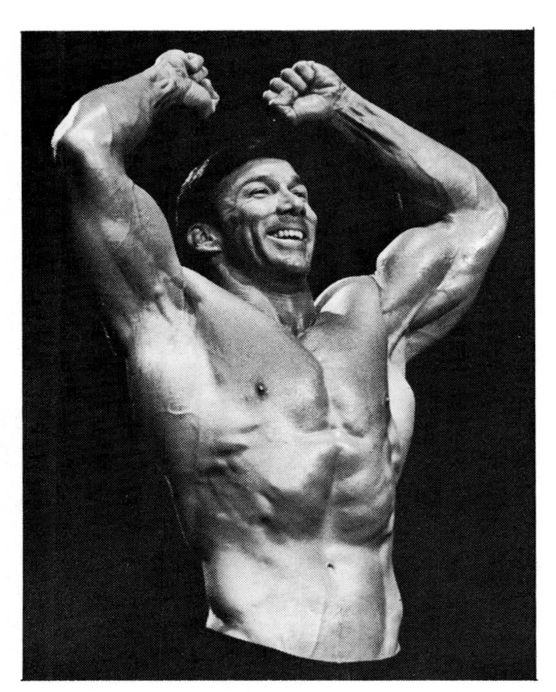

Boyer Coe.

Boyer Coe

Other than the legendary Bill Pearl, no bodybuilder has competed at the highest levels of the sport longer than Boyer Coe. Since 1963 he has competed at least four times and as many as 14 times per year. And he has won virtually every title available—Teenage Mr. America, Junior Mr. America, Mr. America, Mr. Universe (five times), Mr. World (six times), the World Cup Championships, and the overall Grand Prix Championships. Only the Mr. Olympia title has eluded him (he's placed third), and he's set his sights on winning it soon.

Boyer's precontest diet is extremely low in fats, moderately weighted in protein content, and relatively high in carbohydrates. The net effect is a daily caloric consumption of approximately 1,800–2,000 calories per day. In addition to his bodybuilding workouts, Coe averages at least an hour per day of aerobic training to etch the deepest possible cuts into his physique. And his combination of huge mass, perfect proportions, and razor sharp cuts is unequaled in the sport.

Boyer Coe has always been noted for his superb upper arm development, so we asked him for an arm program. Here's his precontest superset routine:

1. Machine Curl: 1 × 15 (warm-up); 5 × 8
2. Triceps Machine: 1 × 15 (warm-up); 5 × 8
3. Incline Dumbbell Curl: 5 × 8
4. Pulley Pushdown: 5 × 8
5. Lying Pulley Curl: 5 × 8
6. One-Arm Dumbbell Triceps Extension: 5 × 8

Boyer is the author of a superb training book, *Boyer and Valerie Coe's Weight Training Book* (Contemporary Books, 1982), and several other bodybuilding books. He's also a consummate businessman, making him one of the most well-rounded athletes in the sport.

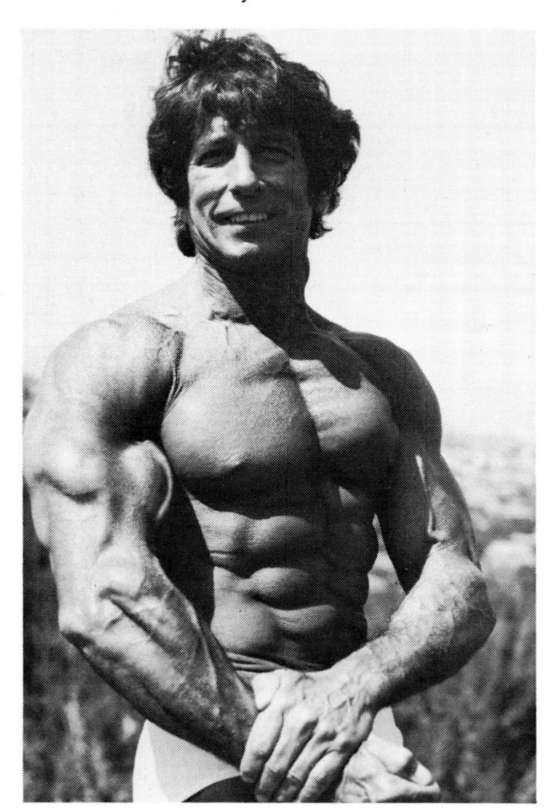

Chuck Collras, at age 46.

Chuck Collras

Chuck has been a long-time member of Gold's, and he's won Mr. Pacific Coast and Mr. West Coast among a host of titles. Chuck has also placed in the top five in the Mr. America competition on two occasions. Collras has even been a regional powerlifting champion. Now in his mid-40s, Chuck is cleaning up in over-40 contests.

Here is a superset shoulder routine that Chuck Collras favored:

1. Upright Rowing: 9 × 8
2. Dumbbell Press: 9 × 8
3. Side Lateral: 9 × 8
4. Pulley Side Lateral: 9 × 8

Chuck is quite an advocate of beach running, particularly while cutting up for a competition. He works as a lighting technician in the film industry.

Franco Columbu

Franco was born into humble surroundings in Sardinia, an island off the coast of Italy. His first job as a youth was as a shepherd. Later he worked in construction and moved to Germany to labor in an automobile factory. During this time he assiduously practiced boxing, becoming amateur champion of Italy in his weight class in 1964. As a pro boxer, he took up weight training to add power to his punches. Unfortunately, he almost killed his next ring opponent and abandoned boxing in favor of powerlifting and bodybuilding.

Columbu has held numerous world records and European championships in powerlifting. He also won the Mr. Italy and Mr. Europe titles before moving to America in 1969. Then his bodybuilding career blossomed as he trained at Gold's. He won Mr. International, Mr. World, and Mr. Olympia twice (1976 and 1981).

While competing, Franco completed rigorous chiropractic medicine studies and was licensed to practice chiropractic. He and his wife have a very successful clinic in Westwood, California, near UCLA. Columbu has also completed studies for a PhD in nutrition science and has authored numerous books on bodybuilding and powerlifting. His *Winning Bodybuilding* (Contemporary Books, 1977) was the first book published written by an established champion bodybuilder.

Dr. Columbu has always been noted for his thick and superstriated pectoral muscles. Here is a typical Columbu superset chest workout.

1. Bench Press: 4–6 × 6–10
2. Incline Barbell Press: 3–4 × 6–10
3. Parallel Bar Dip: 3–4 × 15–20 }
4. Cable Crossover: 3–4 × 15 }

Although past the age of 40, Franco plans one more assault on the Mr. Olympia title. And don't think he won't reach his lifetime best condition for it!

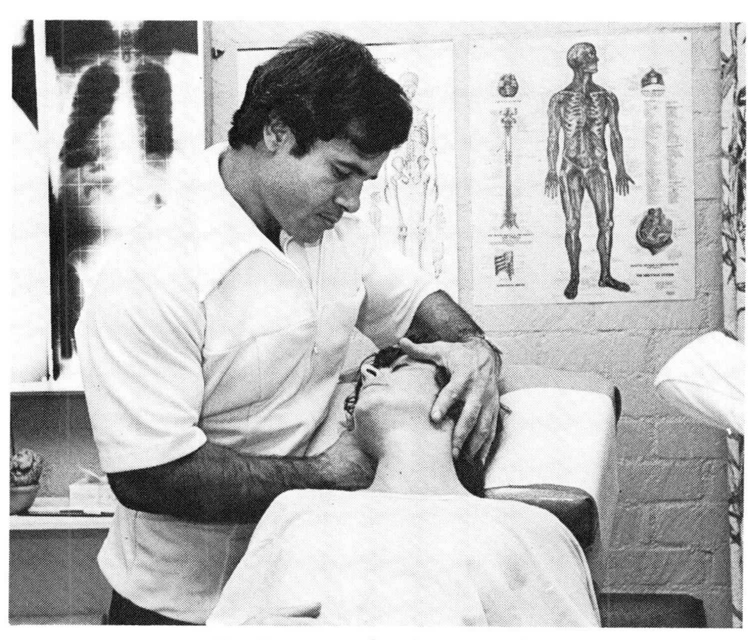

Dr. Franco Columbu at work.

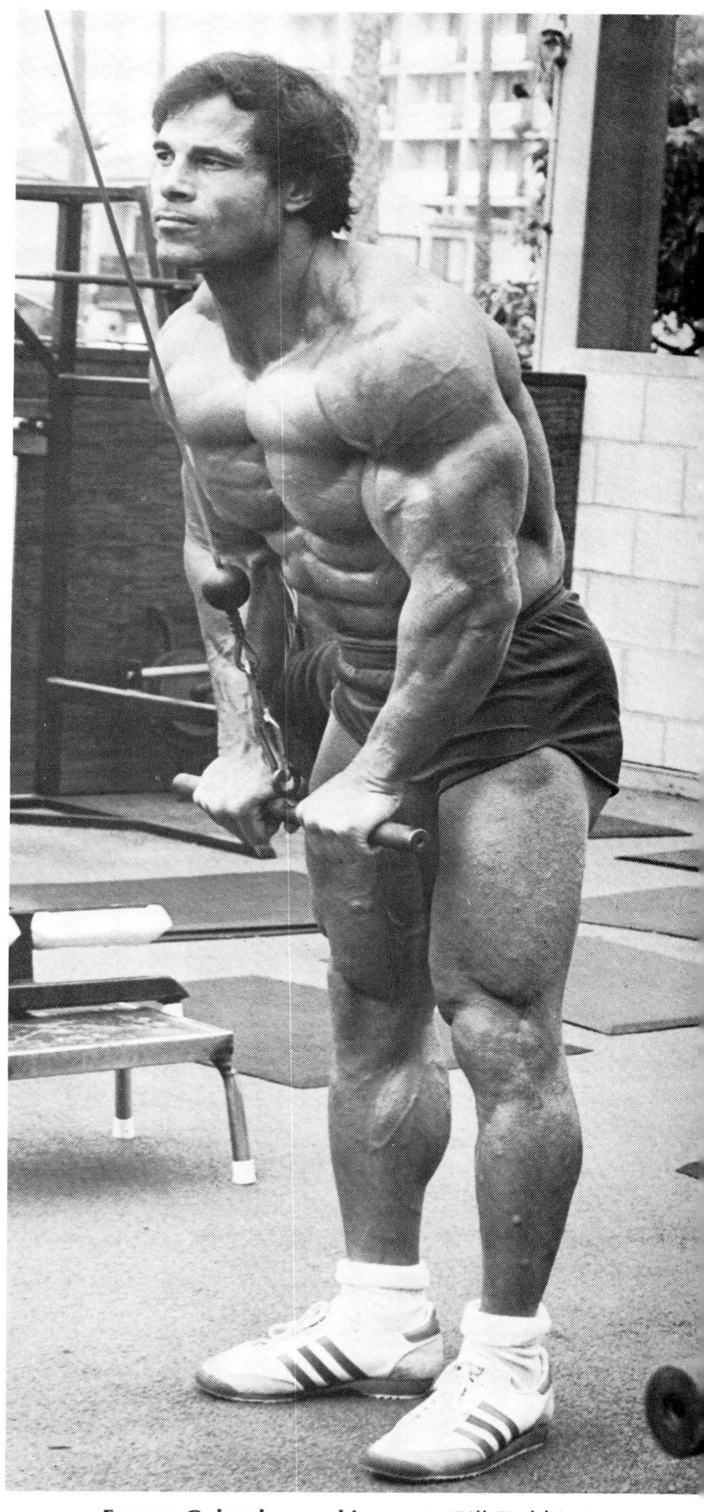

Franco Columbu working out. *(Bill Dobbins)*

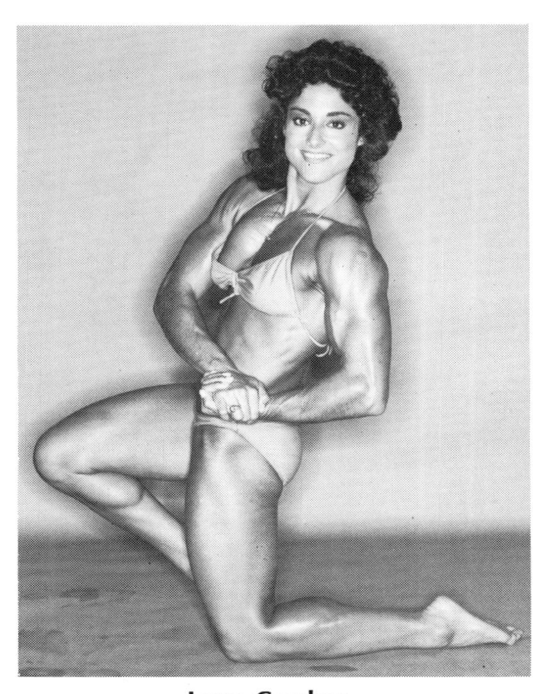

Laura Combes.

Lynn Conkwright.

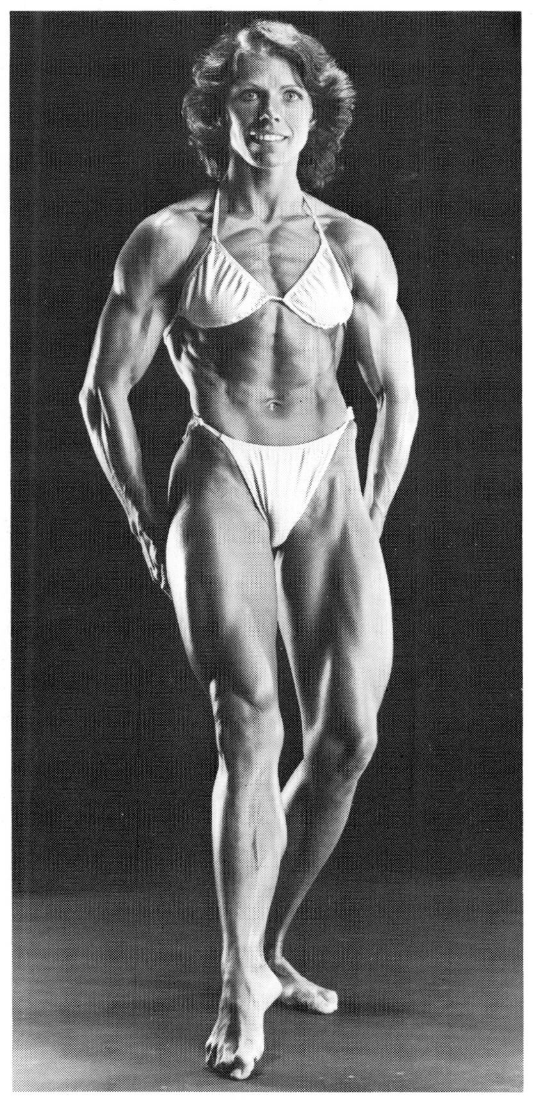

Laura Combes

The first Ms. America winner in 1980, Laura has set a standard for superb muscle mass, balanced body proportions, and finely tuned muscularity that has inspired an entire generation of women bodybuilders. Her onstage charisma and femininity also have helped her win the Ms. Tampa and Ms. Florida titles, as well as fourth place in her first Ms. Olympia appearance. No doubt it will be just a matter of time before she annexes the Ms. Olympia title, since Laura is one of the most dedicated and determined women bodybuilders who's ever pumped iron at Gold's Gym.

Ms. Combes has been training with weights off and on since 1974, initially as an adjunct to her athletic activities. She has been a collegiate national champion in both rugby and water skiing, but she turned to serious bodybuilding training in 1977 and never looked back. Laura does most of her training in her well-equipped home gym but works out at Gold's a month or two each year to peak out completely for major shows.

Laura has written a number of well-received training articles for *Muscle & Fitness* magazine. And her book, *Winning Women's Bodybuilding* (Contemporary Books, 1983), will soon be required reading for all serious women bodybuilders.

Rather than reveal a training program for a particularly strong muscle group, Laura Combes submitted the training schedule that brought her once weak calves up to equal the development of the rest of her superb physique. It's essentially a very simple three-day cycle. On Day 1 she does 6–8 very heavy sets of 8–10 repetitions of Toe Raises on a seated calf machine, followed on Day 2 by 5–6 lighter sets of 20–30 reps of Toe Raises on a standing calf machine. Day 3 is one of complete rest from calf training, and the cycle repeats itself on Day 4. This routine was so effective that it put a full inch on Laura's calves in only nine months.

Lynn Conkwright

A former collegiate gymnast, Lynn has been quite successful as a bodybuilder. On one day in early 1981 she won the World Women's Professional World Championships and the World Couples' Championships (teamed with Chris Dickerson). Lynn has also placed in the top three at the Ms. Olympia and other pro women's competitions.

Lynn has particularly good leg and abdominal development, so we present her ab routine:

1. Wall Crunch: 3 × 20–25
2. Hanging Leg Raise: 3 × 15–20
3. Jackknife Crunch: 3 × 20–25
4. Cable Crunch: 3 × 20–25
5. Seated Twisting: 3 × 25

Lynn has a unique method of performing her Hanging Leg Raises. As she raises her legs upward she extends them in a wide "V" and swings them under the bar until her torso is parallel to the floor and her inner thighs are touching her arms. Try it sometime!

Ed Corney

Known as "The Master Poser," Ed Corney was still placing respectably in the Mr. Olympia competition at nearly 50 years of age. Along the way he's won a host of major titles—Mr. California, Mr. America, Mr. International, and Mr. Universe. Surprisingly, Eddie didn't compete as a bodybuilder until the age of 31, preferring initially to train only for his own health, fitness, and enjoyment. But he had by then developed such a fine physique that friends goaded him into competing.

While training extensively at Gold's, this was one of Ed Corney's favorite biceps workouts:

1. Standing Barbell Curl: 3–4 × 8–10
2. Barbell Preacher Curl: 3–4 × 8–10
3. Wide-Grip Machine Curl: 3–4 × 8–10
4. Dumbbell Concentration Curl: 3–4 × 8–10
5. Barbell Reverse Curl: 3–4 × 8–10

Eddie preferred to train relatively quickly with moderate weights and a maximum degree of mental concentration.

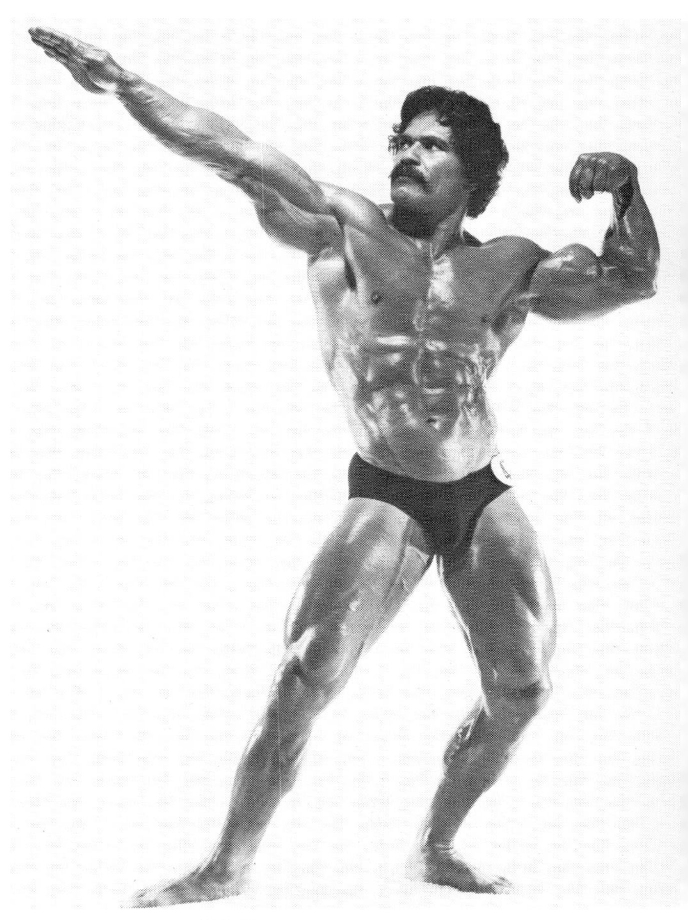

Ed Corney.

Candy Csencsits

Candy, a Pennsylvania native, won the Ms. Eastern America and then turned pro with a vengeance, placing sixth in the 1981 Ms. Olympia, second in the 1981 World Grand Prix, and second in the 1982 Pro World Championships. When on the West Coast, she occasionally trains at Gold's Gym.

Here is one of Candy's successful back training programs:

1. Dumbbell Bent Rowing: 3 × 8–10
2. Behind the Neck Lat Pulldown: 3 × 8–10
3. Seated Pulley Rowing: 3 × 8–10
4. Upright Rowing: 3 × 8–10
5. Hyperextension: 3 × 12–15

Candy Csencsits.

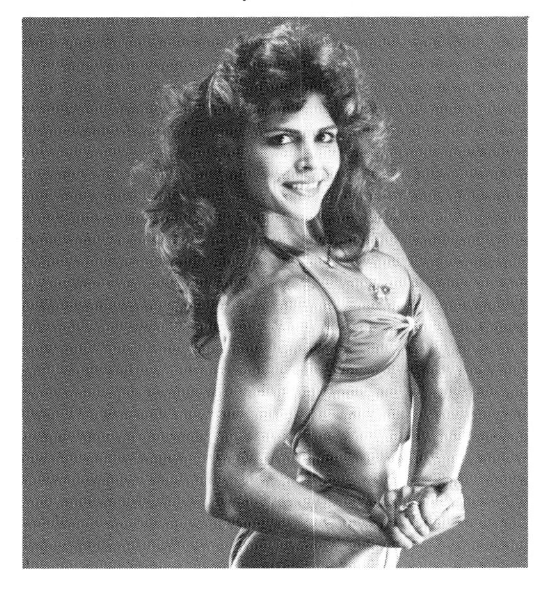

Mario daSilva

Mario is originally from Uruguay, and while living in South America he won the Mr. Uruguay title and an Argentine Championship open to foreign athletes. In America he has placed second in the Mr. Western America show and won the "Best Poser" award at the Mr. World contest. Mario is, indeed, one of the best posers you will ever be fortunate enough to see. A physical trainer and therapist, daSilva has done yeoman work promoting bodybuilding and physical fitness on Spanish-language television and radio programs in America, Mexico, and the rest of Latin America.

Mario gave the authors his precontest lat routine, which is performed three times a week:

1. Front Chin: 6–8 × 8–10
2. Lat Pulldown (Front and Back): 6–8 × 8–10
3. Seated Pulley Rowing (with differing grips): 6–8 × 8–10
4. One-Arm Low Pulley Rowing: 5 × 10–15

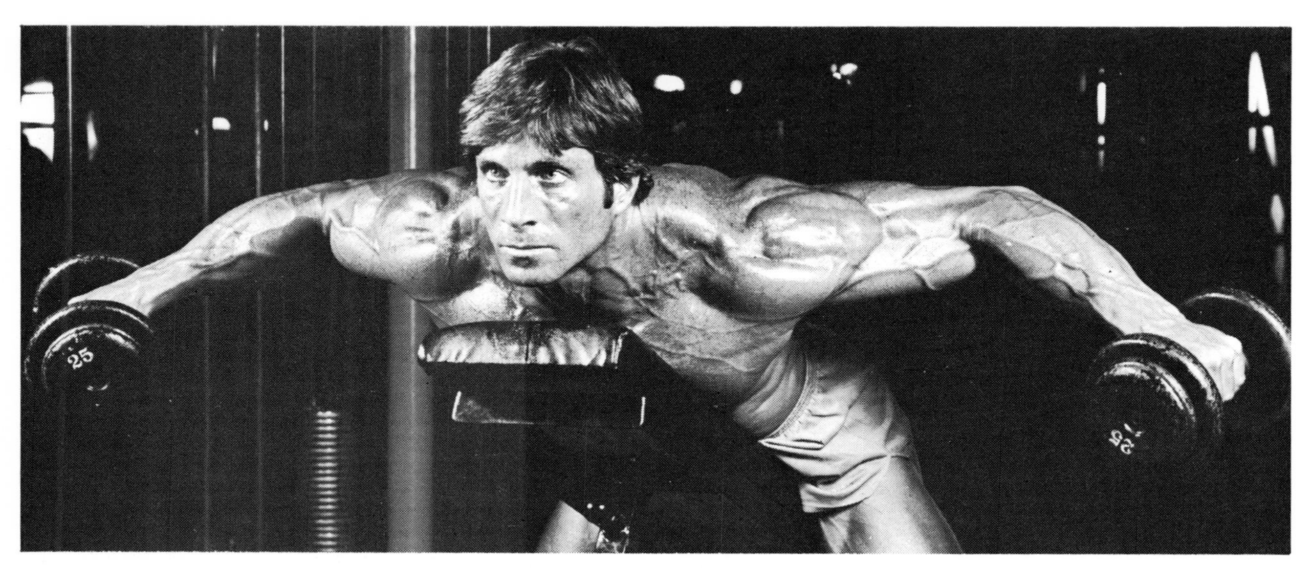

Steve Davis.

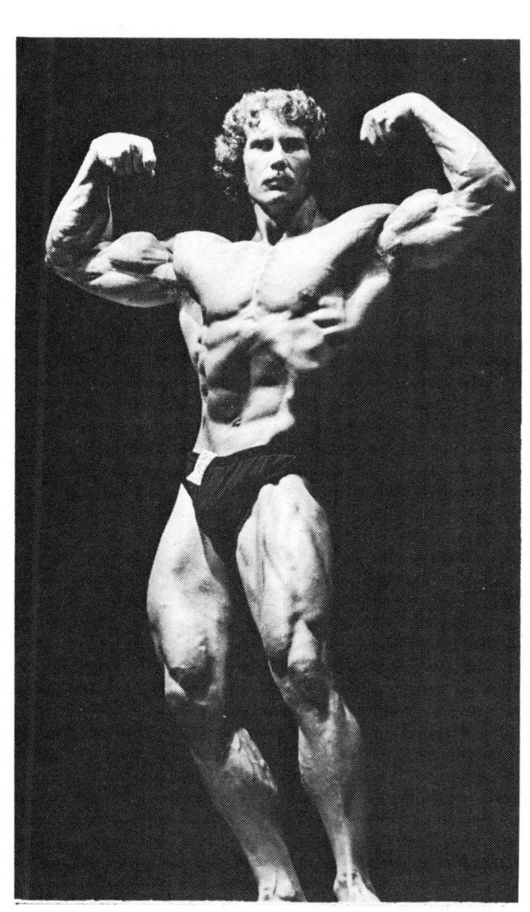

Mike Dayton. *(Art Zeller)*

Steve Davis

Steve Davis will probably be remembered most for training down from being a 285-pound blob to a 200-pound supersymmetrical Mr. World winner. He has also won Mr. California and several other titles, and he operates two gyms in southern California. Steve has trained for extended periods of time at Gold's.

Involving reps of 12–10–8–7–7–6–12 on each exercise, here is a Steve Davis delt workout:

1. Dumbbell Press (up to 100s)
2. Side Lateral Raise (up to 65s)
3. Bent Lateral Raise (up to 65s)

Steve's formula for fast bodybuilding gains is: Intensity Training + Sound Nutrition + Motivation to Win = Bodybuilding Gains. You won't find a better success formula than that!

Mike Dayton

Mike Dayton has won more than 25 bodybuilding titles and over 200 trophies in a long career. Among his titles are Mr. Golden West, Mr. Western America, Mr. Western USA, Mr. Heart of California, Mr. Iron Man (which combines powerlifting and physique), Teenage Mr. America, and Pro. Mr. America. Now an outstanding professional strongman, Dayton has frequently been manacled with regulation police handcuffs onstage and broken them. He can also bend a quarter using only his thumbs and forefingers. Try that one someday!

Since he's occasionally trained at Gold's when passing through Los Angeles, we solicited this Mike Dayton chest routine:

1. Bench Press: 8–10 × 15–5 (up to 400 lbs.)
2. Flat-Bench Flye: 5–6 × 8–10 (up to 100s)
3. Incline Dumbbell Press: 5–6 × 8–10 (up to 150s)
4. Parallel Bar Dip: 5–6 × 8–10 (up to 200 lbs. tied around his waist)

Dayton attributes much of his success as a bodybuilder and strongman to his mastery of *chi,* the internally focused concentration and power of Oriental martial arts masters.

John DeFendis

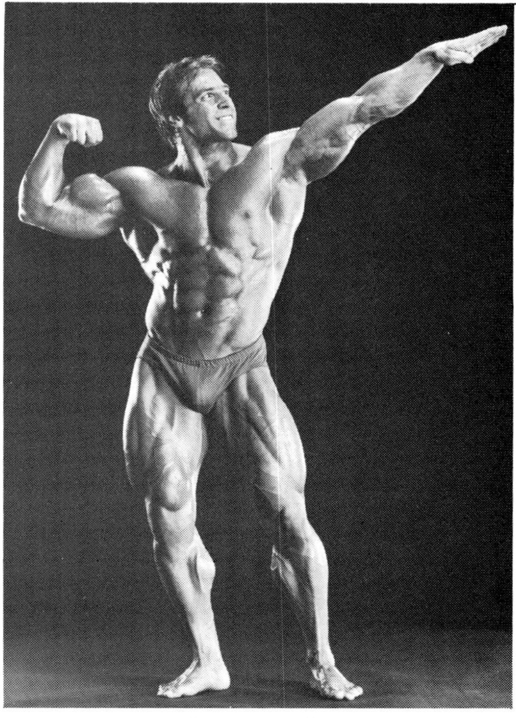

John DeFendis.

John has won numerous titles on the East Coast, but now lives in Arizona and has become one of the best young bodybuilders on the amateur scene. His naturally good symmetry and proportions are magnified by huge muscle mass and very sharp muscularity at contest time. John also is a superb poser, having won the "Best Poser" trophy in the Mr. USA competition.

DeFendis began serious bodybuilding training under the direction of Steve Michalik and has both embraced and further refined Steve's "Intensity or Insanity" training philosophy. John averages 50–60 sets per muscle group each training session, and sometimes he goes as high as 70–80 total sets with quite heavy weights.

Here is a typical John DeFendis precontest chest training routine:

1. Incline Barbell Press: 8–10 × 8–10
2. Incline Dumbbell Press: 8–10 × 8–10
3. Incline Flye: 8–10 × 8–10
4. Bench Press to Neck: 8–10 × 8–10
5. Flat-Bench Flye: 8–10 × 8–10
6. Parallel Bar Dip: 8–10 × 10–15
7. Cable Crossover: 8–10 × 10–15
8. Cross-Bench Dumbbell Pullover: 8–10 × 10–15

John not only *survives* this type of workout, but actually *thrives* on it!

Greg DeFerro

Greg DeFerro.

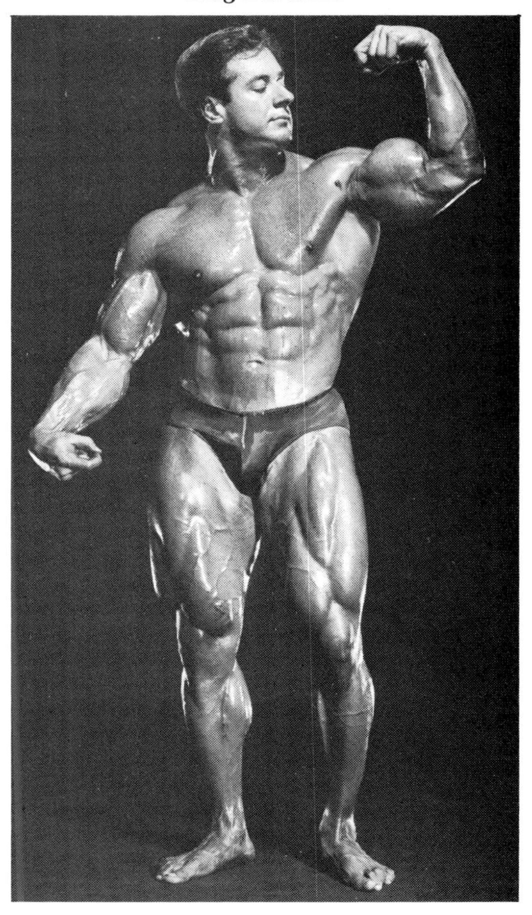

Winner of the prestigious IFBB Mr. International title, DeFerro bears a striking facial resemblance to Sylvester Stallone, leading to his nickname, "Rocky." At 5′8″ in height and weighing 215 pounds in contest shape, Greg sports 21-inch upper arms, a 53-inch chest, a 32-inch waist, and 27½-inch thighs. Currently competing as a pro bodybuilder, Rocky is a threat in every contest he enters. *DeFerro,* incidentally, means *of iron* in Italian, making Greg's family name particularly appropriate for a bodybuilder.

Rocky's back is quite impressive. Here's one of his superset routines for that body part:

{ 1. Wide-Grip Front Lat Pulldown: 3 × 8–12
{ 2. Bench Row: 3 × 8–12
{ 3. Medium-Grip Front Lat Pulldown: 3 × 10
{ 4. T-Bar Row: 3 × 10
5. Low Pulley Row: 3 × 10
6. High Pulley Row: 3 × 10
7. Hyperextension: 4 × 10–12

Greg DeFerro does all of his exercises in very strict form and with maximum mental concentration, factors that all bodybuilders should heed.

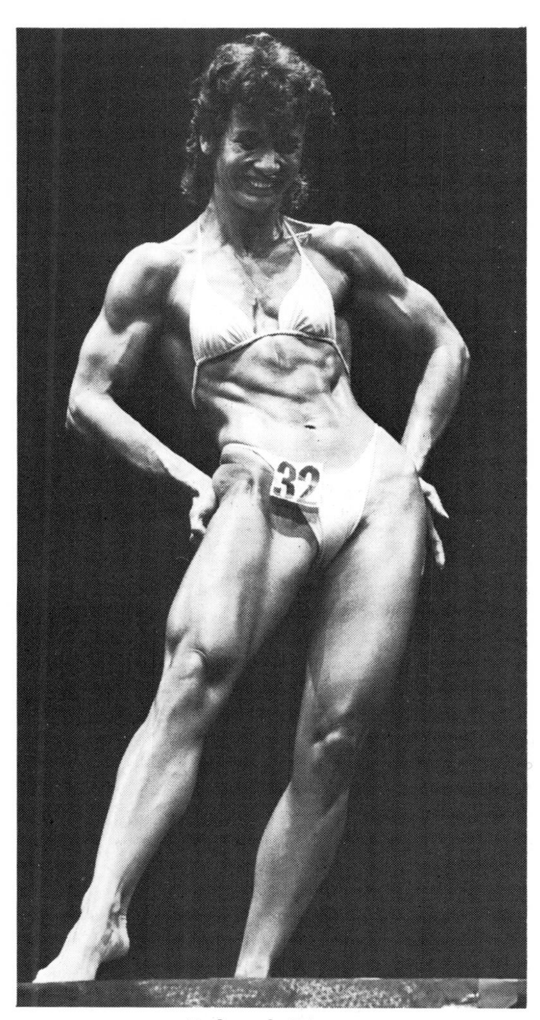

Deborah Diana.

Deborah Diana

Deborah is originally from Pennsylvania, but she now lives in southern California and periodically trains at Gold's Gym. Debbie has won the Ms. USA title and placed in the top three in the Ms. America competition as an amateur. As a professional bodybuilder, Ms. Diana has placed in the final five at the Pro World Championships.

Debbie trains only three days per week on a high-intensity routine, and this is her thigh program (which is done as a giant set):

1. Leg Press: 1 × 10–15
2. Leg Extension: 1 × 10–15
3. Leg Curl: 1 × 10–15
4. Squat: 1 × 10–15

With her classic symmetry and foxy appearance, Deborah Diana has the potential to rise much higher in the ranks of professional women bodybuilders.

Chris Dickerson

Chris is the most successful pro bodybuilder of all time, having won more pro titles and prize money than any other athlete. With his supersymmetrical physique, he has won such titles as Mr. USA, Mr. America, Mr. World, Mr. Universe (twice), the World Couples Championships (twice), and more than 10 pro competitions. Twice he has placed second in the Mr. Olympia competition, both times in controversial decisions and both times when past the age of 40.

Dickerson's deltoids are particularly impressive. This is one routine he has used while training at Gold's Gym:

1. Seated Press Behind the Neck: 6 × 12–8 (up to 180 lbs.)
2. Standing Side Lateral: 6 × 8–10 (up to 55s)
3. Seated Dumbbell Press: 6 × 8 (up to 90s)
4. Seated Bent Lateral: 6 × 12–15 (up to 35s)
5. Upright Rowing: 4 × 10–12 (up to 130 lbs.)

A paragon of perseverance, Dickerson didn't begin bodybuilding until he was 24 and has achieved all of his pro wins since he turned 40!

In late 1982, Chris Dickerson became the sixth bodybuilder to win the Olympia title in its 18-year history.

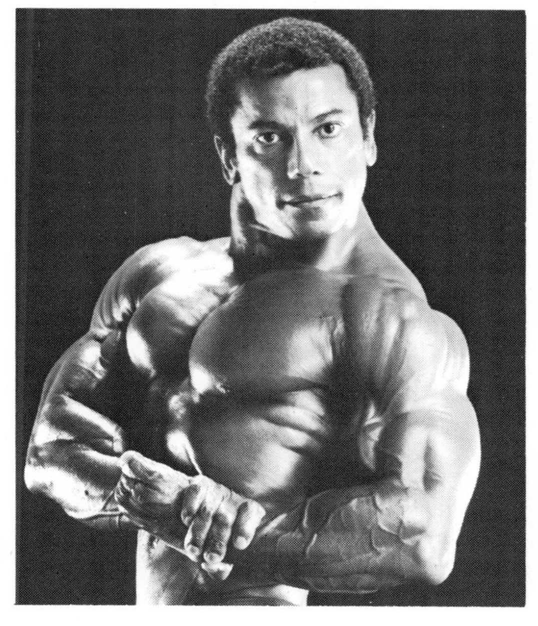

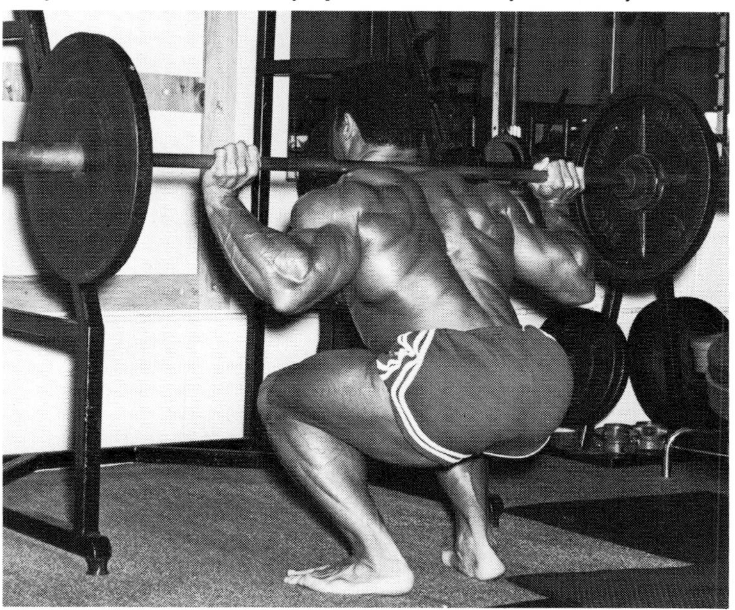

Dave Draper

Known as "The Blond Bomber," Dave was a dominant force in international bodybuilding during the late 1960s and early 1970s. He won the Mr. America, Mr. World, and Mr. Universe titles and placed quite high in the Mr. Olympia competition. With heavy personal publicity in *Muscle & Fitness* magazine, Dave became the idol of millions of bodybuilding aficionados.

In addition to bodybuilding, Draper enjoyed a flourishing acting career. He made numerous films, most notably *Don't Make Waves* with Tony Curtis, Claudia Cardinale, and Sharon Tate. Eventually Dave grew weary of the Hollywood scene and moved to the Santa Cruz Mountains in northern California, where he makes avidly sought furniture from native woods and animal hides. Each piece that Dave constructs takes approximately a week and is a work of art.

Draper's back development was particularly outstanding. Here is one of the lat routines he used while training at Gold's:

1. Front Chin: 5 × 10–15
2. Barbell Bent Rowing: 5 × 10–15
3. Narrow-Grip Chin: 5 × 10–15
4. Behind the Neck Lat Pulldown: 5 × 10–15

Dave Draper was extremely strong. He could routinely do reps with 450 in the Bench Press and perform his Barbell Bent Rows with more than 300 pounds.

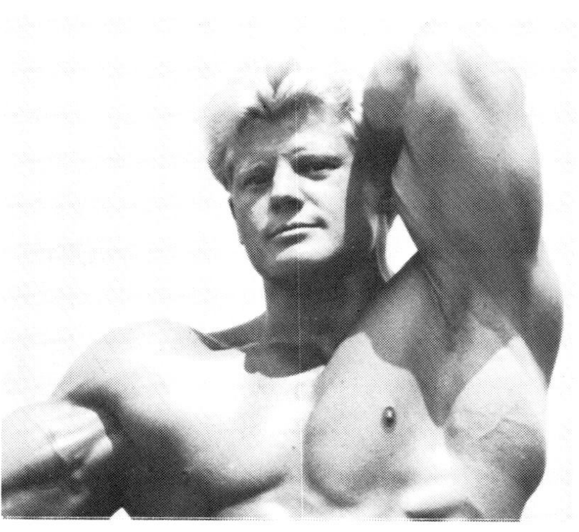

Dave Draper.

Lance Dreher

A former college football player, Lance Dreher has become one of the most massive bodybuilders of the current time. A native of Illinois, he has won the heavyweight Mr. America and Mr. Universe titles. And it is certain that Lance will be a formidable pro competitor in future years.

Dreher's upper arms are phenomenally massive and cut. Here is one routine he has used to build them up to their current impressiveness:

1. Incline Dumbbell Curl: 5 × 6–10
2. Dumbbell Concentration Curl: 5 × 6–10
3. Nautilus Curl: 5 × 6–10
4. Lying Triceps Extension: 5 × 6–10
5. Seated Triceps Extension: 5 × 6–10
6. Pulley Pushdown: 5 × 6–10

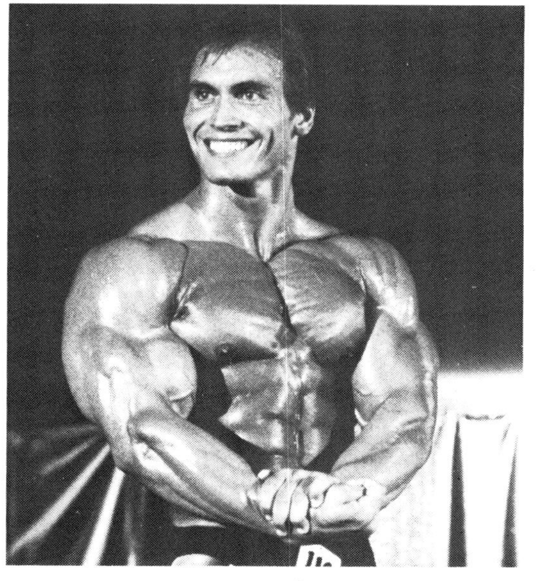

Lance Dreher.

Carla Dunlap

Carla Dunlap is one of the most exciting posers ever to step onstage at a bodybuilding competition. A former synchronized swimming champion, she has won Ms. Atlantic States, the Eastern Cup Championships, the Bodybuilding Expo Championships, and the 1981 and 1982 Ms. America titles. Carla was third in the 1980 Ms. America competition and has placed second in the Ms. USA championships. She's worked out at Gold's several times.

Here's one of Carla Dunlap's favorite chest exercise programs:

1. Incline Dumbbell Press: 4 × 8–10 (up to 55s)
2. Decline Dumbbell Press: 4 × 8–10 (up to 45s)
3. Decline Pullover: 4 × 8–10 (up to 70 lbs.)
4. Pec Deck Flye: 4 × 8–10 (weight varies from machine to machine)

On each exercise Carla prefers to do one light warm-up set, and then uses moderately heavy weights for the remaining sets.

Carla Dunlap.

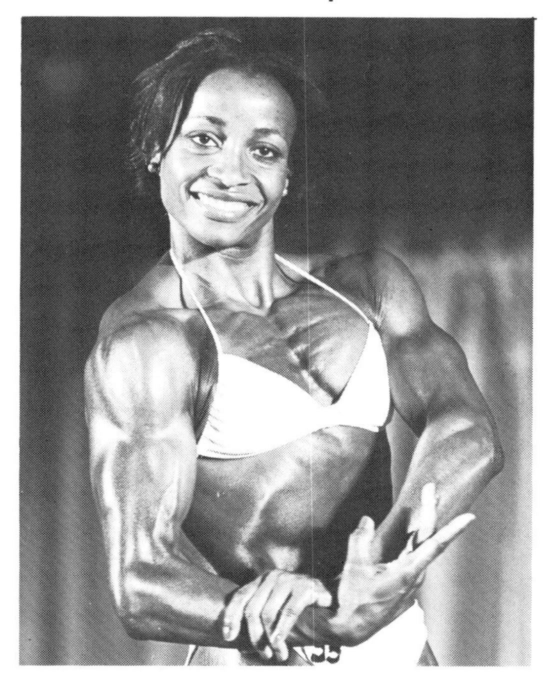

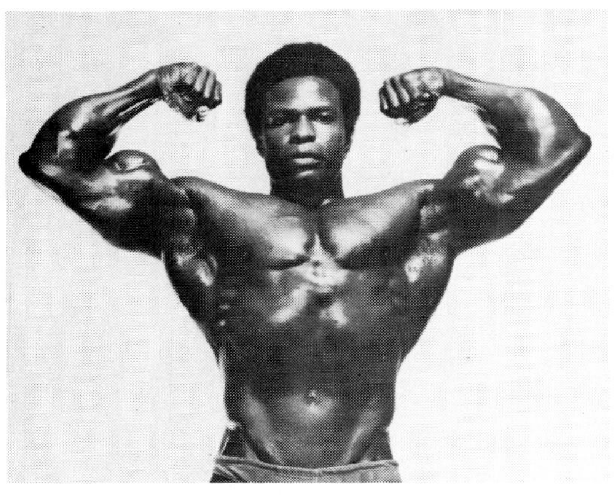

David DuPre. *(Jimmy Caruso)*

David DuPre

Dave DuPre has won a variety of state and regional titles over the years and has placed well in the America. Much of his training has been done at Gold's Gym. Dave's extremely strong, having done such feats as a full Stiff-Leg Deadlift with 705 pounds. In a public Deadlift contest with Franco Columbu, Dave repped 675 (all they could get on the bar) rather easily.

DuPre has often stated that he idolized Steve Reeves as a youth, so it's logical that Dave's calves would tape 18½ inches at 205 pounds body weight. And here's one of the calf programs Dave has used:

1. Donkey Calf Raise: 6 × 20
2. Standing Calf Machine: 6 × 20
3. Seated Calf Machine: 6 × 20

This program is done three days per week, and on three other days he walks on his toes until his calves cramp. Dave also does a lot of free flexing of his calves throughout the day.

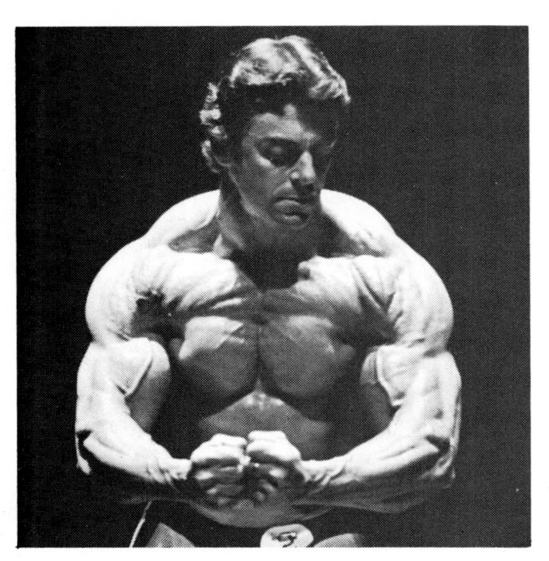

Roy Duval.

Roy Duval

Roy is one of the best bodybuilders ever to come out of Britain, though he now lives in South Arica. He has won Mr. Britain, Mr. Europe, and the 1979 IFBB Middleweight Mr. Universe title.

According to Duval, "I train six times a week at 6:00 a.m. on a split routine; and my sessions last about two hours. I do from 12–20 sets per body part and 6–20 reps each set. As I believe that all body parts respond differently, I do not train each muscle group the same."

Here is a favorite chest routine that Roy Duval contributed:

1. Incline Press: 5–6 × 10–15
2. Decline Press: 5–6 × 10–15
3. Flat-Bench Flye: 5–6 × 10–15

"I concentrate more on the style and feel of the movement than on the actual weight I'm using," Duval concluded.

Lisa Elliott

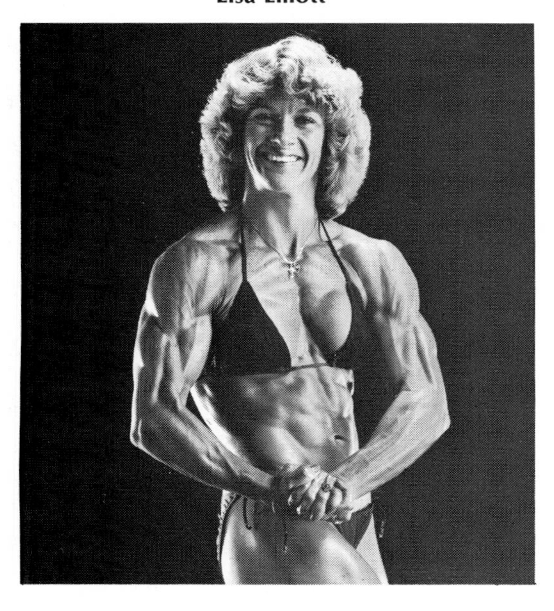

Lisa Elliott

In only two years of competition Lisa has won a host of titles, including Ms. Eastern America, Ms. Southeastern USA, and the Gold's Classic Championships. She has also placed fifth in the Ms. America contest, and many of the sport's cognoscenti believe that only her extreme muscularity has kept Ms. Elliott from placing even higher. Certainly she has all of the physical tools necessary to win both national and international titles.

Lisa is quite a personable woman. And she is exceedingly strong, as evidenced by her ability to do 6–8 reps in the Bench Press with 175 pounds while weighing only 122.

Since Lisa Elliott has absolutely phenomenal deltoids, we asked her for her shoulder routine, which follows:

1. Rotating Dumbbell Press: 4 × 6 (up to 45s)
2. Machine Press Behind the Neck: 4 × 6 (up to 110 lbs.)
3. Dumbbell Side Lateral: 4 × 6 (up to 40s)
4. Seated Bent Lateral: 4 × 6 (up to 35s)
5. Upright Rowing: 4 × 6 (up to 100 lbs.)
6. Cable Side Lateral (mainly just prior to a competition): 4 × 6–8 (up to 25 lbs.)

This routine has given Lisa a roundness with deep striations in her deltoids that is simply mind-blowing.

Kike Elomaa

During 1981 Kike (pronounced *key-key*) Elomaa traveled from her native Finland to sweep to victory in three consecutive major competitions—the European Championships, World Games Championships, and Miss Olympia competition. To say that her victories—and physique—stunned the bodybuilding world would be an understatement.

For several weeks Kike trained periodically at Gold's Gym, and this was one of her thigh workouts:

1. Squat (warm-up): 1 × 20
2. Nautilus Leg Press: 3 × 12–15
3. Nautilus Leg Extension: 3 × 12–15
4. Nautilus Leg Curl: 3 × 12–15

Kike also includes Lunges in her thigh routine prior to a contest, and she credits bicycling for much of her leg muscularity.

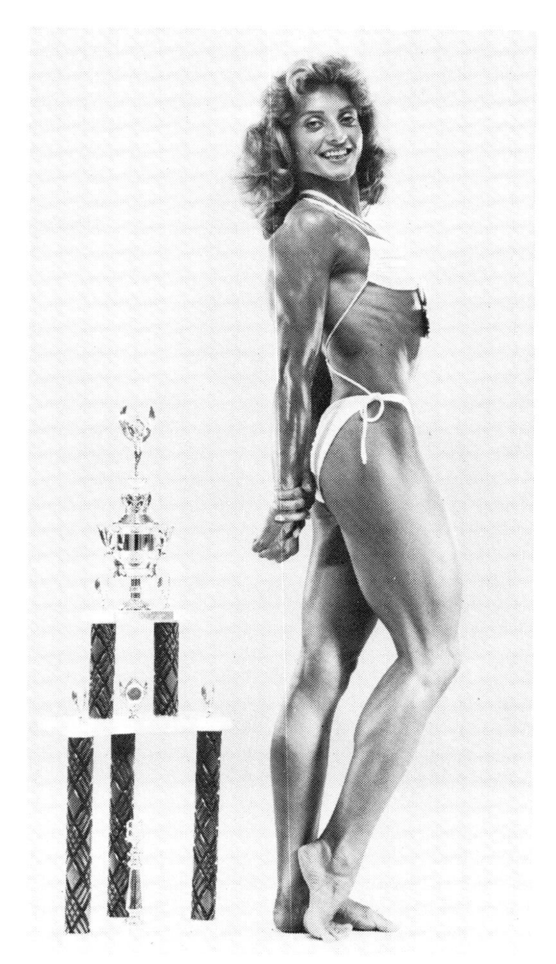

Kike Elomaa and her '81 World Games cup.

Tony Emmott

Now living in southern California, Tony Emmott originally hailed from Ilkley, England. He's won the Mr. United Kingdom, Mr. World, and Mr. Universe titles. Past the age of 40, he is still improving his physique and regularly enters pro competitions.

Tony spent considerable time training at Gold's Gym, and here is one of his favorite lat routines (the first three exercises were performed as a triset):

1. Pulldown behind the Neck: 4 × 15
2. Barbell Bent Rowing (to neck): 4 × 15
3. Wide-Grip Front Chins: 4 × 10
4. Close-Grip Chins: 3 × 12

Tony trains thighs and calves on Monday, Wednesday, and Friday mornings, with abs, chest, and lats later in the day. In one single Tuesday–Thursday–Saturday workout, he hits shoulders, arms, and forearms.

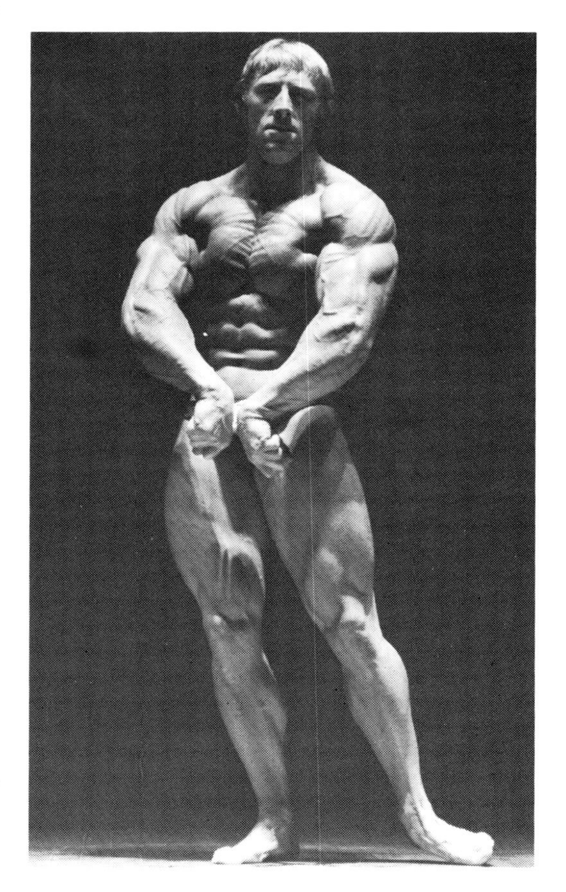

Tony Emmott.

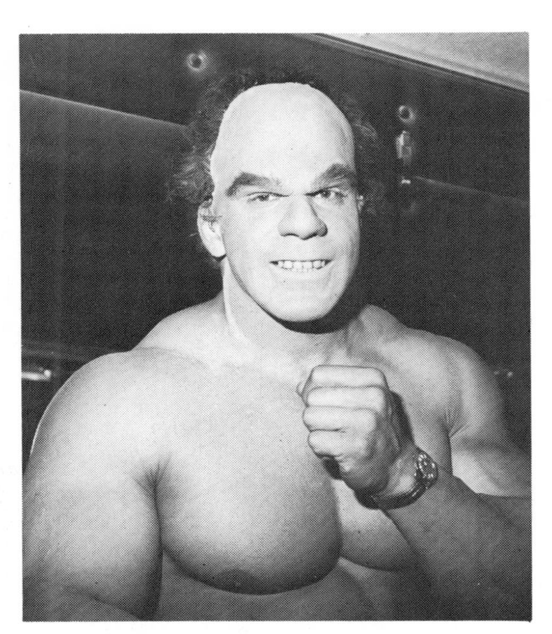

Halfway to Hulk, Lou Ferrigno.

Lou Ferrigno

The success story of Lou Ferrigno is one of the most inspiring in the history of bodybuilding. Virtually deaf from a childhood ear infection, painfully introverted, possessing very poor diction, and as skinny as a rail, Lou began bodybuilding training at the age of 15 in his basement in Brooklyn, New York. Slowly he gained muscle mass, until he eventually weighed a ripped-up 270 pounds at 6′5″ in height.

Lou had an extremely successful competitive career, winning the Teenage Mr. America, Mr. America, Mr. International, and Mr. Universe (twice) titles by the age of 22. But he has gained undying fame with hundreds of millions of television viewers worldwide by being painted green and playing "The Incredible Hulk." Louie has also been involved in remaking the *Hercules* film shot by Steve Reeves in the late 1950s.

Ferrigno has always preferred to do a wide variety of bodybuilding movements for each muscle group, seldom doing the same routine twice for any body part. Here is a typical biceps routine that helped him crash the 23-inch barrier in upper arm measurement:

1. Barbell Preacher Curl: 4 × 8–10
2. Incline Dumbbell Curl: 4 × 8–10
3. Seated Dumbbell Curl: 4 × 8–10
4. Dumbbell Concentration Curl: 4 × 8–10

In addition to his acting career, Lou has written a book on his life and training called *The Incredible Lou Ferrigno* (Simon & Schuster, 1982). Several other books and film projects are in the works.

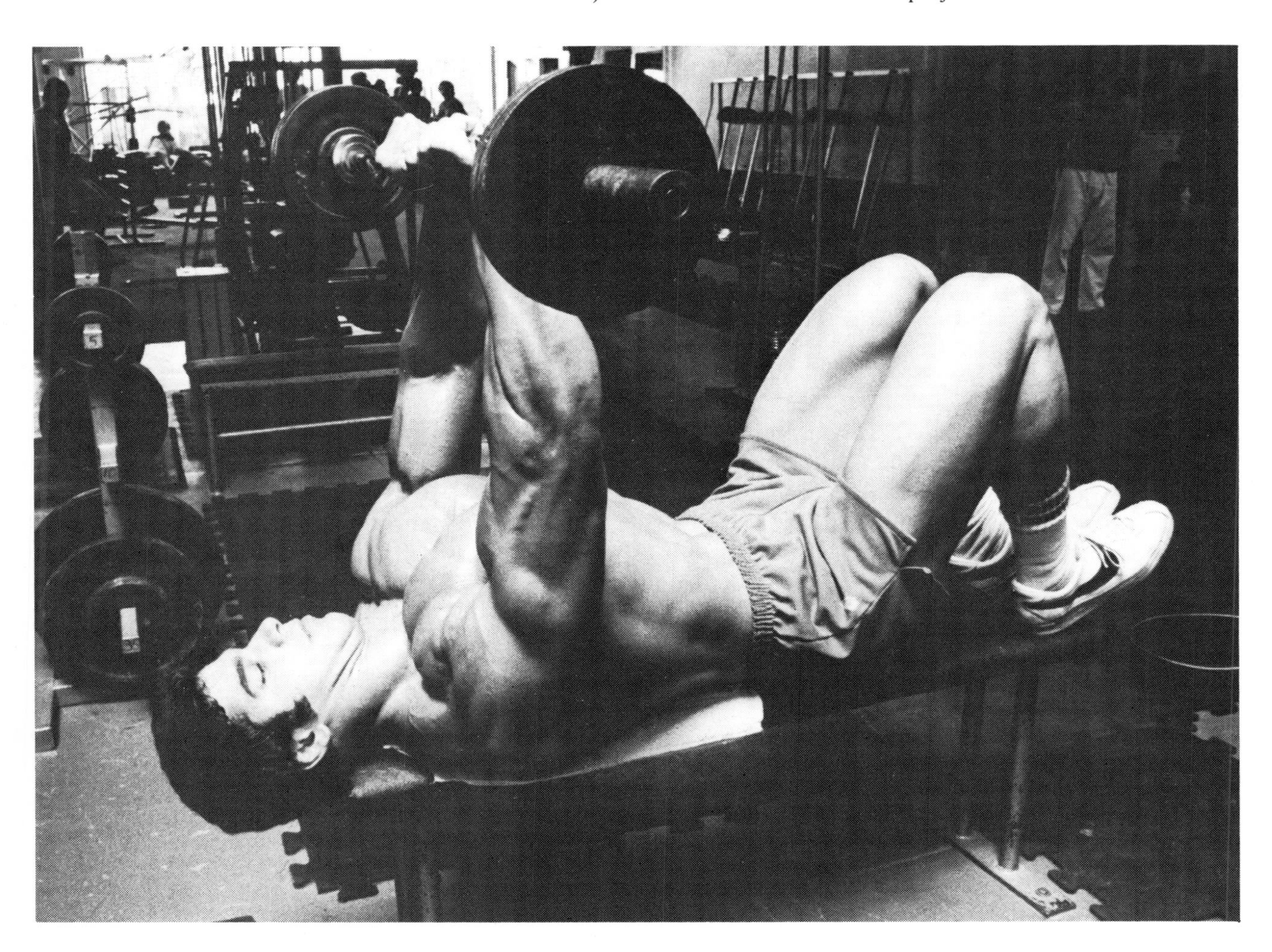

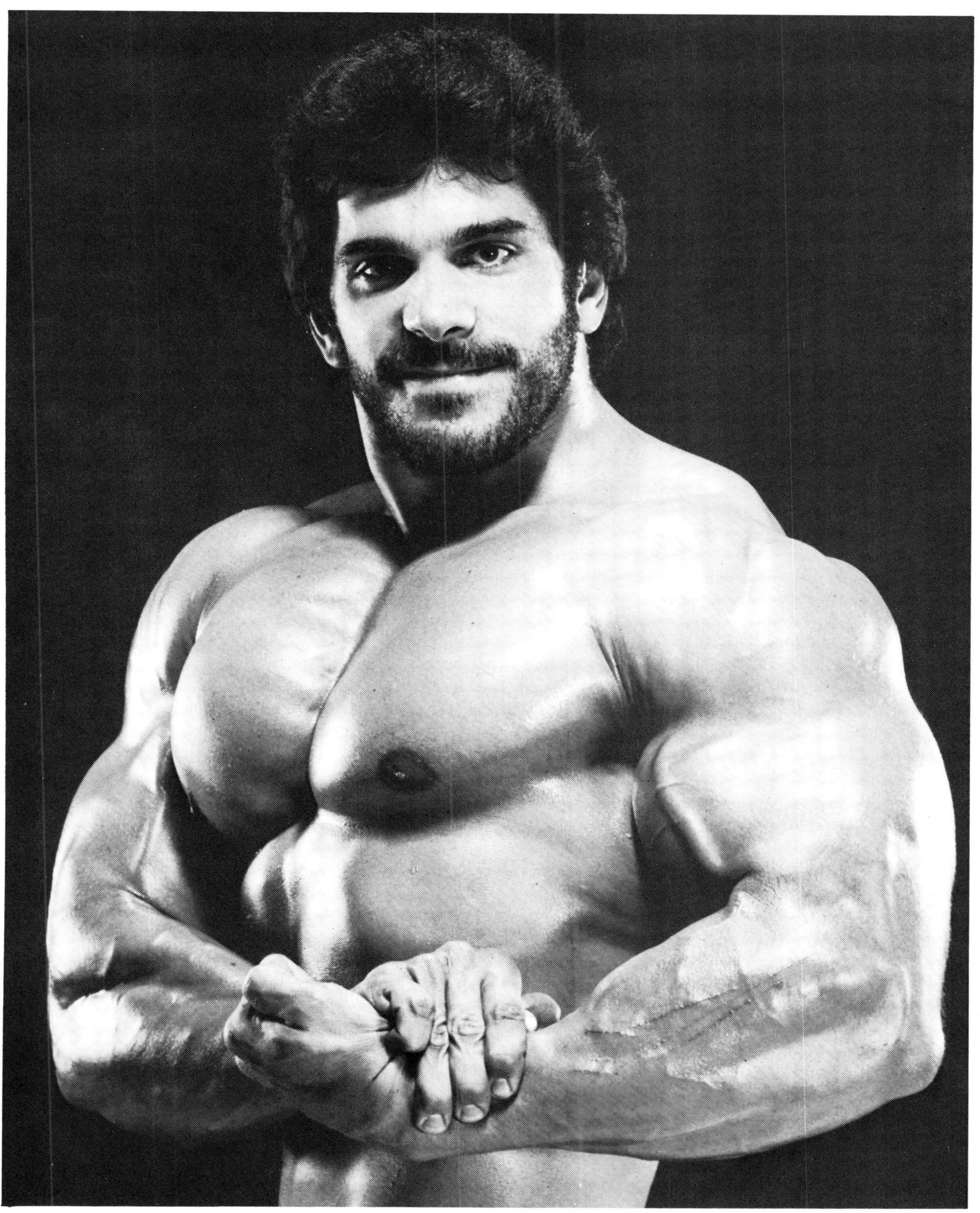

Although he hasn't competed for years, Lou has kept in remarkable shape and has grown a beard for his role as HERCULES.

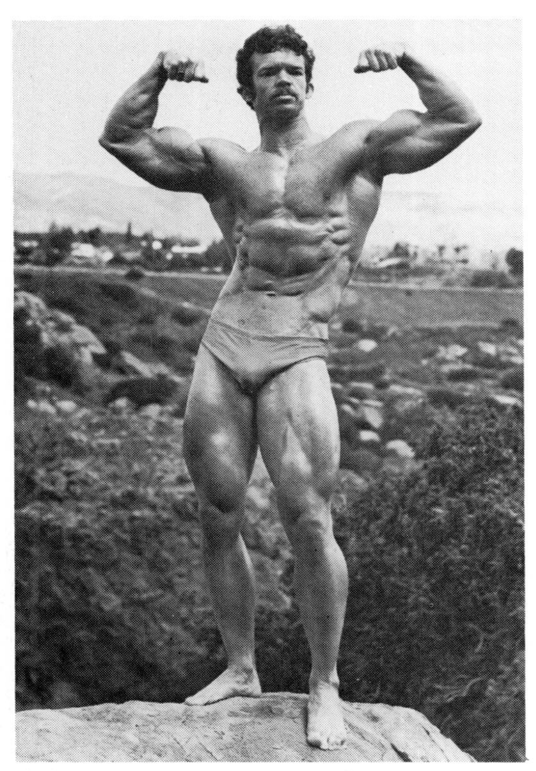

Jim Flaherty.

Jim Flaherty

Jimmy Flaherty has been a member of Gold's Gym for more than 10 years. He's been a training partner of Bill Grant, Danny Padilla, and numerous other Gold's superstars. Flaherty has competed only twice, but placed second and won the "Most Muscular" subdivision both times in the hotly contested Junior Mr. California competition.

Here is a Jim Flaherty off-season thigh program (it is performed twice per week):

1. Leg Extension: 5 × 10–12
2. Squat: 5 × 15–6
3. Leg Press (45-degree angled machine): 5 × 8–10
4. Leg Curl: 5–6 × 8–10

Jim works as a bartender and is looking forward to competing in the Mr. America show.

Cliff Ford

A resident of Virginia, Ford didn't begin training until he was past the age of 30, but once he was in the gym he made up for lost time. He has won over 20 past-35 and past-40 competitions around America, and has twice won his class in the Past-40 Mr. America.

Cliff's waist is quite small and well-muscled. Each day as a warm-up to his main workout, he does this abdominal giant set:

1. Hanging Leg Raise: 4–5 × 15–20
2. Incline Sit-up: 4–5 × 25–30
3. Seated Twisting: 4–5 × 50
4. Bench Leg Raise: 4–5 × 30
5. Roman Chair Sit-up: 4–5 × 25–30

"To display optimum abdominals, you must also follow a tight precontest diet," Cliff cautions. "I diet for 6–8 weeks for a competition and follow a regimen very low in calories. At times I am down to as few as 1,000–1,200 calories per day. It's tough to stick to such a diet when training hard, but if you are able to do so you'll be incredibly ripped at contest time."

Bertil Fox.

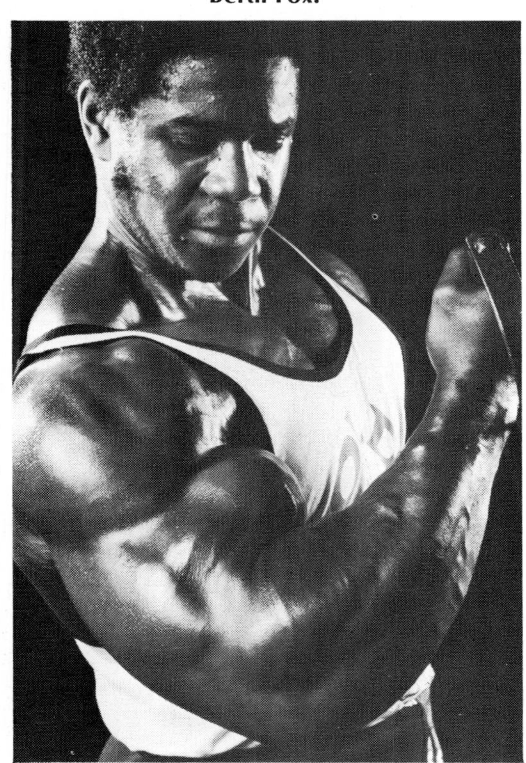

Bertil Fox

Originally from St. Kitts in the Caribbean, Fox lived for most of his life in London, winning Junior Mr. Britain (several times), Mr. Britain, Mr. Europe, and Mr. Universe (twice). At 5′8″ in height, his upper arms are more than 21 inches in girth. Interestingly, Bertil had 16-inch arms at 16, 17-inch arms at 17, 18-inch arms at 18, and 19-inch arms at 19. Fox moved to southern California in 1981 and periodically trains at Gold's Gym.

Having done six reps in the Bench Press with 525 pounds, Fox uses this superset chest routine:

1. Barbell Bench Press: 5–7 × 4–8
2. Dumbbell Bench Press: 5 × 6–8
3. Barbell Incline Press: 5 × 6–8
4. Parallel Bar Dip: 5 × 8–10
5. Flye: 5 × 6–8

Without a doubt, Bertil Fox is already one of the world's greatest bodybuilders. Perhaps one day he will be considered *the* greatest bodybuilder of all time!

Dan Franklin

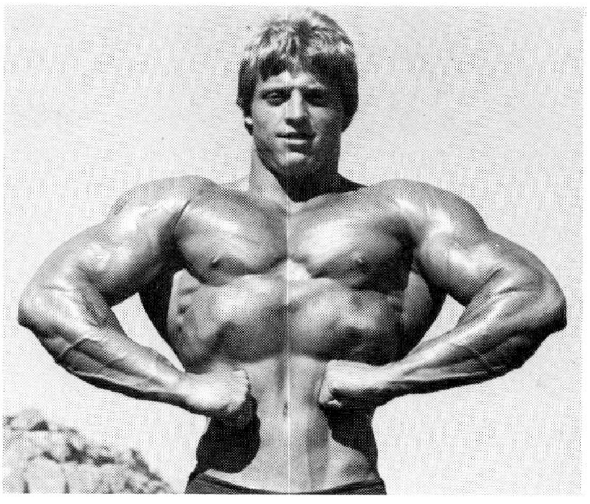

Dan Franklin.

Dan is originally from the Seattle area, where he has won the Mr. Seattle, Mr. Washington, Junior Mr. Pacific Northwest, and Mr. Pacific Northwest titles. He's also won his class in the hotly contested Mr. Western America show and has been a finalist in the Heavyweight Class of the Mr. America competition. A former training partner of Lou Ferrigno, Franklin is 6′2″ tall and weighs 225 pounds in contest shape. Dan has won "Best Legs" subdivision trophies in virtually every competition he's entered.

Franklin's calves tape over 19 inches, and they were built with routines like this:

Monday-Wednesday-Friday

1. Standing Calf Machine Toe Raise: 5 × 10
2. Seated Calf Machine Toe Raise: 5 × 10
3. Nautilus Calf Press: 5 × 10

Tuesday-Thursday-Saturday

1. Donkey Calf Raise: 5 × 20–30

"I believe in heavy low-rep training three days per week with a light pumping day between them," Dan concluded. "And it's vitally important to use a full range of motion on all calf exercises."

Georgia Miller Fudge

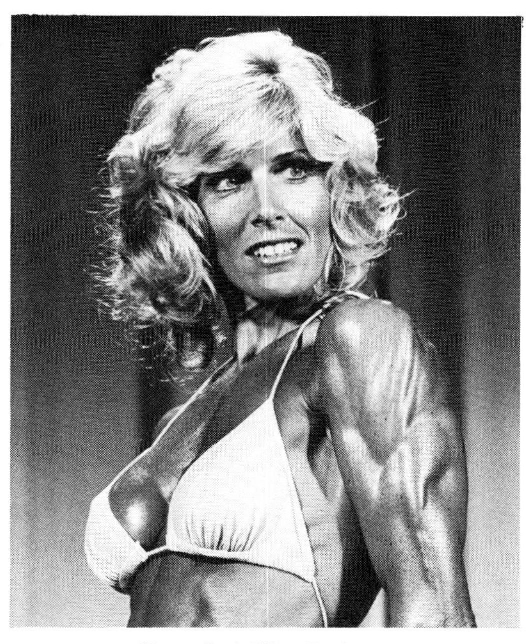

Georgia Miller Fudge.

Georgia lives in St. Petersburg, Florida, where she runs her own gym (The Rare Breed Gym) for women. At 5′7½″ in height she weighs 120 pounds in ripped condition. Georgia has placed high in several pro championships, winning the Pro Women's USA Invitational Cup Championships in 1981. Long, lean, and foxy, Georgia is in her mid-30s and is one of the most popular women bodybuilders on the IFBB pro tour.

Since Georgia Miller Fudge has such well-developed and well-shaped biceps, we secured her routine for that body part. Here it is:

1. Incline Dumbbell Curl: 4 × 6–7
2. High-Pulley Preacher Curl: 4 × 6–7
3. Low-Pulley Preacher Curl: 4 × 6–7

Johnny Fuller

Johnny Fuller

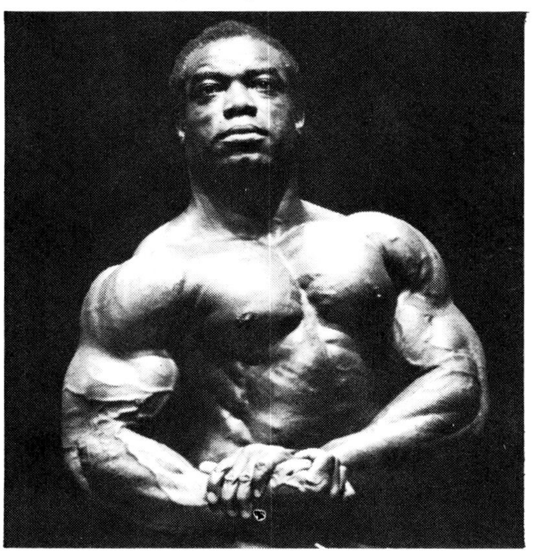

The 1980 IFBB Mr. Universe winner, England's Johnny Fuller is 5′6½″ tall and weighs a superhard 195 pounds for competition. When he first began bodybuilding after a pro boxing career, he weighed only 145 pounds. As a 185-pound powerlifter, Fuller has Squatted with 650 pounds, Benched 440 pounds, and Deadlifted 665 pounds. Johnny has even run a marathon. Obviously, Johnny Fuller is a very versatile athlete.

Every facet of Fuller's physique is fully developed, so it's difficult to pick a particularly strong point. But, we finally asked him for his forearm program, which follows:

1. Narrow-Grip Barbell Reverse Curl: 4–5 × 10–15
2. Barbell Wrist Curl: 4–5 × 15–20
3. Barbell Reverse Wrist Curl: 4–5 × 15–20

Fuller does this simple and effective forearm workout three or four days per week.

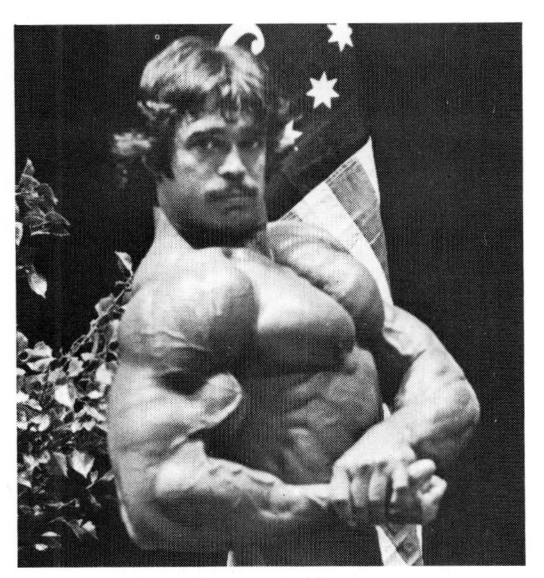

Denny Gable.

Denny Gable

During the middle 1970s Denny Gable was a sensation in California, winning the Mr. Western America title and only narrowly missing a Mr. America win. He was also the training partner of Robby Robinson when "The Black Prince" first moved from Florida to California. Of course, massive Denny trained exclusively at Gold's Gym.

Denny Gable's upper arms were ultimately a well-shaped and muscular pair of 19½-inchers. Here is the arm routine he followed:

1. Seated Dumbbell Curl: 5 × 10
2. Barbell Preacher Curl: 5 × 10
3. Dumbbell Concentration Curl: 5 × 10
4. Pulley Pushdown: 5 × 10
5. Lying Triceps Extension: 5 × 10
6. One-Arm Dumbbell Triceps Extension: 5 × 10

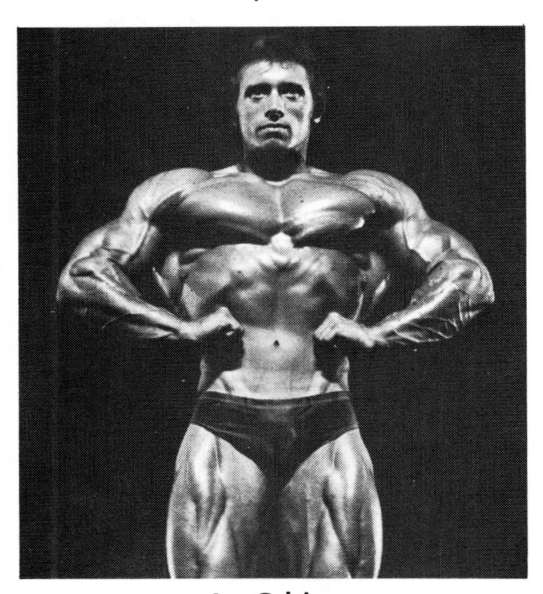

Les Galvin.

Les Galvin

One of the brightest young stars in bodybuilding, Les moved out from his native Ohio to train for a couple of years at Gold's. For much of that time he was Danny Padilla's training partner. Les has won the Mr. Los Angeles title, placed second in the Mr. USA contest, and finished second in the IFBB Mr. International competition. If he continues to train as vigorously as in the past, he will no doubt soon win national and international titles.

Les contributed this forearm program to this book:

Monday-Wednesday-Friday

1. Barbell Reverse Curl: 4–5 × 8–10
2. Barbell Wrist Curl: 4–5 × 10–15

Tuesday-Thursday-Saturday

1. One-Arm Dumbbell Wrist Curl: 4–5 × 10–15
2. Barbell Reverse Wrist Curl: 4–5 × 10–15

"Consistency is the real key to developing large, muscular forearms," Les Galvin advises. "Stick with this routine and you'll experience good results."

Cassandra Gaviola. *(Peter Brenner)*

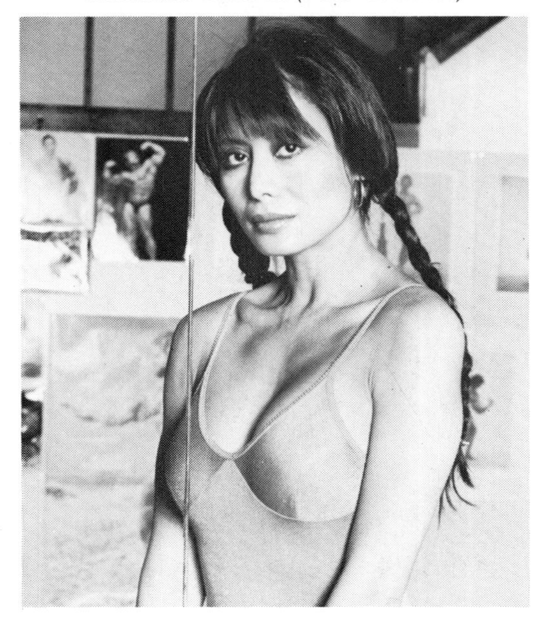

Cassandra Gaviola

Cassandra is the successful actress who played the Wolf Witch in *Conan, the Barbarian* with Arnold Schwarzenegger. (The photo of her is one of many exercises she demonstrated for *The Weider Book of Bodybuilding for Women,* Contemporary Books, 1981.) Through Arnold's persuasive influence, she began weight training to tone her body and improve her energy levels. Cassandra was so successful in achieving these goals that she continues to train.

Here is a calf routine that Cassandra Gaviola performs three times per week:

1. Donkey Calf Raise (on Nautilus multi machine with a hip belt): 2–3 × 15–20

2A. Seated Calf Machine Toe Raise: 2–3 × 15–20

2B. Standing Calf Machine Toe Raise: 2–3 × 15–20

This routine has given Cassandra admirably firm and well-shaped calf muscles.

Donny Gay

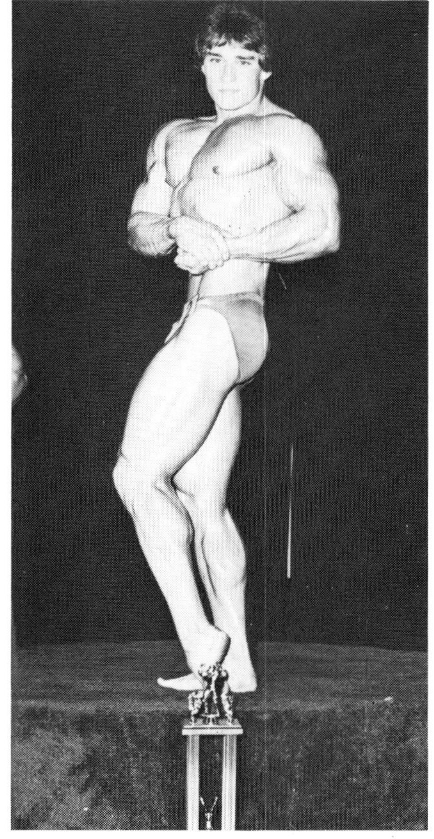

Donny Gay. *(doc sports)*

Donny won the 1981 Mr. Ohio competition, then trained for several weeks at Gold's Gym in preparation for the 1982 Mr. USA contest. He won the light-heavyweight class and placed a strong second overall in the USA. Donny has a tremendous future in bodybuilding.

Here is Donny Gay's precontest, superset, deltoid program, which we observed him using at Gold's:

1. Seated Press Behind the Neck: 4 × 6–8
2. Seated Bent Lateral: 4 × 8–10
3. Seated Dumbbell Press: 4 × 6–8
4. Dumbbell Side Lateral: 4 × 8–10
5. Cable Bent Lateral: 4 × 8–10
6. Cable Side Lateral: 4 × 8–10

Ron Gibson

Ron is an Ohio native who has spent considerable time pumping heavy iron at Gold's Gym. Among his titles are Mr. Ohio, Mr. Heart of America, Mr. Eastern States, Mr. Northern Hemisphere, and Mr. North America. With his thickly developed, dense, and muscular physique, Ron has the potential to go quite far in the sport.

Here is a typical Ron Gibson back routine, which is done on Mondays, Wednesdays, and Fridays:

1. Barbell Bent Rowing: 5 × 8–10 (up to 250 lbs.)
2. Lat Machine Pulldown: 5 × 8–10 (up to 240 lbs.)
3. T-Bar Rowing: 5 × 8–10 (up to 350 lbs.)

Ed Giuliani

Originally from New York, Eddie Giuliani won a variety of titles while training at Gold's. Among these were Mr. Western America, Mr. Eastern America, and class wins in the Mr. America and Mr. USA competitions.

Commenting on abdominal development, Giuliani stated, "Whenever I train any body part, I finish off my routine with abs. I think abdominals should always be done last, because then there's less food in the stomach and they seem to burn more when you do them. People will want to spend an hour or more on a body part like the arms and less than 10 minutes on abdominal training. Then they wonder why their abs are unimpressive. The waist should be worked like any other body part, hard and long. I do Roman Chair Sit-ups for 15–20 consecutive minutes, which is 500–600 reps for the upper abdominals. Then I do Lying Kickouts on a bench for 500 reps to hit my lower abs. Without such regular hard work, I'd never have developed such a good midsection."

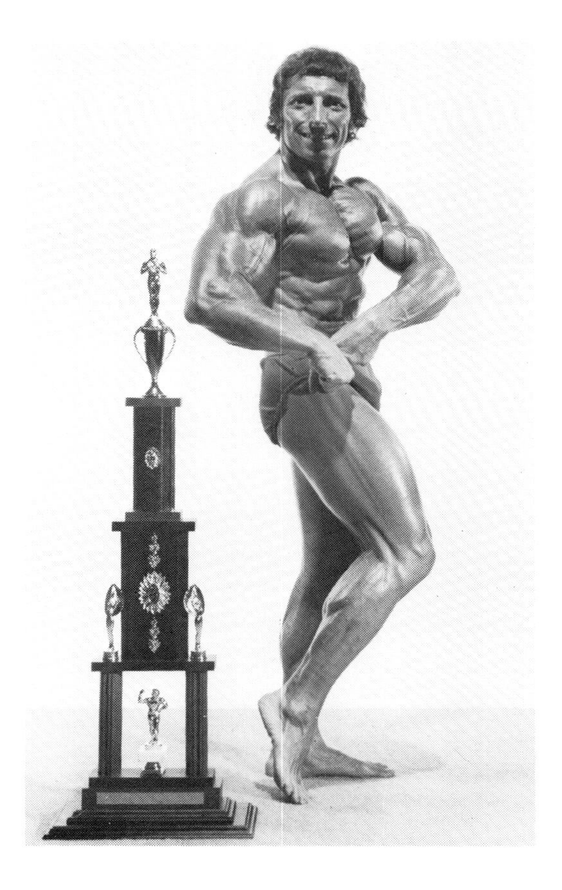

Ed Guiliani. *(Russ Warner)*

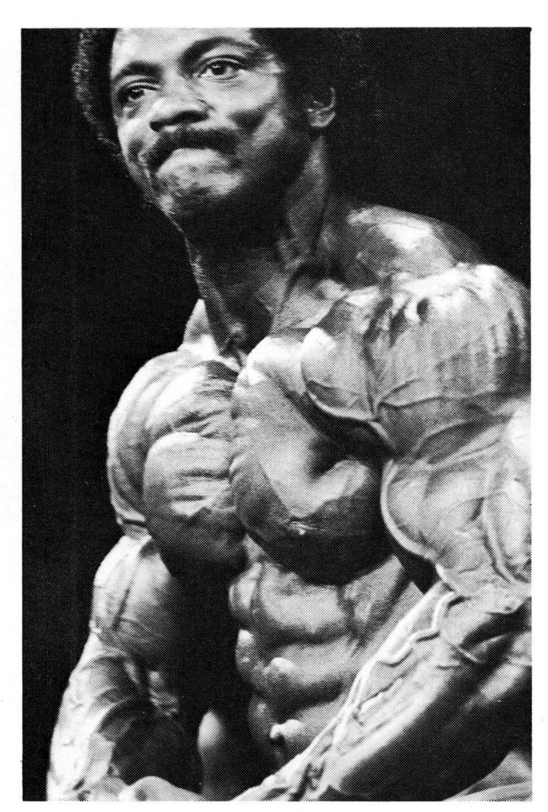

Charles Glass.

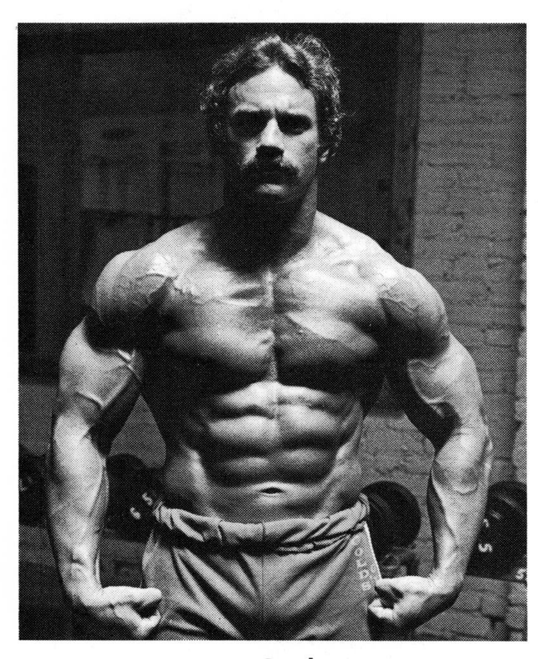

Larry Gordon.

Charles Glass

Charles was captain of the University of California (Berkeley) gymnastics team before turning to bodybuilding, and he still includes a spectacular back flip in his posing routine. Incredibly powerful, he's benched 500 pounds in fairly strict form at under 200 pounds body weight. A top-five finisher in two Mr. America contests, Charles has also won Novice Mr. California, Mr. Western America, and Mr. Southern California.

Charles trains thighs on Tuesdays and Fridays. Here's the Tuesday routine (Note: he allows a maximum rest interval between sets of only 60 seconds):

1. Squat: 6 × 10 (250–400 lbs.)
2. Front Squat: 5 × 6 (275–335 lbs.)
3. Leg Extension: 5–7 × 10 (150–220 lbs.)
4. Leg Curl: 5–7 × 10 (130–170 lbs.)
5. Hack Squat: 10 × 10 (150–200 lbs.)

On Fridays the routine is substantially the same. He does no Hacks and substitutes Leg Presses (10 × 10 with 400–500 lbs.) for Front Squats.

Maria Gonzalez

The training partner of John Balik (the principal photographer for this book), Maria has won the California Expo Women's Championships and placed high in several other competitions. She shows great promise for the future and will soon enter national-level competitions.

Maria contributed the following off-season calf workouts:

Monday-Thursday

1. Standing Calf Machine Toe Raise: 4–5 × 10–15
2. Nautilus Calf Press: 4–5 × 10–15

Tuesday-Friday

1. Seated Calf Machine Toe Raise: 3–4 × 10–15
2. Nautilus Donkey Calf Raise: 3–4 × 10–15

"Consistency in training and the accumulation of several years of regular high-intensity workouts is the key to success in women's bodybuilding," Ms. Gonzalez declared.

Larry Gordon

Larry began his involvement in the iron sport as a powerlifter, officially Benching 475 pounds as a 198-pound lifter. Then he turned to bodybuilding and won the Mr. Ohio competition before getting down to serious business at Gold's Gym. Bearing a remarkable facial and physical resemblance to Mike and Ray Mentzer, Gordon managed to place in the top five of his class in several national and international competitions.

Larry's three-times-per-week thigh workout at Gold's generally looked like this:

1. Squat: 5 × 15
2. Front Squat: 5 × 15
3. Nautilus Leg Extension: 10 × 12–15
4. Nautilus Leg Curl: 10 × 12–15

Larry rested 30–40 seconds between sets, and also believed in doing a lot of wind sprints to add muscularity to his thighs and calves.

One of the most interesting things about Larry Gordon was his appetite. During the off-season, he routinely ate 40–50 pieces of chicken at a restaurant near Gold's where they foolishly advertised "all you can eat in a single sitting." Awesome, even for a bodybuilder!

Bill Grant

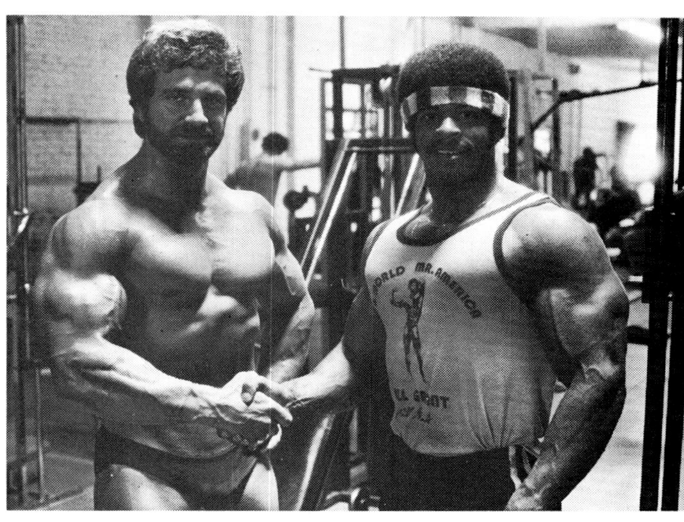

Bill Grant (right) and Jusup Wilkosz. *(Bill Reynolds)*

A native of New Jersey, Bill Grant moved to California specifically to train at Gold's Gym. Known as "The Man of Steel," his superhard physique allowed him to win the Pro Mr. America and Pro Mr. World titles. And Bill also has placed quite respectably in a number of pro competitions.

Grant has appeared in several television and theatrical films and is a consummate showman onstage at any competition or posing exhibition. He travels with a variety of special lighting equipment and smoke generating machines, all of which combine with his fine physique and showmanship to create a memorable performance.

Bill Grant has always been noted for his huge and well-shaped upper arm development, so we sought out his superset arm routine. This is one he used at the time he won Mr. World:

{1. Nautilus Curl: 3 × 8–10
 2. Pulley Pushdown: 3 × 8–10

{3. Incline Dumbbell Curl: 3 × 8–10
 4. Nautilus Triceps Extension: 3 × 8–10

{5. Barbell Preacher Curl: 3 × 8–10
 6. Standing Barbell Triceps Extension: 3 × 8–10

Paul Grant

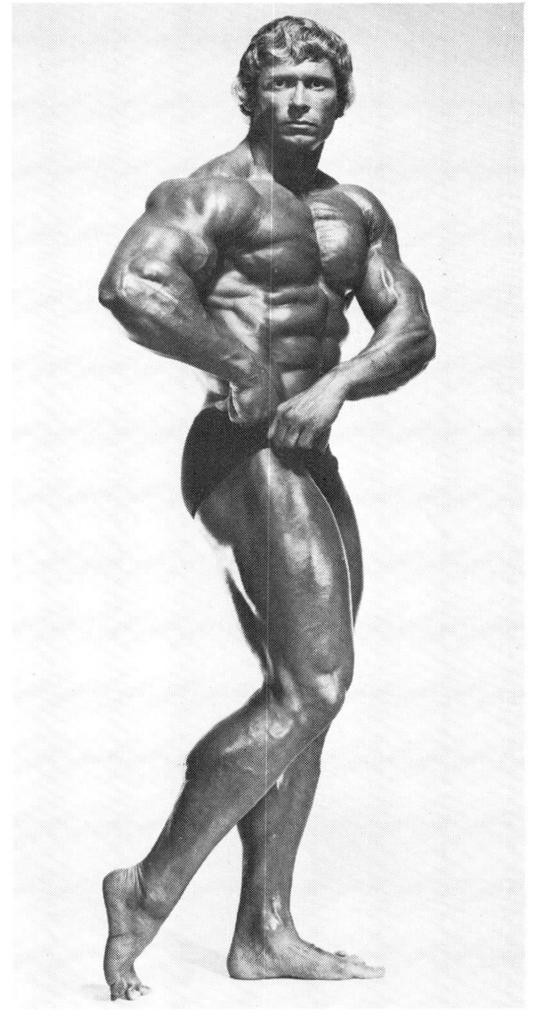

Paul Grant. *(Jimmy Caruso)*

A Welshman, Grant won the Mr. Europe title and placed in the top three in the Mr. Universe competition several times. During the mid-1970s he and his wife (herself a beauty contest winner) lived in southern California, and Paul trained regularly at Gold's. Currently, Paul is again residing in Wales, where he sponsors high-quality bodybuilding shows.

Paul Grant's back was particularly impressive, and this was one of the lat workouts he used while training at Gold's:

1. Behind the Neck Lat Pulldown: 5 × 10–12
2. T-Bar Rowing: 5 × 10–12
3. Seated Pulley Rowing: 5 × 10–12
4. Chin Behind the Neck (with a wide grip): 2 × 10–12

Grant also advocated doing lat stretches between sets of back exercises. This was accomplished by grasping a sturdy vertical upright with either one or both hands and dipping his knees to stretch the lats.

Incidentally, Paul Grant has a great sense of humor and does a very good impression of Arnold Schwarzenegger's voice.

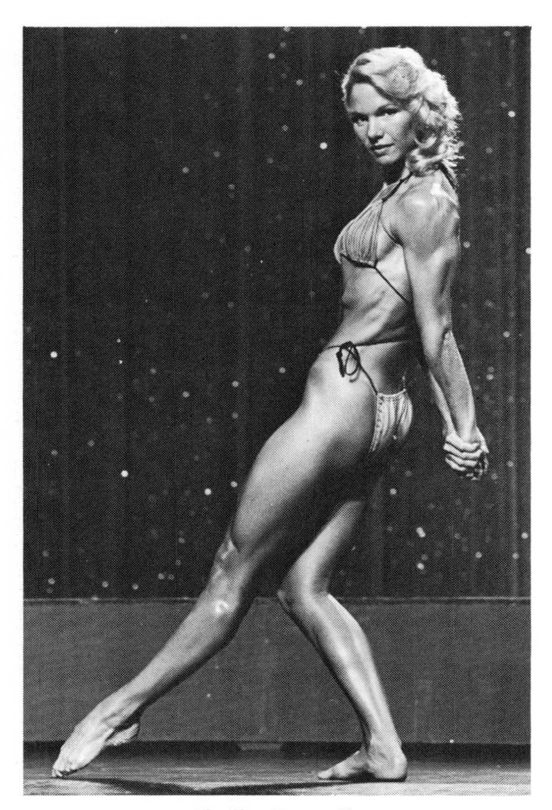

Shelly Gruwell.

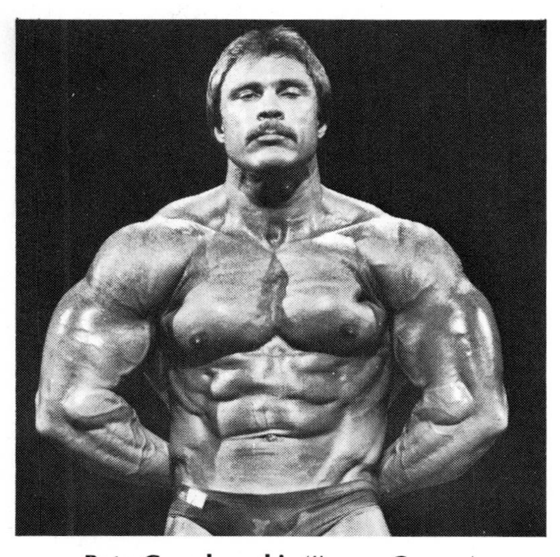

Pete Grymkowski. *(Jimmy Caruso)*

Shelley Gruwell

Even though she lives and trains mainly in Fresno, California, foxy Shelly Gruwell works out at Gold's occasionally when in L.A. Few women have lent as much glamor to the sport of bodybuilding. In 1980 she teamed with John Brown to win the Americn Mixed Pairs Championships. A year later she won the World Women's Professional Grand Prix competition in Montreal, Quebec. And in 1982 she teamed with Tony Pearson to triumph in the World Couples Championships.

Shelley normally does about 10–12 total sets per muscle group in the off-season and a few more prior to a competition. Here is a sample Shelley Gruwell precontest chest workout:

1. Flat-Bench Flye: 3 × 8–10 (up to 45s)
2. Dumbbell Bench Press (flat bench): 3 × 8–10 (up to 55s)
3. Machine Bench Press: 3 × 8–10 (up to 100 lbs.)
4. Incline Barbell Press: 2–3 × 8–10 (up to 75 lbs.)
5. Cable Crossover: 2–3 × 10–15 (up to 30 lbs. per side)

Without a doubt, Shelley Gruwell's gymnastics background has contributed greatly to her success as a bodybuilder, both in terms of her posing style and in that it built a solid foundation for future muscular development.

Pete Grymkowski

Massive Pete wrote the introduction to this book, so you already know he has won the IFBB Mr. World title. He's also won the Junior Mr. USA and Junior Mr. America titles, plus the heavyweight class of the Mr. America competition. And, as previously noted, he is one of the owners of Gold's Gym.

At a height of 5′11″ Grymko has competed in very hard condition at a body weight of 238 pounds. Every muscle group was massively developed, cut to the bone, and in remarkably good proportion with the rest of his physique. The total picture was awesome.

Grymko contributed the following chest training schedule to the authors:

1. Barbell Incline Press (45-degree incline): 10 × 8 (up to 320 lbs.)
2. Barbell Incline Press (65 degrees): 7 × 7–10
3. Decline Press: 6 × 7–9
4. Decline Flye: 5 × 15 }
5. Incline Flye: 5 × 15 }
6. Incline Dumbbell Press: 4 × 12–15
7. High Cable Crossover: 6 × 15–20 }
8. Low Cable Crossover: 6 × 15–20 }

Pete trains rather slowly, taking rest intervals of approximately two minutes between sets. It's little wonder that he trained up to six hours a night prior to a contest. But the results were superb!

Ben Herder

A resident of Holland, big Ben Herder trains at Gold's when in California. One of the most massively developed bodybuilders in IFBB pro competition, Herder has won Mr. Holland, Mr. Europe, and Mr. International. He has been a finalist in both the Amateur and Professional Mr. Universe competitions.

Ben has experienced difficulty in getting his calves up to par with the rest of his physique, and he guarantees that the following calf routine will do the job for any bodybuilder:

Day 1

1. Seated Calf Machine Toe Raise: 5 × 8–10
2. Standing Calf Machine Toe Raise: 5 × 8–10

Day 2

1. Donkey Calf Raise: 3 × 20–30
2. Calf Press: 3 × 20–30

Day 3

Rest

This cycle is repeated every three days, even though it frequently means that Ben must work his calves on Sunday, his normal day of rest from training.

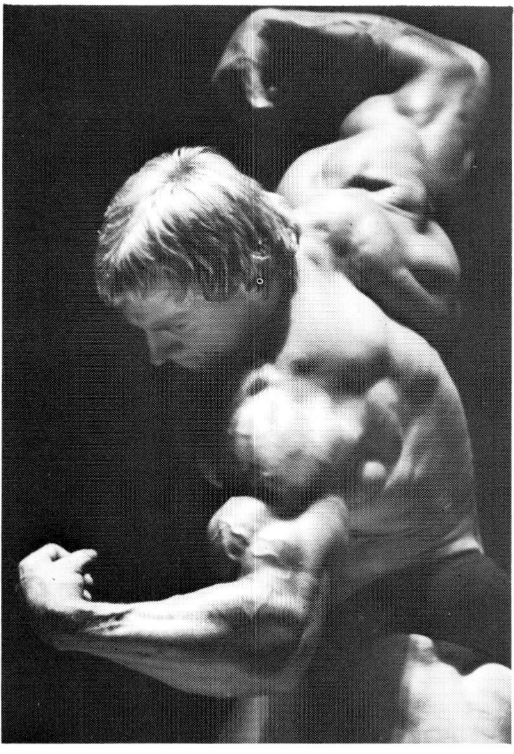

Ben Herder.

Rudy Hermosillo

Rudy has won the Teenage Mr. America and Teenage Mr. USA titles, but he is perhaps more famous as Sylvester Stallone's bodyguard and part-time trainer. Indeed, Hermosillo helped train Stallone for *Rocky II* in which the actor was ripped to the bone. Rudy's no slouch himself, packing 170 pounds of rock-hard, well-proportioned muscle on his 5′5″ frame.

A Gold's Gym regular, Rudy Hermosillo contributed this chest workout:

1. Bench Press: 5 × 10–12
2. Incline Barbell Press: 5 × 10–12
3. Flat-Bench Flye: 5 × 10–12
4. Cable Crossover: 5 × 10–12

To reach peak muscularity for competitions, Hermosillo has dieted on as few as 500–600 calories a day for 4–6 weeks!

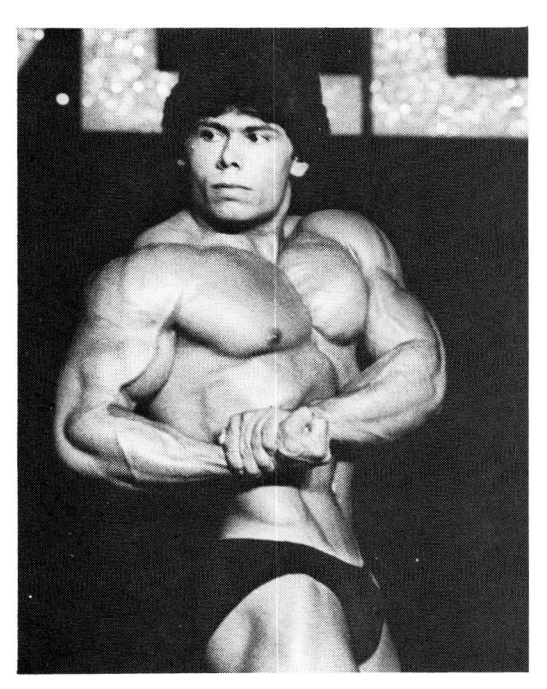

Rudy Hermosillo. *(Jimmy Caruso)*

Paul Hill

Paul was a superb bodybuilder during the early to mid-1970s, and he trained for quite a while at Gold's during his competitive days. Among his titles were Mr. Pacific Coast, Junior Mr. USA, and Mr. USA. Hill's physique had exceptional balance and symmetry, which allowed him to place as high as second in the Mr. America contest.

Here's a Paul Hill abdominal routine which we observed him using at Gold's:

1. Hanging Leg Raise: 3–4 × 15–20
2. Incline Sit-up: 3–4 × 25–30
3. Bench Leg Raise: 3–4 × 25–30
4. Crunch: 3–4 × 25–30

This was more of a precontest abdominal routine, and it was performed six days per week at the beginning of Paul's workout. And it was obviously a productive program, since Paul Hill had exceptional abdominals for a massively developed bodybuilder.

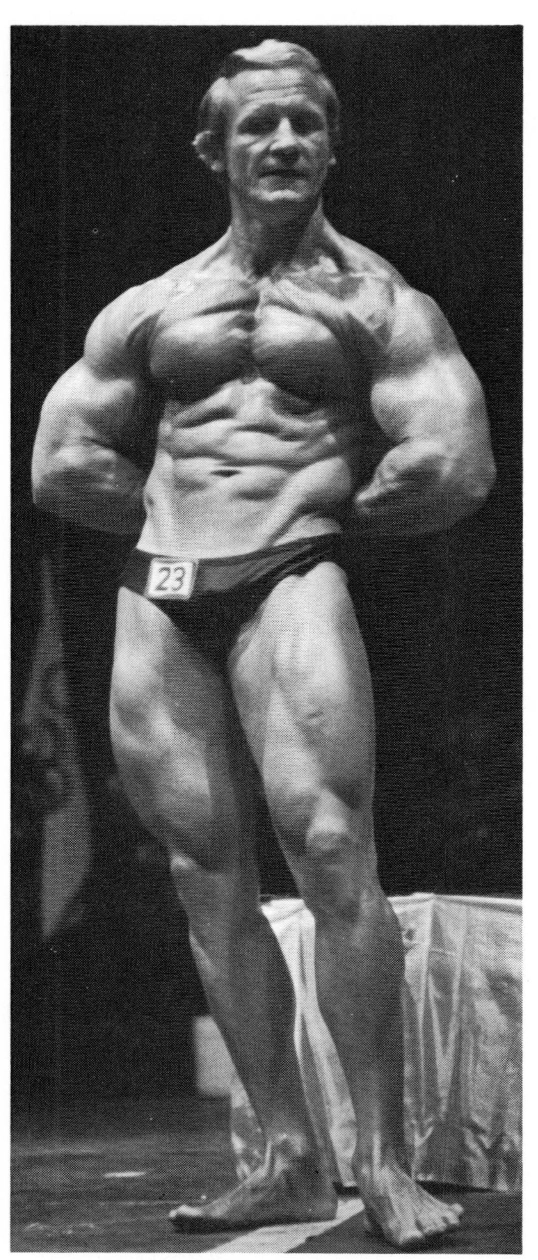

Bill Howard. *(Jimmy Caruso)*

Hulk Hogan

A professional wrestler, Hogan is best known for his excellent portrayal of "Thunderlips," the pro wrestler who tries to destroy Sylvester Stallone during a charity fight in the popular *Rocky III* film. Hulk has trained frequently at Gold's to keep up his power and body bulk between wrestling tours to Japan, Europe, Canada, and Latin America, as well as around the United States.

Less interested in developing a bodybuilding-type physique than in building huge muscle mass and great power, Hogan uses this type of chest routine twice per week at Gold's Gym:

1. Bench Press: 6–8 × 12–2
2. Barbell Incline Press: 5 × 10–2
3. Flat-Bench Flye: 5 × 6–8

"In the flesh, Baby!" Hulk "Thunderlips" Hogan roars in *Rocky III*. And the flesh was largely built by pumping iron at Gold's Gym.

Ed Holmes

Over the past 10 years, Eddie Holmes has trained at a variety of gyms in southern California, including at Gold's. Holmes has won the Novice Mr. Los Angeles and Mr. Central California titles, among others. At a body weight of 175 pounds, he has Bench Pressed 450 pounds, making him one of the stronger bodybuilders currently competing. Recently, Ed has entered mixed pairs competition and won several titles in that discipline.

Ed has a very good arm development, so we secured this precontest upper arm routine, which is done three days per week:

{ 1. Seated Dumbbell Curl: 4–5 × 8–10
{ 2. Lying Triceps Extension: 4–5 × 8–10
{ 3. Barbell Preacher Curl: 4–5 × 8–10
{ 4. Pulley Pushdown: 4–5 × 8–10
{ 5. Dumbbell Concentration Curl: 4–5 × 8–10
{ 6. Dumbbell Kickback: 4–5 × 8–10

No more than 60 seconds rest is allowed between supersets.

Bill Howard

A long-time California bodybuilder, Bill Howard trained from time to time at Gold's. Among his many titles are Mr. Venice Beach, Novice Mr. California, Mr. Western America, and Past-40 Mr. America. Bill also is a successful doctor of chiropractic.

Bill Howard's back was particularly impressive, and this was one of his favorite routines:

1. Front Chin: 5 × 8
2. Barbell Bent Rowing: 5 × 8
3. Seated Pulley Rowing: 5 × 8
4. Behind Neck Lat Pulldown: 5 × 8
5. Close-Grip Chin: 5 × 8

Dan Howard

An all-conference football player at Tulsa University, Dan turned to bodybuilding following a lower back injury sustained on the gridiron. He won the Mr. Oklahoma title and placed high in numerous other competitions before becoming a practicing chiropractor. While in chiropractic college, Howard managed Gold's Gym. Today he owns his own gym in Fountain Valley, California, where he also practices chiropractic medicine.

While training at Gold's, Dan frequently used this calf program three or four days per week:

1. Donkey Calf Raise: 5 × 20
2. Standing Calf Machine Toe Raise: 5 × 15
3. Seated Calf Machine Toe Raise: 5 × 15

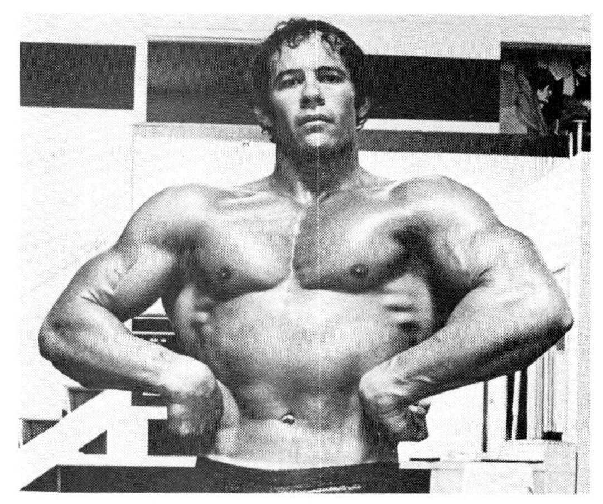

Dan Howard. *(Art Zeller)*

Don Howorth

A Mr. America winner in the late 1960s, Don occasionally worked out at Gold's Gym. He was particularly noted for his narrow waist and broad shoulders. His chest was a stubborn muscle group, but using the following routine, he was finally able to bring it up to par:

1. Bench Press: 5 × 5
2. Decline Flye: 5 × 8
3. Incline Dumbbell Press: 5 × 8
4. Incline Pulley Flye: 5 × 8
5. Dip: 4 × 15

Past the age of 40, Don Howorth retains most of his Mr. America development and trains as hard as ever.

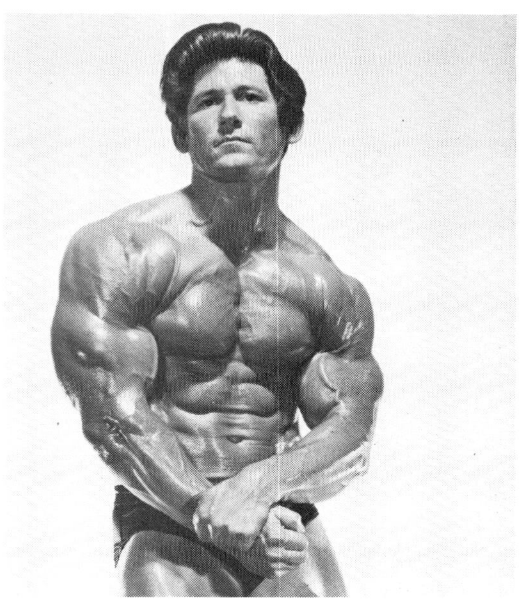

Don Howorth.

Larry Jackson

The 1979 Mr. California winner, Larry has trained at Gold's Gym for many years and won a host of other titles. Most recently, he placed third in the 1981 IFBB Mr. International competition. At 5′9″ in height, Jackson is very massive and ripped to shreds at his 212-pound contest body weight.

Larry Jackson's back is particularly impressive, and he's won the "Best Back" award at the Mr. America competition. Therefore, we solicited this back workout from him:

1. Chin: 5 × 12 (with added resistance)
2. T-Bar Rowing: 5 × 12
3. Seated Pulley Rowing: 5 × 12
4. One-Arm Dumbbell Bent Rowing: 4 × 12
5. Hyperextension: 3 × 25–30

Larry consistently uses over 300 pounds in his T-Bar Rowing. At contest time, Jackson's tightest diet consists of skinned and broiled chicken breasts, fish, two grapefruits per day, and water.

Larry Jackson.

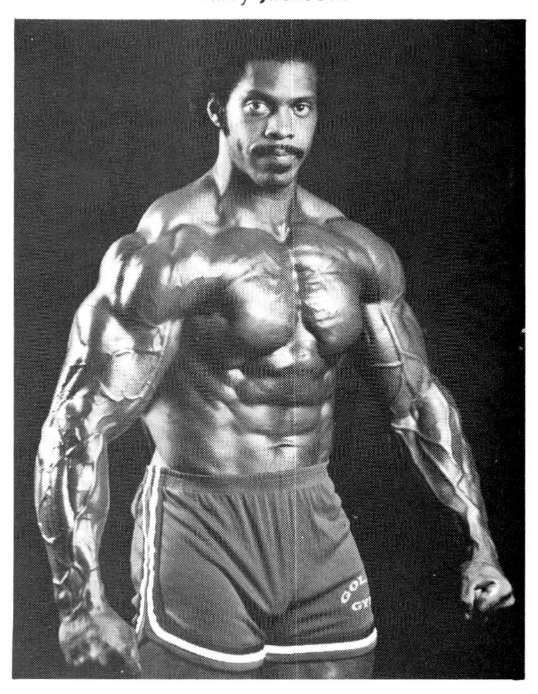

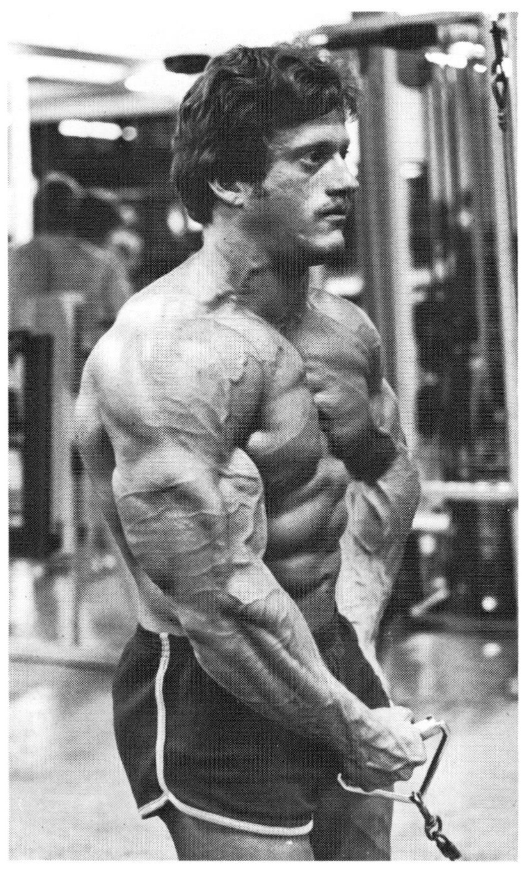

Bob Jodkiewicz.

Serge Jacobs

A resident of Belgium, Serge spent most of a year during the early 1970s at Gold's training for the Mr. Universe competition, in which he was a finalist. Jacobs has won the Mr. Belgium and Mr. Europe titles, and he's also made the top three at the Mr. International competition.

Here is a typical Serge Jacobs deltoid training program:

1. Seated Press Behind the Neck: 4–5 × 6–8
2. Seated Bent Lateral: 4 × 8–10
3. Dumbbell Side Lateral: 4 × 8–10
4. Cable Side Lateral: 4 × 8–10

Bob Jodkiewicz

Bobby Jodkiewicz was somewhat of a prodigy in bodybuilding. By the time he turned 20 he had already won the Teenage Mr. America and Open Mr. Virginia titles. Then he moved briefly to Santa Monica to train at Gold's for the 1977 Mr. America contest. He returned later and became one of the hardest trainers in the gym. Frequently he'll be pumping iron as early as 5:30 in the morning. All of his hard work finally paid off with a Junior Mr. America title in 1979 and several subsequent high placings in national and international competition.

Since Bob's back is so massively developed and supercut, we asked him for his back routine. He trains traps with delts by doing five or six sets of heavy Dumbbell Shrugs, and he does his lower back work with five or six sets of Hyperextensions on his leg day. Here is his lat routine:

1. Front Chin (warm-up): 3–4 × 15–20
2. One-Arm Dumbbell Row: 4–5 × 8–10 (up to 150 lbs.)
3. Seated Pulley Rowing: 4–5 × 8–10 (up to 300 lbs.)
4. Behind the Neck Lat Pulldown: 4–5 × 8–10 (up to 220 lbs.)
5. Front Lat Pulldown: 4–5 × 8–10 (up to 220 lbs.)

To bring out maximum back cuts, Jodkiewicz does a great deal of isotension contraction posing for the last two or three weeks before competing.

Dave Johns. *(Art Zeller)*

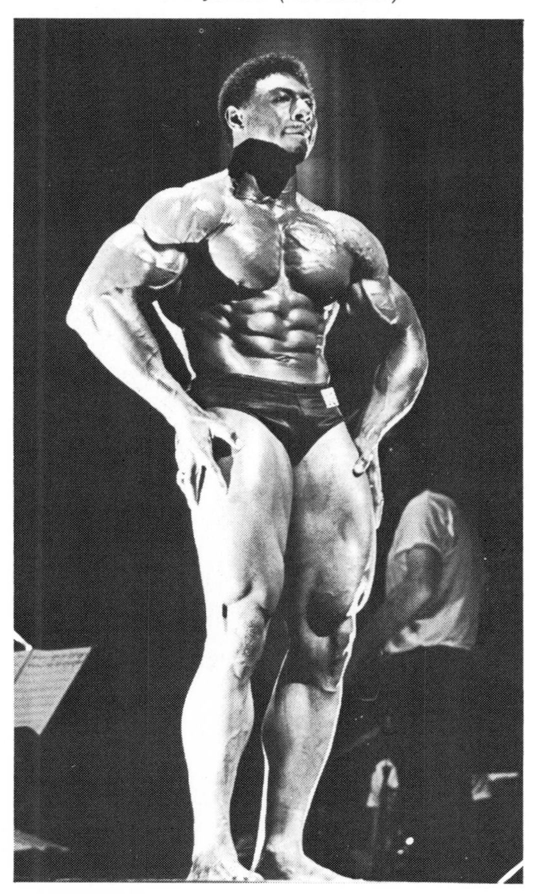

Dave Johns

A probation officer by profession, Dave hit it big by winning the Junior Mr. America contest and placing second in the America in 1976. Then, in 1977, he won Mr. California and Mr. America to establish himself firmly as one of the greats. Dave Johns has also won the NABBA Mr. Universe title and placed high in numerous other international competitions. He currently competes as an IFBB pro bodybuilder.

Dave trains with very heavy weights at all times. While training at Gold's to win his Mr. America title, his chest routine was as follows:

1. Bench Press: 8–10 × 15–4 (up to 430–440 lbs.)
2. Incline Barbell Press: 8–10 × 15–4 (up to 340 lbs.)
3. Parallel Bar Dip: 4–6 × 8–10 (up to 180 lbs. added weight tied around his waist)

With such heavy training, Dave Johns has developed one of the world's most massive physiques.

Mike Katz

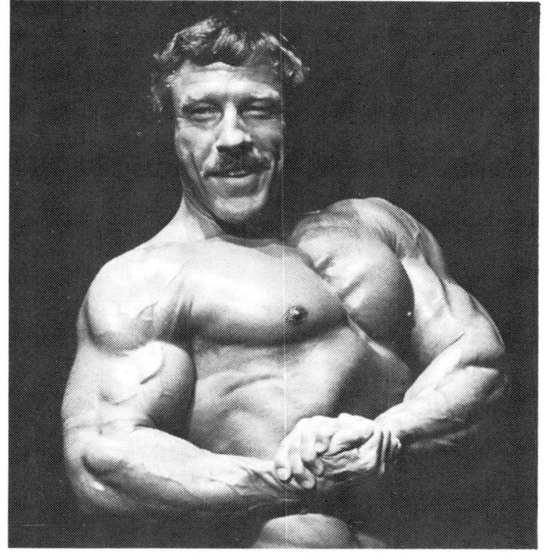

Kent Keuhn.

Genial Mike Katz, a schoolteacher from Connecticut, has a Mr. America title to his credit and has placed high in several Mr. Olympia competitions. He also played pro football for the New York Jets prior to getting serious about bodybuilding. In recent years he has run a series of very popular and successful bodybuilding camps.

Standing over six feet in height, Mike's expanded chest measurement approached 60 inches. Many bodybuilding cognoscenti believe that Katz's chest was the largest and best developed of all time. Here is the off-season, superset pectoral program that he followed at the time he was winning his Mr. America title (he did it on Mondays and Thursdays):

1. Bench Press: 8 × 6–8
2. Barbell Incline Press: 5 × 6–8
3. Flat-Bench Flye: 5 × 8
4. Parallel Bar Dip: 5 × 8

Mike always prefers to do his exercises in very strict form and with maximum possible poundages. And his dedication paid off handsomely with a Mr. America title.

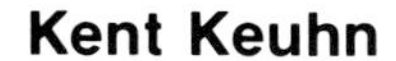

Kent Keuhn

Kent Keuhn, originally from Michigan, has become one of the most popular Gold's Gym members over the years. He's also served for a considerable period of time as the gym's manager. Among Kent's more than 30 bodybuilding titles are Mr. North America, Mr. USA, Past-40 Mr. America, and Past-40 Mr. Universe. Now in his mid-40s, Kent concentrates most of his efforts on educating young upcoming bodybuilders.

Kent had a well-balanced physique with particularly good triceps development. Here is one of his three-times-per-week triceps workouts:

1. Pulley Pushdown: 5 × 10–12
2. Triceps Push-up: 5 × 10–12
3. Lying Triceps Extension: 5 × 10–12
4. One-Arm Triceps Extension: 5 × 10–12

"Be sure to keep up your exercise pace if you desire good gains," Kent Keuhn advises. "There's no excuse for resting more than 45–60 seconds between sets."

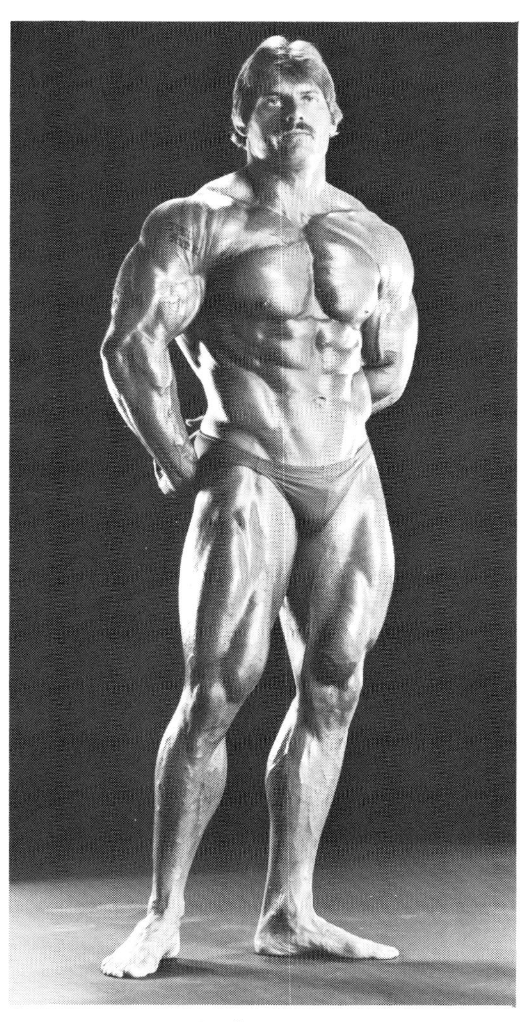

Rod Koontz.

Rod Koontz

Rod has been an outstanding bodybuilder for many years, winning the Mr. USA and Natural Mr. America titles at his peak. He currently competes successfully as an IFBB pro bodybuilder and trains occasionally at Gold's, though he lives 30 miles away in Orange County, California.

Koontz has successfully competed as a powerlifter, recording lifts of 600 pounds in the Squat, 460 pounds in the Bench Press, and 620 pounds in the Deadlift at under 220 pounds body weight. His gym lifts are even higher.

Here is a shoulder routine that Rod used prior to winning the Mr. USA title:

1. Side Lateral: 4 × 10–12
2. Heavy Partial Side Lateral: 4 × 12–15
3. Press Behind the Neck: 4 × 8–10
4. Dumbbell Shrug: 4 × 12–15
5. Partial Front Raise: 4 × 8–10

Exercises 1–3 were performed as a triset with 45–60 seconds rest between trisets. Exercises 4 and 5 were a superset with 30–45 seconds rest between supersets. The routine was done on Mondays, Wednesdays, and Fridays.

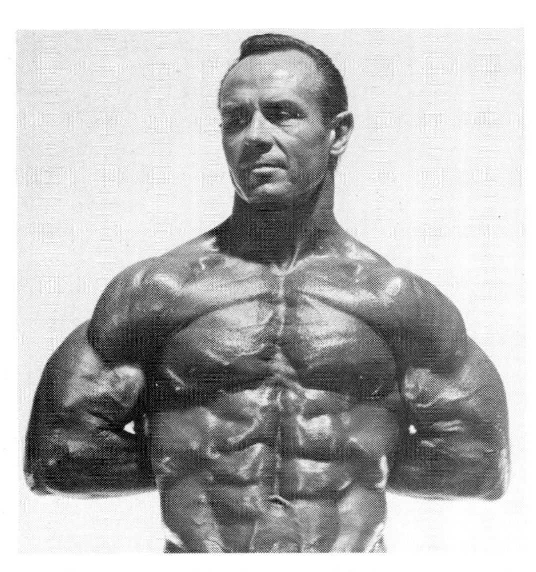

Zabo Koszewski (above) and Gary Leonard (below).

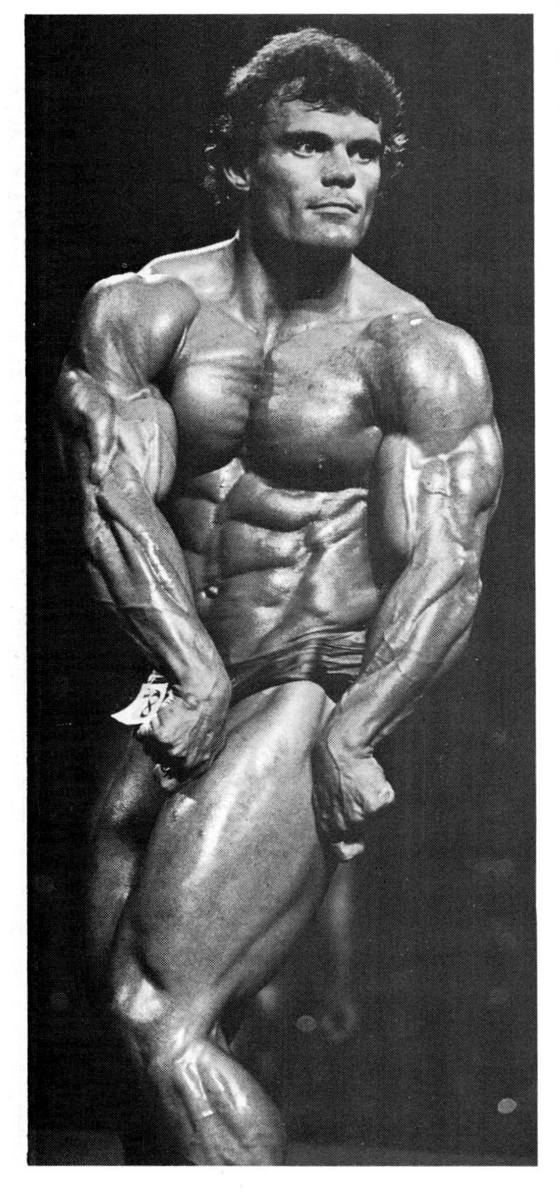

Zabo Koszewski

Originally from New Jersey, Zabo was placing high and winning the "Best Abdominals" subdivision in the Mr. America competition during the late 1940s. Then, while in his mid-40s, he was in such amazing shape that he won "Best Abs" and "Most Muscular" in the Mr. America competition. In his late 50s, Zabo retains his superb muscular definition and physical vigor.

A long-time member of Gold's Gym, Zabo followed a very simple routine to keep his superb abdominals in peak condition. Five or six times per week he would do 500 Incline Sit-ups and 500 Incline Leg Raises. Certainly this was a very simple routine, but it was also a very effective abdominal training program.

Rory Leidelmeyer

Rory is one of the most exciting young bodybuilders to burst onto the sport's posing platform. In 1980 he scored a smashing victory in the Mr. California contest, then placed second in his class to the eventual overall winner in the 1981 Mr. America competition. A superb poser, Rory has every quality of physical development, character, attitude, and charisma necessary to become one of the true greats of the sport.

Since Rory's triceps are so outstanding, we solicited from him a triceps program, which follows:

1. Pulley Pushdown: 4 × 10–12
2. One-Arm Pushdown (reverse grip): 4 × 10–12
3. Lying Triceps Extension: 4 × 8–10
4. Pulley Triceps Extension: 4 × 10–15

Rory and his wife have one child, and he is involved in the gym management business.

Gary Leonard

Gary rocketed to prominence in the sport in 1979 when he placed second to Ray Mentzer in the Mr. America contest. Then in 1980 he won the title, having had less than five years of training under his belt. Unfortunately, Leonard subsequently injured his shoulder quite badly while skiing, necessitating a complete layoff from training. At the time of writing this book, however, Gary's shoulder is fully healed and he is back training hard. With his ripped and perfectly proportioned physique, Leonard could easily make some heads roll in future IFBB pro competition.

Gary Leonard was using the following biceps routine prior to his Mr. America win:

1. Incline Dumbbell Curl: 5 × 6–8 (up to 85s)
2. Barbell Preacher Curl: 5 × 6–8 (up to 160 lbs.)
3. Seated Dumbbell Concentration Curl: 5 × 6–8 (up to 65 lbs.)

"Unlike many bodybuilders, I actually get stronger as a show approaches, even though I'm on a low-calorie diet," Gary revealed. "This is largely because I get so crazy about winning. There's definitely a degree of obsession and desperation. Close to a contest I get so berserk that I lose a lot of sleep, but that just helps me to get more cut."

John Lloyd

A native of Spokane, Washington, John was an All-State high school wrestler before turning to bodybuilding. Lloyd has won the Heavyweight Mr. California, Mr. Iron Man (which combines powerlifting with bodybuilding), and Gold's Classic Championship titles. At 6′2″ in height, John weighs a massive 235 pounds in contest shape. And he is exceedingly powerful, as attested by his ability to Squat with 650 pounds, Bench Press 500, Deadlift 715, Power Clean 360, and do eight reps in the Front Squat with 515 pounds.

John Lloyd's thighs are phenomenally massive and cut to the bone, so we asked him for his thigh workout. John does this thigh program twice per week during the off-season:

1. Leg Extension: 3 × 12 (warm up)
2. Leg Curl: 3 × 12 (warm up)
3. Front Squat: 5–6 × 12–5 (up to 500+ pounds)
4. Lunge (on block): 3 × 15
5. Hack Machine Squat: 3 × 12
6. Standing Leg Curl: 3 × 12

"I do my Hack Squats differently than most bodybuilders," Lloyd explained. "As I begin to straighten my legs, I thrust my hips and knees forward away from the machine's sliding platform, so I'm in a position much like I would be when doing Sissy Squats. Done in this manner, Hacks are great for slicing up the front thighs."

John Lloyd works as the manager of Gold's/San Francisco.

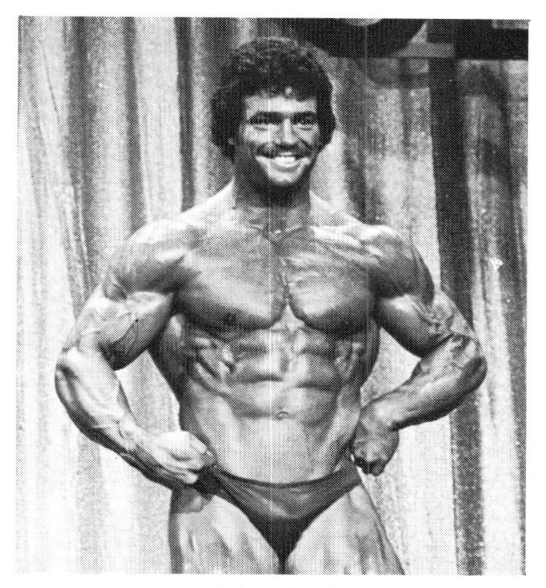

John Lloyd.

Lisa Lyon

Lisa was one of the real pioneers of women's bodybuilding. With a strong background in dance and martial arts (particularly kendo), she turned to weight training to further improve her fitness, self-discipline, and physical impressiveness. Indeed, she was training like a true bodybuilder at Gold's Gym for a couple of years before there was even such a thing as women's bodybuilding.

Ms. Lyon was the outstanding winner of the first World Women's Bodybuilding Championships promoted by Gold's in Los Angeles in June 1979. And from there she did yeoman work popularizing the sport by appearing regularly on television and in other media, promoting women's competitions, and writing a popular book, *Lisa Lyon's Body Magic* (Bantam, 1981). She is currently married to a well-known French rock singer and lives in Paris.

At the peak of her bodybuilding condition, Lisa claimed to train up to 3½ hours a day six days each week. Here is one of her favorite superset thigh workouts:

1. Squat: 4–5 × 10–12
2. Leg Press: 4–5 × 10–12
3. Leg Extension: 4–5 × 12–15 } superset
4. Leg Curl: 4–5 × 12–15 }

Lisa also believes in doing a considerable amount of stretching for her legs, particularly as a warm-up before her weight workout, but occasionally after training as well. She also did a considerable amount of posing practice to further deepen the cuts in her thighs.

Lisa Lyon.

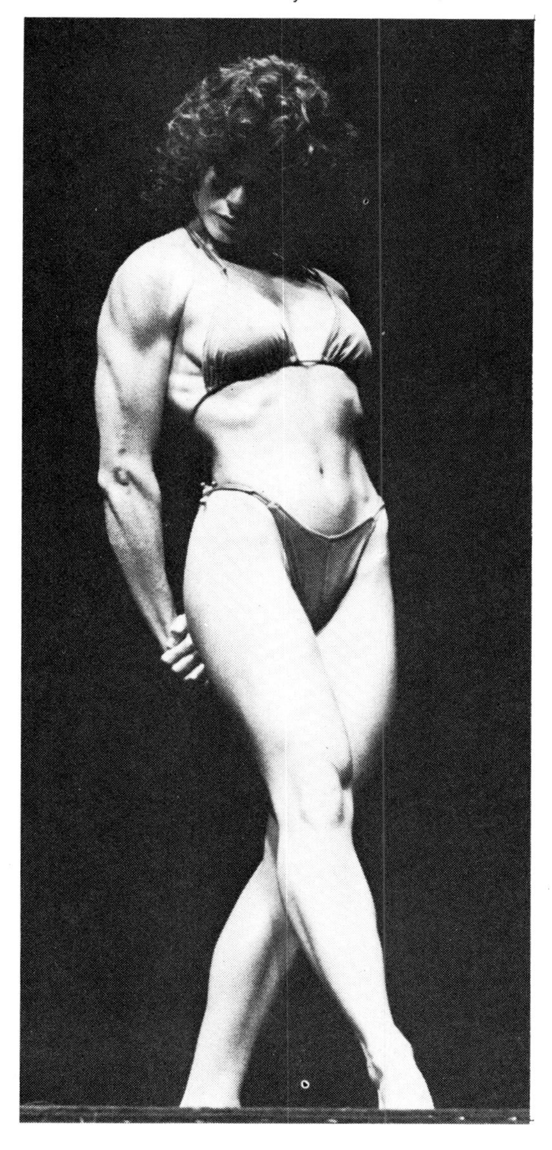

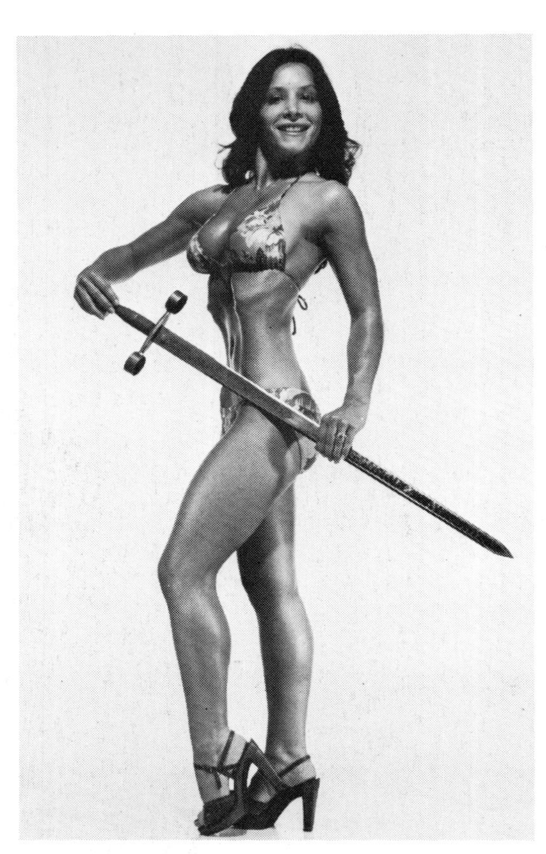

Corinne Machado-Ching. *(Russ Warner)*

Corrine Machado-Ching

Corrine lives in the San Francisco Bay Area, but has worked out periodically at Gold's Gym. Her husband Brian Ching also is an excellent bodybuilder, who has won the Mr. Oakland title and placed in the top three in several other contests. Corrine has won the Ms. Western America title and placed in the top three at both the Women's Pro World Championships and Pro World Couples' Championships (with Boyer Coe as her partner). And, she has been a finalist in the Miss Olympia competition. Of Portuguese descent, Ms. Machado-Ching has a tremendous future in professional women's bodybuilding.

We asked for Corrine's chest routine. She does the following off-season pec workout twice per week:

1. Incline Dumbbell Press: 4 × 6–10 (increasing the weights each set)
2. Flat-Bench Flye: 3 × 8–10
3. Parallel Bar Dip: 3 × 8–10
4. Cross-Bench Dumbbell Pullover: 3 × 8–10

Mohamed Makkawy

Makkawy created a sensation when he charged out of his native Egypt ripped to the bone to devastate Danny Padilla at the 1976 Mr. Universe competition. Now living in Canada, personable Mohamed is in even better shape and has placed extremely well in IFBB pro competitions.

Cautioning that a bodybuilder must have a very low degree of body fat to display sharp abdominals, Mohamed suggests training abdominals as hard as any other muscle group. "Good abdominal muscles should actually be built up and fairly thick looking," he claims.

When he was training at Gold's, Makkawy hit his abdominals five days per week at the conclusion of his regular workout with this routine:

1. Hanging Leg Raise: 3–5 × 20–30
2. Incline Sit-up: 3–5 × 20–30 (holding a 25-pound plate behind his head)
3. Roman Chair Sit-up: 3–5 × 100

This routine gave Mohamed Makkawy sensational abdominal development, which added considerably to his classic physique.

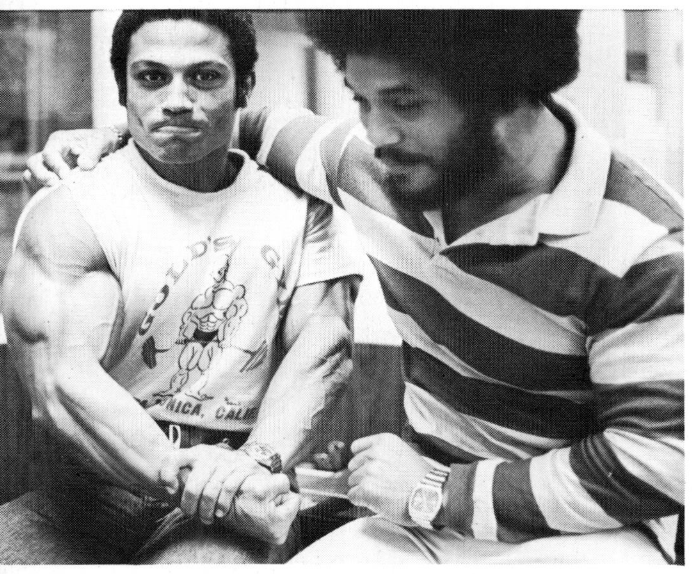

Mohamed Makkawy forcefully shows his arm development to bodybuilding writer (and former Mr. World) Rick Wayne. *(Bill Reynolds)*

Ali Malla

Ali Malla was born, and grew up, in Lebanon. For a time he lived and trained in Denmark, but since early 1981 he has been in California training at Gold's Gym. With his thick and dense physique, Ali has won his class in the 1981 IFBB Mr. International competition, narrowly losing out to Scott Wilson for the overall title.

Ali Malla believes in training his forearms four days per week with these routines:

Monday-Thursday

1. Reverse Curl: 4–5 × 8–10
2. Barbell Wrist Curl: 4–5 × 10–15
3. Barbell Reverse Wrist Curl: 4–5 × 10–15

Tuesday-Friday

1. Zottman Curl: 4–5 × 8–10
2. Dumbbell Wrist Curl: 4–5 × 10–15
3. Dumbbell Reverse Wrist Curl: 4–5 × 10–15

Jim Manion

Best known as national chairman of the American Physique Committee, Inc., Manion owns a gym in Carnegie, Pennsylvania, and has been a very successful competitive bodybuilder over the years. He has won more than 10 titles, including Mr. Pennsylvania. Jim promotes contests today, and he has been one of the most consistently accurate bodybuilding judges in America over the past 10 years.

Jim Manion's triceps development is particularly good, so we asked him for his triceps routine. He does this program three days per week.

1. Pulley Pushdown: 4 × 10–12
2. Nautilus Triceps Extension: 4 × 8–10
3. Dumbbell Kickback: 4 × 8–10

"I would recommend bodybuilding workouts to all men and women," enthused Jim Manion. "It's the safest and least expensive 'high' I know of, since exercise releases endorphins into your blood stream to make you feel good after a training session has been completed."

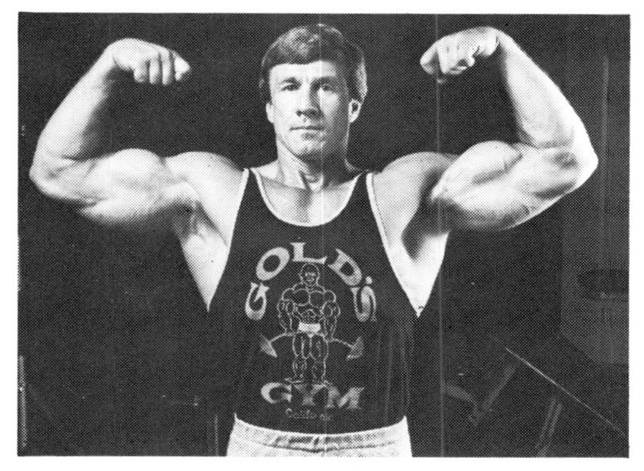

Jim Manion.

Stella Martinez

A former powerlifter who lives in San Francisco, Stella placed well in the first true women's bodybuilding competition, the 1979 Women's World Championships promoted by Gold's Gym. For the next three years, Stella competed infrequently, but peaked out perfectly to easily win the 1982 Ms. USA title with her well-proportioned and tightly muscled physique. She spent a month prior to the USA training at Gold's Gym to totally peak.

Here is a precontest abdominal routine that we observed Stella using at Gold's Gym prior to her Ms. USA win:

{ 1. Hanging Leg Raise: 3 × 15–20
{ 2. Incline Sit-up: 3 × 20–30
{ 3. Incline Leg Raise: 3 × 20–30
{ 4. Wall Crunch: 3 × 20–30
{ 5. Bench Leg Raise: 3 × 20–30
{ 6. Cable Crunch: 3 × 20–25

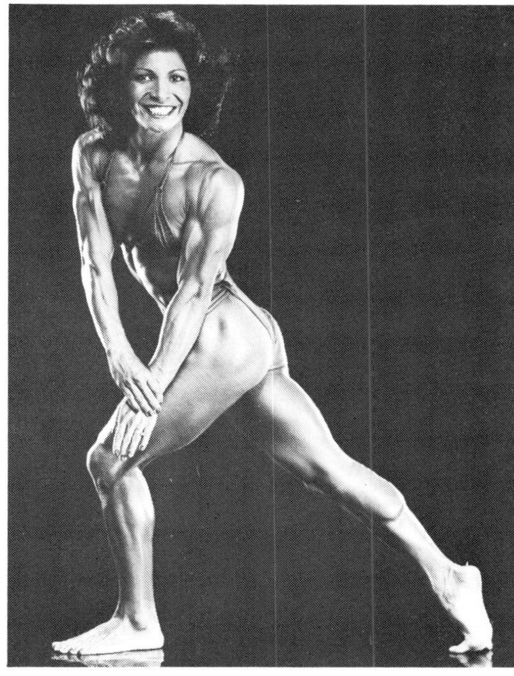
Stella Martinez.

Dave Mastorakis

One of the real child prodigies in the sport, Dave was competing in the *Senior* Mr. America competition (and doing quite well, thank you!) at the age of 16! Among his numerous titles are Mr. East Coast, Mr. New England, and Mr. Massachusetts. An enthusiastic proponent of high-intensity training done primarily on Nautilus machines, Mastorakis has frequently trained at Gold's Gym, often with his friend, Mike Mentzer.

Here is a typical off-season thigh workout used by Dave (it is done as a giant set and is over in less than five minutes!):

{ 1. Leg Extension: 1 × 10–12 (280–300 lbs.)
{ 2. Leg Curl: 1 × 10–12 (120–130 lbs.)
{ 3. Hack Machine Squat: 1 × 10–12 (250–270 lbs.; negative reps only)
{ 4. Leg Extension: 1 × 10–12 (270–280 lbs.)

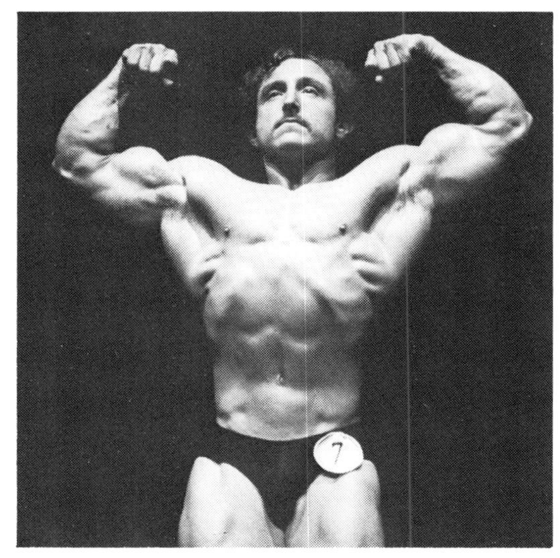

Dave Mastorakis.

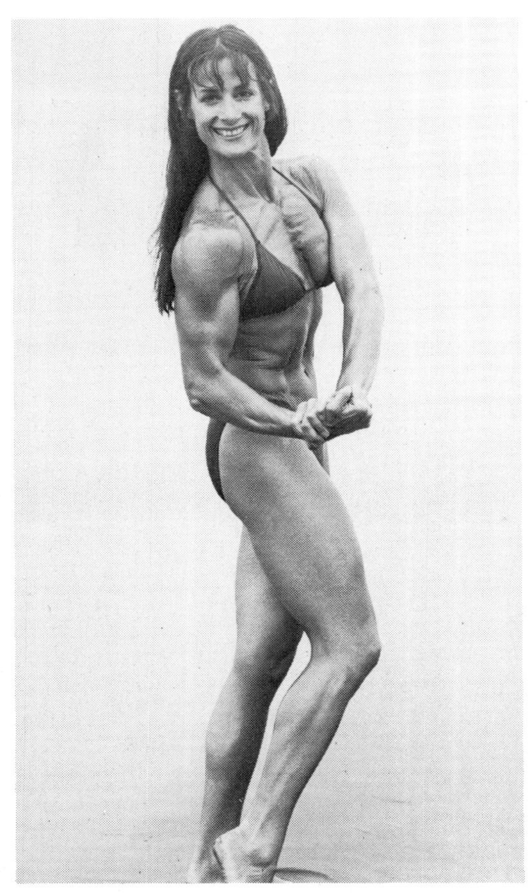

Valerie Mayers. *(Arturo Valenzuela)*

Ron McBeath.

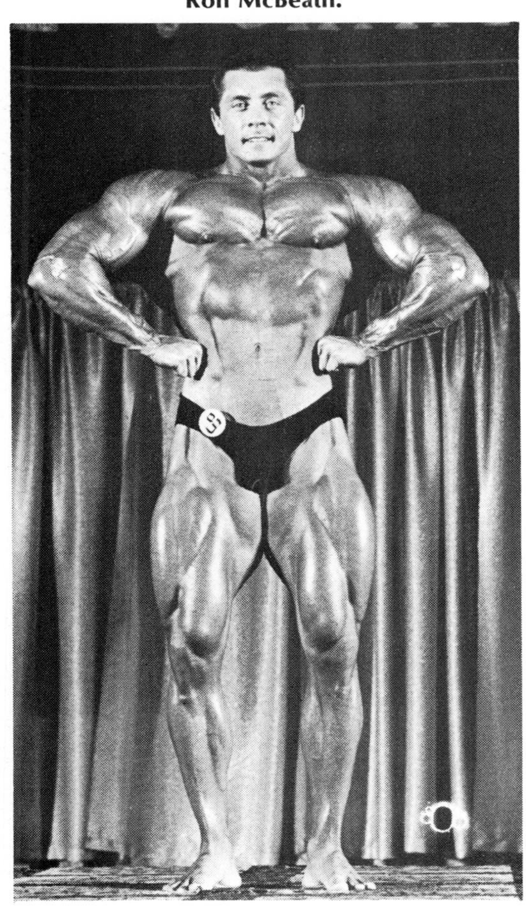

Valerie Mayers

Valerie has won four bodybuilding titles (including Ms. Eastern Seaboard and Ms. Northeast) and was eighth in her class at the American Championships after less than one year of training. With a perfect skeletal structure for bodybuilding, the ability to become extremely defined for competition, a knack for adding balanced muscle mass all over her body, a consummately foxy appearance, and with a rare degree of onstage charisma, Valerie Mayers is one of the future greats of the sport. No doubt by the time some individuals read this book she will have won additional high-level titles.

Ms. Mayers contributed the following lat training routine, which she does three times per week:

1. Wide-Grip Chin (to the back and front of neck on alternate sets): 4–5 × max possible reps
2. One-Arm Dumbbell Bent Rowing: 4–5 × 10–8 (up to 65 lbs.)
3. Behind Neck Lat Pulldown: 4–5 × 8–10 (up to 130 lbs.)
4. Narrow-Grip High Pulley Row: 4–5 × 8–10 (up to 110 lbs.)
5. Bent-Arm Pullover (EZ-curl bar): 3–4 × 8–10 (up to 80 lbs.)

Ron McBeath

Ron is a native of Cincinnati, Ohio, but he has trained extensively at Gold's. For several months in 1978 he was Lou Ferrigno's training partner. A six-footer who weighs 218 pounds in contest condition, McBeath has won Mr. Ohio, Mr. Mid-West, and his class in the Junior Mr. America competition. Ron has also been a finalist in the Mr. USA and Mr. America contests.

McBeath's lat development is particularly outstanding, so here is one of his precontest routines for that muscle group. (It is done three times per week.)

1. Front Chin: 5 × 10–15 (with added weight)
2. Seated Pulley Rowing: 5 × 10–15
3. One-Arm Dumbbell Bent Rowing: 5 × 10–15
4. Nautilus Pullover: 5 × 10–15
5. Behind Neck Lat Pulldown: 5 × 10–15

Ron has a superb frame on which to build an even more impressive physique. He is definitely Mr. America material!

Jerry McCall

Originally from San Francisco, Jerry McCall relocated in Santa Monica so he could train at Gold's Gym with Mike and Ray Mentzer. Long a proponent of high-intensity training, Jerry has won Mr. West Coast, Mr. Greater Bay Area, Mr. Golden West, and a variety of other titles. He has also placed in the top five of his class at the Mr. America contest.

Here is a typical Jerry McCall precontest thigh routine (it's done two days per week):

1. Nautilus Leg Press: 1–2 × 10–15
2. Nautilus Leg Extension: 1–2 × 10–15
3. Squat: 1 × 15–20
4. Nautilus Leg Curl: 2–3 × 10–15

Every set is carried at least to failure, and most are done with additional forced reps and negatives.

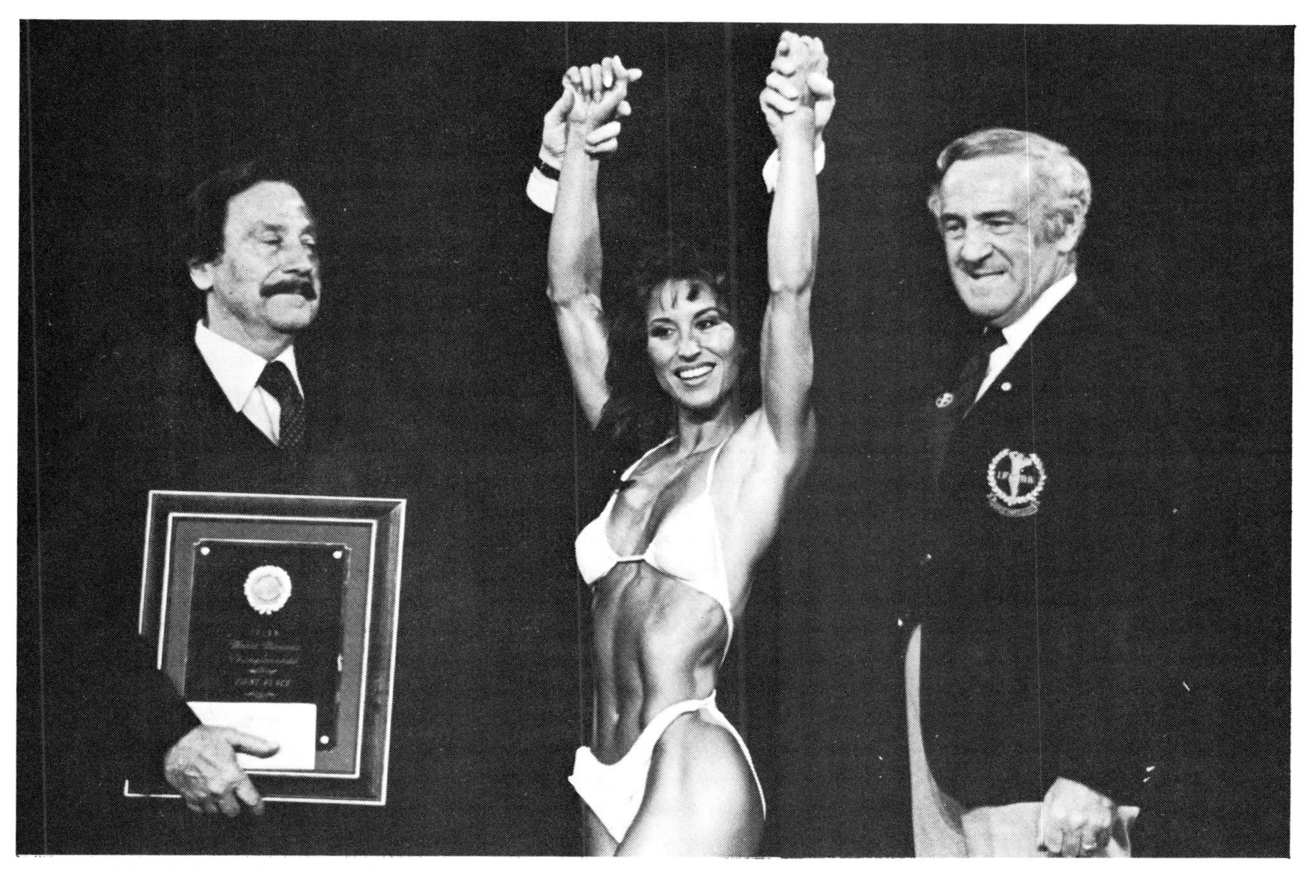

Joe Weider (left) and Ben Weider declare Rachel McLish the winner of the 1982 Women's World Championships. She later went on to win her second Miss Olympia title, making 1982 her most successful year yet.

Rachel McLish

Rachel, a native of Texas, has become the most successful woman bodybuilder to date. She won the United States Championships in 1980 in her first competitive effort, Miss Olympia in 1980, and the World Professional Championships in 1982. Rachel was second in the Zane Pro Invitational in 1980, the Miss Olympia runner-up in 1981, and Miss Olympia in 1982. Rachel works out frequently at Gold's Gym, using a high-intensity, low-set training philosophy.

Here is the superset deltoid workout Rachel McLish used prior to winning her Miss Olympia title:

1. Side Lateral: 3 × 6–8
2. Overhead Press: 3 × 6–8 }
3. Dumbbell Bent Lateral: 3 × 6–8 }

Rachel also frequently does this type of workout on machines, such as performing Side Laterals and Presses on a Nautilus double-shoulder machine and Rear Laterals on a Nautilus rowing machine. Either way, she has an impressive shoulder development, which will no doubt carry her to more pro bodybuilding titles in the future.

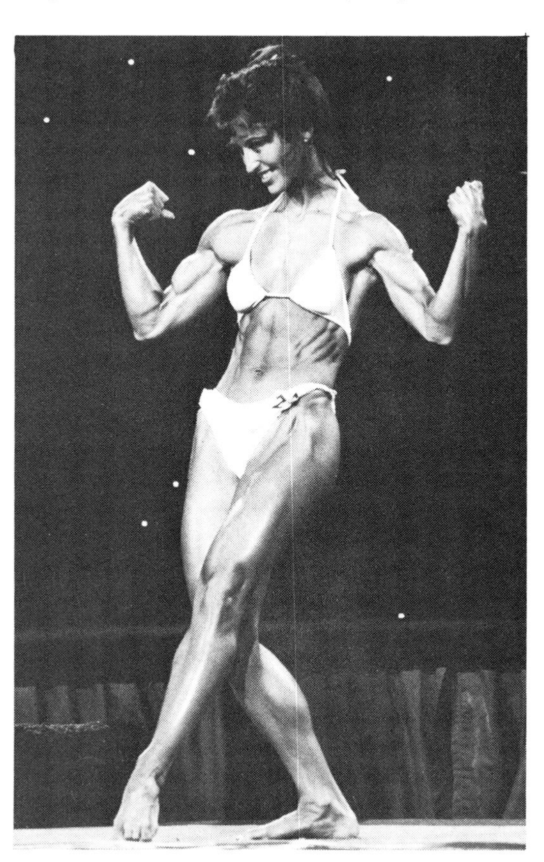

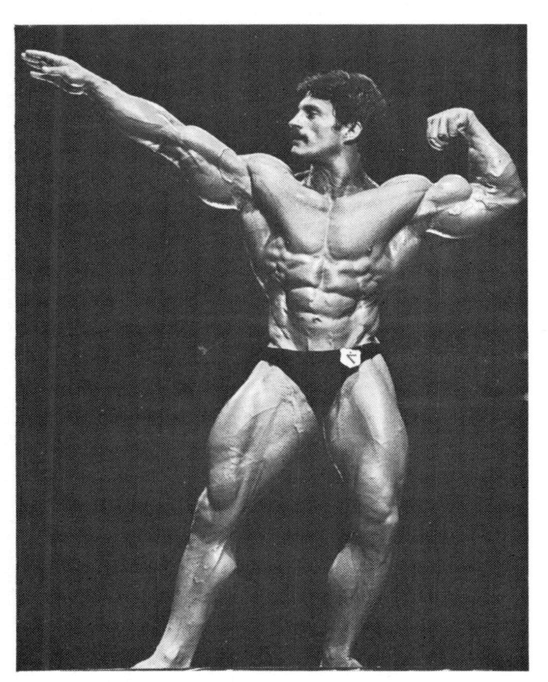

Mike (above) and Ray Mentzer.

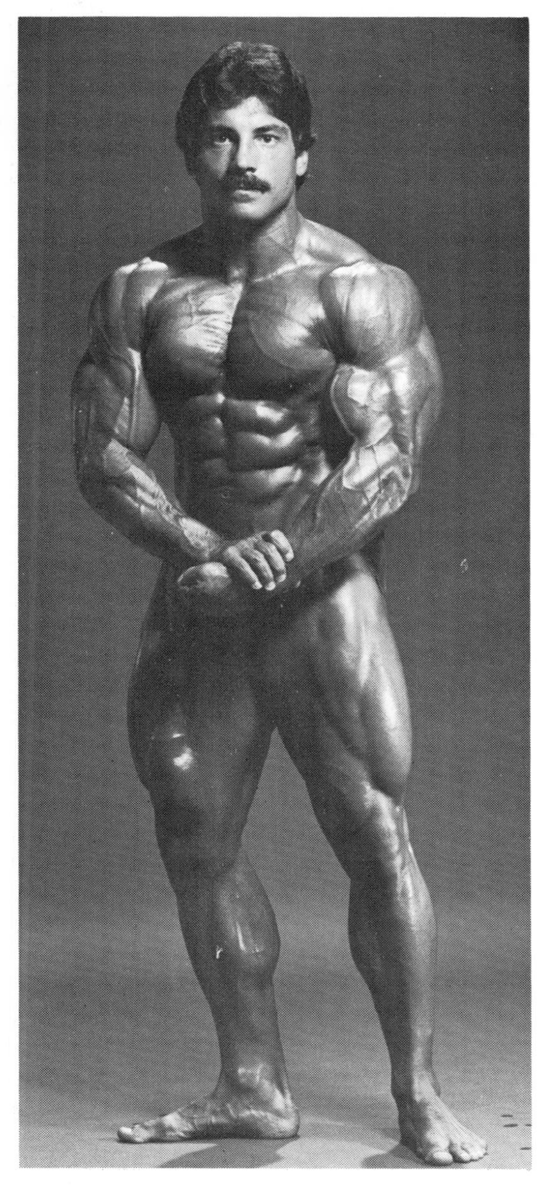

Mike Mentzer

A Pennsylvania native, Mike moved to California to train at Gold's Gym shortly after winning the Mr. America title in 1976. And since then he has won Mr. North America, Mr. Universe, and two pro Grand Prix titles. Mike also took second in the 1979 Mr. Olympia contest behind Frank Zane. He did, however, win the heavyweight Mr. Olympia title. Mike is currently retired from competition and works as an executive assistant to Joe Weider at *Muscle & Fitness* magazine.

Mike Mentzer popularized his Heavy-Duty system of training via two books, a series of training courses, and scores of magazine articles. His system consists of high-intensity, low-set training for each muscle group. He makes use of forced reps, negative reps, and rest-pause training in his workouts.

This is a superset thigh routine that Mike used after a warm-up while training at Gold's:

1. Leg Extension: 1 × 10 (plus 2–3 forced reps)
2. Leg Press: 1 × 10–15 reps to failure with 900 lbs.
3. Squat: 1 × 10–20 (up to 500 lbs.)
4. Leg Curl: 2 × 10–12 (with forced reps)

Mike always uses slow and controlled reps in all of his movements, even with his heaviest weights. To train in a jerky and cheating fashion with such monstrous poundages would certainly result in joint, tendon, and muscle injuries, not in the 27-inch thighs Mike's developed!

Ray Mentzer

The younger brother of Mike Mentzer, Ray won the Mr. USA title in 1978 and the Mr. America title in 1979. At 5′10½″ in height and weighing 230 pounds in contest shape, Ray has also placed second (behind Jusup Wilkosz) in the IFBB Mr. Universe competition and placed high in several recent professional competitions. While there have been several good "brother acts" in bodybuilding, none has ever equaled that of the Mentzer brothers, both of whom have won Mr. America titles.

Like his brother, Ray follows a high-intensity, low-set training philosophy. Prior to winning Mr. America, Ray used the following pectoral workout: "I did Flyes on the Nautilus double-chest machine, one arm at a time, with the whole stack plus a 75-pound plate for 3–4 reps each arm, going very strict and holding the contracted position of each repetition for several counts. Then I did one set of pure negatives and a set with both arms for eight positive reps. Finally, I did Barbell Incline Presses with 375 pounds for three reps, two very strict and the last one with a bit of a bounce. All of this was done within four minutes, and it was a super chest workout!"

Steve Michalik

Even though he owns his own gym in the East (Mr. America's Gym in Farmingdale, New York), Steve has spent quite a bit of time on the West Coast, training at Gold's. The 1972 Mr. America winner and a top pro bodybuilder, Steve was so seriously injured in an auto accident several years ago that he was paralyzed from the waist down for a year. But Steve fought back until he was in better shape than ever before. Due to lingering injury pain, he has devised an "intensity or insanity" workout philosophy in which he does up to 70–80 total sets per body part during each workout with moderate weights.

Here's a typical Steve Michalik "true grit" back training program:

1. Seated Pulley Rowing: 10 × 8–10
2. Close-Grip Lat Pulldown: 8–10 × 8–10
3. Nautilus Pullover: 8–10 × 8–10
4. Parallel-Grip Pulldown: 8–10 × 8–10
5. Seated Lat Pulldown: 8–10 × 8–10
6. Bent Lateral: 8–10 × 8–10

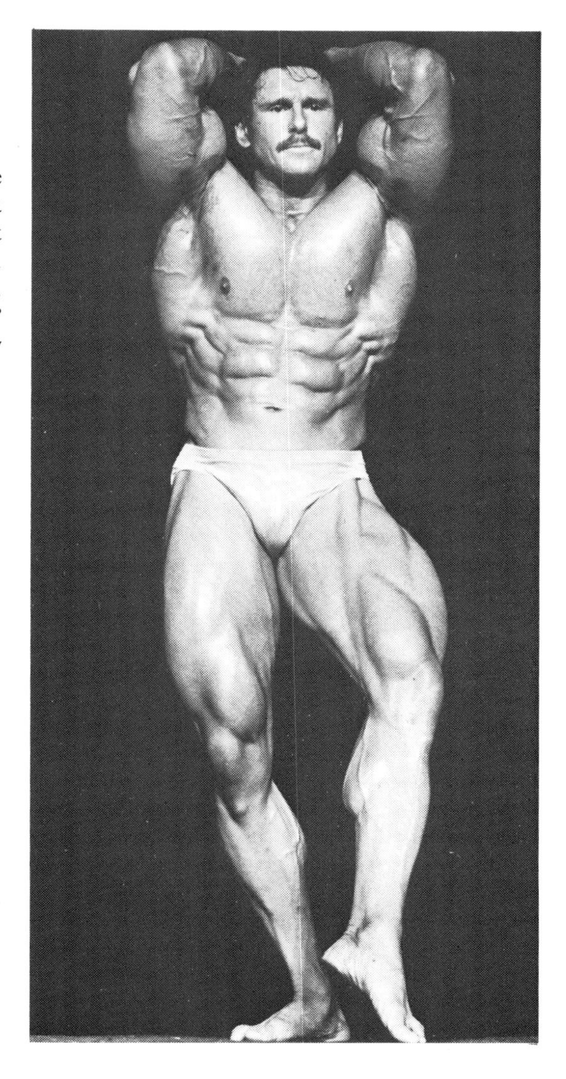

Steve Michalik (above) and Joe Nazario.

Rogelio Pio Montenegro

Montenegro created a sensation with his esthetic physique when he placed second in the NABBA Mr. Universe competition in 1963. He had already won Mr. Argentina and Mr. South America. After a long layoff to concentrate on his business affairs—and at 44 years of age—Rogelio moved to California for a year to train at Gold's Gym. He competed successfully on the IFBB pro tour in 1980 and then retired from competition.

Rogelio trained his forearms six days per week at the conclusion of his daily workouts. Here are his routines for forearm development:

Monday-Wednesday-Friday

1. Reverse Curl: 5 × 8–10
2. Barbell Wrist Curl: 5 × 10–15

Tuesday-Thursday-Saturday

1. One-Arm Dumbbell Wrist Curl: 5 × 10–15
2. Barbell Reverse Wrist Curl: 5 × 10–15

Joe Nazario

Joe grew up in New York, but ultimately moved to the West Coast like so many other superb bodybuilders to train with the best in the sport at Gold's Gym. Among Joe's titles are Mr. Eastern America and the IFBB Mr. International. In top shape, Nazario is very thick and cut-looking, and his proportions are excellent. Only his posing has been criticized in recent years.

Here is the superset deltoid workout Joe followed just prior to winning his Mr. International title in 1978.

{ 1. Press Behind Neck: 5 × 8–10
{ 2. Side Lateral: 5 × 8–10
{ 3. Dumbbell Press: 5 × 8–10
{ 4. Front Lateral: 5 × 8–10
{ 5. Nautilus Side Lateral: 5 × 8–10
{ 6. Bent Lateral: 5 × 8–10

"I was never really able to attain a high degree of muscularity and muscle density until I began doing a high number of sets for each muscle group during my precontest cycle," Nazario noted. "But in the off-season, when I'm trying to build muscle mass, I average a lot less sets, usually in the range of 15–18 total sets per muscle group."

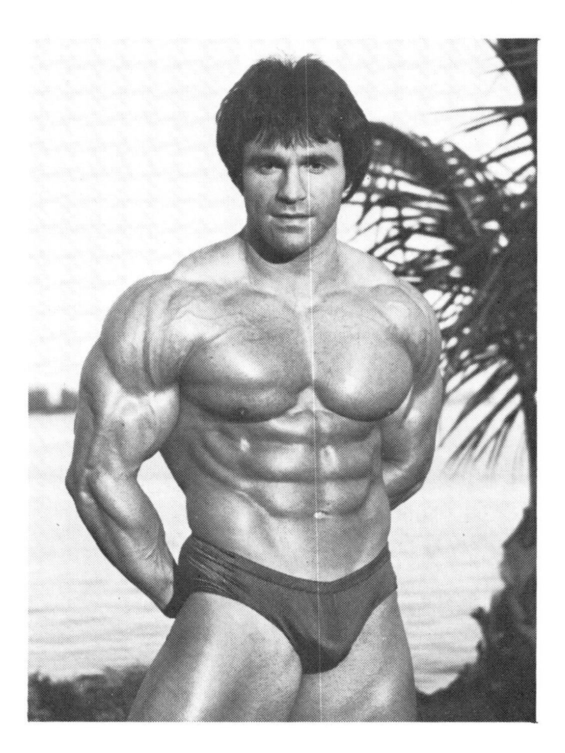

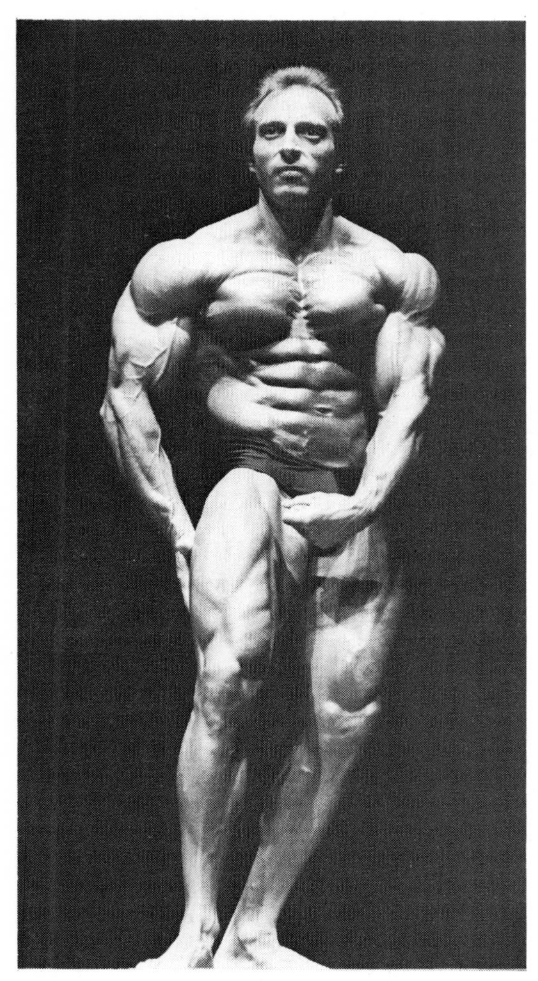

Pat Neve.

Jacques Neuville

Neuville, a resident of Ales, France, is the 1981 IFBB Mr. Universe in the light-heavyweight division. He has also won Mr. France, Mr. Europe, and the World Games Championships. At 5′9″ in height, Jacques packs 200 superhard pounds of muscle on his frame for contests.

Here is one of Jacques Neuville's favorite deltoid programs:

1. Seated Press Behind the Neck: 5 × 10–12
2. Seated Bent Lateral: 5 × 10–12
3. Cable Side Lateral: 5 × 10–12
4. Upright Rowing: 5 × 10–12

"It's best for most bodybuilders to do only one or two basic exercises per muscle group and use heavy weights in each movement," Jacques advises. "Some of the routines I see relatively inexperienced bodybuilders using would almost kill me, even if I was in my peaking phase!"

Pat Neve

Pat has won Mr. USA and his height class in the Mr. America contest twice, as well as a host of national-level "Best Arms" and "Best Chest" awards. He has also set numerous world records as a powerlifter, most notably a 468-pound Bench Press record that stood for more than five years in the 181-pound division.

Although Pat owns his own gym in Phoenix, Arizona, he has frequently trained at Gold's when passing through L.A. He has a degree in physical therapy, and he and his wife Vickie have two sons.

Here's one of Pat Neve's favorite superset, upper arm routines.

{ 1. Incline Dumbbell Curl: 4 × 8–12
{ 2. Dumbbell Triceps Extension: 4 × 8–12
{ 3. Barbell Curl: 4 × 8–12
{ 4. Lying Triceps Extension: 4 × 8–12
{ 5. Barbell Preacher Curl: 4 × 8–12
{ 6. Pulley Pushdown: 4 × 8–12

Joe Nista. *(Bill Reynolds)*

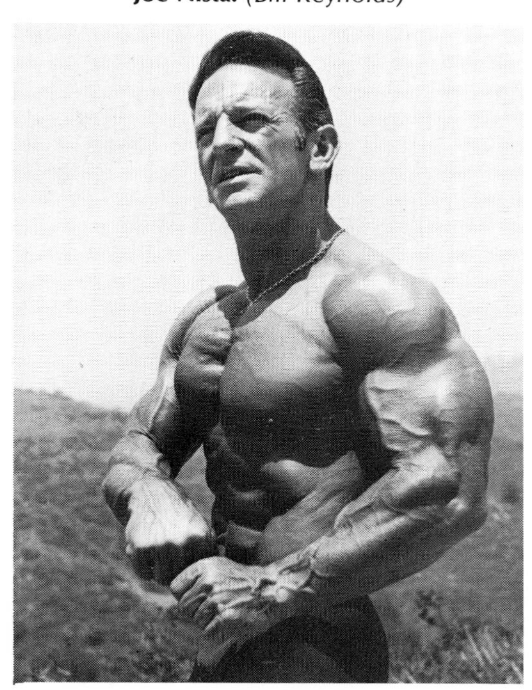

Joe Nista

Although he formerly owned a gym in Cerritos, California, Joe has taken periodic workouts at Gold's Gym over the years. Originally from New York, he came into his own after moving to California. He won the Mr. California title and his height class several times at the Mr. America, Mr. World and Mr. Universe competitions. When near the age of 50, he climaxed his career by winning the Past-40 Mr. America and Past-40 Mr. Universe titles.

Joe's biceps were particularly well shaped, and here was one of his favorite routines:

1. Incline Dumbbell Curl: 4 × 6–8
2. Barbell Preacher Curl: 4 × 8
3. Dumbbell Concentration Curl: 3 × 10–12

"Follow a healthy diet, exercise regularly, and maintain a positive attitude toward life, and you can look 20 when you're in your 50s," explained Joe.

Erwin Note

A resident of Brugge, Belgium, Erwin Note has periodically visited California to train at Gold's Gym, as do so many other international bodybuilders. Erwin has won either the Junior or Senior Mr. Belgium title a total of eight times, and he's also been a Junior and Senior Mr. Europe winner. He's placed in the final three or four at several Mr. International and Mr. Universe contests. At the Universe in 1980, he won the Ben Weider Trophy as the IFBB's most improved amateur athlete for the year.

Here is a simple forearm development routine that Erwin Note recommends for use three days per week:

1. Narrow-Grip Reverse Curl: 5 × 8–10
2. Barbell Wrist Curl (palms up): 5 × 15–20

"A lot of inexperienced bodybuilders neglect their forearm training," Note notes. "But to become a champion, you must develop each body part equally. Never go easy on your forearms."

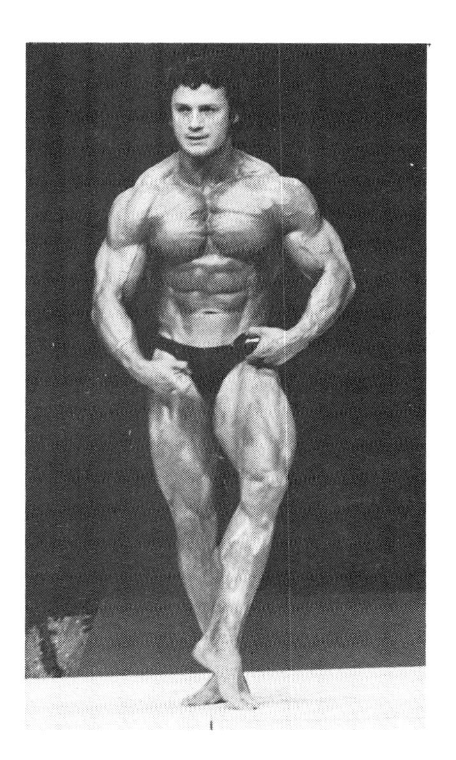

Erwin Note (above) and Serge Nubret.

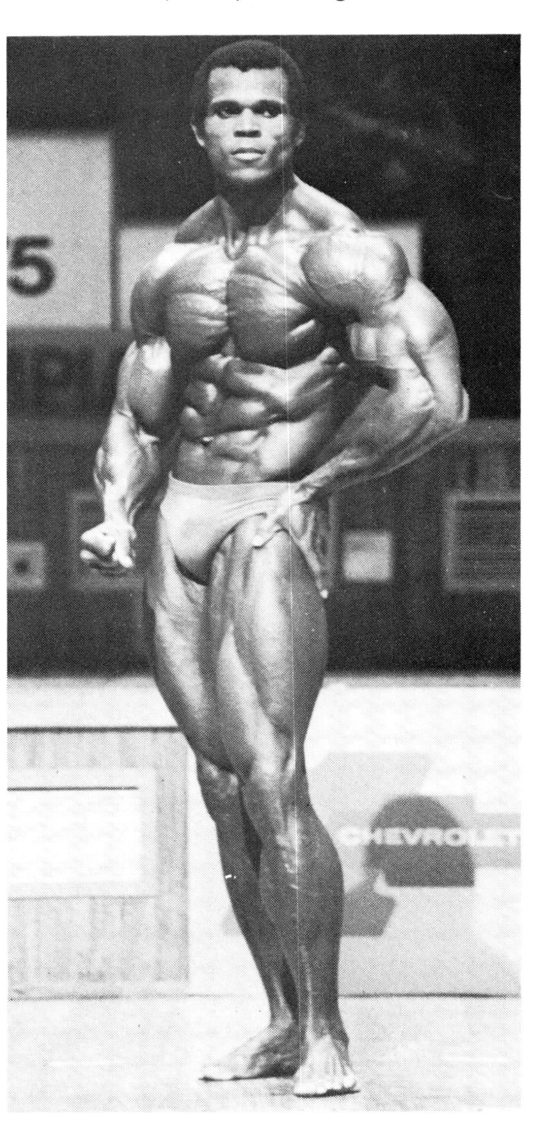

Serge Nubret

Even though he has won only one major title (the NABBA Mr. Universe), the Black Panther of Paris is justifiably one of the world's greatest bodybuilders. Nubret's massive, clearly defined, and esthetic physique is the envy of millions. And with a 550-pound Bench Press to his credit while weighing only 200 pounds, he is one of the more powerful athletes in the sport.

Born in 1939 in Guadeloupe, an island in the Caribbean, he moved to Paris at an early age and studied both law and business administration. His wife Jacqueline is herself a practicing attorney.

Serge frequently visits California and always trains at Gold's, occasionally with his wife as his training partner. Despite his great strength and muscle mass, Nubret relies on a program of high sets and moderately high reps with relatively light weights for each muscle group. He usually works out twice per day and often takes a 15-minute rest between body parts.

Nubret doesn't count sets but relies instead on the clock, usually training a body part for one hour. While it is impossible to give an exact Serge Nubret chest routine, here is approximately how he trains his superb chest:

1. Barbell Incline Press: 10–12 × 12–15 (165–185 lbs.)
2. Barbell Bench Press: 15–20 × 12–15 (185–205 lbs.)
3. Flye (on a slight decline): 10–12 × 12–15 (35s)

Serge rests for approximately 45–60 seconds betweeen sets, seething to go again on a set when he feels he has sufficiently recuperated from the last one. He never does supersets or forced reps and goes to only about 35% of failure on each set. Generally, Nubret does no more than two or three exercises per muscle group, and he seldom changes routines. He feels that once he's designed a productive workout, it's worth sticking to.

Even when dieting, Serge Nubret's appetite is prodigious. He routinely eats 7–10 pounds of various types of meats while on his low-carbohydrate precontest diet. His favorites are horse meat, lobster, and various types of fish. Otherwise, he consumes only water, coffee, and food supplements.

The end result from such long training sessions and heavy eating is a classically beautiful physique.

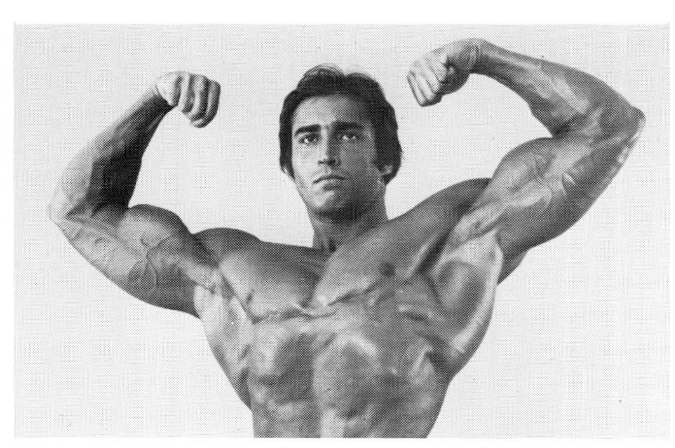

Bill Nuchols. *(Joe Valdez)*

Bill Nuchols

Bill has won the Mr. Western America competition and placed well in the Mr. America contest with his ripped 5′11″ and 206-pound physique. He has also done considerable work as an actor and was a regular as "Wally" the gym instructor on the defunct television series "Supertrain." Bill diets for 6–8 weeks on fish, skinned chicken breasts, a little salad, and water to achieve his superb muscular definition.

Here's a precontest-phase delt workout that Nuchols used when training at Gold's:

1. Press Behind Neck: 4 × 6–8
2. Side Lateral: 4 × 10–12
3. Upright Rowing: 4 × 8–10
4. Bent Lateral: 4 × 10–12
5. Cable Side Lateral: 4 × 10–12

Sergio Oliva

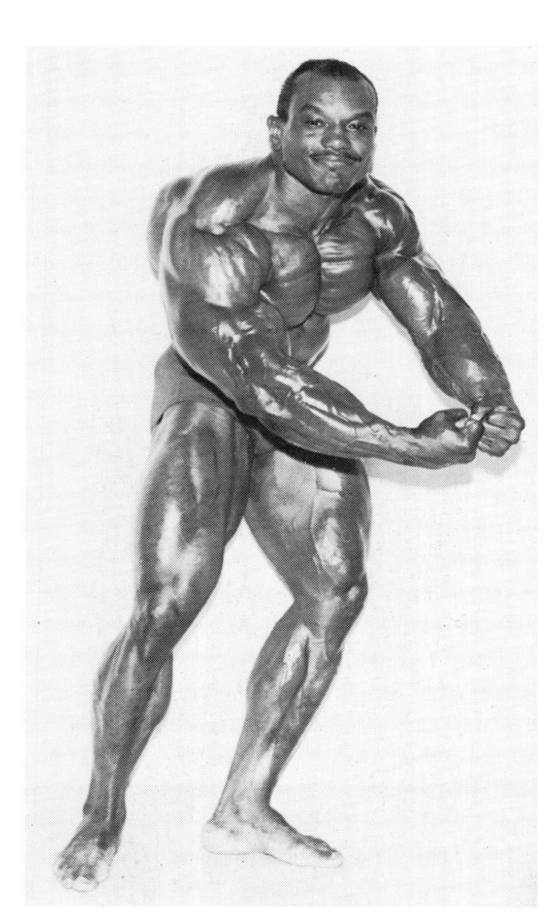

Sergio Oliva. *(Benno Dahmen)*

Many consider Sergio Oliva, a Cuban living in Chicago, the equal of Arnold Schwarzenegger. Certainly, few bodybuilders have been as massive as Sergio and none have had his enormous degree of natural potential. Oliva has won three Mr. Olympia titles (1967–1969), Mr. World, Mr. Universe, Mr. Olympus, and a wide variety of other high-level titles. In his mid-40s, Sergio is still one of the most dominant figures in international bodybuilding.

Oliva has always trained hard and heavy, but oddly enough has such superb metabolism that he can swill soft drinks and gobble burgers all day and still retain good cuts. Indeed, he only diets strictly for two or three weeks prior to a competition in order to rip his massive physique to shreds.

Sergio occasionally trained at Gold's Gym, and his awesome 21-inch upper arms were developed with superset routines like this:

{ 1. Barbell Curl: 6 × 8 (185 lbs.)
{ 2. Standing Barbell Triceps Extension: 6 × 8 (110 lbs.)
{ 3. Preacher Curl (EZ-curl bar): 6 × 8 (130 lbs.)
{ 4. Pulley Pushdown: 6 × 8 (140 lbs.)
{ 5. Dumbbell Preacher Curl: 6 × 8 (80s)
{ 6. Cable Kickback: 6 × 8 (60–70 lbs.)

Known in bodybuilding circles as "The Myth" due to his superhuman development, Sergio Oliva is still the idol of millions. He works in community relations for the Chicago Police Department and still trains full-time. Awesome is the only word for the man!

Danny Padilla

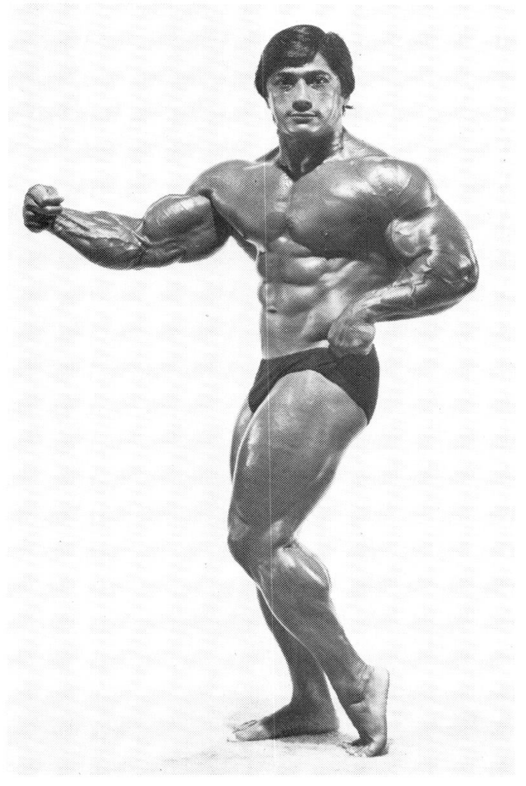

Danny Padilla.

Known affectionately as "The Giant Killer" by his legion of rabid fans, 5′2″ Danny has indeed slain his share of bodybuilding giants. Among his titles are Mr. USA, Mr. World, Mr. America, and Mr. Universe. He has also placed in the top five in the Olympia. When he is in peak condition Danny's symmetry and proportions are unparalleled in bodybuilding.

It's extremely difficult to pick a strong body part on Padilla's physique, since his *is* so perfectly proportioned. We did, however, solicit the following thigh workout:

1. Squat: 6 × 15–8 (135–425 lbs.)
2. Leg Press: 5 × 12 (up to 550 lbs.)
3. Leg Extension: 5 × 15 (150 lbs.)
4. Leg Curl: 5 × 15 (up to 120 lbs.)

When training at Gold's, Danny eschews the use of supersets, preferring instead to do straight sets with approximately 60 seconds of rest between sets. He does every exercise in very strict style and tends to move the weights relatively slowly, feeling resistance throughout the complete range of motion of an exercise.

In the past, Danny has had difficulty gaining deep cuts at contest time, but by dieting on only 800–1,000 calories per day and riding a bicycle for at least an hour per day he has solved this problem. At about 155 pounds, he is now ripped to shreds for every important pro contest. And when he humorously poses to Randy Newman's parody "Short People," his fans virtually tear the roof off the contest venue!

Tony Pandolfo

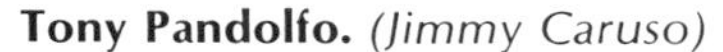

Tony Pandolfo. *(Jimmy Caruso)*

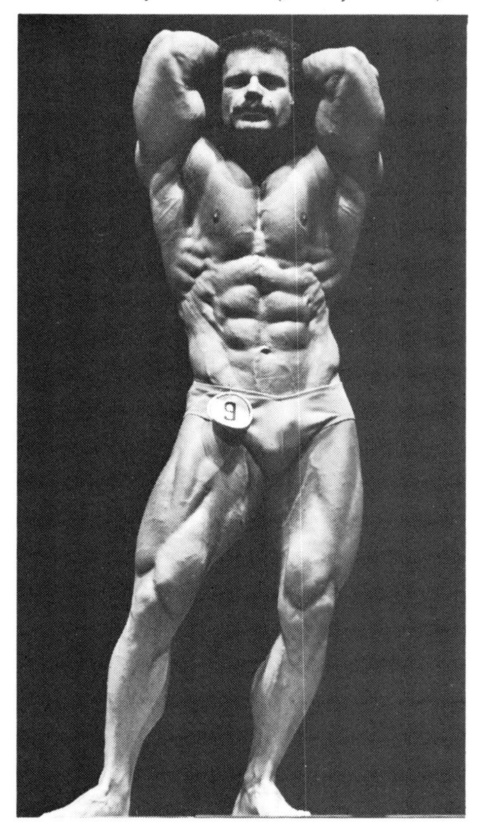

Tony lives in New York and works both as a gym manager and for a moving company. He was inspired to take up competitive bodybuilding by his friends Dennis Tinerino and Chris Dickerson. Pandolfo has won virtually every title open to him on the East Coast (e.g., Mr. New York, Mr. Empire State, Mr. East Coast, Mr. Eastern America, etc.) and has placed in the top three of his class at both the Mr. America and Mr. USA competitions. Now over 40 years of age, Tony is looking forward to competing in the Past-40 Mr. America contest.

The authors asked Tony Pandolfo for his precontest thigh program, which is as follows (it is done three times per week):

{ 1. Leg Extension: 5 × 10–15
{ 2. Squat: 5 × 10–15
{ 3. Hack Machine Squat: 5 × 10–15
{ 4. Leg Curl: 5 × 10–15
5. Lunge: 5 × 10–15

Along with supersetting the first four exercises, everything is done with minimum rest between sets and maximum possible poundages. "I try to kill myself in the gym," Tony explained. "Prior to a contest, I have to put every possible ounce of energy into my workouts in order to reach peak condition."

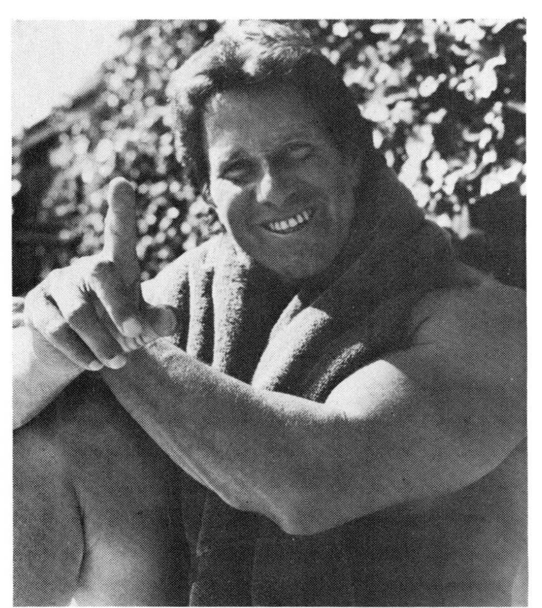

Reg Park.

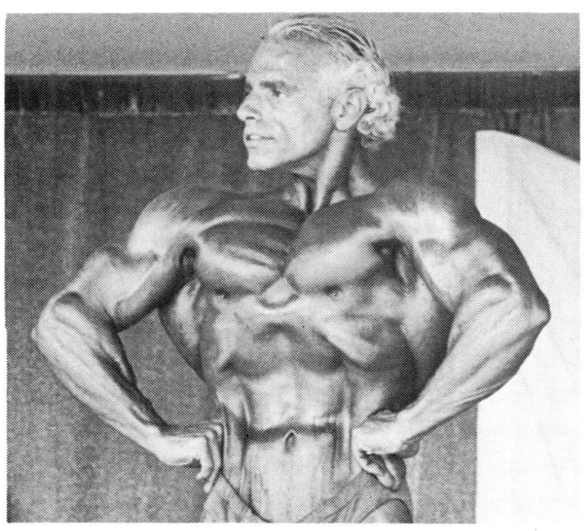

Ken Passariello.

Tony Pearson.

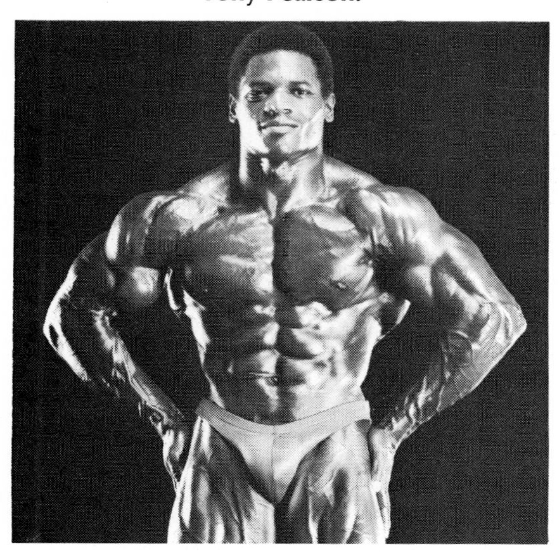

Reg Park

Currently a resident of South Africa, Park was Britain's greatest bodybuilder. Reg won Mr. Britain, Mr. Europe, Mr. World, and Mr. North America, and he was the first man to win the NABBA Mr. Universe title three times. He was also the third man in history to Bench Press 500 pounds. He sells gymnasium equipment in Johannesburg.

During the early 1960s Reg Park made a number of muscle movies in Italy. Unlike Steve Reeves, who was forced by film producers to reduce his body weight for films, Park insisted that his contract specify he could maintain a truly Herculean body weight (230 pounds at a height of 6′1″). So, if you are lucky enough to see one of his films on a television late show, you'll be seeing Hercules in the flesh!

Occasionally Reg trains at Gold's when in Los Angeles, as does his son John-John. Here's a Reg Park deltoid workout:

1. Military Press: 5 × 5
2. Press Behind the Neck: 5 × 5
3. High-Incline Dumbbell Press: 5 × 5
4. One-Arm Dumbbell Press: 5 × 5
5. Handstand Push-Up: 1–2 sets to finish off

Park could routinely use 300 pounds and more for his Presses Behind the Neck when at the peak of his career.

Ken Passariello

Ken lives in Massachusetts and is walking testimony to the benefits of the bodybuilding lifestyle. When Passariello started training and dieting he weighed a corpulent 260 pounds at 5′4″ in height, but six years later he won the 1981 IFBB Mr. Universe title weighing a rockhard 154 pounds. He has tested out being as low in body fat as 1.8% of his body weight. Ken was runner-up in the 1980 Mr. Universe competition and he won the Lightweight Mr. America title in 1980 and 1981. He currently competes professionally.

Here is a Ken Passariello precontest, superset, abdominal routine, which is done six days per week:

{ 1. Hanging Leg Raise: 3–4 × 15–20
{ 2. Roman Chair Sit-up: 3–4 × 30
{ 3. Bench Leg Raise: 3–4 × 30
{ 4. Incline Sit-up: 3–4 × 20–25
{ 5. Incline Leg Raise: 3–4 × 20–25
{ 6. Crunch: 3–4 × 25–30

Tony Pearson

Originally from St. Louis, Missouri, Tony had an incredible season while training at Gold's Gym in 1978. He won Mr. Los Angeles, Junior Mr. USA, Junior Mr. America, and Mr. America. Later he won the NABBA Mr. Universe and WABBA Mr. World titles, but he is again competing in IFBB shows, vying against the best pro bodybuilders in the world.

One of Pearson's most impressive muscle groups is his ripped-to-shreds thighs. Following a warm-up of light Leg Extensions, this is his thigh routine:

1. Squat: 4–6 × 10–20
2. Leg Press: 4–6 × 10–15
3. Leg Curl: 4–6 × 10–15
4. Lunge (precontest only): 4–6 × 10–15

Alois Pek

A member of the Czechoslovakian bodybuilding team, Alois Pek has won a European Heavyweight Championship and placed in the top three at the IFBB Mr. Universe contest. Domestically, he has won Mr. Czechoslovakia three times. In an unprecedented athletic switch, Pek dropped bodybuilding in mid-1978 to become a brakeman on a bobsled team. Despite his inexperience in the sport, Alois made the 1980 Czech Olympic Team in his bobsled.

While in Los Angeles to enter the 1978 World Cup Championships, Pek trained at Gold's Gym. His over 20-inch upper arms were built with biceps routines like this:

1. Standing Barbell Curl: 5 × 8–10 (up to 180 lbs.)
2. Incline Dumbbell Curl: 5 × 8–10 (up to 75)
3. Dumbbell Concentration Curl: 5 × 10–12 (up to 65)

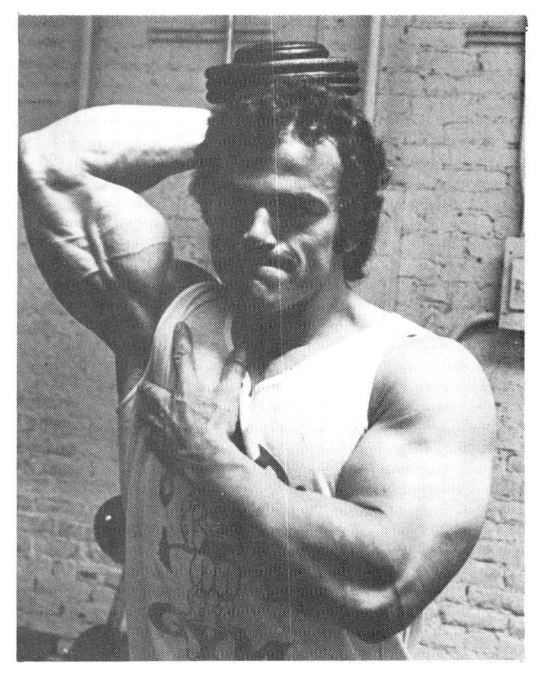

Alois Pek.

Manuel Perry

With less than three years of heavy Gold's style training under his belt, Massachusetts native Manuel Perry won the Mr. USA title and placed second twice in the Mr. America contest. At 6′1″ in height and at a contest body weight of 230 pounds, Manny's massive upper arms stretched a tape to just a tad less than 22 inches. Indeed, he was so massive and muscular that he spent four years as Lou Ferrigno's stunt double on television's "The Incredible Hulk" series.

Massive Manny trained his upper arms three days per week using this type of routine:

1. Barbell Curl: 5 × 12–15
2. Standing Dumbbell Curl: 5 × 12–15
3. Dumbbell Concentration Curl: 5 × 12–15
4. Cable Concentration Curl: 5 × 12–15
5. Pulley Pushdown: 5 × 12–15
6. Standing Triceps Extension: 5 × 12–15
7. One-Arm Dumbbell Triceps Extension: 5 × 12–15
8. Cable Triceps Extension: 5 × 15–20

Perry didn't exactly use baby weights on this strenuous routine, since his Barbell Curls were done in very strict form with up to 170 pounds. It's little wonder that his arms were so huge!

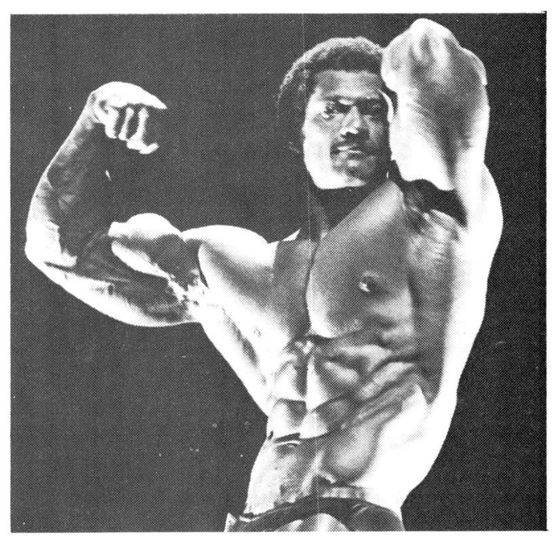

Manuel Perry. *(Art Zeller)*

Don Peters

Now the owner of his own gym in Reseda, California, Don has trained off and on at Gold's Gym since about 1970. Among his many titles are Mr. Texas, Mr. Los Angeles, Mr. Southern California, Mr. Western America, Mr. International, and a host of recent Past-40 titles. Peters has also placed first in his class twice in the Mr. America contest and once in the Mr. Universe show.

A symmetrical six-footer, Peters contributed this advanced-level forearm routine to the authors (do it three days per week following your biceps training):

1. Reverse Curl: 3–4 × 8–10
2. One-Arm Dumbbell Wrist Curl (Supported): 3–4 × 10–15
3. Standing Barbell Wrist Curl (Behind Back): 3–4 × 10–15

"I heartily recommend a fast workout pace," concluded Don Peters. "It shouldn't be so fast that you become hopelessly out of breath, but keep moving at a good pace and you'll get more out of your workouts. The guys who talk a lot between sets at the gym get good jaw muscles, but little else!"

Don Peters.

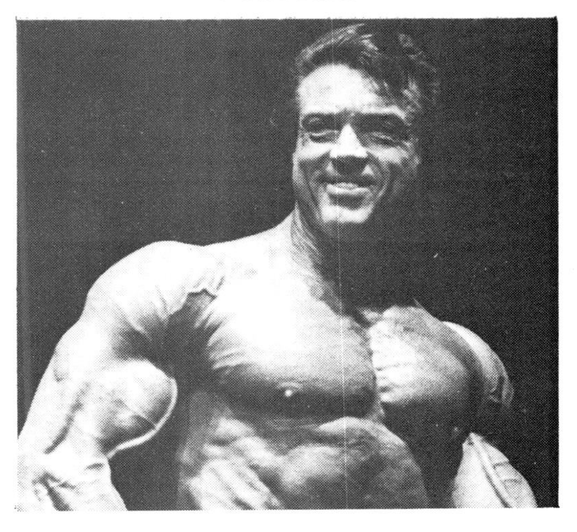

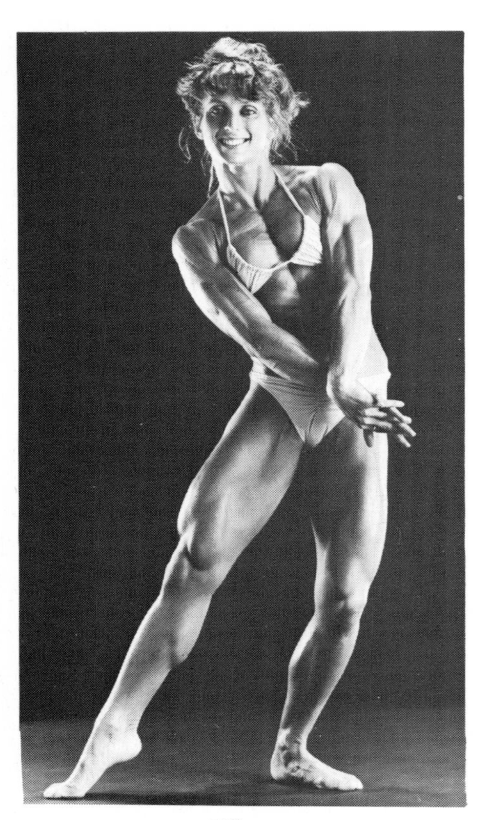

Pillow.

Pillow

One of the most remarkably muscular women to ever step on a stage at a bodybuilding competition, Pillow (the only name she uses) won the Ms. Alaska title, then moved to southern California both for the sun and to train at Gold's Gym. She was a finalist in the 1981 Ms. America competition, and many bodybuilding cognoscenti had her as the winner. But some of the judges felt she was too extremely developed.

Pillow gave us the following off-season thigh routine, which is done twice a week:

1. Angled Leg Press: 5 × 12–6
2. Leg Extension: 4–5 × 8–10
3. Hack Machine Squat: 4–5 × 8–10
4. Lying Leg Curl: 5–8 × 8–10
5. Standing Leg Curl: 5–8 × 8–10
6. Cable Abduction: 4–5 × 8–10
7. Cable Adduction: 4–5 × 8–10

"I'm doing a lot more Leg Curls now than ever before, because I'm attempting to add mass and greater detail to my hamstring muscles," Pillow stated. "The more sets I do for a muscle group, the better it seems to become."

Dr. Lynne Pirie

Dr. Lynne Pirie, an orthopedic surgeon living in Phoenix, Arizona, frequently visits Gold's Gym for a workout or two. And, of course, she is one of the world's greatest women bodybuilders in addition to being chairperson of the AFWB Medical Committee.

A former world-class 800-meter runner, Lynne grew up in Canada and received her medical degree from Michigan State University. Turning to competitive bodybuilding, she has enjoyed considerable success, winning eight titles and placing third (as an amateur) in the 1982 Professional World Championships.

Lynne's training is very heavy and extremely high in intensity, and she trains her entire body in one session on three nonconsecutive days per week. She eats natural foods primarily and consumes approximately 1,000 calories per day when peaking for competition.

Dr. Pirie contributed a good intermediate-level chest routine, which she suggests doing three days per week:

1. Incline Dumbbell Press: 3–4 × 6–10
2. Nautilus Flye: 2–3 × 8–10
3. Parallel Bar Dip: 2–3 × 8–10
4. Flat-Bench Flye: 2–3 × 8–10

Lynne notes that an advanced bodybuilder who can correctly use high-intensity training techniques will actually do fewer sets than an intermediate trainee. She herself does only four or five total sets of chest training during each workout!

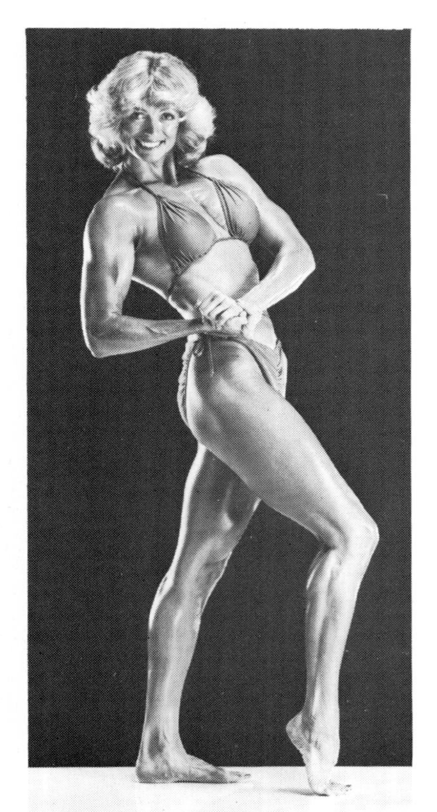

Dr. Lynne Pirie.

Tom Platz

Considered by many of bodybuilding's cognoscenti to be the most massively muscular bodybuilder of all time, Tom has won the Mr. Universe title and placed third in the Mr. Olympia extravaganza. No less an authority than Arnold Schwarzenegger feels that Platz will be the dominant bodybuilder of the 1980s.

Tom trains exceedingly hard and with great mental intensity. Some of the training poundages he routinely uses in his workouts are nearly impossible to believe: Squat, 600 × 10–15; Parallel Bar Dip, 200 × 8–10; Seated Pulley Rowing, 350 × 10–12. And all of these movements are done in superstrict form. To watch Platz train is a truly inspiring experience.

Tom Platz is most noted for his thigh development, and this is a routine he used to achieve his Herculean thigh mass:

1. Squat: 8–10 × 20–5 (working up in weight to well over 600 lbs.)
2. Hack Squat: 5 × 10–15
3. Leg Extension: 5–8 × 10–15
4. Leg Curl: 6–10 × 10–15

With such a strenuous leg workout, it's little wonder that Tom's thighs are unparalleled in their huge and striated development!

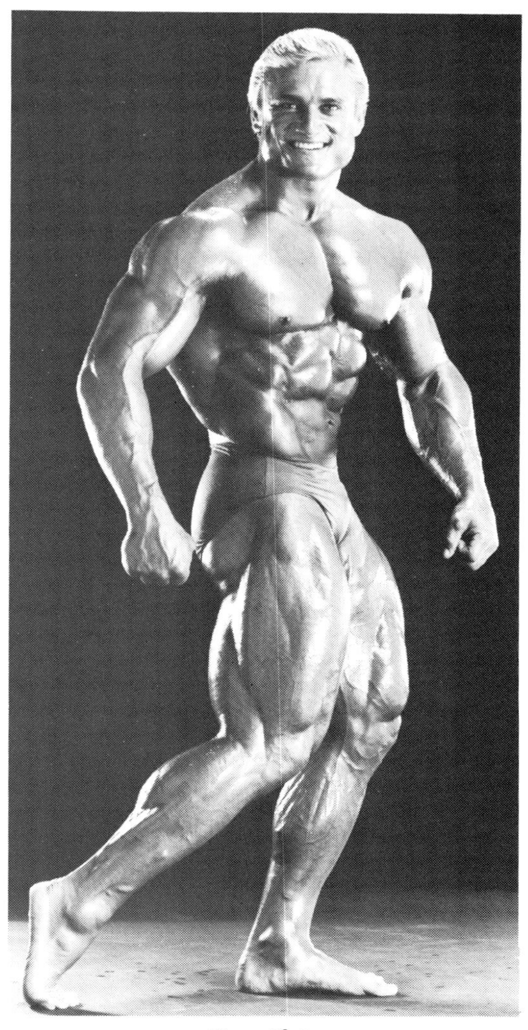

Tom Platz.

Damon Poole

Formerly known as Harold Poole, Damon was an outstanding high school athlete in his native state of Indiana. He was also a bodybuilding prodigy, placing in the top 10 at the AAU Mr. America contest at only 17 years of age. Eventually, Damon won the Mr. America, Pro Mr. America, and Mr. Universe titles. He also placed second in the Mr. Olympia competition on two occasions.

Then for a decade, Poole wrestled professionally and worked as one of New York City's most respected bouncers. Finally, in 1979 Damon made a comeback to bodybuilding, and he currently competes on the IFBB pro circuit.

Here is one typical Damon Poole thigh routine, as we observed him performing it at Gold's:

1. Squat: 6 × 15–6
2. Hack Machine Squat: 4 × 10–12
3. Leg Extension: 4 × 10–12
4. Leg Curl: 5–6 × 10–12

Damon Poole is a staunch advocate of steroid-free bodybuilding.

Jorma Räty

Jorma distributes bodybuilding gym equipment and food supplements in his native Helsinki, Finland. He has won Mr. Finland and Mr. Scandinavia several times, plus Mr. Europe. Prior to winning his 1980 IFBB Middleweight Mr. Universe title in Manila, Philippines, he trained for the entire summer at Gold's Gym. A former competitive weightlifter, Jorma is very strong on all bodybuilding movements.

Räty's latissimus dorsi development is among the best in the sport. Here's one lat workout he used while training at Gold's:

1. Front Chin: 5–8 × 10–15 (with added weight)
2. Seated Pulley Rowing: 4–5 × 8–10
3. Nautilus Pullover: 4–5 × 8–10
4. Behind the Neck Lat Pulldown: 4–5 × 8–10

Jorma likes to do a lot of isotension posing of his back muscles to bring out peak muscularity just prior to a competition.

Jorma Räty.

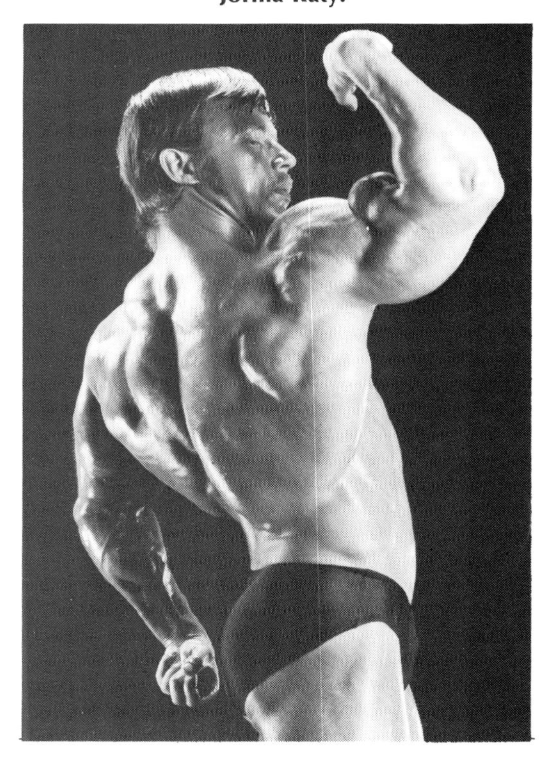

Steve Reed

A former Mr. Eastern America winner, Reed trained at Gold's for a couple of years in the late 1970s, then apparently dropped out of competition. A firm believer in heavy training primarily on basic exercises, Steve was noted for his Herculean mass. Here's his forearm workout (done on Mondays, Wednesdays, and Fridays):

1. Barbell Wrist Curl: 4–5 × 15–20
2. Barbell Reverse Wrist Curl: 4–5 × 15–20

"I probably do less forearm training than most good bodybuilders," Reed revealed. "This is because constantly gripping the heavy barbells and dumbbells that I use in my workouts helps to keep my forearms fully muscled and well cut up."

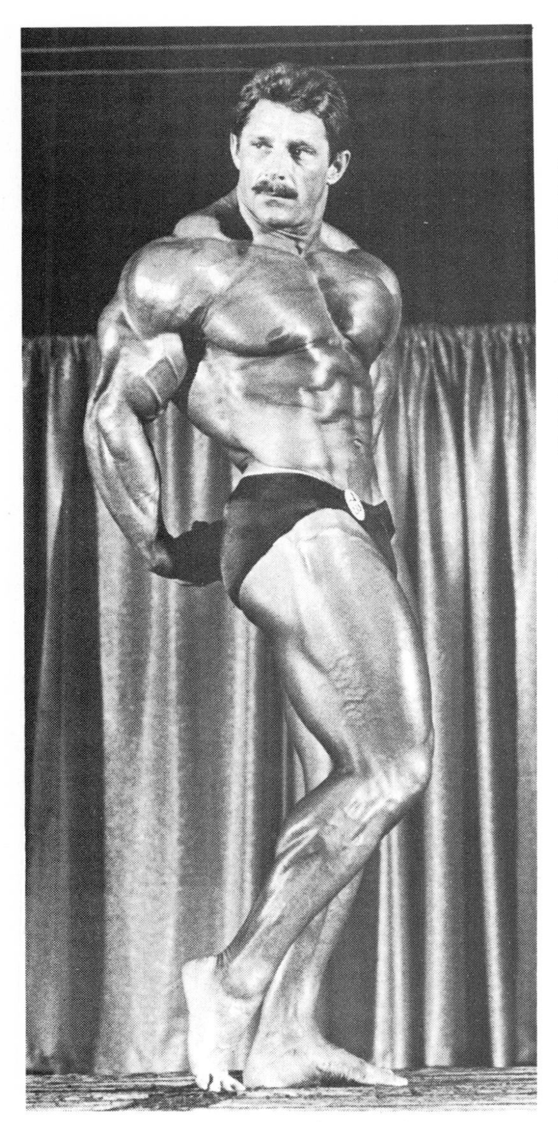

Bob Reis.

Bob Reis

Bob has been a super-successful bodybuilder over the years and once managed the San Francisco Gold's Gym. Among Reis's titles are Mr. Wisconsin, Mr. Mid-West, Mr. Gold Cup, Mr. Western States and Mr. USA. At 5′9″ and 215 pounds in hard contest shape, Bob is incredibly impressive onstage. He also is phenomenally strong, having Bench Pressed 515 pounds for eight reps and 580 for a single at a body weight of approximately 225 pounds.

Here is a typical Bob Reis precontest chest workout:

1. Bench Press: 5 × 10–6 (up to 500+ lbs.)
2. Barbell Incline Press: 3–4 × 10 (up to 325 lbs.)
3. Flye: 3–5 × 10 (up to 135-pounders)

In his early 30s, Reis feels that his best competitive years lie ahead of him. "I've improved significantly every year that I've trained," Bob said. "I don't intend retiring from competition until I've reached my potential, so I'm going to be around for quite a while!"

Bill Reynolds. *(John Balik)*

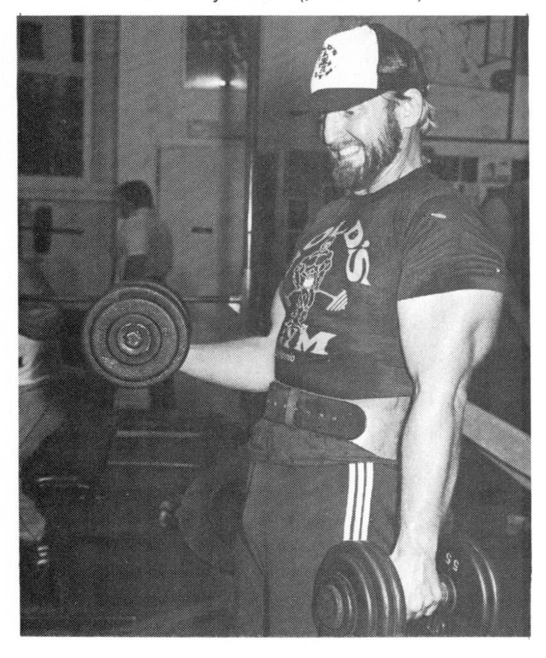

Bill Reynolds

One of the co-authors of this book, Bill has won six bodybuilding titles and over 50 trophies while competing during the late 1960s and early 1970s. He's also been a college and military football star and javelin thrower. The editor-in-chief of *Muscle & Fitness* magazine since 1978, Bill has written more than 20 books and over 1,500 magazine articles on bodybuilding and weight training. For his bodybuilding reportage over the last 12 years, Bill was awarded the IFBB Certificate of Merit in 1982.

"Looking back in my old training diaries, I noted that I used to win 'Best Abdominals' subdivision awards doing three sets of 25–30 reps on Incline Sit-ups and the same sets and reps on Incline Leg Raises each workout day," Reynolds noted. "While working on this book, I got psyched up to train hard again, and after two months of training and dieting my weight went down from 240 to 205 pounds and my waist measurement fell from 39″ to 32½″!

"My abdominal routine now consists of two or three trisets of Hanging Leg Raises (15 reps), Twisting Roman Chair Sit-ups (30 reps), and Side Bends (50 reps each way), plus two or three supersets of Bench Leg Raises (30 reps) and Crunches (30 reps). This routine hits every facet of my abdominals, and I do it all at the beginning of my workout. It was suggested to me by Laura Combes, Ms. America.

"My diet was made up by Valerie Mayers, Ms. Eastern Seaboard. It consists of an average of 1,500 calories per day, mainly from fish, broiled chicken breasts, brown rice, baked potatoes, melons, and iced tea. The diet really works great for me, and it's easy to follow!"

Frank Richard

Reg Park notwithstanding, Frank Richard was one of the greatest of all British bodybuilders. In the late 1960s and early 1970s he won Mr. Britain, Mr. Europe and his height class at the NABBA Mr. Universe. For quite a period of time he trained at Gold's with Arnold Schwarzenegger and Franco Columbu. Richard is currently a bodybuilding administrator in his native England.

Here is a typical Frank Richard superset back training program:

1. Chin: 5–6 × 10–15
2. Barbell Bent Rowing: 5–6 × 8–10
3. One-Arm Rowing: 5–6 × 8–10
4. Seated Pulley Rowing: 5–6 × 8–10
5. Stiff-Leg Deadlift: 5–6 × 10–15

Robby Robinson

Known as "The Black Prince," Robby is one of the most successful bodybuilders ever to train at Gold's Gym. Among his titles are Mr. America, Mr. North America, Mr. World, Mr. Universe, and a raft of pro championships. His unique combination of superhuman muscle mass, sharp muscularity, and awesome proportions has made him a legend in his own time. Few, if any, bodybuilders can duplicate his front double biceps shot.

An advocate of low-carbohydrate and low-calorie dieting, Robby professes his favorite foods to be all types of broiled fish, broiled chicken breasts, and honeydew melons. These melons, he has discovered, are not only delicious but very low in carbohydrate and caloric count.

To build his awesome biceps, Robby uses a variety of training routines, all with an emphasis on peak contraction and continuous tension. "Using these techniques, I can make a 70-pound barbell feel like it weighs 150," he claims. Here is a typical three-day-per-week, Robby Robinson biceps training program:

1. Standing Barbell Curl: 4 × 10–12
2. Barbell Concentration Curl: 4 × 10–12
3. One-Arm Cable Curl: 4 × 10–12

Robby, incidentally, is a superb natural athlete. With very little specific track training, he has sprinted 100 yards in 9.5 seconds!

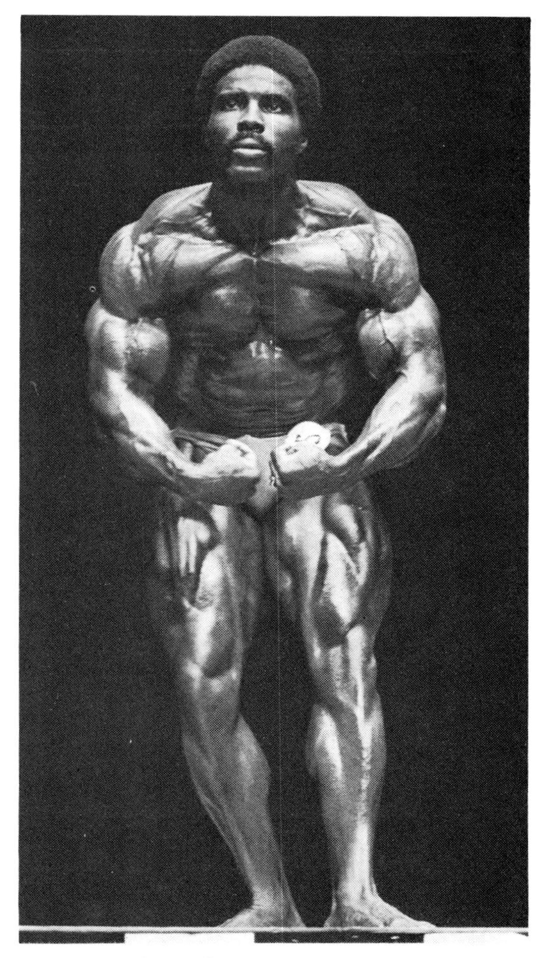

Robby Robinson. *(Jimmy Caruso)*

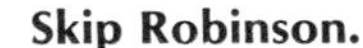

Skip Robinson.

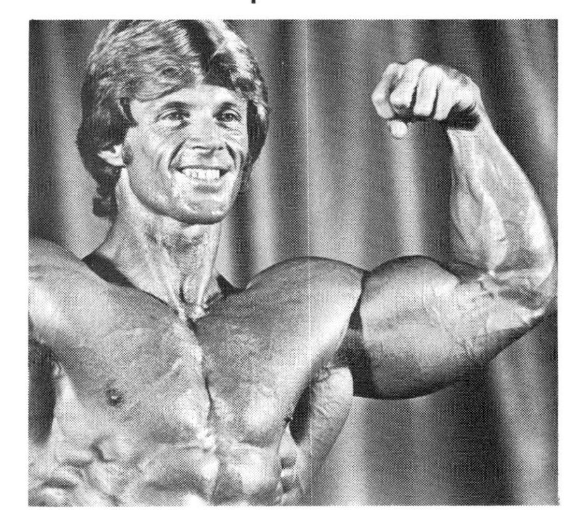

Skip Robinson

A high school teacher by profession, Skip has won the Mr. Maine, Mr. New England, Mr. East Coast, and Mr. Eastern America titles. He has also been a finalist in the Mr. America show. A Regional Champion powerlifter, Robinson has deadlifted over 700 pounds, or more than 3½ times his body weight! For a couple of summers Skip Robinson trained at Gold's Gym in preparation for the fall national and international bodybuilding competitions.

Six days per week, Skip would perform this routine as a triset for his abdominals:

1. Roman Chair Sit-up: 5 × 50
2. Twisting Incline Sit-up: 5 × 50
3. Bench Leg Raise: 5 × 50

No rest was allowed between exercises of the triset, and a rest interval of less than 60 seconds was taken between trisets.

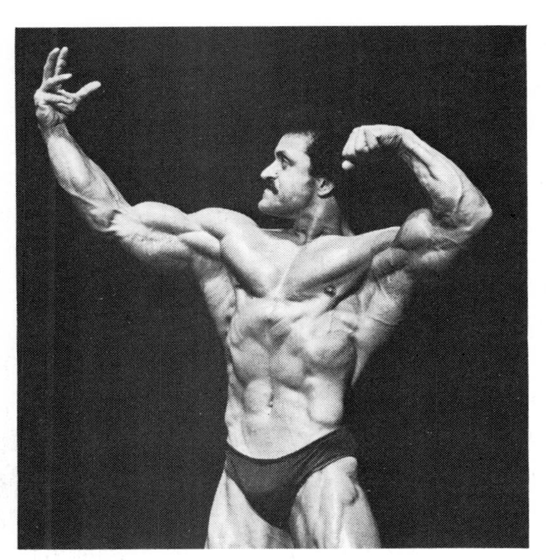

Carlos Rodriguez.

Carlos Rodriguez

Carlos operates his own gym in Tucson, Arizona, but trains at Gold's when in Los Angeles. He has won a host of titles, among them Mr. USA, Mr. North America, Mr. Latin America, and Mr. Universe. Known as "El Rey" or "The King" by his Latino fans, Carlos is tremendously popular worldwide. A part-time rodeo cowboy, he occasionally walks onstage for pro shows wearing his ten-gallon hat and casually carrying a saddle on his shoulder.

Rodriguez's physique is evenly developed so it's difficult to single out a particularly strong muscle group. He did, however, give us this precontest deltoid routine, which he does three times per week:

1. Military Press (warm-up): 1–2 × 15–20
2. Seated Machine Press: 4–5 × 6–8
3. Seated Dumbbell Press: 4–5 × 6–8
4. Dumbbell Side Lateral: 4–5 × 8–10
5. Cable Side Lateral: 4–5 × 8–10
6. Dumbbell Bent Lateral: 4–5 × 8–10

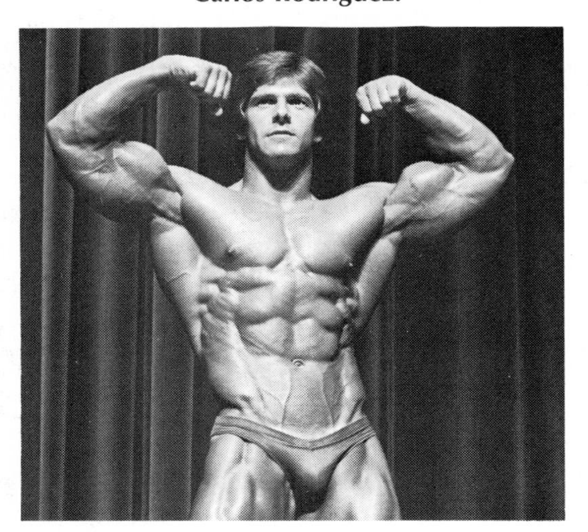

David Rogers.

David Rogers

A six-footer who weighs 220 pounds in hard contest shape, Rogers is originally from Tennessee, but lives and trains now in Georgia. David was the first Gold's Classic winner, has been second in his class in the Mr. America competition and won both the Junior and Senior Mr. USA titles. Dave trains five days per week in the off-season, averaging about 20 sets per muscle group, and works out six days per week prior to competition.

Rogers has incredible abdominals for a big man. When asked about how he trains them, Dave replied, "I actually have three different workouts, and I rotate them daily throughout the week. I do 4–6 supersets of maximum possible reps on one or the other of these three routines:

1. Roman Chair Sit-up + Hanging Leg Raise
2. Weighted Crunch + Bench Leg Raise
3. Incline Sit-up + Hanging Leg Raise

"These simple routines plus a low degree of body fat allow me to display very sharp abdominals when in contest condition," Rogers concluded.

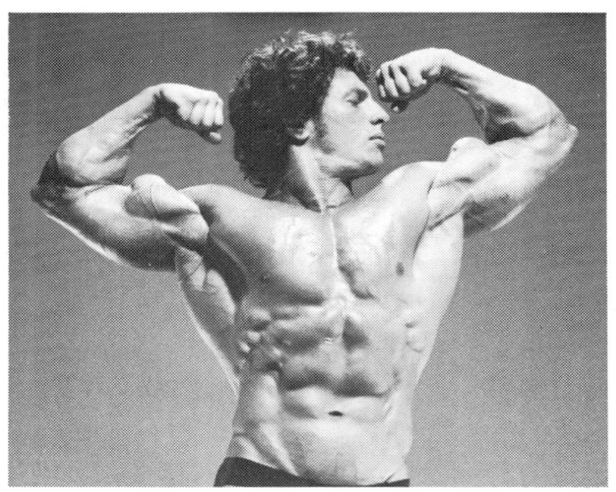

Don Ross.

Don Ross

Originally from Detroit, Michigan, Don Ross lives in Oakland, California and manages a gym. He's previously been a pro wrestler, and like so many top bodybuilders he's frequently worked out at Gold's. Among Don's titles are Mr. Michigan, Mr. USA, Mr. North America, and Pro Mr. America. Ross currently competes on the IFBB pro bodybuilding circuit.

Don has great delts, so we solicited this precontest shoulder routine from him (performed on Mondays, Wednesdays, and Fridays):

1. Side Lateral: 8 × 8
2. Front Raise: 8 × 8
3. Bent Lateral: 6 × 8

"Persistence and consistency in putting in hard, heavy workouts is the key to success," Don stated. "A missed workout can *never* be made up!"

Doug Ross

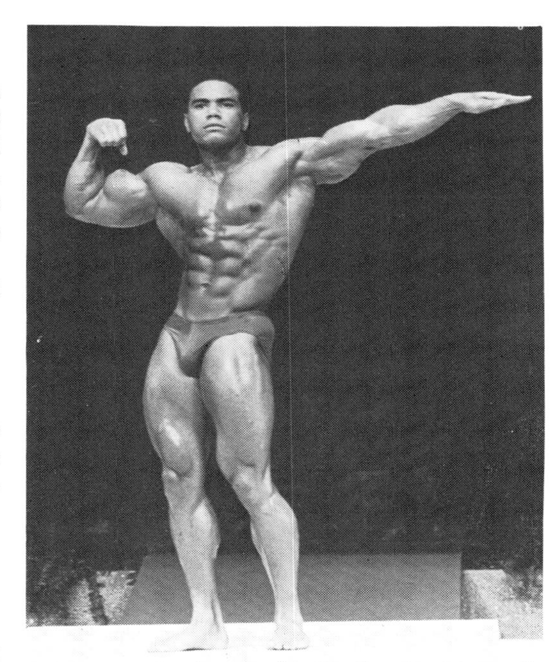

Doug Ross.

Doug is a young bodybuilder from Winnipeg, Manitoba, who has won two Mr. Canada titles. He has also placed in the top five at the IFBB Mr. Universe competition. A former provincial champion high school wrestler, he has developed a well-proportioned and massive physique. Ordinarily, Ross works out in Winnipeg with Reid Schindle as his training partner, but he's spent a couple of months training with the superstars at Gold's Gym.

Here is the off-season pectoral routine we observed Doug using at Gold's (he performs it twice per week):

1. Barbell Incline Press: 6–8 × 12–4
2. Flat-Bench Flye: 5 × 6–8
3. Parallel Bar Dip: 5 × 8–10 (with added weight)

"Visiting Gold's Gym was a dream come true to me," said an enthusiastic Doug Ross. "While training there I was able to compare notes with all of the champions who train at Gold's. Chris Dickerson—as great as he is—went out of his way to help me."

Pat Ruelle

Pat Ruelle is a former Mr. Michigan winner who trained off and on at Gold's Gym for several years. "Before a contest I train twice a day six days per week and once on Sundays just to hit calves and abdominals," Pat revealed. "Monday, Wednesday, and Friday I train legs in the morning, then chest and back later in the day. Tuesday, Thursday, and Saturday I do shoulders in the morning and biceps and triceps in the afternoon. Abs and calves are done every day."

Pat contributed this chest routine, which he followed prior to contests:

1. Bench Press: 5–6 × 10–12
2. Incline Press: 5 × 10–12
3. Flat-Bench Flye: 5 × 10–12
4. Cable Crossover: 5 × 10–12

"I get my best results from the Bench Press when I use a variety of grip widths," Ruelle said. "I do some sets with a wide grip, some with a medium grip and some with a relatively narrow grip."

Dale Ruplinger

Dale lives in Bettendorf, Iowa, and trains mainly at Joe's Gym in Moline, Illinois, but he has occasionally pumped iron at Gold's Gym while passing through Los Angeles. He has won the Mr. Iowa, Mr. Central USA, Mr. USA, Mr. America (Class III), and Mr. Universe titles, and he is one of the brightest prospects on the bodybuilding scene today.

Ruplinger's upper arms are quite well-developed, so we asked him for his arm workout. He follows this routine three times per week in the off-season:

1. Standing Barbell Curl: 3–4 × 6–10
2. Incline Dumbbell Curl: 3–4 × 6–10
3. Lying Triceps Extension: 4–5 × 6–10
4. Pulley Pushdown: 4–5 × 8–12

Dale Ruplinger and his wife Ginny have two young sons, and he works in an Alcoa Aluminum plant.

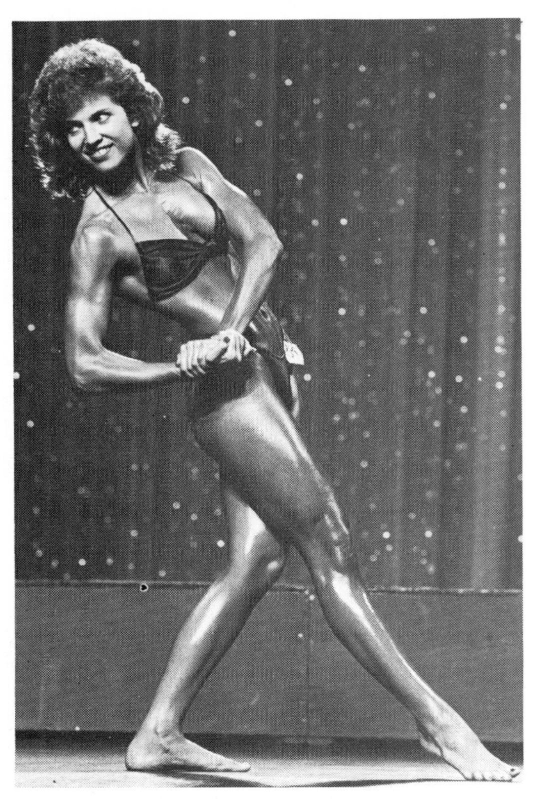

Peggy Russell.

Peggy Russell

Peggy has trained for quite some time at Gold's Gym. She has won the Ms. Central California title and placed high in several state and regional contests. She was also on the cover of the *Women of Iron* book, which gave her considerable national exposure.

Here is a typical Peggy Russell calf training program during an off-season cycle at Gold's:

Monday-Thursday

1. Seated Calf Machine Toe Raise: 4–5 × 10–15
2. Donkey Calf Raise (on Nautilus multi machine): 3–4 × 10–15

Tuesday-Friday

1. Standing Calf Machine Toe Raise: 4–5 × 10–15
2. Calf Press (on Nautilus Leg Press): 3–4 × 10–15

Mike Sable

Few bodybuilders have had as little physical potential as Mike Sable, yet succeeded so handsomely. Both fat *and* skinny during his youth and with a terrible skeletal structure, Mike built a superb physique by dint of eight years of hard and dedicated training, plus strict adherence to a carefully calculated bodybuilding diet. Among Mike's more than 20 titles are Mr. Golden West, Mr. Western America, Mr. Central California, Mr. Cal Expo, Mr. West Coast, and Mr. Western USA. Mike has also been a finalist in his class at the Mr. America event and has competed honorably in the NABBA Mr. Universe show. Sable has trained at numerous gyms all over southern California, including at Gold's.

Since Mike Sable has won numerous "Best Legs" trophies, we asked him for this thigh workout. This is his precontest routine, done three days per week on a double-split routine:

1. Leg Extension: 5 × 10–15 }
2. Angled Leg Press: 5 × 10–15 }
3. Hack Machine Squat: 5 × 10–15 }
4. Leg Curl: 5 × 10–15 }
5. Squat: 5 × 10–15
6. Lunge: 5 × 10–15

The first two pairs of exercises are supersetted, while the remaining two movements are done singly with 30–40 seconds rest between sets.

Mike Sable.

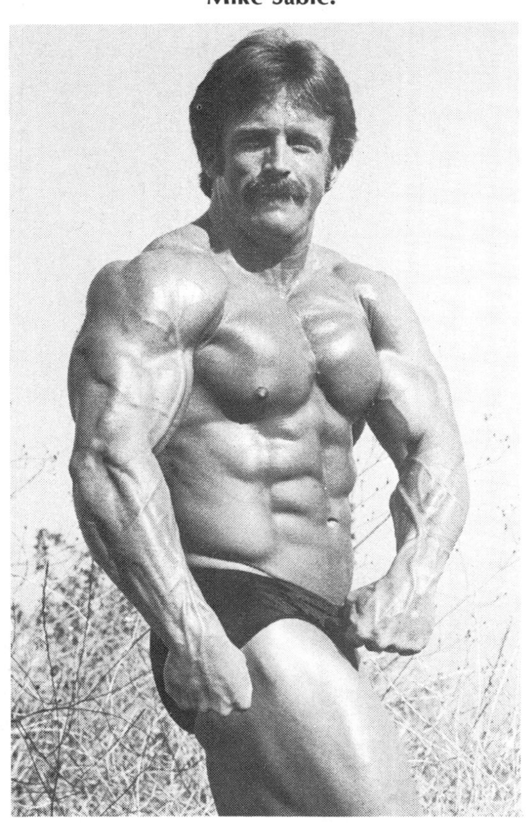

Ernie Santiago

An ex-Marine, Ernie lives in Hawaii. He has won the Mr. Hawaii, Junior Mr. USA, and Junior Mr. America titles. Handsome and superbly developed, Ernie has also been a finalist in the Mr. America competition.

Ernie's thighs are fully developed and exceptionally well separated. Here's a suggested off-season thigh program. (Do it two days per week.)

1. Squat: 6 × 15–6 (upping the weight each set)
2. Leg Press: 4 × 8–10
3. Leg Extension: 4 × 8–10
4. Leg Curl: 5–8 × 8–10

Reid Schindle

Awesome is the only way to describe the potential of Reid Schindle, a game warden from the province of Manitoba in Canada. Massive Reid has won Mr. Canada three times and placed in the top three at two Mr. Universe contests. From time to time he shows up at Gold's to peak out for a major contest.

A typical Reid Schindle biceps routine includes these exercises:

1. Standing Dumbbell Curl: 5 × 8 (up to 75 lbs.)
2. Dumbbell Concentration Curl: 4 × 12 (up to 55 lbs.)
3. Standing Barbell Curl: 4 × 8 (up to 160 lbs.)

Once Reid Schindle successfully cuts up his supermassive physique, he will become one of the sport's real greats!

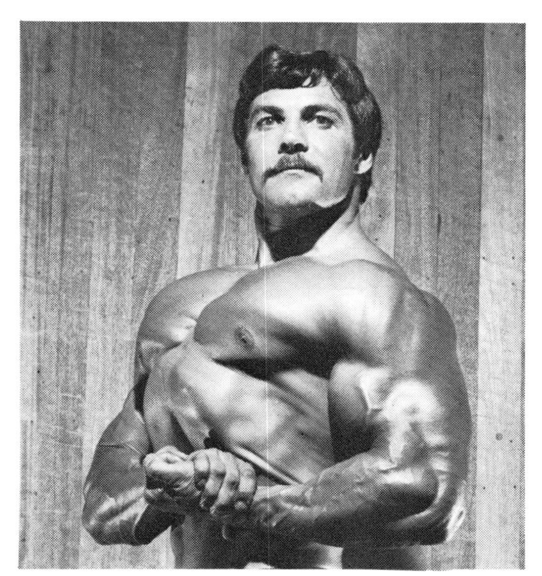

Reid Schindle.

Arnold Schwarzenegger

Arnold Schwarzenegger is undoubtedly the greatest bodybuilder of all time. He has won 13 world championships, including an unprecedented seven Mr. Olympia titles (1970–1975, 1980), the last one after a five-year retirement from competition. Arnold also became a successful actor—starring in such films as *Stay Hungry, Pumping Iron,* and *Conan the Barbarian*—and a best-selling author.

In top contest condition, the 6′2″ Austrian Oak packed 230 pounds of ripped-up muscle on his body. His upper arms measured well over 20 inches in girth and his chest taped larger than 55 inches. He was noted for his gigantic muscles, perfect body proportions, and esthetic body shape and symmetry. The world may never see another bodybuilder to equal him.

Arnold's huge, Everest-peaked biceps were greatly admired by bodybuilders all over the world. Bill Reynolds interviewed him in late 1979 to determine how he developed such incredible biceps. Early in his career, Arnold did up to 20–25 total sets for his biceps during each workout, but toward the end of his competitive career he did only a little more than half that number. This was because he "could train with more intensity, and (he) also didn't want to exaggerate (his) biceps and throw off overall proportions."

Late in his career, Arnold Schwarzenegger preferred to do three exercises, with four sets of 10 reps on each movement. "Typically, this would be Barbell Curls, Dumbbell Curls, and Concentration Curls," he said. "Almost always, I would use a 'stripping method' for Barbell and Dumbbell Curls. This consisted of three sets within each set, done with a quick weight reduction between them. In other words, I would do several reps with a heavy barbell, then have some plates stripped off while I took a short rest-pause. Immediately after the plates were off, I would do a few more reps, strip off more plates, and finally force out a last few very hard repetitions."

Arnold Schwarzenegger. *(Robert Gardner)*

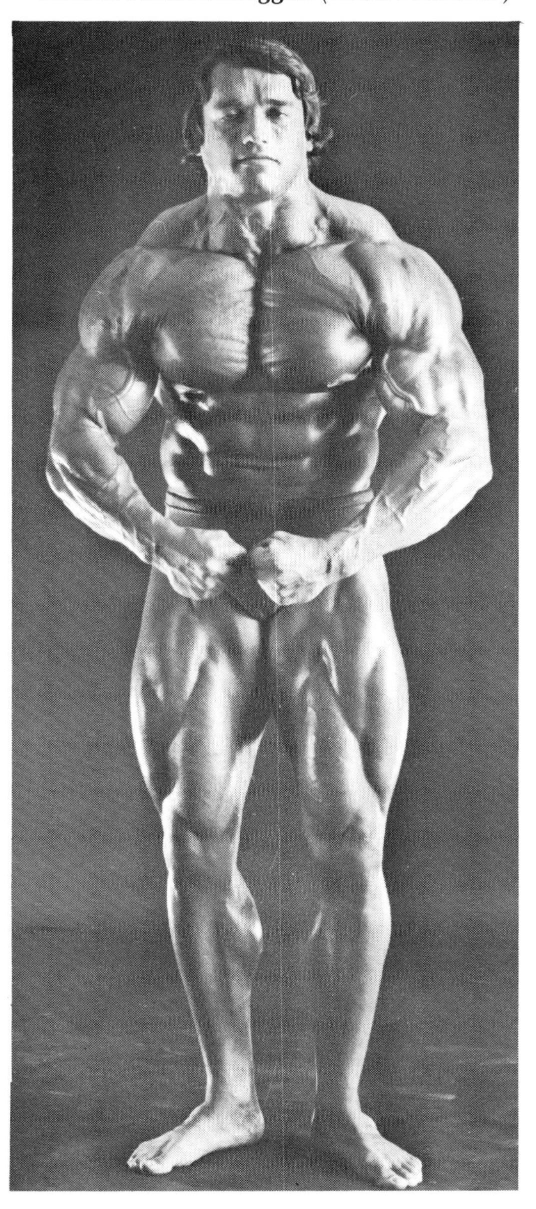

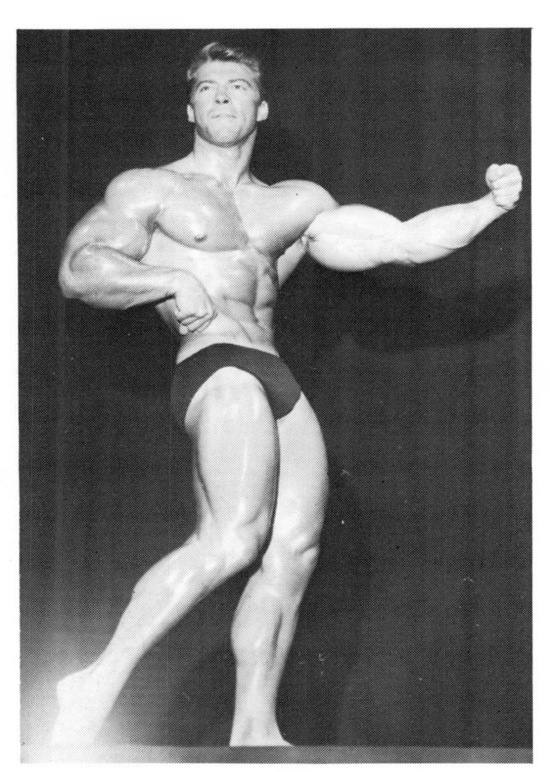

Larry Scott.

Larry Scott

A native of Idaho, Larry Scott lived for many years in southern California, training in a variety of gyms. He now lives in Salt Lake City, Utah, where he has his own $1,000,000 gym and racquetball complex. During his tenure as the most popular athlete in the sport he won the first two Mr. Olympia titles in 1965 and 1966. Prior to that, Scott had won the Mr. California, Mr. America, and Mr. Universe titles.

Larry worked hard and fast year-round, averaging about 45 seconds of rest between sets. And through hard, consistent training and a huge consumption of milk products, he was able to develop a massive and well-balanced physique on a below-average skeletal structure.

At approximately 5′8″ in height and weighing slightly over 200 pounds, Larry Scott's widely envied arms taped over 20 inches. Here is a typical Scott upper arm, superset workout, as reported by Gene Mozee:

1. Dumbbell Preacher Curl: 6 × 6
2. Barbell Preacher Curl: 6 × 6
3. Reverse Barbell Curl: 4 × 8
4. Lying Triceps Press: 6 × 8
5. High Pulley Triceps Extension: 6 × 8
6. Dumbbell Kickback: 4–6 × 8–10

Since Larry Scott popularized the Preacher Curl, many bodybuilders now honor him by calling it the "Scott Curl."

Vic Seipke

A fireman from Michigan, Seipke won the first Past-40 Mr. America competition, a good 20 years after he had been chosen Junior Mr. America in 1957. Vic's victory inspired a legion of mature bodybuilders to train for competition, until now Past-40 events are very popular features of virtually any bodybuilding show.

Vic Seipke suggests that intermediate bodybuilders use this thigh program three nonconsecutive days per week:

1. Squat: 4–5 × 12–6 (increasing weight each set)
2. Leg Extension: 4 × 8–10
3. Leg Curl: 5 × 8–10

"My own thighs respond rather easily, so this is basically the same routine I follow in the off-season," Vic commented. "I also include a lot of aerobic work in my training philosophy, most frequently in terms of a two- or three-mile run each night."

Jim Seitzer.

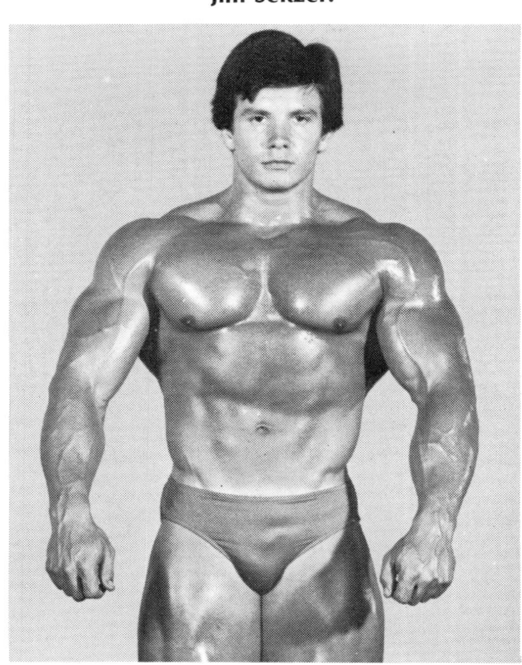

Jim Seitzer

A former Ohio State University gymnast, Jim has won the Mr. Ohio, Mr. Mid-West, and Junior Mr. USA titles. He has also been a finalist in his class at several Mr. USA and Mr. America competitions. A talented powerlifter, Seitzer has also achieved his Master's Rating in that sport.

Jim Seitzer's thighs are very massive, deeply cut, and well-shaped. Here is his precontest thigh program:

1. Squat: 5–6 × 15–6 (up to 500+ lbs.)
2. Leg Extension: 5 × 10–15
3. Lunge: 5 × 10–15
4. Leg Curl: 5 × 10–15

Jim has a master's degree in business administration and was an All Big 10 gymnast in college.

C. F. Smith, M.D.

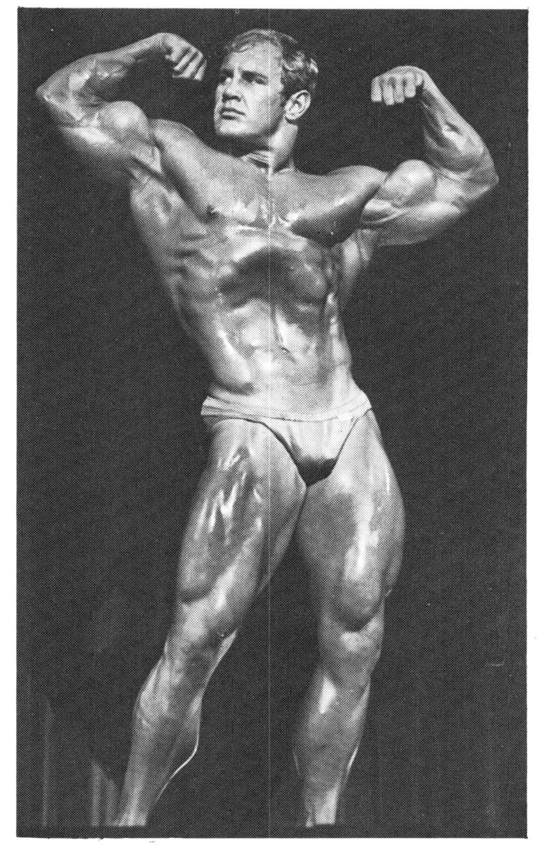

C. F. Smith. *(Jimmy Caruso)*

Intellectual brilliance and eccentricity often go hand in hand, and Dr. C. F. Smith is a good example of a champion bodybuilder with such a combination of qualities. He's a former Mr. Tennessee winner who has placed in the top five in the Mr. America competition. And Charlie Frank is a threat in any bodybuilding competition he deigns to enter.

Dr. Smith reaches peak condition doing a mere 3–6 total sets per muscle group, and he's able to cut his physique to ribbons eating hamburgers, fries, and a coke for lunch. "It's all a matter of calories," he revealed. "When I'm cutting up, I can eat anything I want as long as I don't exceed an average daily food intake of 2,000 calories. A 2,000-calorie diet results in a steady fat loss of 1½–2 pounds per week in my case."

Here's a typical C. F. Smith precontest arm training program:

1. Seated Alternate Dumbbell Curl: 1 × 10 (80-pound dumbbells)
2. Lying Dumbbell Triceps Extension: 1 × 10 (80 lbs.)
3. Pulley Pushdown: 1 × 8–10 (150 lbs.)
4. Nautilus Curl: 2 × 8–10
5. Nautilus Triceps Extension: 2 × 8–10

Charlie Frank's bodybuilding philosophy can be summed up in one statement: "If you control your head, you control everything!"

Ken Sprague

One of the co-authors of this book, Ken Sprague is a former owner of Gold's Gym. An all-around athlete in high school and college (he was a particularly good discus thrower, football player, and boxer), Sprague won the Mr. Cincinnati and Mr. Mid-America titles. He has also placed in the top three of his class in the Mr. America contest. Ken Sprague has written three previous books—*The Gold's Gym Weight Training Book* (J. P. Tarcher, 1976), *The Gold's Gym Strength Training Book* (Berkeley, 1981), and *The Athlete's Body* (J. P. Tarcher, 1981). Sprague currently is a strength training coach for a wide variety of college and professional athletes, and he conducts bodybuilding training camps.

Ken Sprague has won numerous "Best Arms" subdivision awards. Here is one of his favorite arm workouts, which is done three days per week:

1. Alternate Dumbbell Curl: 5 × 8–10
2. Pulley Pushdown: 5 × 8–10
3. Incline Dumbbell Curl: 5 × 8–10
4. Lying Barbell Triceps Extension: 5 × 8–10
5. Dumbbell Concentration Curl: 5 × 10–12
6. Dumbbell Kickback: 5 × 10–12

A maximum of 60 seconds rest should be allowed between supersets.

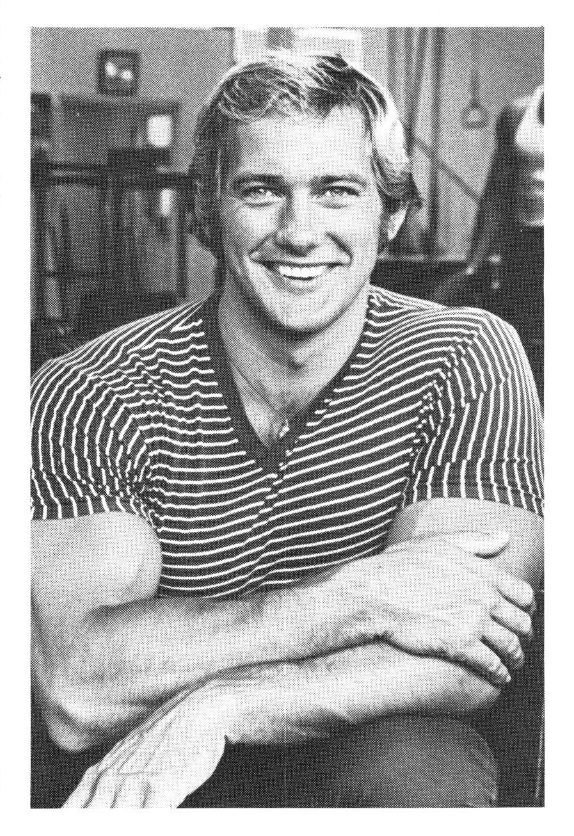

Ken Sprague. *(Art Zeller)*

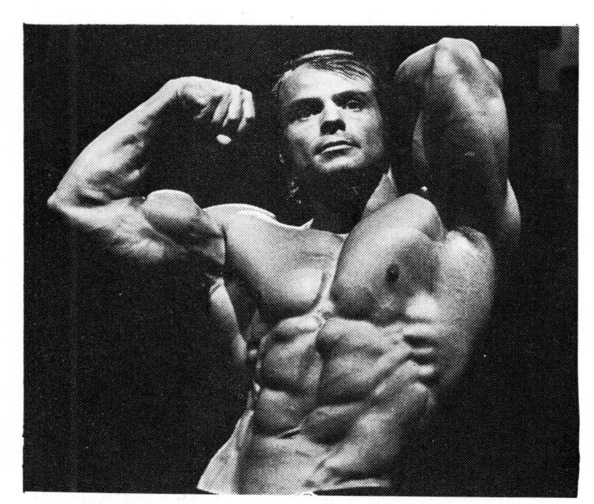

Petr Stach. *(Jimmy Caruso)*

Petr Stach

Stach is undoubtedly the best bodybuilder to come out of Czechoslovakia to date. He's won Mr. Czechoslovakia numerous times and Mr. Europe (twice), and he has placed in the top three in two IFBB Mr. Universe competitions. Petr is among the world's most innovative posers and one of only two or three who have mastered the use of every square inch of space on a posing platform.

When in California for the 1978 World Cup Championships, Stach trained every day at Gold's. This is how he worked his calves:

Monday-Wednesday-Friday (Heavy Days)

1. Seated Calf Machine: 5–6 × 8–10
2. Standing Calf Machine: 5–6 × 10–12

Tuesday-Thursday-Saturday (Light Days)

1. Calf Press: 3–4 × 15–20
2. One-Leg Calf Raise: 3–4 × 15–20

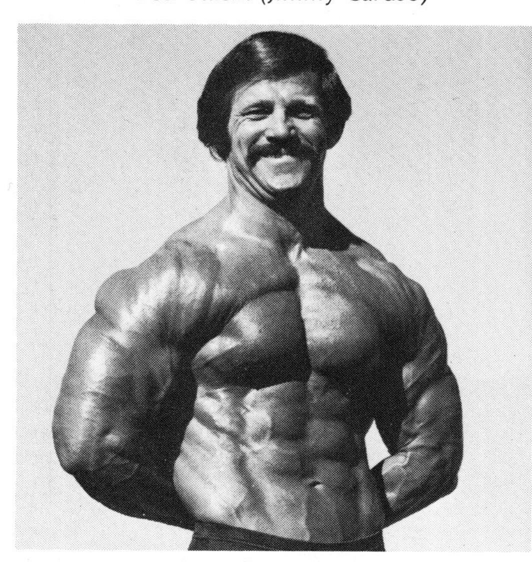

Pat Stewart.

Pat Stewart

Pat Stewart is interesting in that he has combined his bodybuilding with a dangerous career as an undercover agent for the U.S. Drug Enforcement Agency. Despite the lingering effects of a gunshot wound in his leg (suffered while undercover) that makes calf work quite painful, Pat has won the Mr. Louisiana, Mr. Virginia, and Mr. Arizona titles. (His work forces him to move around a lot!) Stewart has also won his class in the prestigious IFBB Mr. North America competition.

Pat Stewart contributed his shoulder workout to the readers of this book:

1. Press Behind Neck: 3 × 8–12 (up to 185 lbs.)
2. Alternate Dumbbell Press: 3 × 8–12 (up to 85)
3. Side Lateral: 2 × 8–12 (up to 55)
4. Cable Bent Lateral: 2 × 10–12 (up to 40 lbs. on each side)
5. Upright Rowing: 3 × 8–10 (up to 165 lbs.)

Also an ordained minister, Stewart claims, "Bodybuilding is the world's toughest sport, but I'll still be pumping iron when they nail me in my coffin!"

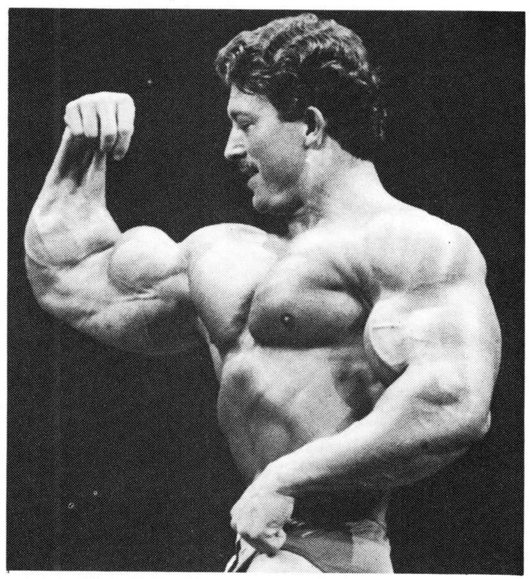

Kalman Szkalak.

Kalman Szkalak

Born in Hungary, Szkalak moved to America with his parents at the age of three following the Hungarian Revolution of 1956. He grew up in Delaware, but the lure of sunny California ultimately brought him to Gold's Gym, where he trained to win the Mr. California and Mr. America titles in 1976. A year later he won the IFBB Mr. Universe title, and he still competes occasionally.

At a height of 5′10″ Kal weighed 220 pounds in hard shape and sported 21-inch upper arms, a 53-inch chest, and a tiny 30-inch waist, but relatively weak thigh and calf development hampered him in pro competition. Here was his biceps workout at the time he won the Mr. America title:

1. Incline Dumbbell Curl: 5 × 8–9
2. Barbell Preacher Curl: 5 × 8
3. Nautilus Curl: 5 × 12
4. Cable Concentration Curl: 5 × 12
5. Reverse Curl: 5 × 12

Mandy Tanny

Mandy is the daughter of Armand Tanny, a former Mr. USA winner and the well-known *Muscle & Fitness* magazine writer. Although Mandy has never competed, she has been a pioneering force in women's bodybuilding through her insightful articles in *Muscle & Fitness*. Ms. Tanny was the first woman to earn an IFBB International Judge's Card, and she is an accomplished judge of both men's and women's bodybuilding contests.

Mandy Tanny contributed the following abdominal routine:

1. Crunch: 1 × 30
2. Lying Jackknife: 1 × 30
3. Cable Crunch: 1 × 15
4. Knee-up: 1 × 20
5. Bent-Over Twisting: 1 × 20
6. Incline Leg Raise: 1 × 20

"This exercise routine should be performed 4–6 times weekly at the beginning of your regular workouts," Mandy advised.

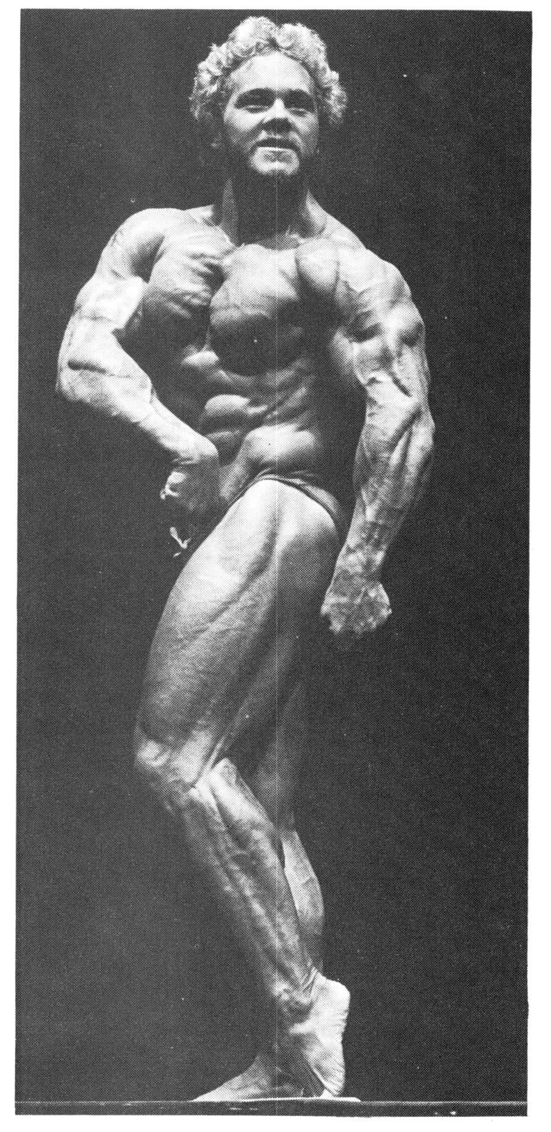

Ron Teufel.

Ron Teufel

Ron Teufel must have been born with huge muscles, because while still only 18 years of age he had won the Teenage Mr. America title and placed fifth in the senior Mr. America show. A year later he had moved up to third in the America and won the Mr. USA title. Today he is one of the most consistent competitors in IFBB pro shows.

"Teuf" has always been able to combine huge muscle mass with startling cuts, largely as a result of consistently training very heavy and doing an average of 15–18 total sets per muscle group. As an example of his strength, Ron has done several strict reps in the Bench Press with 440 pounds while weighing only 185 himself.

Teuf has frequently trained for extended periods of time at Gold's, even though he is a resident of Prospect Park, Pennsylvania. Here is a typical off-season chest workout that Ron contributed:

1. Bench Press: 5 × 6–8 (working up in weight)
2. Barbell Incline Press: 5 × 8–10
3. Dumbbell Incline Press: 4 × 10
4. Parallel Bar Dip: 4 × 10–12 (with added weight)

Ron Teufel's advice to teenage bodybuilders: "Hang in there and never let anyone discourage you. In bodybuilding you get out of it exactly what you put into it in terms of hard training and strict dieting."

Dennis Tinerino.

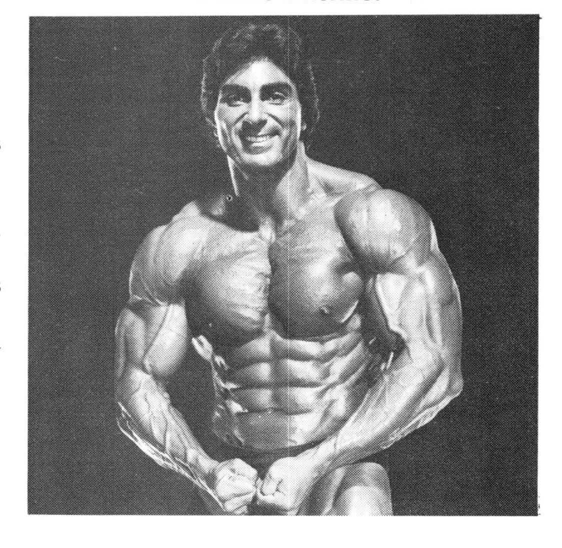

Dennis Tinerino

One of the most successful bodybuilders of the past decade or two has been Dennis Tinerino. Among his titles are Teenage Mr. America, Mr. USA, Junior Mr. America, Natural Mr. America, Mr. America, Mr. World, Mr. International, and Mr. Universe (four times). He is, indeed, the only major champion to win a steroid-free contest (the Natural Mr. America). Only the Mr. Olympia title has eluded Tinerino, but he's placed in the top five and continues to seek the title.

One of Dennis's most exceptional body parts is his deltoids. Here's a favorite Tinerino shoulder workout:

1. Machine Front Press: 6 × 6 (up to 200 lbs.)
2. Seated Dumbbell Press: 4 × 6–8 (up to 85s)
3. Bent Lateral: 4 × 8–10 (up to 50s)
4. Dumbbell Side Lateral: 4 × 8–10 (up to 55s)
5. Cable Side Lateral: 4 × 8–10 (up to 40 lbs.)

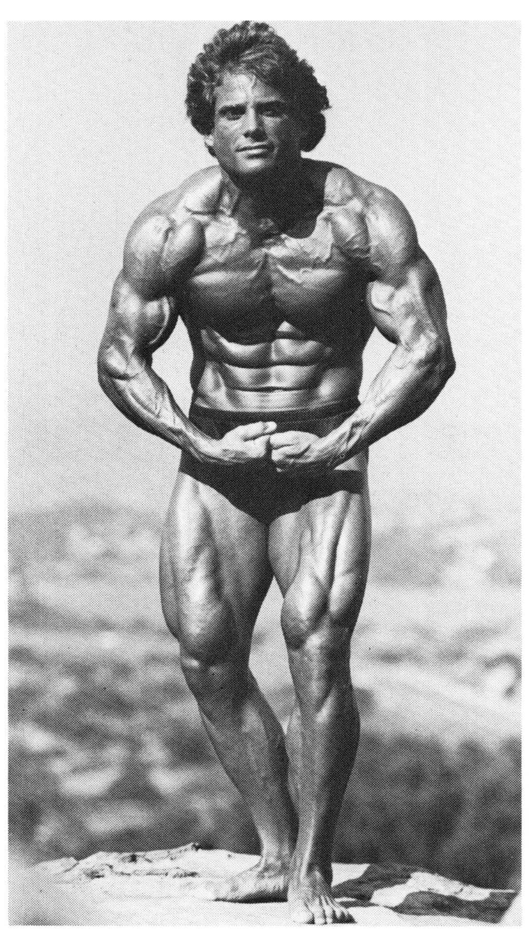

Mike Torchia.

Mike Torchia

Mike is a former Teenage Mr. America winner who frequently trains at Gold's. Mike once was an overweight teenager (he weighed 250 pounds at 5′6″ in height before beginning bodybuilding training). A sensible diet and hard workouts, however, changed his life and physique dramatically.

One of Mike Torchia's best body parts is his back, and here's one routine he uses at Gold's Gym:

1. One-Arm Dumbbell Bent Rowing: 2 × 8–10 (up to 125 lbs.)
2. Seated Pulley Rowing: 2 × 8–10 (up to 300 lbs.)
3. Behind Neck Pulldown: 2 × 8–10 (up to 250 lbs.)
4. Hyperextension: 2 × 8–10 (up to 135 lbs.)

One of Mike's secrets of success is that he frequently changes routines to maintain greater interest in his training.

Pierre Van Den Steen

Pierre, a Belgian bodybuilder who frequently trained at Gold's was—and still is—one of the world's most incredibly defined bodybuilders. His abdominals, in particular, couldn't have been carved any more sharply with a razor blade. He has won numerous titles, including Mr. International, Mr. Europe, his class at the Mr. Universe competition several times, and most recently the Senior Mr. Universe title for athletes over 40 years of age.

Since Van Den Steen's abdominals were so superb, we present you with the ab routine he used while training at Gold's. Using very intense concentration and slow movements, he would do this program six days per week:

1. Roman Chair Sit-up: 1 × 200
2. Hanging Leg Raise (Twisting): 2 × 25
3. Incline Sit-up: 1 × 50 (with a 50-pound plate held behind his head)
4. Twisting Leg Raise: 2 × 80–100

Overall, Pierre Van Den Steen is one of the sport's hardest trainers. Other than for his abs, he routinely does 30–40 total sets per muscle group and trains each major body part three times per week on a six-day split routine prior to competing!

Pierre Van Den Steen. *(Art Zeller)*

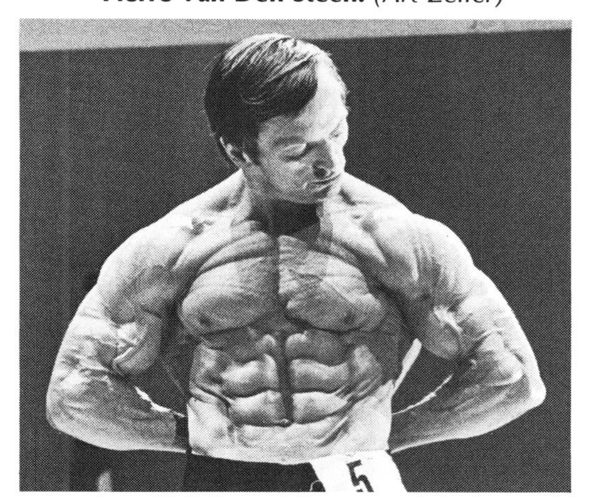

Casey Viator

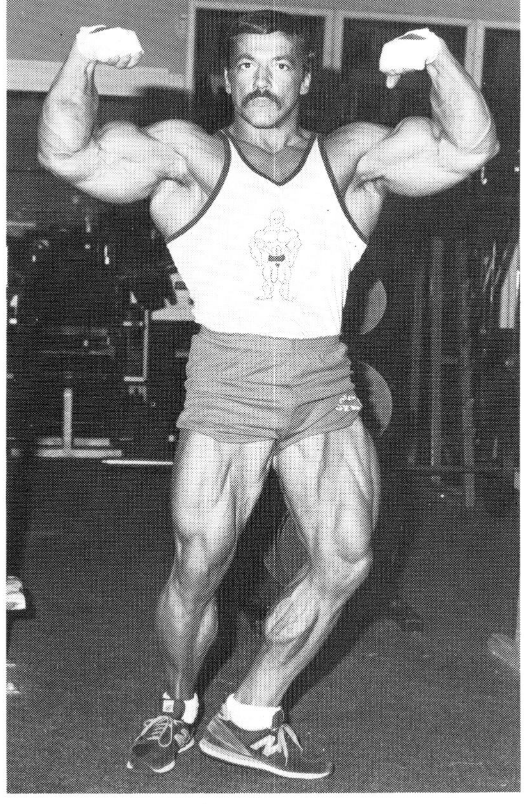

Casey Viator.

Casey Viator became history's youngest Mr. America when he won the title in 1971 at the age of 19. Prior to that he had won the Mr. USA and Teenage Mr. America titles. And in recent years he has won two professional titles on the IFBB Grand Prix circuit. In top shape, Casey is an awesome sight to see.

Casey also is one of the world's strongest bodybuilders. He routinely uses 650 pounds for reps in the Squat, 540 pounds for reps in the Bench Press, 475 pounds for reps in the Incline Press, and 245 pounds for strict reps in the Barbell Curl. Obviously, overload training is the name of the game for Casey Viator.

Casey trains an average of 3–4 hours a day, six days each week. And even when following a precontest 1,500-calorie-per-day diet, he is able to keep up a fast pace and use fairly substantial poundages in all of his workouts.

Because his physique is so well balanced, it is difficult to pick a strong point. Impressed with his superb shoulder development, however, we asked him for his deltoid routine. This is his normal shoulder workout three times per week:

1. Nautilus Side Lateral Raise (one arm at a time with up to 75 pounds added to the machine's weight stack): 3–5 × 15–20
2. Barbell Press Behind the Neck: 5–6 × 10–12 (up to 270 pounds)
3. Dumbbell Side Lateral: 4–5 × 10–12 (up to 70-pound dumbbells in strict form)
4. Dumbbell Bent Lateral: 4–5 × 10–12 (up to 75-pound dumbbells, again in strict form)
5. Barbell Upright Rowing: 4–5 × 10–15 (up to 225 pounds)

And that, sports fans, is how to build delts the size of honeydew melons!

Roger Walker

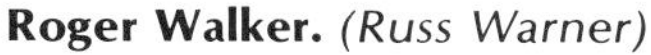

Roger Walker. *(Russ Warner)*

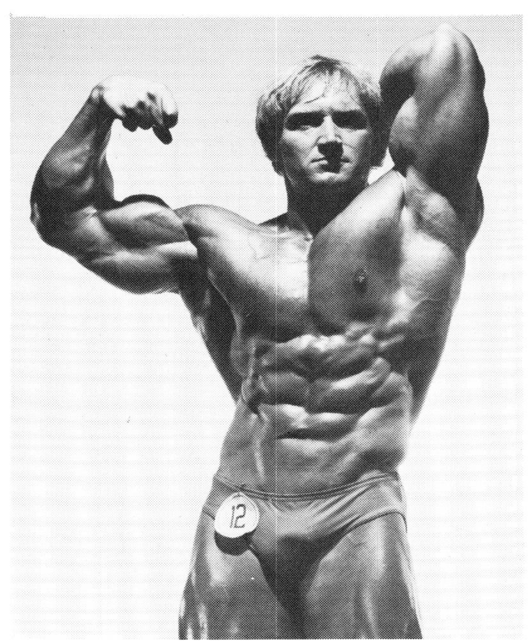

Originally from England, Roger is in the gym business in Sydney, Australia. When in America, he consistently trains at Gold's Gym. Among Walker's titles are Mr. Australia, Mr. Asia, Mr. Southern Hemisphere, and Mr. Universe. He has also been a Mr. Olympia finalist. He continues to compete internationally in IFBB professional contests.

Roger Walker's back development is particularly impressive. Here is one of his favorite precontest, superset back programs:

{ 1. Chin Behind the Neck: 5 × 10–12
{ 2. Barbell Bent Rowing: 5 × 10–12
{ 3. Seated Pulley Rowing: 5 × 10–12
{ 4. Front Lat Pulldown: 5 × 10–12
5. T-Bar Rowing: 5 × 10–12
6. One-Arm Dumbbell Bent Rowing: 5 × 10–12

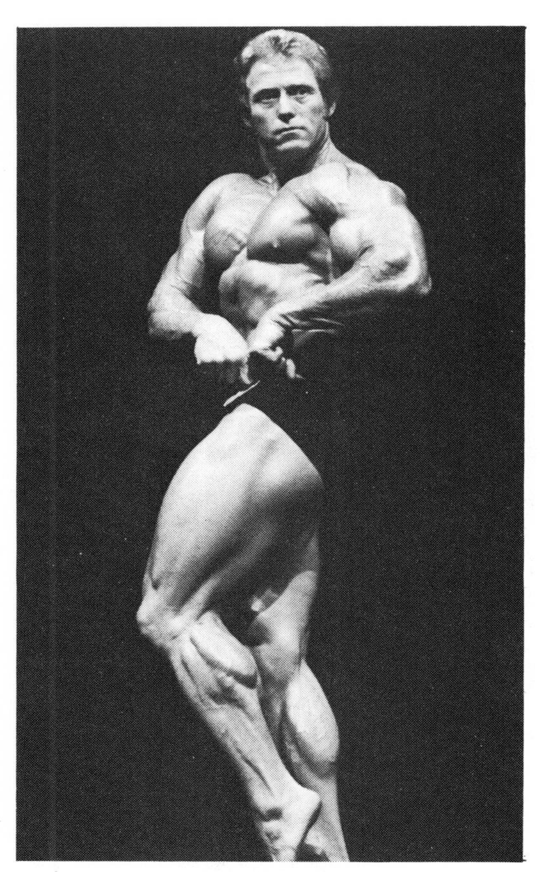

Ken Waller.

Ken Waller

A genial former pro football player from Kentucky, Waller has trained at Gold's for more than 10 years. He's won the YMCA Mr. America, Mr. USA, Mr. America, Mr. World, NABBA Mr. Universe, and IFBB Mr. Universe titles. His training and competition for this later title formed a significant segment of the film *Pumping Iron.* If you've seen the film, you'll recall a mischievous Ken Waller hiding Mike Katz's favorite T-shirt during the prejudging session of the Universe. Waller has also twice won the heavyweight class of the Mr. Olympia competition.

Kenny is also one of the strongest bodybuilders to work out at Gold's. He routinely did Squats with 600 pounds, 10–12 reps in the Incline Dumbbell Press with a pair of 170s, and Barbell Bent Rows with more than 300 pounds. Obviously, he came by his physique honestly—via long, hard, and heavy training.

Ken Waller's calves are particularly impressive, and through incredible mental concentration he was able to develop them with this abbreviated daily routine:

1. Donkey Calf Raise: 5 × 15–20
2. Seated Calf Raise: 3 × 15–20
3. One-Leg Calf Raise: 2–3 × 15–20

Without a doubt, Ken's extensive college and pro football experience was also responsible to a degree for his calf development, since most football players have large, well-shaped calves.

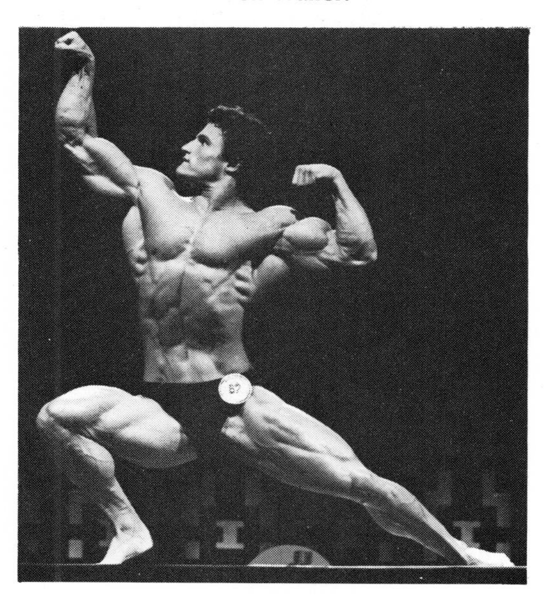

Mike Watson.

Mike Watson

A resident of Hamilton, Ontario, Watson has won two Mr. Canada titles and twice placed in the top five at the IFBB Mr. Universe competition. He's trained at Gold's Gym two different summers to prepare for international shows. Mike's physique has tremendous muscle density and vascularity, combined with fine physical proportions. To see him in person doing a "Most Muscular" pose is an awesome experience!

Since Mike had the most trouble getting his calves up to par, he submitted this grueling calf program:

Monday-Wednesday-Friday (Heavy Days)

1. Seated Calf Machine (Toe Raise): 5 × 10–12
2. Donkey Calf Raise: 5 × 15–20
3. Standing Calf Machine (Toe Raise): 5 × 10–15

Tuesday-Thursday-Saturday (Light Days)

1. Calf Press: 3–4 × 15–20
2. One-Leg Calf Raise: 3–4 × 15–20

"The stretch at the bottom of every rep of calf work is vital," Mike stated. "Without a complete stretch at the bottom of every rep of every set of every exercise, you won't reach your potential for calf development."

Rick Wayne

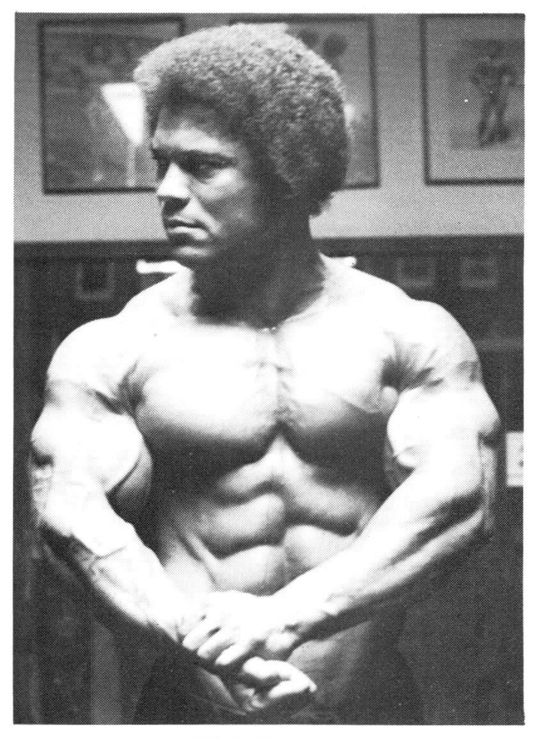

Rick Wayne.

Originally from St. Lucia in the Caribbean, Rick Wayne lived for many years in England, then moved to America about 15 years ago. Along the way he became a Pro Mr. America and Mr. World winner and one of the most respected writers in the sport. For many years he was editor-in-chief of *Muscle Builder* magazine (now called *Muscle & Fitness*). When training to win Mr. World (he also took the "Best Arms" subdivision in that competition), Rick worked out at the original Gold's Gym on Pacific Avenue in Venice, California.

Since his upper arm development was so phenomenal, we present Rick Wayne's precontest arm program (done after a warm-up of four supersets of Chins and Standing Barbell Presses):

1. Barbell Cheat Curl: 3–4 × 8–10
2. Pulley Pushdown: 3–4 × 10–12
3. Seated Dumbbell Curl (curling forward): 3–4 × 8–10
4. Dumbbell Concentration Curl: 3–4 × 10–12
5. Close-Grip Barbell Curl: 3 × 8–10
6. Seated Barbell Triceps Extension: 3 × 10–12
7. Seated Dumbbell Curl (curling outward): 3–4 × 8–10

Exercises 1–4 were performed as a giant set, while exercises 5–7 were done as a triset.

"To further muscularize your physique," Rick Wayne advises, "practice posing between exercises. If you happen to be bombing your arms, practice posing and controlling the biceps and triceps. Get into those poses which you will hit at contest time. Learn to master the art of muscle control, and in the process you'll develop amazing muscular definition!"

Joe Weider

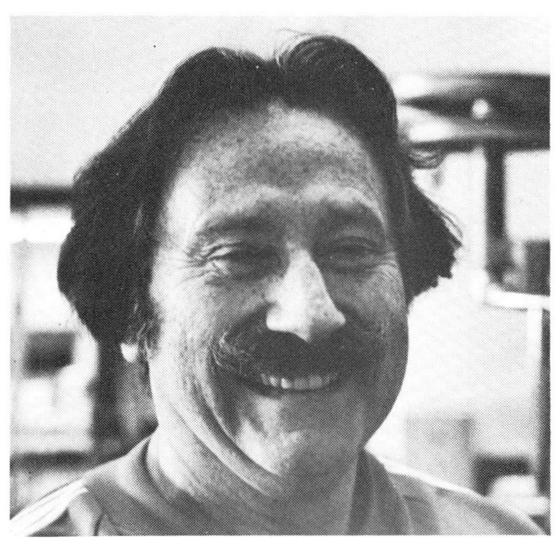

Joe Weider.

Joe Weider is the publisher of *Muscle & Fitness*, the bible of bodybuilding. He has been continuously publishing muscle magazines since 1940 and has written numerous books on bodybuilding. Since 1936, he has been known as "The Trainer of Champions." In short, Joe Weider has had the greatest impact on bodybuilding of any man in history. And, we are proud to say that he often trains at Gold's Gym.

The Master Blaster's knowledge of bodybuilding is vast, but to keep within the scope of this chapter, we asked him for the following intermediate-level chest routine. (Do it twice per week on a four-day split routine.)

1. Incline Dumbbell Press: 4 × 10–6 (increasing weight each set)
2. Flat-Bench Flye: 4 × 8–10
3. Parallel Bar Dip: 4 × 10–15

"This routine stresses all of the major areas of your chest muscles," Joe Weider said. "Use it for six weeks without missing a workout, and you'll notice a marked improvement in your chest musculature."

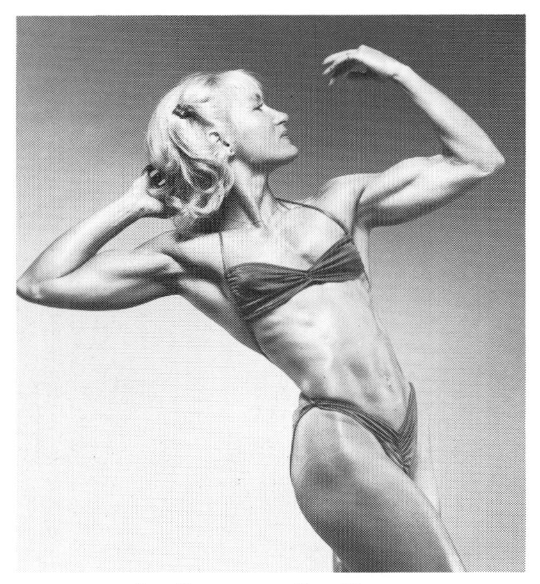

Claudia Cornwell Wilbourn.

Claudia Cornwell Wilbourn

Claudia, one of the most important pioneers in women's bodybuilding, did much of her training at Gold's, commuting more than an hour each way from her home in San Juan Capistrano. In June 1979, she placed second to Lisa Lyon in the first World Women's Bodybuilding Championships held by Gold's Gym in Los Angeles. A third-place finish in the U.S. Championships in 1980 solidified Claudia's reputation in the sport. Later, in 1980, she won the Ms. California title and placed a close second to Laura Combes in the inaugural Ms. America contest.

Currently retired from competition, Ms. Wilbourn still trains hard and stays quite active in the women's bodybuilding movement as a national and international judge and official. And she works as an editor on Joe Weider's *Flex* magazine.

Claudia contributed the following back routine:

1. Lat Pulldown: 3 × 6–10 (100–120 lbs.)
2. Seated Pulley Rowing: 3 × 6–10 (100–120 lbs.)
3. One-Arm Dumbbell Bent Rowing: 3 × 8 (60 lbs.)
4. Barbell Shrug Pull: 3 × 8 (150 lbs.)
5. One-Arm Low Pulley Rowing: 2 × 8 (60 lbs.)

This routine helped to build a widely envied back for Claudia, adding much to her symmetrical, esthetic, and muscular physique.

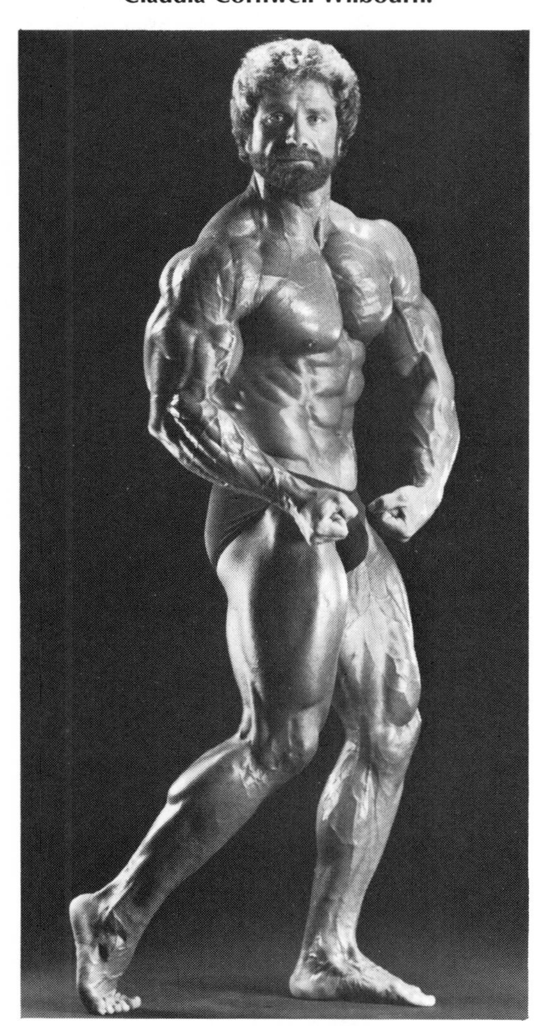

Jusup Wilkosz.

Jusup Wilkosz

A government communications specialist from Stuttgart, Germany, Wilkosz was good enough as an Olympic lifter to win the German Junior Championships. But Jusup has distinguished himself as a bodybuilder by winning Mr. Germany, Mr. Europe, Amateur Mr. Universe, and Pro Mr. Universe. Additionally, he has placed within the top six in the Mr. Olympia competition.

Jusup has trained for extended periods of time at Gold's Gym. Here are two alternative Wilkosz shoulder routines:

Routine A

{1. Alternate Front Dumbbell Raise: 5 × 10–12
{2. Side Lateral: 5 × 10–12
3. Seated Bent Lateral: 5 × 10–12
4. Seated Military Press: 5 × 10–12
5. Cable Side Lateral: 5 × 10–12

Routine B

{1. Side Lateral: 5 × 10–12
{2. Seated Press Behind the Neck: 5 × 10–12
3. Bent Lateral: 5 × 10–12
4. Barbell Upright Rowing: 5 × 10–12
5. Cable Side Lateral: 5 × 10–12

Jusup credits his wife, Ruth, for being "my main inspiration and source of support in my quest for the Mr. Olympia title."

Scott Wilson

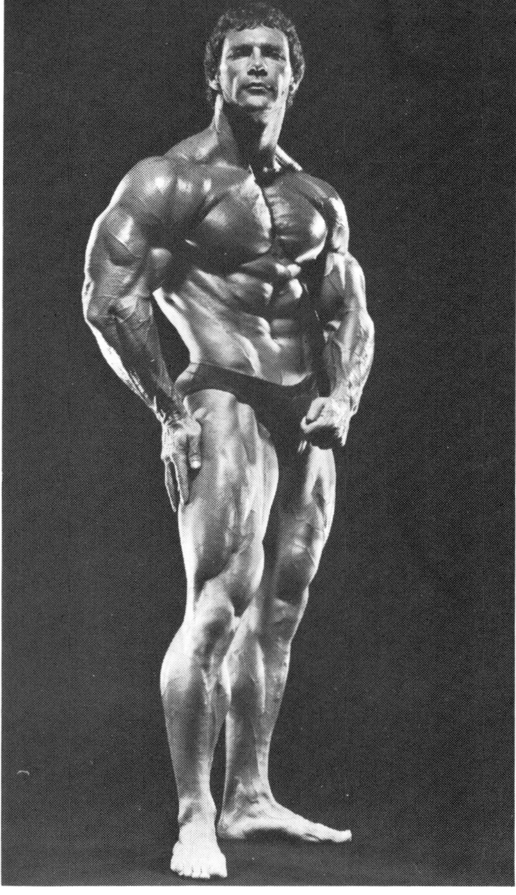

Scott Wilson. *(Russ Warner)*

An instructor and manager at Gold's/San Jose, Scott is the 1981 IFBB Mr. International winner. He has also won Mr. Southern California, Mr. California, and Pro Mr. America during a long but sporadic bodybuilding career. A very good powerlifter in the off-season from bodybuilding competition, Wilson has done a 625-pound Squat, 470-pound Bench Press, and 665-pound Deadlift at a body weight of 235 pounds.

Here is the precontest back routine that Scott used prior to winning his Mr. International title:

1. Deadlift: 5 × 5
2. Barbell Bent Rowing: 5 × 6–8
3. T-Bar Rowing: 5 × 6–8
4. Lat Machine Pulldown: 5 × 8
5. One-Arm Dumbbell Bent Rowing: 5 × 8
6. Barbell Shrug: 5 × 8
7. Upright Rowing: 5 × 8

Scott is married and has three sons, with whom he plays a lot of basketball.

Jim Yasenchock

Jim won the 1977 Teenage Mr. America competition while training at Gold's Gym, and he is a threat in any competition he enters. A six-footer, he weighs 218 pounds in top shape. Yasenchock is very good at endurance work on basic exercises, as evidenced by his ability to do 100 repetitions nonstop with 225 pounds in the Bench Press.

Here is a precontest, superset shoulder routine that Jim used at Gold's (it was done three days per week):

1. Seated Press Behind the Neck: 5 × 8–10
2. Standing Side Lateral: 5 × 10–12
3. Seated Dumbbell Press: 5 × 8–10
4. Cable Bent Lateral: 5 × 10–12
5. One-Arm Cable Side Lateral: 5 × 10–12

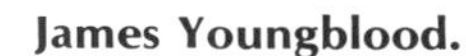

James Youngblood.

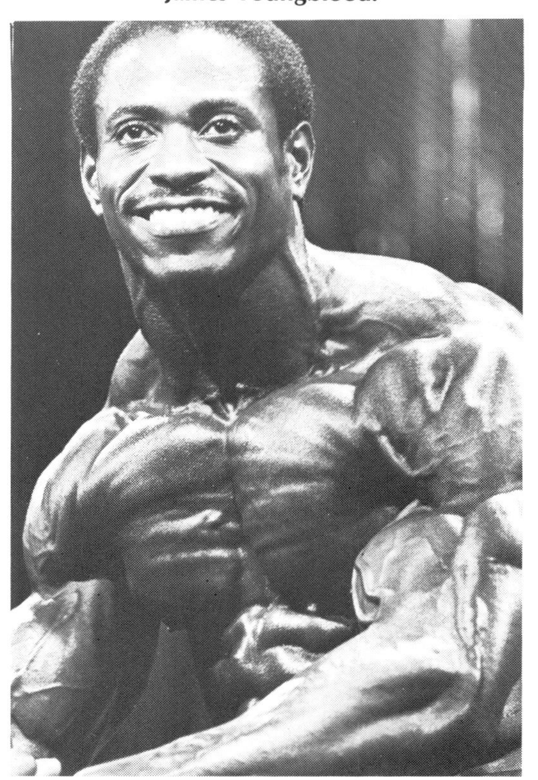

James Youngblood

James is a resident of Houston, Texas, and he's won nearly 20 physique titles, including Mr. Texas, the Gold's Classic (two times), and his class at the 1981 Mr. America contest. Youngblood also placed a strong second in the '81 IFBB Mr. Universe competition at Cairo, Egypt. "I prefer to compete regularly, because it keeps my training enthusiasm and intensity consistently high," James revealed.

Youngblood follows a double-split routine almost year-round, with each workout lasting 45–60 minutes. Here's a typical precontest abdominal workout:

1. Hanging Leg Raise: 3–4 × 15–20
2. Twisting Incline Sit-up: 3–4 × 25–30
3. Bench Leg Raise: 3–4 × 25–30
4. Roman Chair Sit-up: 3–4 × 25–30
5. Crunch: 3–4 × 25–30
6. Cable Crunch: 3–4 × 20–25

This routine is done as a giant set with no rest between exercises and less than a minute pause between giant sets.

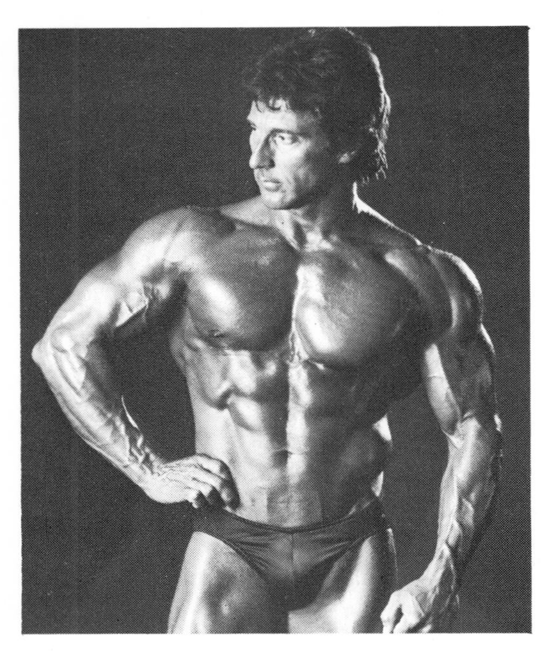

Frank Zane

Born and raised in Pennsylvania, Zane was a teacher in Florida when he moved to California to train at Gold's with a galaxy of other superstars. With more than 20 years of training behind him, Frank has won every major title—Mr. America, Mr. North America, Mr. World, Mr. Universe (four times), and Mr. Olympia (three times). And he was the pioneer in popularizing the super-ripped and highly defined type of physique that is popular today.

Zane's back in particular is amazingly striated and completely developed. Here's a back routine he used at Gold's:

1. Barbell Bent Rowing: 4 × 10
2. Chin Behind the Neck: 5 × 10
3. Front Lat Pulldown: 4 × 10
4. One-Arm Dumbbell Rowing: 4 × 10
5. T-Bar Rowing: 4 × 10

With his wife Christine, Frank Zane runs Zane Haven, a bodybuilding training resort in Palm Springs, California. The Zanes have also authored two bestselling exercise books.

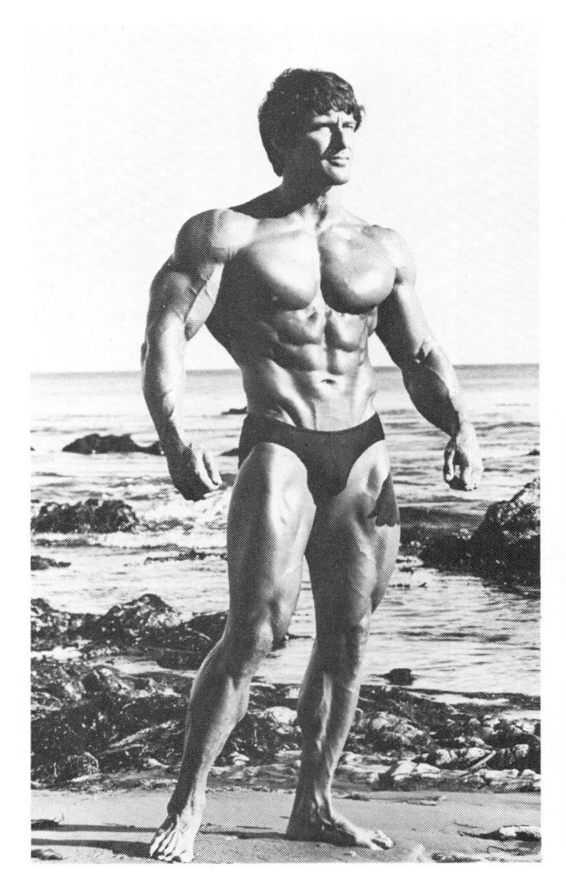

Frank Zane.

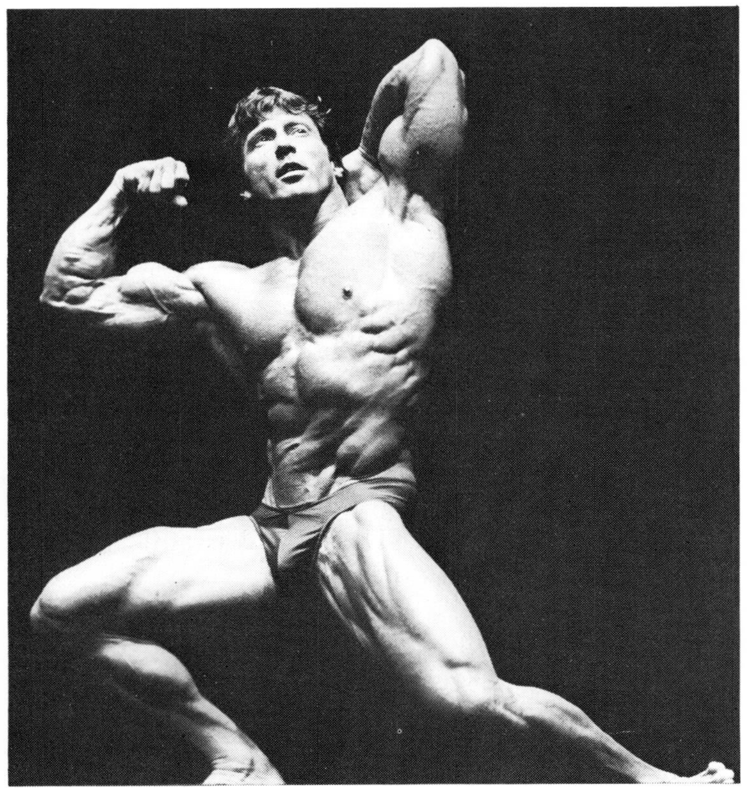

APPENDIX I: GLOSSARY

AEROBIC EXERCISE—Long-lasting, low-intensity exercise that can be carried on within the body's ability to consume and process enough oxygen to support the activity. The word *aerobic* means literally *with air*. Typical aerobic exercise activities include running, swimming, and cycling. Aerobic exercise leads to cardiorespiratory fitness.

AFWB—The American Federation of Women Bodybuilders, the sports federation responsible for administering women's amateur bodybuilding in America. The AFWB is affiliated internationally with the IFBB.

AMDR—The Adult Minimum Daily Requirement for various nutrients, as established by the U.S. Food and Drug Administration.

ANAEROBIC EXERCISE—High-intensity exercise that exceeds the body's aerobic capacity and builds up an oxygen debt. Because of its high intensity, anaerobic exercise can be continued for only a short time. A typical anaerobic exercise would be full-speed sprinting on a track.

APC—The American Physique Committee, Inc., the sports federation responsible for administering men's amateur bodybuilding in America. Like the AFWB, the APC is affiliated internationally with the IFBB.

BALANCE—Referring to even body proportions, as in, "He has nice balance to his phyique."

BAR—The iron or steel shaft that forms the handle of a barbell or dumbbell. Barbell bars vary in length from about four to seven feet, while dumbbell bars are 12–16 inches long. Bars are usually one inch in diameter, and they are often encased in a revolving sleeve.

BARBELL—This is the basic piece of equipment for weight training and bodybuilding. It consists of a bar, sleeve, collars, and plates. The weight of an adjustable barbell without plates averages five pounds per foot of bar length. The weight of this basic barbell unit must be considered when adding plates to the barbell to form a required training poundage. Barbells in large gyms are usually "fixed," with the plates welded or otherwise semipermanently fastened to the bars in a variety of poundages. These poundages are designated by numerals painted or engraved on the sides of the plates of each barbell.

BMR—The Basal Metabolic Rate, or the natural speed at which the body burns calories when at rest to provide its basic survival energy needs.

BODYBUILDING—A subdivision of the general category of weight training in which the main objective is to change the appearance of the human body via heavy weight training and applied nutrition. For most men and women bodybuilding consists merely of reducing a fleshy area or two and/or building up one or two thin body parts. In its purest form, bodybuilding for men and women is a competitive sport, both nationally and internationally, in amateur and professional categories.

BODYSCULPTING—This term is occasionally used in a feminine context to mean *bodybuilding.*

BURN—The feeling a muscle gets when it has really been pushed to its limits.

CHEATING—A method of swinging the weights or body to complete a rep that would have otherwise been impossible.

CIRCUIT TRAINING—A specialized form of weight training that develops body strength and aerobic endurance simultaneously. In circuit training a bodybuilder plans a circuit of 10–20 exercises covering all of the body's major muscle groups, then proceeds around the circuit in order while resting minimally between sets. Many bodybuilders use circuit training to improve their muscularity prior to a competition. As such, it is a good form of quality training.

CLEAN—The act of raising a barbell or dumbbell to shoulder height.

COLLAR—The cylindrical metal clamp used to hold plates in position on a barbell. Usually these collars are secured in place with a "set screw" threaded through the collar and tightened against the bar with a wrench. *Inside collars* keep plates from sliding inward and injuring a bodybuilder's hands, while *outside collars* keep the plates from sliding off the end of the bar. For safety's sake, you should never lift a barbell unless the collars are tightly fastened in place.

COUPLES' COMPETITION—Sometimes called "Mixed Pairs Competition," this is a new form of bodybuilding competition in which man-woman teams compete against each other. Couples' competition is becoming very popular with bodybuilding fans all over the world. It is now part of competitions even on the international level.

CUT UP—A term used to denote a well-defined bodybuilder. Usually this is a complimentary term, as in saying, "He's really cut up for this show!"

DEFINITION—This term is used to denote an absence of body fat in a bodybuilding competitor, so that every muscle is fully delineated. When a competitor has achieved ideal definition, his or her muscles will show striations, or individual fibers visible along a muscle mass. Definition is often called *muscularity.*

DENSITY—The hardness of muscle tissue, denoting complete muscularity, even to the point where fat within a muscle mass has been eliminated.

DUMBBELL—This is simply a shorter version of a barbell, which is intended for use in one hand, or more commonly with equally weighted dumbbells in each hand. All of the characteristics and terminology of a barbell are the same in a dumbbell.

EXERCISE—Used as a noun, this is the actual bodybuilding movement being done (e.g., a Bench Press or a Concentration Curl). An exercise is often called a *movement.* Used as a verb, *to exercise* is to work out physically and recreationally with weight training or any number of other forms of exercise (e.g., running, playing softball, etc.).

FLEXIBILITY—A suppleness of muscles and connective tissue that allows any man or woman to move his or her limbs and torso over a complete—or even exaggerated—range of motion.

FORCED REPS—A method of training whereby a training partner helps lift a weight just enough so the movement can be completed for two or three repetitions once the trainee has reached a point where he cannot complete it on his own.

HYPERTROPHY—The increase due to an overload on a muscle in that muscle's mass and strength. This is usually referred to by bodybuilders as *muscle growth,* though muscles do not grow in the sense of adding new cells to their mass.

IFBB—The International Federation of Bodybuilders, which was founded in 1946 by Ben and Joe Weider. It is the parent international federation overseeing worldwide men's and women's amateur and professional bodybuilding. More than 115 national bodybuilding federations are affiliated with the IFBB, making bodybuilding the world's fifth most popular sport.

INTENSITY—The degree of difficulty built into weight training exercise. Intensity can be increased by adding resistance, increasing the number of repetitions done of an exercise, or decreasing the rest interval between sets. The greater the intensity of bodybuilding exercise placed on a muscle, the greater will be that muscle's rate of hypertrophy.

JUDGING ROUNDS—In the internationally accepted IFBB system of bodybuilding judging, three judging rounds are contested, plus a final posedown in which the top five contestants compete in a free-posing manner for added points. In Round I each bodybuilder is viewed standing relaxed with his or her front, left side, back, and right side toward the judging panel. Round II consists of a set of standardized "compulsory poses," while Round III is devoted to creative individual "free posing" to each contestant's own choice of music.

LIFTING BELT—A leather belt four to six inches wide at the back that is worn around the waist to protect a trainee's lower back and abdomen from injuries. The six-inch belt can be used in training, but only the four-inch belt can be used in actual weightlifting competition.

MASS—The size or fullness of muscles. Massiveness is highly prized in bodybuilding competition, especially by the male competitors.

MUSCULARITY—Another term for *definition,* it denotes an absence of body fat, so that every muscle is fully delineated.

NUTRITION—The various practices of taking food into the human body. Bodybuilders have made a science of nutrition by applying it either to add muscle mass or to totally strip fat from their bodies to achieve optimum muscle definition.

OLYMPIAN—An appellation given to those men and women who have competed in the Mr. Olympia or Miss Olympia contests. Olympians are elite bodybuilders.

OLYMPIC BARBELL—A highly specialized and finely machined barbell used in weightlifting competition and heavy bodybuilding training. An Olympic barbell weighs 20 kilograms (slightly less than 45 pounds), and each of its collars weighs 2½ kilograms (5.5 pounds).

OLYMPIC LIFTING—A form of competitive weightlifting included in the Olympic Games program since the revival of the modern Olympics at Athens in 1896. Until 1972 this form of weightlifting consisted of three lifts: the Press, Snatch, and Clean and Jerk. Because of officiating difficulties, however, the Press was dropped from use following the 1972 Olympic Games, leaving the Snatch and Clean and Jerk as the two competitive Olympic lifts.

OVERLOAD—A degree of stress placed on the muscle that is over and above the amount the muscle is ordinarily used to handling. In bodybuilding this overload is applied by lifting heavier and heavier weights.

PEAK—Used two ways in bodybuilding jargon—to indicate the top of a muscle (usually the biceps) and to describe the process of reaching top physical condition before a contest.

PHA—An abbreviation for *peripheral heart action,* in which each skeletal muscle acts as an auxiliary heart by milking blood past one-way valves in the arterial system. Without PHA the heart itself would have difficulty circulating blood throughout the body. PHA is also a term assigned to a system of circuit training in which shorter series of four to six exercises are used in circuits. This system was pioneered by Bob Gajda, the 1966 Mr. America winner.

PLATES—The flat discs pierced with holes in the middle that are fitted on barbells and dumbbells to increase the weight of these apparatus. Plates are made of either cast metal or vinyl-covered concrete. They come in a wide range of graduated weights from as little as 1¼ pounds to more than 100 pounds each.

POUNDAGE—The actual weight of a barbell, dumbbell, or weight machine resistance used in an exercise.

POWER LIFTING—A form of competitive weightlifting using three lifts: the Squat, Bench Press, and Deadlift. The sport has both national and international competitions. Unlike in Olympic lifting, special women's competitions are held in powerlifting.

PROGRESSION—The act of gradually and steadily adding to the resistance used to overload a muscle group stressed by an exercise.

PROPORTION—A competitive bodybuilding term referring to the size relationships between various body parts. A contestant with good proportions will have no over- or underdeveloped muscle groups.

PUMP—To achieve a *pump* or to get *pumped* is to exercise a muscle until it is heavily engorged with blood.

QUALITY TRAINING—A type of workout in which the rest intervals between sets are drastically shortened prior to a competition. Quality training in combination with a low-calorie diet results in the best possible combination of muscle mass and muscle density.

REPETITION—Often abbreviated as *rep,* this is each individual full cycle of an exercise from the starting point of the movement to the midpoint and back again to the starting point. Usually, a series of several repetitions are done for each exercise.

RESISTANCE—As with poundage, this is the actual weight being used in an exericse.

REST INTERVAL—The pause between sets of an exercise during which the worked muscles are allowed to recuperate partially before the succeeding set is begun. Rest intervals vary from as little as 10–15 seconds to as much as five minutes. An average rest interval is about 60 seconds.

RIPPED—A term synonymous with *cut up,* as in "He's really ripped."

ROUTINE—Sometimes called a *program* or *schedule*, this is the complete accumulation of exercises, sets, and reps done in one training session. A routine is usually repeated two or three times each week.

SET—A distinct grouping of repetitions, followed by a brief rest interval and another set. Usually, several sets are done for each exercise in a training program.

SLEEVE—A hollow metal tube fitted over the bar of a barbell. The sleeve allows a bar to rotate more freely in your hands. Ordinarily, grooved knurlings are scored into the sleeve to aid in gripping the barbell when the hands have become sweaty during a training session.

SPOTTERS—Training partners who stand by as a safety factor to prevent you from being pinned under a heavy barbell during an exercise. Spotters are particularly necessary when you are doing limit Bench Presses and Squats.

STEROIDS—Prescription artificial male hormones that some bodybuilders use to increase muscle mass. Anabolic steroids are very dangerous drugs, however, and we do not recommend that anyone use them.

STICKING POINT—Any part of a movement that is very difficult to get past in order to complete the movement.

STRETCHING—A type of exercise program used to promote body flexibility. It involves assuming and then holding postures in which certain muscle groups and body joints are stretched.

STRIATIONS—This is the ultimate degree of muscle definition. When a muscle mass like the pectoral is fully defined, it will have myriad small individual grooves across it, almost as if a cat had repeatedly scratched the surface of a wax statue's pectoral muscles. These tiny muscular details are called striations.

SUPPLEMENTS—Concentrated vitamins, minerals, and proteins, usually in tablet/capsule or powder form. Food supplements are widely used by competitive bodybuilders, weightlifters, and other athletes to optimize their overall nutritional intake.

SYMMETRY—In competitive bodybuilding parlance, this is the shape or general outline of the body, as if it were seen in silhouette. Symmetry is enhanced in both male and female bodybuilders by a wide shoulder structure; a small waist-hip structure; small knees, ankles, and wrists; and large muscle volumes surrounding these small joints.

TRAINING TO FAILURE—Method of training whereby the trainee has continued a set to a point where it is impossible for him to complete another rep without assistance.

VASCULARITY—The appearance of surface veins and arteries in any bodybuilder who has achieved a low level of body fat. Women tend to have vascularity primarily in their arms, while male bodybuilders can have surface vascularity all over their bodies.

WEIGHT—Another term for *poundage* or *resistance*. Sometimes this term is used generally to refer to the apparatus (barbell, dumbbell, etc.) being used in an exercise, versus the exact poundage being used in an exercise.

WEIGHT CLASS—So that smaller athletes are not overwhelmed by larger ones, both competitive bodybuilding and weightlifting use weight classes. In women's bodybuilding the classes (at the time of this writing) were under 52½ kilograms (114 lbs.) and over 52½ kilos, while men's bodybuilding weight classes are set at 70 kilograms (154 pounds), 80 kilograms (176 pounds), 90 kilograms (198 pounds), and over 90 kilograms, or "unlimited." Powerlifting and Olympic lifting are contested in a much wider variety of weight classes. Converted to pounds from international metric equivalents, these are 114, 123, 132, 148, 165, 181, 198, 220, 242, 275, and over 275 pounds.

WEIGHTLIFTING—The subdivision of weight training in which men and women compete in weight classes both nationally and internationally to see who can lift the heaviest weights for single repetitions in prescribed exercises. Two types of weightlifting—Olympic lifting and powerlifting—are contested.

WEIGHT TRAINING—The various acts of using resistance training equipment either to exercise the body or for competitive purposes.

WORKOUT—A bodybuilding training session. "To work out" is to take a bodybuilding training session.

YOGA—An Eastern physical discipline that promotes body flexibility. Yoga also is a particularly tranquil philosophy of life.

APPENDIX II: ADDITIONAL SOURCES

BIBLIOGRAPHY

Anatomy

Gray, Henry. *Anatomy, Descriptive and Surgical.* London: Crown Publishers, 1968.

Bodybuilding Books

Bass, Clarence. *Ripped.* Albuquerque, NM: Ripped Enterprises, 1980.

Coe, Boyer and Valerie, with Reynolds, Bill. *Boyer and Valerie Coe's Weight Training Book.* Chicago: Contemporary Books, Inc., 1982.

Coe, Boyer, and Summer, Bob. *Getting Strong, Looking Strong.* New York: Atheneum, 1979.

Coe, Boyer, and Morey, Dr. Stan. *Optimal Nutrition.* Huntington Beach, CA: Boyer Coe Enterprises, 1979.

Columbu, Dr. Franco. *Franco Columbu's Complete Book of Bodybuilding.* Chicago: Contemporary Books, Inc., 1982.

Columbu, Franco, and Fels, George. *Coming on Strong.* Chicago: Contemporary Books, Inc., 1978.

Columbu, Franco, and Fells, George. *Winning Bodybuilding.* Chicago: Contemporary Books, Inc., 1977.

Ferrigno, Lou, and Hall, Douglas Kent. *The Incredible Lou Ferrigno.* New York: Simon and Schuster, 1982.

Gaines, Charles, and Butler, George. *Pumping Iron.* New York: Simon and Schuster, 1974.

Kennedy, Robert. *Hardcore Bodybuilding.* New York: Sterling Publishing Co., Inc., 1982.

Kennedy, Robert. *Natural Body Building for Everyone.* New York: Sterling Publishing Co., Inc., 1980.

Lurie, Dan, and Lima, John J. *Dan Lurie's "Instant Action" Body-Building System.* New York: Arco Publishing, Inc., 1980.

Mentzer, Mike, and Friedberg, Ardy. *Mike Mentzer's Complete Weight Training Book.* New York: William Morrow and Company, Inc., 1982.

Mentzer, Mike, and Friedberg, Ardy. *The Mentzer Method to Fitness.* New York: William Morrow and Company, Inc., 1980.

Murray, Jim. *Inside Bodybuilding.* Chicago: Contemporary Books, Inc., 1978.

Pearl, Bill. *Keys to the Inner Universe.* Pasadena, CA: Physical Fitness Architects, 1979.

Schwarzenegger, Arnold, with Dobbins, Bill. *Arnold's Bodybuilding for Men.* New York: Simon and Schuster, 1981.

Schwarzenegger, Arnold, and Hall, Douglas Kent. *Arnold: The Education of a Bodybuilder.* New York: Simon and Schuster, 1977.

Snyder, George, and Wayne, Rick. *3 More Reps (Books 1, 2, 3).* Warrington, PA: Olympus Health and Recreation, Inc., 1979, 1981.

Weider, Joe. *Bodybuilding: The Weider Approach.* Chicago: Contemporary Books, Inc., 1981.

Weider, Joe. *The IFBB Album of Bodybuilding All-Stars.* New York: Hawthorne Books, Inc., 1979.

Weider, Joe (Editor). *Champion Bodybuilders' Training Strategies and Routines.* Chicago: Contemporary Books, Inc., 1982.

Weider, Joe (Editor). *More Bodybuilding Nutrition and Training Programs.* Chicago: Contemporary Books, Inc., 1982.

Weider, Joe (Editor). *More Training Tips and Routines.* Chicago: Contemporary Books, Inc., 1982.

Weider, Joe (Editor). *The World's Leading Bodybuilders Answer Your Questions.* Chicago: Contemporary Books, Inc., 1981.

Weider, Joe (Editor). *Training Tips and Routines.* Chicago: Contemporary Books, Inc., 1981.

Zane, Frank and Christine. *The Zane Way to a Beautiful Body.* New York: Simon and Schuster, 1979.

Bodybuilding Drugs

Coe, Boyer, and Morey, Dr. Stan. *Steroids.* Huntington Beach, CA: Boyer Coe Enterprises, Inc., 1979.

Wright, James E., Ph.D. *Anabolic Steroids and Sports.* Nattick, MA: Sports Science Consultants, 1978.

Flexibility

Anderson, Bob. *Stretching.* Fullerton, CA: Anderson, 1975.

Foreign Language Bodybuilding Books

Szekeley, Dr. Laszlo. *Culturism.* Romania: Editura Sport-Turism, 1977.

Wilkosz, Jusup. *Was Würde bloss die Emma dazu sagen?* Stuttgart: Ha We-Verlag, 1980.

General Resistance Training

Carnes, Ralph and Valerie. *Playboy's Book of Fitness for Men.* Chicago: Playboy Press, 1980.

Darden, Ellington. *The Nautilus Book* (Revised). Chicago: Contemporary Books, Inc., 1982.

Dobbins, Bill, and Sprague, Ken. *The Gold's Gym Weight Training Book.* Los Angeles: J. P. Tarcher, Inc., 1977.

Ferrigno, Carla. *For Women Only: Carla Ferrigno's Total Shape-Up Program.* Chicago: Contemporary Books, Inc., 1982.

Murray, Jim. *Contemporary Weight Training.* Chicago: Contemporary Books, Inc., 1978.

Ravelle, Lou. *Bodybuilding for Everyone.* New York: Pocket Books, 1977.

Reynolds, Bill. *Complete Weight Training Book.* Mountain View, CA: Anderson-World, Inc., 1976.

Reynolds, Bill. *Weight Training for Beginners.* Chicago: Contemporary Books, Inc., 1982.

Sing, Vanessa. *Lift for Life!* New York: Bolder Books, 1977.

Sprague, Ken. *The Gold's Gym Book of Strength Training.* Los Angeles: J. P. Tarcher, Inc., 1979.

Injury Treatment and Rehabilitation

Mirkin, Gabe, and Hoffman, Marshall. *Sports Medicine Book.* Boston: Little, Brown & Co., 1978.

Kinesiology

Wells, Katharine E., and Luttgens, Kathryn. *Kinesiology: Scientific Basis of Human Motion.* Philadelphia: W. B. Saunders Co., 1976.

Nutrition

Darden, Ellington. *The Nautilus Nutrition Book.* Chicago: Contemporary Books, Inc., 1981.

Neve, Vickie. *Pat Neve's Bodybuilding Diet Book.* Phoenix, AZ: Phoenix Books, 1980.

Nutrition Almanac. New York: McGraw-Hill Book Co., 1977.

Physiology

Astrand, Per-Olof and Rohdahl, Kaare. *Text Book of Work Physiology.* New York: McGraw-Hill Book Co., 1977.

Women's Bodybuilding

Barrilleaux, Doris, and Murray, Jim. *Inside Weight Training for Women.* Chicago: Contemporary Books, Inc., 1978.

Schwarzenegger, Arnold, with Hall, Douglas Kent. *Arnold's Bodyshaping for Women.* New York: Simon and Schuster, 1979.

Weider, Joe (Editor). *Women's Weight Training and Bodybuilding Tips and Routines.* Chicago: Contemporary Books, Inc., 1982.

Weider, Joe, and Weider, Betty. *The Weider Book of Bodybuilding for Women.* Chicago: Contemporary Books, Inc., 1982.

Bodybuilding Magazines

Bodybuilder. Charlton Publications, Charlton Building, Derby, CT 06418.

Body & Power. Family Publications, P. O. Box 1984, Reseda, CA 91335.

Flex. 21100 Erwin Street, Woodland Hills, CA 91367.

Iron Man. Box 10, Alliance, NE 69301.

Muscle Digest. 10317 East Whittier Blvd., Whittier, CA 90606.

Muscle & Fitness. 21100 Erwin St., Woodland Hills, CA 91367.

Muscle Mag International. Unit Two, 270 Rutherford Rd. S., Brampton, Ontario L6W 3K7, Canada.

Muscle Training Illustrated. 1665 Utica Ave., Brooklyn, NY 11234.

Muscle Up. Charlton Publications, Charlton Building, Derby, CT 06418.

Muscle World. Charlton Publications, Charlton Building, Derby, CT 06418.

Muscular Development. Box 1707, York, PA 17405.

Strength & Health. Box 1707, York, PA 17405.

AUTHORITATIVE BODYBUILDING COURSES

Balik, John: Four courses—*You Can't Flex Fat; Total Muscularity; The Complete Cycle;* and *Anabolic Steroids.* Address: John Balik, Box 337, Santa Monica, CA 90406.

Cahling, Andreas: Four courses—*Viking Power Arms and Shoulders; Viking Power Chest and Back; Viking Power Legs and Abs;* and *Viking Power Training Secrets.* Address: Andreas Cahling, Box 988, Santa Monica, CA 90406.

Coe, Boyer: Seven courses—*Massive, Ripped Thighs & Calves; Arm Perfection; Dynamic Deltoids; Complete Chest Development; Advanced Back Training; Intensified Waist Training;* and *Power Posing.* Address: Boyer Coe, Box 5877, Huntington Beach, CA 92646.

Columbu, Franco: Ten courses—*Power; Chest and Abdominals; Shoulders; Arms and Forearms; Back; Thighs, Calves and Abdominals; Photo Album; Nutrition; Definition;* and *Spinal Problems and Injuries.* Address: Franco Columbu, Box 415, Santa Monica, CA 90406.

Davis, Steve: Four courses—*Achieving Total Muscularity; Foundation of Training; Gaining Muscle Size and Density;* and *Best of the New Breed—Volume 1.* Address: Steve Davis Fitness Center, 23115 Lyons Ave., Newhall, CA 91321.

Dickerson, Chris: Seven courses—*Calves; Thighs; Back; Deltoids; Arms; Chest;* and *Abdominals.* Address: Chris Dickerson, Box 1123, Santa Monica, CA 90406.

Ferrigno, Lou: Twelve courses—*The Mind; Basic Principles; Intermediate and Advanced Principles; Legs; Abdominals and Serratus; Super-Wide Shoulders; The Back; Arms; Chest; Muscular Size & Power; Contest Training;* and *Photo Album.* Address: Lou Ferrigno, Box 1671, Santa Monica, CA 90406.

Mentzer, Mike: Eight courses—*Heavy Duty Training System; Building Heavy Duty Arms; Heavy Duty Leg Training; Heavy Duty Torso Training; Heavy Duty Shoulders; The Heavy Duty Journal; Heavy Duty Nutrition;* and *Heavy Duty Training for Women.* Address: Mike Mentzer, Box 67276, Los Angeles, CA 90067.

Pearl, Bill: Five courses—*Your Key to Broad Shoulders; Building Bulk and Power; Complete Chest Development; Build Big Arms;* and *Fabulous Forearms.* Address: Physical Fitness Architects, 100 South Michigan Ave., Pasadena, CA 91106.

Platz, Tom: Two courses—*Leg Training Manual* and *Upper Body Mass and Power.* Address: Tom Platz, Box 1262, Santa Monica, CA 90406.

Schwarzenegger, Arnold: Ten courses—*Arnold's Own Conditioning Course; Build Massive Arms; Building a Giant-60-inch Chest!; Building a Wide, Powerful Back!; Building Legs of an Oak!; Developing a "Mr. Universe" Body!; The Art of Posing!; Massive Size, Muscular Weight!; Muscular Mass, Sharp Definition!;* and *Doorway-Wide Shoulders!* Address: Arnold Schwarzenegger, Box 1234, Santa Monica, CA 90406.

Scott, Larry: Thirteen courses—*How to Build 20" Arms; Building a Mr. America Chest; Massive Thick Lats; Herculean Thighs; Cannon Ball Deltoids; Mr. America Body; Photo Album; Slice Your Physique for Definition; Secrets of Bulking Up Quick; Instinctive Training; Posing; Mighty Forearms;* and *Abdominal Training.* Address: Larry Scott, Box 934, Salt Lake City, UT 84110.

Tinerino, Dennis: Six courses—*Natural Champion Training Philosophy; Secrets of Building Muscular Bulk and Power; Shoulders & Back; Championship Legs; Chest & Arms;* and *Waist Trimming & Muscularizing.* Address: Dennis Tinerino, Box 299, Northridge, CA 91328.

Zane, Frank: Eight courses—*How to Build Championship Legs and a Small Waistline; Develop a Classic Upper Body; Total Training for the Total Body; Secrets of Advanced Bodybuilding; The Mind in Bodybuilding; On Posing; The Zane Supernutrition Cookbook;* and *At a Zane Seminar.* Address: Frank Zane, Box 366, Santa Monica, CA 90406.

SEMINAR CASSETTE TAPES

Bass, Clarence. "Ripped Seminar Cassette." Ripped Enterprises, 205 Sandia Savings Building, 400 Gold St., S.W., Albuquerque, NM 87102.

Cahling, Andreas. "Vegetarian Bodybuilding Seminar." Andreas Cahling, Box 929, Venice, CA 90291.

Coe, Boyer. "Boyer Coe Seminar Tape." Boyer Coe, Box 5877, Huntington Beach, CA 92646.

Davis, Steve. "Raw Muscularity." Steve Davis Fitness Center, 23115 Lyons Ave., Newhall, CA 91321.

Ferrigno, Lou. "The Incredible Muscle-Up Seminar." Lou Ferrigno, Box 1671, Santa Monica, CA 90406.

Mentzer, Mike. "Heavy Duty Seminar." Mike Mentzer, Box 67276, Los Angeles, CA 90067.

Siegel, Peter. Numerous tapes on mental aspects of bodybuilding and self-hypnosis. Fitness Research Institute of Hypnosis, Suite 753, 2210 Wilshire Blvd., Santa Monica, CA 90403.

Viator, Casey. "The Unreal Seminar Tape." Casey Viator, Box 826, Santa Monica, CA 90406.

TRAINING FILMS

Columbu, Franco: Four 50-foot Super-8 films—*Posing; Training the Chest, Lats and Abs; Training the Shoulders, Arms and Forearms;* and *Training the Thighs and Calves.* Address: Franco Columbu, Box 415, Santa Monica, CA 90406.

FEDERATION ADDRESSES

American Federation of Women Bodybuilders. Doris Barrileaux, Box 937, Riverview, FL 33569.

American Physique Committee, Inc. Jim Manion, 1050 Lafayette St., Bridgeville, PA 15017.

International Federation of Bodybuilders, 2875 Bates Rd., Montreal, P.Q. H3S 1B7, Canada.

INDEX

U–V

W–Z